Diagnosis and Treatment of Rare Gynecologic Cancers

Diagnosis and Treatment of Rare Gynecologic Cancers

Edited By

Michael Frumovitz, MD, MPH
Department of Gynecologic Oncology and Reproductive Medicine
The University of Texas MD Anderson Cancer Center
Houston, TX
United States

Mario M. Leitao, Jr., MD
Department of Surgery
Memorial Sloan Kettering Cancer Center
New York, NY
United States

Preetha Ramalingam, MD
Department of Pathology and Laboratory Medicine
The University of Texas MD Anderson Cancer Center
Houston, TX
United States

ELSEVIER

Elsevier
Radarweg 29, PO Box 211, 1000 AE Amsterdam, Netherlands
The Boulevard, Langford Lane, Kidlington, Oxford OX5 1GB, United Kingdom
50 Hampshire Street, 5th Floor, Cambridge, MA 02139, United States

Notices

Knowledge and best practice in this field are constantly changing. As new research and experience broaden our understanding, changes in research methods, professional practices, or medical treatment may become necessary.

Practitioners and researchers must always rely on their own experience and knowledge in evaluating and using any information, methods, compounds, or experiments described herein. In using such information or methods they should be mindful of their own safety and the safety of others, including parties for whom they have a professional responsibility.

To the fullest extent of the law, neither the Publisher nor the authors, contributors, or editors, assume any liability for any injury and/or damage to persons or property as a matter of products liability, negligence or otherwise, or from any use or operation of any methods, products, instructions, or ideas contained in the material herein.

ISBN: 978-0-323-82938-0

For information on all Elsevier publications
visit our website at https://www.elsevier.com/books-and-journals

Publisher: Dolores Meloni
Acquisitions Editor: Nancy Duffy
Editorial Project Manager: Sam Young
Production Project Manager: Poulouse Joseph
Cover Designer: Vicky Pearson Esser

Typeset by STRAIVE, India

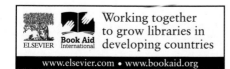
Working together to grow libraries in developing countries

www.elsevier.com • www.bookaid.org

Dedication

Michael: For my partners and colleagues who are dedicated to treating women with gynecologic cancers and my wife Karen whose support seems limitless.

Mario: I want to dedicate this work to my wife, Toula, and my children, Marco, Alexa and Zoe. They are the reason I wake up every morning and are my everything. I want to thank them for their love, support and patience which is what has made it so much easier for me to do the things I do.

Preetha: For my family, mentors and colleagues who have supported me through the years and made this journey more rewarding than I could have hoped for.

Contents

Contributors

Emeline Aviki, MD, MBA, Department of Surgery Memorial Sloan Kettering Cancer Center, New York, NY, United States

Ross S. Berkowitz, MD, Department of Obstetrics and Gynecology and Reproductive Biology, Brigham and Women's Hospital, Harvard Medical School, Boston, MA, United States

Vance Broach, MD, Department of Surgery Memorial Sloan Kettering Cancer Center, New York, NY, United States

Leigh A. Cantrell, MD, MSPH, Department of Obstetrics and Gynecology, University of Virginia, Charlottesville, VA, United States

M. Herman Chui, MD, FRCPC, Department of Pathology and Laboratory Medicine, Memorial Sloan Kettering Cancer Center, New York, NY, United States

William Cliby, MD, Virgil S. Counseller, M.D., Professor of Surgery, Department of Obstetrics and Gynecology, Mayo Clinic, Rochester, Minnesota, United States

Kevin M. Elias, MD, Department of Obstetrics and Gynecology and Reproductive Biology, Brigham and Women's Hospital, Harvard Medical School, Boston, MA, United States

Lora Hedrick Ellenson, MD, Department of Pathology and Laboratory Medicine, Memorial Sloan Kettering Cancer Center, New York, NY, United States

Amanda N. Fader, MD, Kelly Gynecologic Oncology Service, Department of Gynecology and Obstetrics, Johns Hopkins School of Medicine, Baltimore, MD, United States

Donato Callegaro Filho, MD, PhD, Department of Medical Oncology, Hospital Israelita Albert Einstein, São Paulo, Brazil

Nicole D. Fleming, MD, Department of Gynecologic Oncology, The University of Texas MD Anderson Cancer Center, Houston, TX, United States

Michael Frumovitz, MD, MPH, Department of Gynecologic Oncology and Reproductive Medicine, The University of Texas MD Anderson Cancer Center, Houston, TX, United States

David M. Gershenson, MD, Department of Gynecologic Oncology and Reproductive Medicine, The University of Texas MD Anderson Cancer Center, Houston, TX, United States

Sushmita Gordhandas, MD, Department of Surgery, Memorial Sloan Kettering Cancer Center, New York, NY, United States

Rachel N. Grisham, MD, Department of Medicine, Gynecologic Medical Oncology Service, Memorial Sloan Kettering Cancer Center and Weill Cornell Medical College, New York, NY, United States

Arthur Herbst, MD, Department of Obstetrics & Gynecology, University of Chicago Medicine, Chicago, IL, United States

R. Tyler Hillman, MD, PhD, Department of Gynecologic Oncology and Reproductive Medicine, The University of Texas MD Anderson Cancer Center, Houston, TX, United States

Emily Hinchcliff, MD, MPH, Department of Obstetrics and Gynecologic, Northwestern University, Chicago, IL, United States

Anjelica Hodgson, MD, FRCPC, Department of Laboratory Medicine and Pathobiology, University of Toronto, Toronto, ON, Canada

Neil S. Horowitz, MD, Department of Obstetrics and Gynecology and Reproductive Biology, Brigham and Women's Hospital, Harvard Medical School, Boston, MA, United States

Elizabeth Kertowidjojo, MD, PhD, MPH, Department of Pathology, University of Chicago, Chicago, IL, United States

Sarah H. Kim, MD, Department of Surgery, Memorial Sloan Kettering Cancer Center, New York, NY, United States

Anne Knisely, MD, Department of Obstetrics and Gynecology, Columbia University College of Physicians and Surgeons, New York, NY

Katherine C. Kurnit, MD, MPH, Department of Obstetrics and Gynecology, University of Chicago Medicine, Chicago, IL, United States

Barrett Lawson, MD, Department of Pathology and Laboratory Medicine, The University of Texas MD Anderson Cancer Center, Houston, TX, United States

Mario M. Leitao, Jr., MD, Department of Surgery, Memorial Sloan Kettering Cancer Center, New York, NY, United States

Douglas A. Levine, MD, Oncology Early Development, Merck Research Laboratories, Rahway, NJ, United States

Ying Liu, MD, MPH, Department of Medicine, Memorial Sloan Kettering Cancer Center, Weill Cornell Medical College, New York, NY, United States

Beverly Long, MD, Department of Obstetrics and Gynecology, Florida State University College of Medicine, Sarasota Memorial Healthcare System, Sarasota, FL, United States

Beryl Manning-Geist, MD, Department of Surgery, Memorial Sloan Kettering Cancer Center, New York, NY, United States

Diana Miao, MD, Kelly Gynecologic Oncology Service, Department of Gynecology and Obstetrics, Johns Hopkins School of Medicine, Baltimore, MD, United States

Jennifer J. Mueller, MD, FACOG, Department of Surgery, Memorial Sloan Kettering Cancer Center, Weill Cornell Medical College, New York, NY, United States

Priyadharsini Nagarajan, MD, PhD, Department of Pathology and Laboratory Medicine, The University of Texas MD Anderson Cancer Center, Houston, TX, United States

Roisin E. O'Cearbhaill, MD, Department of Medicine, Memorial Sloan Kettering Cancer Center, Weill Cornell Medical College, New York, NY, United States

Katherine Peng, MD, Department of Obstetrics and Gynecology, University of Virginia, Charlottesville, VA, United States

Preetha Ramalingam, MD, Department of Pathology and Laboratory Medicine, The University of Texas MD Anderson Cancer Center, Houston, TX, United States

Ravin Ratan, MD, Department of Sarcoma Medical Oncology, The University of Texas MD Anderson Cancer Center, Houston, TX, United States

Gloria Salvo, MD, Department of Gynecologic Oncology and Reproductive Medicine, The University of Texas MD Anderson Cancer Center, Houston, TX, United States

Alessandro D. Santin, MD, Department of Obstetrics, Gynecology and Reproductive Sciences, Yale University, New Haven, CT, United States

Aaron Shafer, MD, Department of Gynecologic Oncology and Reproductive Medicine, The University of Texas MD Anderson Cancer Center, Houston, TX, United States

Pamela Soliman, MD, MPH, Department of Gynecologic Oncology and Reproductive Medicine, The University of Texas MD Anderson Cancer Center, Houston, TX, United States

Sahana Somasegar, MD, Department of Obstetrics and Gynecology, University of Chicago Medicine, Chicago, IL, United States

Joan R. Tymon-Rosario, MD, Department of Obstetrics, Gynecology and Reproductive Sciences, Yale University, New Haven, CT, United States

Jason D. Wright, MD, Department of Obstetrics and Gynecology, Columbia University College of Physicians and Surgeons, New York, NY, United States

S. Diane Yamada, MD, Department of Obstetrics and Gynecology, University of Chicago Medicine, Chicago, IL, United States

Oliver Zivanovic, MD, Department of Surgery, Memorial Sloan Kettering Cancer Center, New York, NY, United States

Foreword

Prior to 2000, and somewhat beyond, almost all gynecologic cancers of the same anatomic site (ovary, endometrium, cervix, vulva, etc.) were treated identically, both within the context of clinical trials and off protocol. A few exceptions included malignant ovarian germ cell tumors, sex cord-stromal ovarian tumors, and sarcomas. As the Human Genome Project was completed in 2003, we were also beginning to witness the refinement of pathological criteria, the dissemination of hypothesis-generating observational studies, and an explosion of information on tumor biology facilitated by technological advances. Coupled with microscopic cell type, genomic profiles allowed us to begin the process of splitting tumors into even smaller cohorts and to study them separately, facilitated by the emerging availability of targeted agents developed by pharmaceuticals. However, this amazing opportunity also underscored the challenges in studying rare tumors, spawned from only somewhat less rare tumors. Even as this process evolved, rare tumors were still considered the Rodney Dangerfield of malignancies: "I don't get no respect." In addition to the obvious dilemmas involved in the study of rare tumors (small numbers of cases, prolonged duration of clinical trial accrual, low levels of evidence supporting a control arm, low funding priority by both pharma and the federal government, and biostatistical methods not conducive to the study of small cohorts), we learned several lessons: (1) there are rare tumors, very rare tumors, and extremely rare tumors (e.g., small cell carcinoma of the ovary, hypercalcemic type, and Sertoli-Leydig cell tumors); (2) the process of attempting to conduct clinical trials of certain rare tumors highlighted the problems with precise histologic diagnosis (e.g., distinguishing mucinous ovarian cancers from gastrointestinal cancers) and feasibility; and (3) for some rare gynecologic tumors, the lack of identifiable actionable mutations or other biomarkers has served as a barrier to progress (e.g., ovarian granulosa cell tumors). That said, the gynecologic cancer community has been able to finally make progress through the conduct of a few innovative clinical trials, continuously improved technologies, increased availability of novel agents via pharma pipelines, greater attention by funding agencies, and promotion of awareness and fundraising by the patient advocacy community. In truth, the future for the study of rare gynecologic cancers has never looked brighter. Over the past decade, the study of rare gynecologic tumors has benefited from various strategies—clinical trials, observational studies, and registries. Also, we have been smarter about playing off clues from more common cancers: malignant ovarian germ cell tumors from testicular cancer, low-grade serous ovarian cancer from ER-positive breast cancer and melanoma, mucinous ovarian cancer from colorectal cancer, clear cell ovarian cancer from renal cell cancer, neuroendocrine gynecologic cancers from the larger neuroendocrine cancer community, and gynecologic sarcomas from the larger sarcoma community, just to name a few examples. Inevitably, as we continue to learn more about the biology of cancer, rare gynecologic cancers will increasingly be split into even smaller subsets.

Into this milieu is introduced *Diagnosis and Treatment of Rare Gynecologic Cancers*. This is by no means the first book of its sort; however, the book screams, "I am special!" Why is that? First, this is a collaboration between two internationally renowned comprehensive cancer centers. MD Anderson Cancer Center and Memorial Sloan-Kettering Cancer Center are consistently ranked the top two hospitals for cancer in the US News & World Report's annual survey. Each is a major tertiary referral center that cares for a high volume of women with rare gynecologic cancers and has been a world leader in the study of rare tumors. Second, the editors—Dr. Michael Frumovitz, Dr. Mario Leitao, and Dr. Preetha Ramalingam—have bona fides and an established track record in rare gynecologic cancer investigations. Michael is a recognized expert in the study of neuroendocrine carcinomas of the cervix and mucinous ovarian cancers; likewise, Mario has devoted a large part of his career to the study of vulvovaginal melanoma. Preetha has published extensively about unique pathological features of a variety of rare gynecologic cancers.

The editors have clearly assembled a remarkable group of contributors to provide critical information on the histologic diagnosis and therapeutic options for women with rare tumors. The authors are among those who see more patients with a specific rare tumor in a month than most oncologists see in an entire career. Each chapter follows a similar format, including epidemiology, pathological assessment, molecular biology, evaluation and treatment options for both newly diagnosed and recurrent tumors. Importantly, readers of this textbook will also have access to a website that will continually update treatment algorithms for these rare tumors every 6 months. All considered, this is a book that should be essential for all who care for women with gynecologic malignancies—gynecologic oncologists, medical oncologists, radiation oncologists, nurses, and allied health professionals.

David M. Gershenson, MD
Professor
Department of Gynecologic Oncology & Reproductive Medicine
The University of Texas MD Anderson Cancer Center

Section A

Ovarian cancers

Chapter 1

Malignant ovarian germ cell tumors

Aaron Shafer, David M. Gershenson, Anjelica Hodgson, and M. Herman Chui

Clinical case

A 22-year-old G0 presents to an emergency department with pain and vomiting. CT scan of the abdomen/pelvis reveals a complex mass with cystic and solid components, including scattered calcifications, which occupies a large portion of the abdomen and pelvis and measuring up to 24 cm (Fig. 1.1). There is also a small amount of pelvic fluid and an enlarged paraaortic lymph node in the aortocaval region measuring 1.5×0.8 cm. Tumor markers were drawn and are as follows: CA-125 127; Inhibin A 9.8; Inhibin B 27; Beta-hCG 3.4; AFP 3506; LDH 200. The patient undergoes an exploratory laparotomy, right salpingo-oophorectomy (RSO) with omentectomy, right paraaortic lymphadenectomy, and pelvic peritonectomy with no gross residual disease. Final pathology reveals a mixed ovarian germ cell tumor [20% high-grade immature teratoma (IT); 20% yolk sac tumor (YST); 60% mature teratoma] with metastatic YST in 1 paraaortic node and in a cul-de-sac nodule. How would you now manage this patient?

Epidemiology

Malignant ovarian germ cell tumors (MOGTs) are overall rare, accounting for only 3%–5% of ovarian cancers. Additionally, the incidence of germ cell tumors varies greatly depending on age. The incidence of MOGTs rises steadily in young girls from age 9 to peak in the late teens between the ages of 15 and 19. This incidence then steadily declines after that, and malignant germ cell tumors are extremely rare after age 40.[1] A SEER database study identified 2451 women with MOGTs between 1978 and 2010. The median age at diagnosis was 22 years old, and 93% of the women were under age 40 at diagnosis.[2] Germ cell tumors make up 75% of ovarian cancers in women less than 20 years old but less than 5% of ovarian cancers in adult women.[3] The most common germ cell tumors are benign mature cystic teratomas which can account for 20% of all ovarian tumors. When looking specifically at malignant germ cell tumors, the most common histologies are dysgerminoma, IT, and YST (Table 1.1). Rarer histologies are mixed tumors, embryonal carcinomas, and nongestational choriocarcinomas.

A major risk factor for development of germ cell tumors is gonadal dysgenesis. Swyer syndrome is a condition in which a woman or girl is phenotypically female but has a 46XY karyotype. These patients generally have intraabdominal streak gonads. There can be an up to a 30% risk of development of germ cell tumors such as gonadoblastoma and dysgerminoma with a much smaller risk of a mixed germ cell tumor.[4] More rarely, germ cell tumors have been described in women with Turner syndrome (45X) and mosaicism which can lead to gonadal dysgenesis. These women appear to be at risk of gonadoblastomas and dysgerminomas, but dysgerminomas are very rare compared to gonadoblastomas, which have a generally benign course.[5,6] MOGTs have no relation to hereditary cancer syndromes, such as BRCA or Lynch syndrome. The only other risk factor may be geographic location. There seems to be an increased risk for development of MOGTs in southeast Asian countries, especially in adolescent girls. The exact mechanism for this, genetic or environmental, is not clear.[3]

Pathology

Dysgerminoma

Gross appearance

Dysgerminomas are usually large ($\sim$15 cm) and have a fleshy, yellow, solid and lobulated appearance. Areas of cystic degeneration, hemorrhage, and necrosis may also be seen. Calcification may indicate the presence of a gonadoblastoma. Bilateral ovarian involvement occurs in relatively small proportion of cases.[7]

Diagnosis and Treatment of Rare Gynecologic Cancers. https://doi.org/10.1016/B978-0-323-82938-0.00001-X

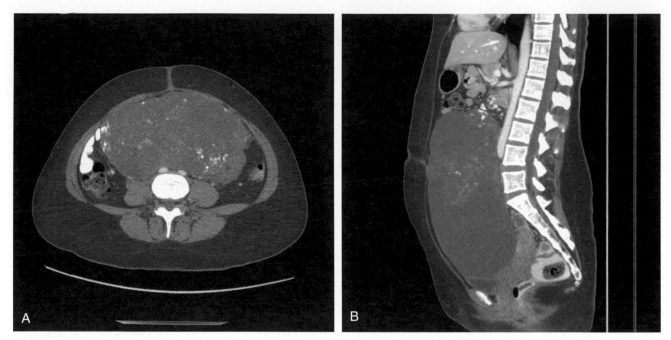

FIG. 1.1 Axial (A) and sagittal (B) views of a mixed germ cell tumor presenting as a 24 cm abdominal-pelvic mass with elevated AFP and beta-hCG.

TABLE 1.1 Common histologies of malignant germ cell tumors[a].

Histology	Percent of malignant ovarian germ cell tumors
Dysgerminoma	33%
Immature teratoma	36%
Yolk sac tumor	15%
Mixed germ cell tumor	5%
Embryonal carcinoma	4%
Choriocarcinoma	2%

[a]From Smith (2006).[1]

Histopathologic features

Dysgerminomas are histologically characterized by sheets, nests, and cords/trabeculae of tumor cells with intervening lymphocyte-rich fibrous septae (Fig. 1.2A and B). Poorly formed granulomas may be present in the surrounding stroma. The tumor cells are monotonous with clear or eosinophilic cytoplasm, well-defined cell borders, and a central nucleus with one or two macronucleoli. Mitotic figures are often conspicuous. Scattered syncytiotrophoblastic cells may be found in a minority of tumors. When seen in cytologic preparations, dysgerminomas classically show a "tigroid" background.[8]

Immunohistochemistry

Immunohistochemical markers of dysgerminoma include SALL4, OCT4, c-kit (CD117), D2-40, and PLAP. They may exhibit focal staining for cytokeratins, and hCG could be used to highlight syncytiotrophoblastic cells, if present. Dysgerminomas are negative for EMA, AFP, Glypican-3, and CD30.[9]

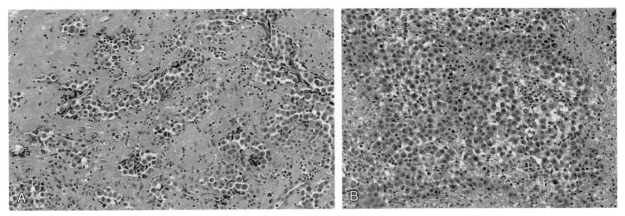

FIG. 1.2 Dsygerminomas showing nests and cords of tumor cells with intervening fibrous septae (A). Tumor cells have abundant cytoplasm and prominent nucleoli. Scattered lymphocytes are present around the tumor nests (B).

Differential diagnosis

The morphological differential diagnosis for dysgerminoma includes other germ cell tumors (YST, embryonal carcinoma, and mixed germ cell tumor), epithelial primary ovarian tumors (clear cell carcinoma, undifferentiated carcinoma), and metastatic/secondary tumors involving the ovary (melanoma, lymphoma). Dysgerminomas, especially when large, must be well sampled to exclude other mixed germ cell components such as YST or embryonal carcinoma. YSTs have variable architecture with papillary, glandular, reticular, and solid patterns, unlike dysgerminomas that are usually solid and monotonous. Immunostains such as AFP and glypican-3 are positive in the former, and OCT4 and CD117 will be positive in the latter. Embryonal carcinoma has higher-grade nuclei and is positive for CD30. Clear cell carcinoma can be particularly challenging on morphology, but markers such as PAX8 and napsin-A (positive in CCC), and SALL4 (positive in dysgerminoma) will help in the differential. Lymphomas and melanomas are distinguished from dysgerminoma using characteristic immunostains of these entities. Distinction between the above entities at the time of intraoperative consultation can be particularly challenging.

Molecular features

Chromosome 12 amplification or isochromosome 12p is present in 80% of dysgerminomas, and *KIT* mutation or amplification is present in 30%–50% of cases.[10,11]

Yolk sac tumor

Gross examination

YSTs are usually unilateral, large (>10 cm), solid and cystic. The external surface is usually smooth. The solid cut surface has a tan yellow appearance, frequently with areas of hemorrhage and necrosis. The polyvesicular vitelline areas may grossly have a spongy/honeycomb-like appearance.

Histopathologic features

There is considerable heterogeneity in the histologic appearance of YST and a number of architectural patterns have been described including microcystic/reticular (most common), (Fig. 1.3A) endodermal sinus (with Schiller–Duval bodies), polyvesicular-vitelline, glandular, papillary, solid, and others. Schiller–Duval bodies (Fig. 1.3B) are characterized by the presence of a cystic space that envelops a central papillary structure with a fibrovascular core that is lined by a layer of tumor cells. The tumor cells usually exhibit clear cytoplasm and large nuclei with prominent nucleoli. Hyaline globules are often present (Fig. 1.3C).[12]

Immunohistochemistry

Immunohistochemical markers of YST include SALL4, AFP, Glypican-3, CDX2 (in tumors with intestinal differentiation), HepPar-1 (in tumors with hepatoid differentiation) and TTF1 (in tumors with foregut/respiratory differentiation). YSTs are negative for EMA, CK7, ER, PR, OCT4, D2-40, and CD30.[9]

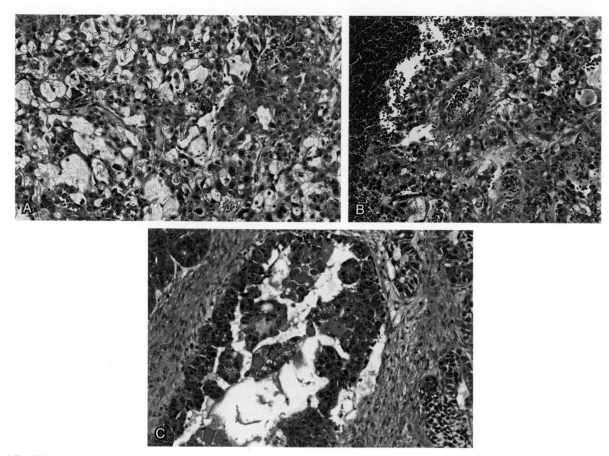

FIG. 1.3 Yolk sac tumor with microcystic/reticular growth pattern (A). Perivascular papillary structures, (i.e., Schiller–Duval bodies), though not always present, are characteristic of yolk sac tumor (B). Yolk sac tumor with glandular differentiation and hyaline globules (C).

Differential diagnosis

Given the extraordinary morphologic variability that YSTs may exhibit, depending on the morphologic appearance of the tumor, the differential diagnosis is quite broad. In addition to other germ cell tumors (dysgerminoma and embryonal carcinoma, in particular), clear cell carcinoma and endometrioid carcinoma can also share significant morphologic overlap with YST. Clear cell carcinomas and YSTs can have papillary, glandular and solid patterns with cytoplasmic clearing. Immunostains such as CK7, napsin-A and above described markers of YST will allow the distinction. YST can have a prominent glandular pattern mimicking endometrioid carcinoma. The presence of squamous morules and lower grade cytology in conjunction with positive staining for PAX8 and hormone receptors (ER and PR) will confirm endometrioid carcinoma. Other tumors that may enter into the differential diagnosis include Sertoli–Leydig cell tumor (intermediate or poor differentiation) or the rare hepatoid carcinoma (which resembles hepatocellular carcinoma). Somatically derived YSTs are admixed with an epithelial tumor and can be difficult to diagnose.[13] Subtle histologic features typical of YST must be looked for to make the correct diagnosis.

Embryonal carcinoma

Gross examination

Ovarian embryonal carcinomas are exceedingly rare and they are usually seen as a component of a mixed germ cell tumor. These tumors are unilateral, large, solid, hemorrhagic and necrotic.

Histopathologic features

Ovarian embryonal carcinoma is morphologically identical to its testicular counterpart and these tumors are characterized by polygonal tumor cells arranged in solid, nested, glandular and papillary arrangements. Primitive nuclei with marked cytologic atypia is the norm, and mitotic activity is usually conspicuous. Scattered syncytiotrophoblastic cells may be seen.

Immunohistochemistry

Immunohistochemical markers of embryonal carcinoma include cytokeratins, SALL4, OCT4, PLAP, and CD30. These tumors are negative for c-kit (CD117), D2-40, AFP, and Glypican-3.[9]

Differential diagnosis

The main differential diagnoses for embryonal carcinoma are dysgerminoma and YSTs, as previously discussed. High-grade ovarian carcinomas may also enter into the differential diagnosis, although these typically occur in older patients. The presence of syncytiotrophoblasts may raise the possibility of choriocarcinoma, but a second population of cytotrophoblasts is not identified.

Molecular features

Like dysgerminoma and YSTs, chromosome 12 abnormalities including 12p amplification or isochromosome formation are common.[14]

Immature teratoma

Gross examination

These tumors are usually unilateral, large (average of 16 cm), fleshy, solid, and cystic with areas of hemorrhage and necrosis. Mature teratomatous elements such as hair, teeth, cartilage, or bone may be present. Adequate sampling of these tumors (at least 1 section/centimeter) is imperative to exclude the presence of other germ cell components.

Histopathologic features

IT is a teratoma containing variable amounts of mature tissues of various lineages and an immature primitive component. The immature component is specific to the presence of neuroepithelial tissue, which commonly takes the form of tubules and rosettes that are composed of mitotically active cells with high nuclear-cytoplasmic ratios and hyperchromatic nuclei. Immature mesenchyme usually is present in association with the neuroectodermal rosettes (Fig. 1.4A–D). The grading scheme for these tumors is shown in Table 1.2. The two-tier grading system is recommended.

Metastases/implants are considered Grade 0 when no immature tissue is present, regardless of the grade of the ovarian tumor. Gliomatosis peritonei is a specific type of Grade 0 implant comprised of mature glial tissue and is associated with good prognosis.[15]

Immunohistochemistry

Immunohistochemical workup is not typically used in the evaluation of ITs, although it may be necessary to definitively identify and characterize immature neuroepithelium which would be expected to express SALL4 and OCT4, in addition to markers of neural differentiation (S100, GFAP, NSE).[16] The Ki-67 proliferation index in the immature component is high.

Differential diagnosis

The diagnosis of a teratomatous neoplasm is usually straightforward, given the distinctive presence of different tissue types not normally found in the ovary. Care should be taken not to confuse normal tissue types in a teratoma including cerebellum and lymphoid aggregates with immature neuroepithelial elements. When the immature component is widespread, distinction should be made with primitive neuroectodermal tumor (PNET), which consists of massive, confluent growth of neuroectodermal tissue, while IT shows a spectrum of neuroepithelial differentiation and an admixture of other tissue types. Carcinosarcoma may also enter into the differential diagnosis but this tumor occurs in older patients and consists of high-grade epithelial and mesenchymal components.

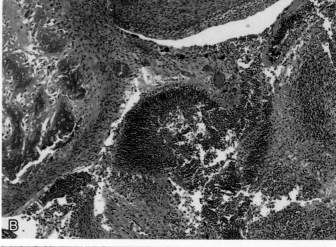

FIG. 1.4 High-grade immature teratoma with sheets of immature neuroepithelium and immature mesenchyme (A). Immature elements are frequently admixed with other mature tissue types such as squamous epithelium and bone (B). Neuroepithelial rosettes (C). Gliomatosis peritonei, characterized by mature glial cells within a fibrillary matrix; a number of reactive astrocytes are noted (D).

TABLE 1.2 Grading criteria for immature teratoma.

Grading criteria	Three-tier grading scheme	Two-tier grading scheme
Immature neural tissue occupying less than one low-power field (40×) in any slide	1	Low
Immature neural tissue occupying >1 but ≤3 low-power fields (40×) in any slide	2	High
Immature neural tissue exceeding three low-power fields (40×) in any slide	3	

Nongestational choriocarcinoma

General review

Nongestational choriocarcinomas are exceedingly rare and may occur in pure form or as a component of a mixed germ cell tumor. These tumors are large with a friable and hemorrhagic cut surface.

Histopathologic features

Choriocarcinoma is a malignant biphasic germ cell tumor composed of an admixture of cytotrophoblast and syncytiotrophoblast cells (Fig. 1.5) and, less frequently, intermediate trophoblast cells. Syncytiotrophoblast cells have abundant eosinophilic cytoplasm and multinucleated smudgy nuclei, while cytotrophoblast cells are smaller with pale cytoplasm and a single nucleus with evident brisk mitotic activity and prominent nucleoli. Intermediate trophoblast cells are also mononuclear, and if present are usually seen clustering around blood vessels. The syncytiotrophoblast component is usually the most prominent, but in some cases, the cytotrophoblast component predominates and shows solid sheet-like growth. Extensive hemorrhage and necrosis are common.

Immunohistochemistry

Choriocarcinomas are positive for hCG, keratin, and inhibin, while negative for OCT4, c-kit (CD117), and CD30.[16]

Differential diagnosis

In its classic form, choriocarcinoma has a characteristic appearance although other germ cell tumors with a syncytiotrophoblastic component, in addition to high-grade ovarian carcinomas may enter into the differential diagnosis. Nongestational and gestational choriocarcinoma cannot be definitively distinguished on histologic grounds alone and correlation with clinical history is necessary, and in addition, genotype analysis may also be necessary depending on the clinical scenario.[17]

Diagnosis and workup

Differential diagnosis

Ovarian germ cell tumors should be suspected in any adolescent or preadolescent girl who presents with a pelvic mass. While the risk of MOGTs decreases dramatically after age 20, the possibility of an ovarian germ cell tumor should be considered in women under the age of 40 with complex adnexal masses.

Signs and symptoms

Evaluation should start with a thorough history and physical exam. Specific questions to ask on history taking are: (1) Any changes to menstrual patterns if the woman is or was having regular menses; (2) Whether the patient has experienced any recent weight change or change in the fit of their clothes; also, (3) Whether she has noticed any new bloating or abdominal discomfort or even whether or not she can palpate an abdominal-pelvic mass. Pain can also be a presenting complaint as these tumors can grow rapidly and also can be associated with internal hemorrhage and rupture. YSTs, in particular, are known to be hemorrhagic, friable, can bleed easily, and often present with pain.[18] Patients may complain of abnormal vaginal bleeding.

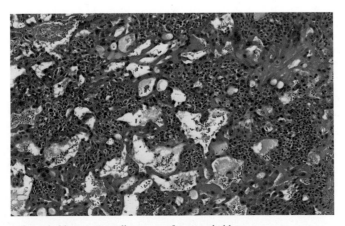

FIG. 1.5 Choriocarcinoma with syncytiotrophoblasts surrounding nests of cytotrophoblasts.

Physical exam findings

On physical exam, there is often a palpable, tender pelvic mass on bimanual exam up to 85% of the time. Sometimes, MOGTs can be quite large and can be palpated on abdominal exam as well. Rarely, there are no specific findings or palpable mass on exam.[18–20] Precocious puberty has been described as a presenting sign, but this is extremely rare and more common with mixed germ cell tumors.[19]

Tumor markers

Tumor markers should be drawn when evaluating a young woman with a complex pelvic mass and a suspicion for MOGTs. In addition to CA-125, young women with any pelvic mass should have alpha-fetoprotein (AFP), lactate dehydrogenase (LDH), and beta-human chorionic gonadotropin (β-hCG) drawn. Often, in malignant germ cell tumors, one or more of these will be elevated, though it is also possible that they can all be within the normal range as well (Table 1.3). CA-125 will often be elevated but not usually to the levels seen in epithelial ovarian cancers, and it is also not as discriminating in premenopausal women.[21] AFP is almost always elevated in YSTs and is a useful marker not only to aid in diagnosis but also for monitoring response to treatment and in surveillance.[21,22] AFP may also be elevated in patients with mixed germ cell tumors and about one-third to one-half of those with pure ITs, though usually to a lower level than those seen in YSTs.[20,21] AFP elevation may be more prevalent in pediatric and adolescent patients with ovarian ITs, and in some centers, AFP level helps in the decision on postsurgical observation vs. chemotherapy in these patients.[23–25] Dysgerminomas will classically have an increase in LDH, but LDH can be nonspecific and milder elevations can be seen in other germ cell tumors.[21] Nongestational choriocarcinomas will have elevated levels of beta-hCG, but again, mixed germ cell tumors can also show a variety of tumor marker elevations including beta-hCG as seen in Table 1.3.

Imaging

Imaging workup is similar to that for any pelvic mass in a young woman. Pelvic ultrasound or MRI are appropriate to characterize the pelvic mass. Whatever modality of imaging one chooses, characteristics to pay particular attention to for any signs of malignancy are architectural complexity (presence of both solid and cystic components), increased blood flow, or invasion into adjacent structures. Benign, mature teratomas are the most common ovarian germ cell tumors and will usually have a significant, and even predominantly, cystic component in addition to a solid or fat component. On CT scan, mature teratomas characteristically have significant fat signal in the solid component and calcifications, if present, are usually not described as "course".[26] ITs, on the other hand, will have a more solid rather than cystic appearance, will have "course calcifications" on CT scan and increased vascularity in the solid components on Doppler ultrasound. Dysgerminomas are predominantly solid, multilobulated, masses with "fibrovascular septa" that show postcontrast enhancement. YSTs are usually mixed solid and cystic masses that will often have areas of hemorrhage and a smooth external surface. There may also be a "bright dot sign" on contrast enhanced CT due to the increased vascularity.[26,27] If suspicion for malignancy is high, CT of the chest, abdomen, and pelvis is warranted to help assess for extra-pelvic disease, lymphadenopathy, as well as to assess for surgical resectability and approach.

Definitive preoperative diagnosis of MOGTs is difficult as this is a pathologic diagnosis. As with adnexal masses in postmenopausal women, preoperative biopsy of an ovarian mass is not recommended. Surgery, for both diagnosis and treatment, is almost always warranted—especially in those women with a large or solitary mass on imaging.

TABLE 1.3 Tumor markers and ovarian germ cell tumors.

Tumor	Beta-hCG	AFP	LDH
Dysgerminoma	+/−	−	+
Yolk sac tumor	−	+	+/−
Choriocarcinoma	+	−	−
Immature teratoma	−	+/−	+/−
Embryonal carcinoma	+	+	+/−
Polyembryoma	+/−	+/−	+/−
Mixed tumor	+/−	+/−	+/−

Staging

MOGTs are staged by either the Children's Oncology Group (COG) or FIGO staging, depending on the woman's age and who has operated on the patient. Generally, adolescents younger than 18 or 20 years of age are staged by the pediatric staging system (Table 1.4), while women in their 20s and older are managed by gynecologic oncologists (Table 1.5).

Management

Surgery

Surgery for MOGTs is the mainstay of treatment, staging, and prognosis. Ideally, women or girls with suspected MOGT, and probably anyone with an enlarging pelvic mass or one with concerning radiologic characteristics, should be referred to a gynecologic oncologist or pediatric surgeon depending on their age and subspecialty availability. These patients often have large, complex masses, and careful attention and skill to minimize surgical spill is important. Specific surgical staging guidelines differ between gynecologic oncologists and pediatric surgeons/oncologists, though there has been a move toward adopting a "less is more" approach among gynecologic oncologists. Pediatric surgery guidelines include intact unilateral salpingo-oophorectomy (USO), biopsy and/or resection of any *abnormal* peritoneal surfaces, omentum, and lymph nodes, removal of any resectable, grossly metastatic disease, and peritoneal cytology or sampling of ascites. Routine, systematic lymphadenectomy of grossly normal pelvic and para-aortic nodes is not performed. This change to a less aggressive approach amongst pediatric surgeons was initially based on a retrospective study of 131 patients with ovarian germ cell

TABLE 1.4 COG staging for malignant ovarian germ cell tumors.

Stage	Extent of disease
	Ovarian malignant germ cell tumors
I	☐ Ovarian tumor removed intact without violation of the tumor capsule. ☐ No evidence of partial or complete capsular penetration. ☐ Peritoneal cytology negative for malignant cells. ☐ Peritoneal surfaces and omentum documented to be free of disease in operative note or biopsied with negative history if abnormal in appearance. ☐ Lymph nodes all <1.0 cm by short axis on multiplanar imaging or biopsy proven negative. (Note: Nodes 1–2 cm, require short interval follow-up in 4–6 weeks. If nodes are unchanged at 4–6 weeks (1–2 cm), consider biopsy or transfer to chemotherapy arm. If growing, transfer to chemotherapy arm).
II	☐ Ovarian tumor completely removed but with preoperative biopsy, violation of tumor capsule in situ, or presence of partial or complete capsule penetration at histology. ☐ Tumor greater than 10 cm removed laparoscopically. ☐ Tumor morcellated for removal so that capsule cannot be assessed for penetration. ☐ Peritoneal cytology must be negative for malignant cells. ☐ Lymph nodes, peritoneal surfaces and omentum documented to be free of disease in operative note or biopsied with negative histology if abnormal in appearance.
III	☐ Lymph nodes ≥2 cm or lymph nodes >1 ≤ 2 cm on short axis by multiplanar imaging CT that fail to resolve on reimaging at 4–6 weeks. ☐ Ovarian tumor biopsied or removal with gross residual. ☐ Positive peritoneal fluid cytology for malignant cells, including immature teratoma. ☐ Lymph nodes positive for malignant cells, including immature teratoma. ☐ Peritoneal implants positive for malignant cells, including immature teratoma.
III-X	Patients otherwise Stage I or II by COG criteria but with the following: ☐ Failure to collect peritoneal cytology. ☐ Failure to sample abnormal peritoneal surfaces or omentum. ☐ Delayed completion of surgical staging at a second procedure for those patients who had only oophorectomy at first procedure.
IV	Metastatic disease to the parenchyma of the liver (surface implants are Stage III) or metastases outside the peritoneal cavity to any other viscera (bone, lung, brain) and pleural fluid with positive cytology

Bilateral ovarian tumors may be any stage as long as other stage criteria are met. Tumor stage according to ovary with most advanced features.

TABLE 1.5 TNM and FIGO staging for ovary, fallopian tube, and primary peritoneal carcinomas.

Primary tumor (T)		
T category	**FIGO stage**	**T criteria**
TX		Primary tumor cannot be assessed
T0		No evidence of primary tumor
T1	I	Tumor limited to ovaries (one or both) or fallopian tube(s)
T1a	IA	Tumor limited to one ovary (capsule intact) or fallopian tube, no tumor on ovarian or fallopian tube surface; no malignant cells in ascites or peritoneal washings
T1b	IB	Tumor limited to both ovaries (capsules intact) or fallopian tubes; no tumor on ovarian or fallopian tube surface; no malignant cells in ascites or peritoneal washings
T1c	IC	Tumor limited to one or both ovaries or fallopian tubes, with any of the following:
T1c1	IC1	• Surgical spill
T1c2	IC2	• Capsule ruptured before surgery or tumor on ovarian or fallopian tube surface
T1c3	IC3	• Malignant cells in ascites or peritoneal washings
T2	II	Tumor involves one or both ovaries or fallopian tubes with pelvic extension below pelvic brim or primary peritoneal cancer
T2a	IIA	Extension and/or implants on the uterus and/or fallopian tube(s) and/or ovaries
T2b	IIB	Extension to and/or implants on other pelvic tissues
T3	III	Tumor involves one or both ovaries or fallopian tubes, or primary peritoneal cancer, with microscopically confirmed peritoneal metastasis outside the pelvis and/or metastasis to the retroperitoneal (pelvic and/or paraaortic) lymph nodes
T3a	IIIA2	Microscopic extrapelvic (above the pelvic brim) peritoneal involvement with or without positive retroperitoneal lymph nodes
T3b	IIIB	Macroscopic peritoneal metastasis beyond pelvis 2 cm or less in greatest dimension with or without metastasis to the retroperitoneal lymph nodes
T3c	IIIC	Macroscopic peritoneal metastasis beyond the pelvis more than 2 cm in greatest dimension with or without metastasis to the retroperitoneal lymph nodes (includes extension of tumor to capsule of liver and spleen without parenchymal involvement of either organ)
Regional lymph nodes (N)		
N category	**FIGO stage**	**N criteria**
NX		Regional lymph nodes cannot be assessed
N0		No regional lymph node metastasis
N0(i+)		Isolated tumor cells in regional lymph node(s) no greater than 0.2 mm
N1	IIIA1	Positive retroperitoneal lymph nodes only (histologically confirmed)
N1a	IIIA1i	Metastasis up to and including 10 mm in greatest dimension
N1b	IIIA1ii	Metastasis more than 10 mm in greatest dimension
Distant metastasis (M)		
M category	**FIGO stage**	**M criteria**
M0		No distant metastasis
M1	IV	Distant metastasis, including pleural effusion with positive cytology; liver or splenic parenchymal metastasis; metastasis to extraabdominal organs (including inguinal lymph nodes and lymph nodes outside the abdominal cavity); and transmural involvement of intestine
M1a	IVA	Pleural effusion with positive cytology
M1b	IVB	Liver or splenic parenchymal metastases; metastases to extraabdominal organs (including inguinal lymph nodes and lymph nodes outside the abdominal cavity); transmural involvement of intestine

tumors showing excellent survival outcomes despite not undergoing true "comprehensive" staging. These were mostly pediatric patients with a median age of 11. In particular, the most commonly omitted procedure in these patients was bilateral lymphadenectomy (97%). Long-term survival was greater than 90% in these patients.[28] A more recent retrospective review of 102 patients with a median age of 22 years revealed no difference in survival or recurrence among those women/girls who had comprehensive surgical staging and those who did not. In this cohort, only 23% of these patients had comprehensive surgical staging. Additionally, in those who did have pelvic and/or paraaortic lymphadenectomy, only 1 patient was found to have positive nodes.[29]

In contrast, gynecologic oncology surgical guidelines state that women/girls with malignant germ cell tumors should have complete surgical staging, including USO, peritoneal cytology, pelvic and paraaortic lymphadenectomy, omentectomy and peritoneal biopsies.[22] Similar to epithelial ovarian cancer, any gross extra-ovarian disease should be resected if surgically feasible.[30–32] A metaanalysis identified an 11% risk of positive nodes in suspected early-stage malignant germ cell tumors of the ovary. In this analysis, the highest risk for nodal metastases appeared to be in dysgerminomas (18%); when dysgerminomas were removed from the analysis, the risk of positive nodes in clinically early stage tumors dropped to <5%.[33] A SEER database study examined women with clinical stage I MOGTs from 1988 to 2006. In this population of 1083 women, lymphadenectomy was performed in only 46%. In those who had lymphadenectomy, only 10% had positive nodes. Again, patients with dysgerminoma had the highest risk at 11%, while other histologies had a <3% risk of positive nodes. In multivariate analysis of this population, the performance of LND did not affect survival, and positive nodes did not affect survival.[34] These data show that there is not an insignificant risk of nodal metastases in apparent early stage MOGTs, even in dysgerminomas. Despite the up to 10% risk of nodal metastases, in women with apparent early stage MOGTs, the performance of lymphadenectomy does not appear to positively impact survival. Because of these data, in patients with clinically negative nodes, either by imaging and/or palpation, many believe that routine lymphadenectomy can most likely be omitted.

When operating on a woman for known or suspected MOGT, or even someone with a solitary adnexal mass, all attempt at a fertility-sparing procedure should be made. Most women with MOGTs are younger, and consideration of future fertility is important. In almost all cases, the contralateral ovary and uterus can be spared in the initial surgical management of germ cell tumors. It is rare for there to be bilateral ovarian involvement of MOGTs, except in the case of pure dysgerminomas, which can be bilateral in 10%–15% of cases.[35,36] Many retrospective studies have shown that fertility-preserving surgery is safe, feasible and has good oncologic outcomes.[37–39] In MITO-9, a retrospective study of rare ovarian tumors in Italy, 144 patients with stage I MOGTs were identified.[33] Eighty-seven percent of these women had fertility-sparing surgery. In Cox regression analysis of risk factors for recurrence, fertility-sparing surgery was not associated with higher recurrence. Only having "no staging," described as no evaluation of and biopsy of the omentum/peritoneum, was associated with higher recurrence. Another retrospective review of 92 patients with MOGTs in China, of whom 46 (50%) had fertility-sparing surgery, also showed no difference in recurrence or survival.[32] Blood loss, operative time and operative complications were higher in the "comprehensive" surgery group. In another retrospective review of 171 patients, all of whom underwent fertility-sparing surgery, 5-year disease-free survival (DFS) was 86%, and overall survival was high at 97%.[34] Incomplete staging, YST histology, and residual disease at initial surgery were associated with higher risk of recurrence in this population. Only yolk sac histology and residual disease were associated with worse overall survival. In select patients, it appears that ovarian cystectomy may also be adequate and safe, especially in those with ITs.[40]

Documentation of the inspection of peritoneal surfaces and nodal basins is important. As mentioned above, care should be taken to avoid surgical spill of ovarian masses. If, on preoperative imaging, there is no evidence of extra-ovarian disease and the surgeon feels that the mass can be safely handled, then a minimally invasive approach is appropriate. For patients who have not had surgery performed by a gynecologic oncologist or pediatric surgeon and comprehensive staging was not done, there is controversy as to whether second-look or staging surgery should be performed. Postoperative imaging should be performed. If postoperative imaging is negative, and the operative report does not describe metastatic disease, then there is probably no benefit to a second surgery.

Surveillance

Traditionally, very few women with MOGTs were treated with close surveillance alone after surgery. Historically, all patients other than those with a stage IA dysgerminoma and stage IA, grade 1 pure IT were given adjuvant chemotherapy. Much like surgical staging, there has been a desire and movement toward a "less is more" approach to adjuvant therapy for younger patients with stage I low-intermediate risk germ cell tumors. This is because the risk of recurrence in some of these patients is low, and the ability to salvage patients that do recur with systemic chemotherapy is so high. More retrospective data is being accumulated that suggests that close surveillance of women with stage I germ cell tumors other than pure dysgerminomas may be safe. Multiple studies with mostly pure IT have shown the safety of surveillance for stage IA disease regardless of grade.[41,42] In a retrospective study of 108 women from Italy and the UK with stage IA, IB, or IC IT, 75% were followed with close surveillance while 25% received adjuvant chemotherapy. There was no difference in recurrence of IT between the two groups and all but one of the patients who recurred in the surveillance group were salvaged with chemotherapy, surgery, or both.[41] Newton and colleagues in the UK also recently published their experience with germ cell tumors in 138 women. In their cohort, 42 patients had pure IT and only 9 received upfront chemotherapy. Giving chemotherapy did not seem to reduce the risk of recurrence of teratoma (33% in the chemotherapy group and 15% in the surveillance group). Recurrences were treated with surgery ± chemotherapy. There were also no deaths in the pure IT patients.[42] A pooled analysis of 179 (98 pediatric and 81 adult) patients with ovarian ITs from 4 clinical trials was performed by the Malignant Germ Cell International Collaborative (MaGIC). In this population, only 8 of the 98 (8.1%) pediatric patients received chemotherapy after surgery. Conversely, all 81 adult patients received adjuvant chemotherapy. Despite this difference in adjuvant therapy, there was little to no difference in 5-year relapse-free and overall survival between the pediatric and adult groups. Only higher tumor grade and stage seemed to correlate with risk of relapse.[43] These and other retrospective studies lend strong support to the "idea" of surveillance for all stage I pure ITs.[43]

The question of whether other non-IT germ cell histologies can be safely observed is less clear but more data is emerging to suggest the safety of surveillance alone. Billmire et al. reported on 25 girls (median age 12 years old) with stage I MOGTs who were managed with close surveillance after initial surgery. Patients had pure yolk sac tumors or mixed histology. None had pure IT. While 12 of the 25 recurred, 11 of those 12 were salvaged with systemic chemotherapy. All the girls who recurred had elevated tumor markers, and the median time to recurrence was 2 months.[44] In the study by Newton et al., a significant number of patients with dysgerminoma, including stage IB, were observed, and despite the fact that 3 of these 15 patients recurred, all were salvaged with chemotherapy and all were alive at the time of last follow-up.[42] These studies suggest the possible safety of close surveillance with frequent tumor markers and imaging in women with stage I non-IT germ cell tumors. As such, the GOG and COG has a prospective trial (AGCT 1531, NCT 03067181), currently enrolling, examining observation in women age 50 and younger with stage I MOGTs. Specifically, all FIGO stage IA and IB (COG stage I) ITs as well as stage IA and IB MOGTs (YSTs, embryonal carcinomas and choriocarcinomas) are eligible if postoperative imaging is negative and tumor markers (AFP, hCG, LDH) are normal or decreasing. These patients can be enrolled on the "low-risk" arm and close surveillance with tumor markers and imaging is initiated (https:/childrensoncologygroup.org/agct1531). We are encouraging all eligible patients with newly diagnosed stage I germ cell tumors to enroll on this trial (Fig. 1.6).

Chemotherapy

Despite the recent trend in increasing active surveillance for patients with stage I MOGTs, most women and adolescents with MOGTs will require adjuvant chemotherapy. Unlike most epithelial ovarian cancers, even advanced stage MOGT have a high chance of cure with systemic chemotherapy. Starting in the 1970s, germ cell malignancies were treated with vincristine, actinomycin-D, and cyclophosphamide (VAC). This regimen was shown to be effective in women with early stage and completely resected disease, but women with advanced and/or incompletely resected disease had a high risk of

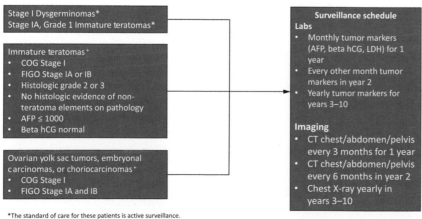

FIG. 1.6 Schema/criteria for observation of low-risk Stage I malignant ovarian germ cell tumors.

*The standard of care for these patients is active surveillance.

+Active surveillance alone for these patients is not yet standard of care and we strongly recommend enrollment on the COG trial AGCT1531 from which this schema is adapted if considering surveillance.

TABLE 1.6 Bleomycin, etoposide, and cisplatin (BEP) regimen for malignant ovarian germ cell tumors.

Bleomycin	30 units IV day 1 or weekly (day 1, day 8, day 15)[a]
Etoposide	100 mg/m^2 IV days 1, 2, 3, 4, and 5
Cisplatin	20 mg/m^2 IV days 1, 2, 3, 4, and 5
Repeated every 21 days	

[a]There is no consensus as to the optimal bleomycin frequency in ovarian germ cell tumors. For low-risk patients, day 1 bleomycin alone is probably sufficient. For women with advanced stage and/or residual disease, we recommend weekly bleomycin.

relapse and death.[31,45,46] Also, those patients with early-stage endodermal sinus tumor also had a significant risk of recurrence with this regimen.[31] The introduction of cisplatin proved a major advancement in the treatment of advanced germ cell tumors, initially being incorporated into testicular germ cell regimens and then into ovarian regimens. This led to the development and study of bleomycin, etoposide, and cisplatin (BEP).[47] Gershenson et al. in 1990 described their experience with twenty-six women with MOGTs treated with BEP at MD Anderson. Twenty-two of these women received BEP as first-line adjuvant therapy and four received BEP for either progressive or recurrent disease. Four patients had measurable disease at the start of treatment. At a median follow-up of 22.4 months, 96% (25/26) of patients remained disease-free.[47] Williams et al. reported in 1994 the results of a GOG trial of BEP in women with MOGTs, stage I–III with completely resected disease.[48] Of 93 patients eligible for evaluation, 91 were alive and free of disease. These studies helped establish BEP as first line adjuvant chemotherapy therapy for women with MOGTs. BEP has continued to be the first-line therapy for early-stage and late stage ovarian germ cell tumors with cure rates over 95% for early-stage disease and as high as 75%–80% in those with Stage III–IV disease.[22,47–49]

BEP chemotherapy is generally given as a 5-day regimen every 21 to 28 days (Table 1.6). For patients with early-stage disease, 3 adjuvant cycles are usually sufficient.[48] For advanced disease, 4 cycles, or 1 cycle past normalization of tumor markers, is our standard practice. Given that bleomycin toxicity is total dose dependent, 4 cycles of bleomycin, especially if given weekly, is the maximum dose. If a patient with advanced disease has tumor markers that are still elevated after 4 cycles of BEP, then continuing with etoposide/cisplatin (EP) until 1 cycle past normalization of markers may be warranted. Bleomycin pulmonary toxicity is of particular concern, and consideration should be given to checking pretreatment pulmonary function tests (PFTs) with specific attention to the diffusion capacity for carbon monoxide (DLCO) which measures the ability of oxygen to diffuse across alveolar membranes and into the pulmonary bloodstream. Pulmonary fibrosis from bleomycin will cause a decrease in DLCO.[50] Some advocate for checking PFTs at the end of treatment as well to have as a baseline, while others only do PFTs if there are symptoms or signs of pulmonary toxicity. There is no established definite decrease of DLCO at which bleomycin should be stopped, but a decrease in 20%–40% should prompt referral to pulmonary medicine, and in patients with a decrease in DLCO of 40%–60% from baseline, consideration of discontinuing bleomycin should be made.[50]

Pure dysgerminomas are exquisitely chemosensitive, and even stage IV disease can often be cured with systemic chemotherapy. There can be significant toxicity with BEP including pulmonary fibrosis, neuropathy, and neutropenia.[48,51] Because of this, there has been a lot of interest in less toxic regimens. For patients with pure dysgerminomas, carboplatin/etoposide alone is probably sufficient treatment with less toxicity. The GOG conducted a prospective Phase II study of women with stage IB–III pure dysgerminoma who had undergone comprehensive surgical staging and presumed complete resection of macroscopic disease.[52] These women were treated adjuvantly with carboplatin (400 mg/m^2 on day 1) and etoposide (120 mg/m^2 on days 1, 2, and 3) every 28 days for 4 cycles. Forty-two women were enrolled, and 39 were eligible for evaluation. Fifty-four percent ($n = 21$) were stage II or III. Of these 39 women, 37 of those patients received carboplatin/etoposide. None of these patients experienced a recurrence of dysgerminoma, and the regimen was overall well-tolerated. Another pooled analysis done by the Malignant Germ Cell Tumor International Consortium (MaGIC) of six germ cell tumor trials identified 126 patients with pure dysgerminoma: 56 treated with carboplatin-based and 70 treated with cisplatin-based regimens.[53] Outcomes were similar between the two groups, with 5-year event-free survival 96% in the carboplatin group and 93% in the cisplatin group. Five-year OS was 96% in both groups. These studies lend support to the use of carboplatin/etoposide as a reasonable alternative to BEP in women with pure dysgerminoma. Interestingly, in testicular seminomas which are analogous to ovarian dysgerminomas, there is evidence to suggest poorer outcomes with carboplatin/etoposide compared to cisplatin/etoposide. Therefore, in testicular cancer, cisplatin/etoposide is preferred in good-risk patients.[54] Of note, the carboplatin dose used in GOG 116 was before AUC dosing of carboplatin. When using the carboplatin/etoposide regimen for dysgerminoma, we recommend a carboplatin dose at an AUC of 5.

Posttreatment surveillance

After completing adjuvant therapy, patients should have baseline imaging in the form of a CT chest, abdomen, and pelvis. This will serve as a comparator for further surveillance and also make sure there is not any persistent or residual disease. Initial surveillance includes monthly tumor markers (AFP, LDH, beta-hCG) if they were elevated at diagnosis. Imaging should be every 3 months for the first 6–12 months. Those patients who experience recurrence almost always recur within the first 24 months after completion of therapy. After 12 months, tumor markers can be checked every 2 months and imaging can be spaced out to every 6 months per NCCN guidelines. Even so, some would still recommend more frequent imaging during year 2 of surveillance. Surveillance should still continue for 5 years after completion of therapy as late recurrences have been described, yet these are almost always in patients with pure dysgerminoma.[55,56]

Recurrent disease

While even those women with stage IV disease will have a >80% chance of long-term remission, failures will occur. Of women who do experience recurrence, most will recur within the first 2 years of initial treatment, and this emphasizes the importance of close initial surveillance.[22,57] The most important prognostic factor in determining response to salvage therapy is whether their disease is platinum sensitive and whether or not they had a complete response to initial therapy. If a patient recurs after surgery alone and has not yet received adjuvant platinum-based chemotherapy, then BEP chemotherapy should be the first consideration. However, once a patient with a MOGT recurs despite BEP chemotherapy, the chance of cure goes down dramatically.[57] Workup of suspected or confirmed recurrence should be measurement of tumor markers as well as imaging with CT of chest/abdomen/pelvis. There is some suggestion that elevated tumor markers at recurrence portend a worse prognosis.[57] If there is any question as to whether a mass or masses represents recurrence or if there has been a long disease-free interval, consideration should be made for biopsy to confirm recurrence. Surgery should be considered for women with a single site of recurrence if it is amenable to resection. Also, in women with biopsy-confirmed recurrence of pure IT, repeat surgery may be warranted as these tumors are notoriously resistant to chemotherapy and there is higher chance of long term remission with surgery.[58]

For those with multifocal disease or disease that is not amenable to resection, salvage systemic chemotherapy should be initiated (Table 1.7). While there are numerous salvage regimens, their response rates are overall poor and women with ovarian germ cell tumors seem to do worse than men with relapsed testicular tumors.[59] There is a paucity of literature evaluating chemotherapy regimens for MOGTs specifically in the relapsed setting. Most prospective studies include a combination of advanced and recurrent patients.[60] Extrapolating again from testicular cancer, the recommendation is to consider early use of high-dose induction chemotherapy with stem-cell transplant (SCT). In a large series of men with recurrent germ cell tumors, use of high-dose chemotherapy (HDC) with SCT as third line or later was associated with a significantly lower 2-year PFS. Those that received HDC as their second line therapy had a 63% 2-year PFS compared to 49% for third line or later.[61] While compared to testicular cancer, there are fewer reports and fewer patients, salvage rates for women with recurrent MOGTs treated with high-dose induction chemotherapy followed by SCT seems to be better than conventional salvage chemotherapy regimens. Women who receive HDC with SCT have a 30%–40% salvage rate. However, in these same series, when HDCT is used as the first salvage regimen, the long-term survival rate for women with MOGTs is 59%–67%.[59,62,63] This suggests the importance of early use of these HDCT regimens in these women (Table 1.8). Salvage rates with standard second-line regimens, though, are probably closer to 10%–20%.[57]

TABLE 1.7 Salvage chemotherapy regimens for malignant ovarian germ cell tumors.

Vinblastine, ifosfamide, cisplatin (VeIP)
Ifosfamide, carboplatin, etoposide (ICE)
Gemcitabine and oxaliplatin
POMB/ACE (cisplatin, vincristine, methotrexate, bleomycin/dactinomycin, cyclophosphamide, etoposide)
TIP (paclitaxel, ifosfamide, cisplatin)
High-dose chemotherapy with stem-cell transplant (HDC/SCT)

TABLE 1.8 Studies of high-dose chemotherapy with stem cell therapy.

Study	No. of patients	No. treated with HDCT and SCT	No. of patients HDCT/SCT given as 2nd line	No. salvaged 2nd line	No. treated 3rd line[c]	No. salvaged 3rd line
Reddy et al. (2005)	13	13	5	3	8	1
Meisel et al. (2015)	24	11	6	4	5	1
De Giorgi et al. (2017)[a]	60[b,c]	51	22[d]	13[d]	38[d]	13[d]

[a]Included both gonadal and extragonadal germ cell patients.
[b]Of the 60 patients, 38 were primary ovarian germ cell tumors.
[c]Nine patients received HDCT as late intensification as opposed to salvage after a prior chemotherapy regimen.
[d]Includes both ovarian and extragonadal patients.

Growing teratoma syndrome

After systemic treatment for IT or mixed germ cell tumors, some patients will experience persistent or recurrent disease. This may be recurrence of MOGTs but may also may represent growing, mature teratoma which can occur after treatment of the immature elements with systemic chemotherapy. This can manifest as growing teratoma syndrome or more rarely, gliomatosis peritonei.[64] Growing teratoma syndrome appears to be more common among older IT patients who were treated with systemic chemotherapy compared to younger women who may have had initial observation.[65] These women usually have normal tumor markers at "recurrence" and generally present within 5 years of their MOGTs diagnosis.[64,65] It is therefore important to biopsy or consider surgery in women treated for pure IT or mixed germ cell tumors who present with new or growing lesions after upfront systemic chemotherapy. Gliomatosis peritonei can be diagnosed at the time of initial surgery/diagnosis for MOGTs or may be found at a second surgery.[15] Recurrent immature teratoma would be approached by salvage chemotherapy ± surgery. Growing teratoma syndrome or gliomatosis peritonei, on the other hand, is not responsive to chemotherapy and is a surgically treated disease. Sometimes, if the patient is asymptomatic, and the mass or masses are not growing rapidly, close surveillance with repeat imaging may be warranted. If the patient has symptoms such as pain or the mass is showing significant growth, then surgical removal should be considered (Fig. 1.7). Even if

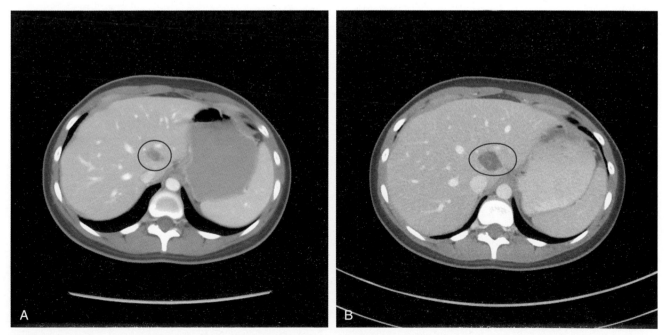

FIG. 1.7 Growing teratoma syndrome in a 22-year-old after treatment for a Stage IIIB immature teratoma. (A) 10 Months after completion of BEP chemotherapy and (B) 16 months after completing adjuvant BEP.

mature teratoma is confirmed on biopsy, close surveillance should continue as dormant lesions can grow or, more rarely, de-differentiate to IT.[64] If surgical resection is undertaken, care should be taken to perform a fertility-sparing surgery at all costs. While both growing teratoma syndrome and gliomatosis peritonei may lead to recurrent treatment and increased surveillance, overall long-term survival for these patients is very high.[15,64]

Case follow-up

Our patient had an exploratory laparotomy with RSO/omentectomy/R paraaortic node dissection and partial pelvic peritonectomy. Final pathology revealed a FIGO stage IIIA2(ii) mixed germ cell tumor of the ovary (20% IT, 20% YST, 60% mature teratoma). One right PA node was positive for YST. Her AFP normalized after cycle #3 (from 3500 to 6.1) so she received 4 cycles of adjuvant BEP chemotherapy. Her posttreatment CT showed no evidenced of disease, and her tumor markers including AFP, beta-hCG and LDH were all normal. She has been placed into surveillance with every other month tumor markers and CT imaging every 3–4 months. At 4 months after completion of therapy, she had not yet resumed her menses.

References

1. Smith HO, et al. Incidence and survival rates for female malignant germ cell tumors. *Obstet Gynecol.* 2006;107(5):1075–1085.
2. Solheim O, et al. Prognostic factors in malignant ovarian germ cell tumours (The Surveillance, Epidemiology and End Results experience 1978–2010). *Eur J Cancer.* 2014;50(11):1942–1950.
3. Hubbard AK, Poynter JN. Global incidence comparisons and trends in ovarian germ cell tumors by geographic region in girls, adolescents and young women: 1988–2012. *Gynecol Oncol.* 2019;154(3):608–615.
4. Piazza MJ, Urbanetz AA. Germ cell tumors in dysgenetic gonads. *Clinics (Sao Paulo).* 2019;74, e408.
5. Matsumoto F, et al. Variation of gonadal dysgenesis and tumor risk in patients with 45,X/46,XY mosaicism. *Urology.* 2020;137:157–160.
6. Tam YH, et al. Tumor risk of children with 45,X/46,XY gonadal dysgenesis in relation to their clinical presentations: Further insights into the gonadal management. *J Pediatr Surg.* 2016;51(9):1462–1466.
7. Warnnissorn M, Watkins JC, Young RH. Dysgerminoma of the ovary: an analysis of 140 cases emphasizing unusual microscopic findings and resultant diagnostic problems. *Am J Surg Pathol.* 2021.
8. Cao D, Vang R. Dysgerminoma. In: WHO Classification of Tumors Editorial Board, ed. Female Genital Tumors. World Health Organization Classification of Tumors. Lyon: IARC Press; 2020:123–124.
9. Rabban JT, Zaloudek CJ. A practical approach to immunohistochemical diagnosis of ovarian germ cell tumours and sex cord-stromal tumours. *Histopathology.* 2013;62:71–88. https://doi.org/10.1111/his.12052.
10. Cheng L, Roth LM, Zhang S, et al. KIT gene mutation and amplification in dysgerminoma of the ovary. *Cancer.* 2011;117:2096–2103.
11. Hoei-Hansen CE, Kraggerud SM, Abeler VM, et al. Ovarian dysgerminomas are characterised by frequent KIT mutations and abundant expression of pluripotency markers. *Mol Cancer.* 2007;6:12.
12. Nogales FF, Preda O, Nicolae A. Yolk sac tumours revisited. A review of their many faces and names. *Histopathology.* 2012;60:1023–1033.
13. McNamee T, Damato S, McCluggage WG. Yolk sac tumours of the female genital tract in older adults derive commonly from somatic epithelial neoplasms: somatically derived yolk sac tumours. *Histopathology.* 2016;69:739–751.
14. Cheng L, Zhang S, Talerman A, et al. Morphologic, immunohistochemical, and fluorescence in situ hybridization study of ovarian embryonal carcinoma with comparison to solid variant of yolk sac tumor and immature teratoma. *Hum Pathol.* 2010;41:716–723. https://doi.org/10.1016/j.humpath.2009.10.016.
15. Liang L, Zhang Y, Malpica A, et al. Gliomatosis peritonei: a clinicopathologic and immunohistochemical study of 21 cases. *Mod Pathol.* 2015;28:1613–1620. https://doi.org/10.1038/modpathol.2015.116.
16. Nogales FF, Dulcey I, Preda O. Germ cell tumors of the ovary: an update. *Arch Pathol Lab Med.* 2014;138:351–362. https://doi.org/10.5858/arpa.2012-0547-RA.
17. Yamamoto E, Ino K, Yamamoto T, et al. A pure nongestational choriocarcinoma of the ovary diagnosed with short tandem repeat analysis: case report and review of the literature. *Int J Gynecol Cancer.* 2007;17:254–258.
18. Gershenson DM, et al. Endodermal sinus tumor of the ovary: the M. D Anderson experience. *Obstet Gynecol.* 1983;61(2):194–202.
19. Gershenson DM, et al. Mixed germ cell tumors of the ovary. *Obstet Gynecol.* 1984;64(2):200–206.
20. Gershenson DM, et al. Immature teratoma of the ovary. *Obstet Gynecol.* 1986;68(5):624–629.
21. Kawai M, et al. Seven tumor markers in benign and malignant germ cell tumors of the ovary. *Gynecol Oncol.* 1992;45(3):248–253.
22. Gershenson DM. Management of ovarian germ cell tumors. *J Clin Oncol.* 2007;25(20):2938–2943.
23. Depani S, et al. Results from the UK Children's Cancer and Leukaemia Group study of extracranial germ cell tumours in children and adolescents (GCIII). *Eur J Cancer.* 2019;118:49–57.
24. Shinkai T, et al. Pediatric ovarian immature teratoma: histological grading and clinical characteristics. *J Pediatr Surg.* 2020;55(4):707–710.
25. Terenziani M, et al. Malignant ovarian germ cell tumors in pediatric patients: the AIEOP (Associazione Italiana Ematologia Oncologia Pediatrica) study. *Pediatr Blood Cancer.* 2017;64(11).

26. Hanafy AK, et al. Imaging in pediatric ovarian tumors. *Abdom Radiol (NY)*. 2020;45(2):520–536.

27. Wang Q, Yu D, Wang F. Clinical and computed tomography features of female pelvic malignant germ cell tumors in children and adolescents: a series of 30 cases. *J Pediatr Adolesc Gynecol*. 2020;33(1):83–88.

28. Billmire D, et al. Outcome and staging evaluation in malignant germ cell tumors of the ovary in children and adolescents: an intergroup study. *J Pediatr Surg*. 2004;39(3):424–429. discussion 424-9.

29. Zhao T, et al. The role of staging surgery in the treatment of apparent early-stage malignant ovarian germ cell tumours. *Aust N Z J Obstet Gynaecol*. 2016;56(4):398–402.

30. Bafna UD, et al. Germ cell tumors of the ovary: is there a role for aggressive cytoreductive surgery for nondysgerminomatous tumors? *Int J Gynecol Cancer*. 2001;11(4):300–304.

31. Slayton RE, et al. Vincristine, dactinomycin, and cyclophosphamide in the treatment of malignant germ cell tumors of the ovary. A Gynecologic Oncology Group Study (a final report). *Cancer*. 1985;56(2):243–248.

32. Williams SD, et al. Cisplatin, vinblastine, and bleomycin in advanced and recurrent ovarian germ-cell tumors. A trial of the Gynecologic Oncology Group. *Ann Intern Med*. 1989;111(1):22–27.

33. Kleppe M, et al. Lymph-node metastasis in stage I and II sex cord stromal and malignant germ cell tumours of the ovary: a systematic review. *Gynecol Oncol*. 2014;133(1):124–127.

34. Mahdi H, et al. Prognostic impact of lymphadenectomy in clinically early stage malignant germ cell tumour of the ovary. *Br J Cancer*. 2011;105 (4):493–497.

35. Bjorkholm E, et al. Dysgerminoma. The Radiumhemmet series 1927–1984. *Cancer*. 1990;65(1):38–44.

36. Gordon A, Lipton D, Woodruff JD. Dysgerminoma: a review of 158 cases from the Emil Novak Ovarian Tumor Registry. *Obstet Gynecol*. 1981;58 (4):497–504.

37. Liu Q, et al. The significance of comprehensive staging surgery in malignant ovarian germ cell tumors. *Gynecol Oncol*. 2013;131(3):551–554.

38. Mangili G, et al. The role of staging and adjuvant chemotherapy in stage I malignant ovarian germ cell tumors (MOGTs): the MITO-9 study. *Ann Oncol*. 2017;28(2):333–338.

39. Park JY, et al. Analysis of outcomes and prognostic factors after fertility-sparing surgery in malignant ovarian germ cell tumors. *Gynecol Oncol*. 2017;145(3):513–518.

40. Beiner ME, et al. Cystectomy for immature teratoma of the ovary. *Gynecol Oncol*. 2004;93(2):381–384.

41. Bergamini A, et al. Can we replace adjuvant chemotherapy with surveillance for stage IA-C immature ovarian teratomas of any grade? an international multicenter analysis. *Eur J Cancer*. 2020;137:136–143.

42. Newton C, et al. A multicentre retrospective cohort study of ovarian germ cell tumours: evidence for chemotherapy de-escalation and alignment of paediatric and adult practice. *Eur J Cancer*. 2019;113:19–27.

43. Pashankar F, et al. Is adjuvant chemotherapy indicated in ovarian immature teratomas? A combined data analysis from the Malignant Germ Cell Tumor International Collaborative. *Cancer*. 2016;122(2):230–237.

44. Billmire DF, et al. Surveillance after initial surgery for pediatric and adolescent girls with stage I ovarian germ cell tumors: report from the Children's Oncology Group. *J Clin Oncol*. 2014;32(5):465–470.

45. Gershenson DM, et al. Treatment of malignant nondysgerminomatous germ cell tumors of the ovary with vincristine, dactinomycin, and cyclophosphamide. *Cancer*. 1985;56(12):2756–2761.

46. Slayton RE, et al. Treatment of malignant ovarian germ cell tumors: response to vincristine, dactinomycin, and cyclophosphamide (preliminary report). *Cancer*. 1978;42(2):390–398.

47. Gershenson DM, et al. Treatment of malignant germ cell tumors of the ovary with bleomycin, etoposide, and cisplatin. *J Clin Oncol*. 1990;8(4): 715–720.

48. Williams S, et al. Adjuvant therapy of ovarian germ cell tumors with cisplatin, etoposide, and bleomycin: a trial of the Gynecologic Oncology Group. *J Clin Oncol*. 1994;12(4):701–706.

49. Gershenson DM, Frazier AL. Conundrums in the management of malignant ovarian germ cell tumors: Toward lessening acute morbidity and late effects of treatment. *Gynecol Oncol*. 2016;143(2):428–432.

50. Sleijfer S. Bleomycin-induced pneumonitis. *Chest*. 2001;120(2):617–624.

51. Maruyama Y, et al. Prognostic impact of bleomycin pulmonary toxicity on the outcomes of patients with germ cell tumors. *Med Oncol*. 2018;35(6):80.

52. Williams SD, et al. Adjuvant therapy of completely resected dysgerminoma with carboplatin and etoposide: a trial of the Gynecologic Oncology Group. *Gynecol Oncol*. 2004;95(3):496–499.

53. Shah R, et al. Is carboplatin-based chemotherapy as effective as cisplatin-based chemotherapy in the treatment of advanced-stage dysgerminoma in children, adolescents and young adults? *Gynecol Oncol*. 2018;150(2):253–260.

54. Kondagunta GV, Motzer RJ. Chemotherapy for advanced germ cell tumors. *J Clin Oncol*. 2006;24(35):5493–5502.

55. Khan O, et al. Late relapse of ovarian germ cell tumour. *J Obstet Gynaecol Can*. 2018;40(10):1329–1332.

56. Bekaii-Saab T, Einhorn LH, Williams SD. Late relapse of ovarian dysgerminoma: case report and literature review. *Gynecol Oncol*. 1999;72(1): 111–112.

57. Murugaesu N, et al. Malignant ovarian germ cell tumors: identification of novel prognostic markers and long-term outcome after multimodality treatment. *J Clin Oncol*. 2006;24(30):4862–4866.

58. Munkarah A, et al. Salvage surgery for chemorefractory ovarian germ cell tumors. *Gynecol Oncol*. 1994;55(2):217–223.

59. Reddy Ammakkanavar N, et al. High-dose chemotherapy for recurrent ovarian germ cell tumors. *J Clin Oncol*. 2015;33(2):226–227.

60. Simone CG, Markham MJ, Dizon DS. Chemotherapy in ovarian germ cell tumors: a systematic review. *Gynecol Oncol.* 2016;141(3):602–607.

61. Adra N, et al. High-dose chemotherapy and autologous peripheral-blood stem-cell transplantation for relapsed metastatic germ cell tumors: the Indiana University experience. *J Clin Oncol.* 2017;35(10):1096–1102.

62. De Giorgi U, et al. Salvage high-dose chemotherapy in female patients with relapsed/refractory germ-cell tumors: a retrospective analysis of the European Group for Blood and Marrow Transplantation (EBMT). *Ann Oncol.* 2017;28(8):1910–1916.

63. Meisel JL, et al. Development of a risk stratification system to guide treatment for female germ cell tumors. *Gynecol Oncol.* 2015;138(3):566–572.

64. Euscher ED. Germ cell tumors of the female genital tract. *Surg Pathol Clin.* 2019;12(2):621–649.

65. Imran H, et al. Growing teratoma syndrome after chemotherapy for ovarian immature teratoma. *J Pediatr Hematol Oncol.* 2020;42(7):e630–e633.

Chapter 2

Sex cord stromal tumors of the ovary

R. Tyler Hillman and Preetha Ramalingam

Clinical case

A 58-year-old G2P2 female presents with a 10 cm complex adnexal mass and postmenopausal bleeding. CT imaging also demonstrates a 4 cm perihepatic tumor implant (Fig. 2.1). Image-guided biopsy of this implant demonstrates an adult granulosa cell tumor (AGCT), and preoperative inhibin A was elevated at 22 pg/mL and inhibin B was elevated at 751 pg/mL. How do you treat this patient?

Epidemiology

Incidence/mortality

The sex cords and stromal compartments collectively comprise the mesenchymal support structures and sites of local and systemic hormone production for both the male and female gonad. Pure sex cord tumors include those arising from granulosa cells and Sertoli cells, as well as the rarer entity sex cord tumor with annular tubules which occur in the setting of Peutz–Jeghers syndrome (PJS) in up to 30% of cases.[1] Pure stromal malignancies of the ovary are generally rare and include fibrosarcomas and malignant steroid cell tumors. Mixed Sertoli–Leydig cell tumors (SLCTs) are uncommon, and although they may be associated with androgenic excess, the majority of such tumors described in large historical series exhibited benign behavior.[2] The World Health Organization classification of sex cord/stromal tumor is shown in Table 2.1. The incidence rate of sex cord/stromal ovarian cancers in the United States has been estimated to be approximately 0.5 per 100,000 using large cancer registries,[3] but this may be an underestimate due to misclassification of early stage disease as nonmalignant. For example, the category "Granulosa cell tumor, adult type" carries a nonmalignant behavior code in the International Classification of Diseases for Oncology (ICD-O) and thus is excluded from many cancer registry analyses.[4] In support of this observation are longitudinal multinational population data from Scandinavia showing that between the years 1953 and 2012, the incidence rate of ovarian granulosa cell tumors alone was between 0.6 and 0.8 per 100,000,[5] a higher rate than has been reported for all sex cord/stromal ovarian cancers in the United States.

The median age for diagnosis of AGCT of the ovary is around 45–50 years with most diagnoses occurring in the fourth of fifth decade of life.[6–8] The juvenile-type of granulosa cell tumor (JGCT) of the ovary is histologically distinct from AGCT of the ovary and arises most often during the prepubertal years. Including both benign and malignant entities, SLCTs tend to arise in the third decade of life but there is wide variance in the reported age of onset.[2] A review of patients in the National Cancer Institute's Surveillance, Epidemiology, and End Results (SEER) database showed women diagnosed with SLCTs were younger than those diagnosed with granulosa cell tumors (median age 32 vs 51).[9] Staging of sex cord/stromal tumors of the ovary uses the same FIGO system employed in the management of more common epithelial malignancies of the ovary.[10] In general, sex cord/stromal tumors are more likely to be stage I at the time of diagnosis (75%–90%) than are the more common epithelial subtype of ovarian cancers. Largely due to the combination of a favorable stage distribution at diagnosis and indolent behavior, 10-year survival rates for SLCT and AGCT of the ovary are generally excellent for completely resected disease. Stage at diagnosis is the clinical factor that has most consistently been linked to recurrence risk and outcomes across sex cord/stromal tumor subtypes.[11] Additionally, poorly differentiated SLCTs or those with heterologous elements are more likely to recur and exhibit malignant behavior following initial surgical resection.[2] Some evidence also suggests that the presence of a retiform pattern may also portend a higher risk of SLCT recurrence.[12] Among AGCT of the ovary, several factors including mitotic rate,[13] cellular atypia,[11] and tumor size, patient body mass index at the time of diagnosis[14] have been variably associated with recurrence risk and survival outcomes.

Diagnosis and Treatment of Rare Gynecologic Cancers. https://doi.org/10.1016/B978-0-323-82938-0.00002-1

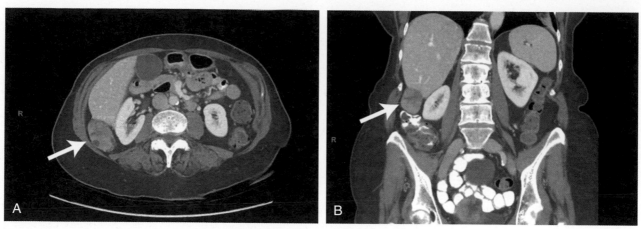

FIG. 2.1 CT images of perihepatic metastasis present at diagnosis in a woman with AGCT of the ovary.

TABLE 2.1 WHO classification of sex cord/stromal tumors of the ovary.

Sex cord/stromal tumors

Pure stromal tumors

- Fibroma
- Cellular fibroma
- Thecoma
- Luteinized thecoma associated with sclerosing peritonitis
- Fibrosarcoma
- Sclerosing stromal tumor
- Signet-ring stromal tumor
- Microcystic stromal tumor
- Leydig cell tumor
- Steroid cell tumor
- Steroid cell tumor, malignant

Pure sex cord tumors

- Adult-type granulosa cell tumor
- Juvenile-type granulosa cell tumor
- Sertoli cell tumor
- Sex cord tumor with annular tubules

Mixed sex cord/stromal tumors

- Sertoli–Leydig cell tumor
  - Well-differentiated
  - Moderately differentiated
    - With heterologous elements
  - Poorly differentiated
    - With heterologous elements
  - Retiform
    - With heterologous elements
- Sex cord/stromal tumors, NOS

Etiology/risk factors

There are no known environmental risk factors for the development of sex cord/stromal tumors. For example, a population-based cohort study in Scandinavia examined the risk of granulosa cell tumor across time and occupation between the years 1953 and 2012.[5] The stability of granulosa cell tumor incidence over the observation period of this study suggests that the usage of hormonal contraceptives, postmenopausal hormone replacement therapy, or fertility treatments do not substantially influence patterns of risk for this disease, since the use of these interventions changed dramatically throughout the 60-year observation period of this study. In the United States, both Sertoli–Leydig and granulosa cell tumors occur more frequently in Black women compared to White women or Asian/Pacific Islanders.[9]

Genetic evidence indicates that germline mutations may account for a subset of sex cord/stromal tumors. Hotspot somatic missense mutations in the RNase IIIb domain of the gene coding for the microRNA processing enzyme *DICER1* are found in approximately 60% of SLCTs, with a smaller subset of affected individuals also carrying truncating germline *DICER1* mutations.[15,16] Evidence from public exome sequencing datasets indicate that at least 1 in 10,000 individuals likely carry such a germline *DICER1* mutation, representing a Mendelian syndrome associated with an increased risk of SLCT as well as a spectrum of other malignancies including pediatric pleuropulmonary blastoma. The association between sex cord tumor with annular tubules and PJS was known from the time this tumor type was first described in 1970.[17] Germline pathogenic mutations in the *STK11* gene, the causative lesion of PJS, account for approximately one-third of all cases of sex cord tumor with annular tubules.[1] In contrast, *STK11* mutations are rare in sporadic sex cord tumor with annular tubules.[18]

Pathology

Adult granulosa cell tumor

Gross

The majority of AGCT are unilateral. The tumor size can vary from microscopic to extremely large (mean 10.0 cm). The tumors can be either entirely solid, solid and cystic or less commonly entirely cystic. The cyst contents may be serous or more typically hemorrhagic and rupture may result in hemoperitoneum. The cut surface of the solid component is usually yellow white in appearance.

Microscopic features

AGCT can demonstrate a variety of patterns including diffuse, microfollicular, macrofollicular, insular (discrete nests), trabecular/corded, gyriform, pseudopapillary, and watered-silk. The diffuse pattern is most common and is composed of fascicles of spindle cells (Fig. 2.2). The Call-Exner body (Fig. 2.3) characterized by the presence of tumor cells around a central space containing eosinophilic secretions, degenerating nuclei or hyaline material, resulting in the microfollicular pattern is the histologic hallmark of these tumors.[19] The background stroma can be either fibromatous or thecomatous and in some cases can largely overrun the granulosa cell component, making it difficult to recognize (Fig. 2.4). The nuclei of AGCT are oval and monotonous with fine chromatin and indistinct nucleoli. The coffee bean appearance secondary to the presence of nuclear grooves (Fig. 2.5) is characteristic. Mitotic activity is variable but is low in most cases (<4/10 hpfs). Of the various pathologic parameters no single one is predictive of adverse outcome for stage IA patients. Pathologic parameters such as tumor size, nuclear atypia, and the predominant histologic pattern of the tumor have not been shown to consistently predict behavior in patients with Stage 1A disease. There is some controversy about the mitotic index in that some authors report worse outcome with mitoses anywhere from >4 to >10/10 hpfs, while others have not found mitotic index to be predictive of behavior.[20]

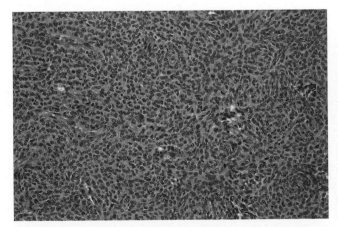

FIG. 2.2 The diffuse pattern of AGCT showing fascicles of spindle cells.

FIG. 2.3 The Call-Exner body is characterized by the presence of tumor cells around a central space containing eosinophilic secretions (*arrows*), resulting in the microfollicular pattern.

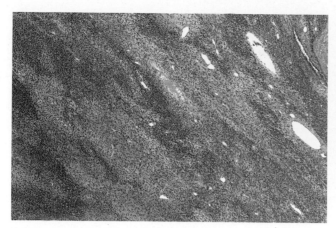

FIG. 2.4 AGCT with prominent fibromatous background mimicking cellular fibroma.

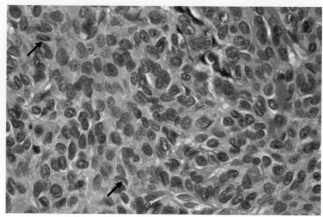

FIG. 2.5 High-power image of AGCT demonstrates oval and monotonous nuclei with indistinct nucleoli and nuclear grooves, giving the classic "coffee bean" appearance.

Ancillary testing

AGCT and all other sex cord tumors described in this chapter are usually positive for SF-1, inhibin (Fig. 2.6), and calretinin. Reticulin stain usually highlights loss of reticulin fibers around individual tumor cells.

Differential diagnosis

Due to the numerous histologic patterns of AGCT the differential diagnosis is quite vast and depends on the dominant pattern. Diffuse AGCT can be misinterpreted as cellular fibroma or endometrial stromal sarcoma. Loss of reticulin fibers around individual tumor cells in AGCT can help distinguish it from cellular fibroma. Endometrial stromal sarcomas have short spindle cells with typical spiral arteriole-like vascular pattern, lack of nuclear grooves and CD10 positivity, while they are negative for inhibin, calretinin and SF-1.

Endometrioid adenocarcinoma, particularly when they have sex cord-like pattern, can closely mimic the microfollicular pattern of AGCT. Areas of conventional pattern of endometrioid carcinoma with squamous and or mucinous differentiation are usually present and should facilitate this diagnosis. Furthermore, an adenofibromatous component and endometriosis will further support this diagnosis. Endometrioid carcinomas are positive for EMA and PAX-8 while negative for inhibin/calretinin/SF-1.

The nested appearance of the insular pattern of AGCT can resemble carcinoid tumor. The latter tumor has salt and pepper chromatin, lacks nuclear grooves and is positive for neuroendocrine markers synaptophysin and chromogranin. Markers of sex cord differentiation such as SF-1, inhibin and calretinin are negative. FOXL2 immunostain is positive in

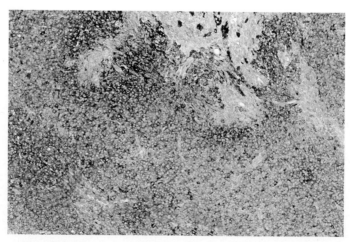

FIG. 2.6 AGCT showing positive staining for inhibin.

majority of sex cord/stromal tumors and can be used as an additional marker to distinguish sex cord/stromal tumors from epithelial tumors and other mimics, though this stain is not routinely available in most laboratories.

Lastly, the macrofollicular pattern of AGCT can mimic a follicular cyst. If the cyst is larger than 10 cm, has loss of theca cells and shows nuclear grooving and organization of tumor cells, a diagnosis of AGCT would be favored.

Molecular alterations

FOXL2 belongs to the family of forkhead/winged-helix transcription factors and has been shown to play an important role in the formation of follicles in the adult ovary. The majority of AGCT harbor a missense mutation c.402C-G (p. C134W) in the Forkhead box L2 (*FOXL2*) gene.[21,22] This mutation is absent in most sex cord tumors as well as epithelial tumors and is fairly sensitive and specific for AGCT. Rarely thecomas and JGCT have been reported to have the *FOXL2* mutation. Molecular testing for *FOXL2* is not typically performed in routine practice but may be helpful in challenging cases such as fibromatous AGCT.[22]

Juvenile granulosa cell tumor

Gross

JGCT are typically unilateral and present with disease confined to the ovary. These tumors can range from small to very large (mean, 12 cm). Similar to AGCT, the cut surface of the tumor can be purely solid, solid and cystic, or only cystic.

Microscopic findings

Histologically JGCT are composed of granulosa cells that can either have a diffuse or nodular pattern. Necrosis and hemorrhage may be present. Follicle-like spaces filled with basophilic or eosinophilic material are a key histologic feature in the diagnosis of JGCT (Fig. 2.7).[23] A subset of cases may have a pseudopapillary pattern. The tumor cells often have abundant pale pink or clear cytoplasm and the nuclei are small, round or oval. Nuclear grooves are rare or absent. Tumors with brisk mitotic activity and bizarre atypia (Fig. 2.7) are seen in about 10% of cases, but these findings do not appear to have an impact on prognosis. Small foci of JGCT can sometimes be admixed with AGCT or Sertoli cell tumors and these cases are classified based on the dominant histotype.

Ancillary testing

JGCT are positive for the usual sex cord markers such as inhibin, calretinin, CD56 and SF-1. A small subset may be positive for FOXL2 immunostain but its use in routine diagnosis is limited.[23]

Differential diagnosis

Differentiating JGCT from AGCT can be difficult particularly when the latter tumor shows prominent luteinization. Young age at presentation, nodular pattern, follicle-like spaces, and lack of nuclear grooves would favor JGCT.

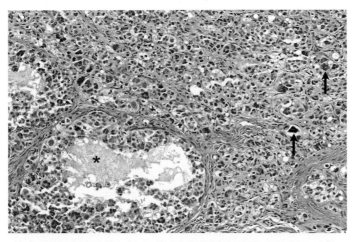

FIG. 2.7 Juvenile granulosa cell tumor showing follicle-like spaces (*) filled with basophilic material, and bizarre atypia (*arrow*).

Small cell carcinoma of the ovary, hypercalcemic type (SCCOHT) can closely mimic JGCT as both tumors are characterized by the presence of follicle-like spaces. SCCOHT is composed of small cells with minimal cytoplasm as well as rhabdoid morphology (large cell variant), and are negative for sex cord markers. Clinically, unlike JGCT, SCCOHT presents with advanced stage disease and a subset of patients have accompanying hypercalcemia. Recently studies have shown that most SCCOHT have either somatic or germline mutations in the *SMARCA4* gene, and lack SMARCA4 (BRG1) expression by immunohistochemistry. This latter finding is virtually diagnostic of SCCOHT and facilitates the correct diagnosis.[24]

Molecular alterations

The molecular mechanisms of JGCT are not that well studied. Trisomy12 is the most frequent cytogenetic abnormality identified and is present in most cases tested so far. *FOXL2* mutations rarely occur in JGCT. Recent studies have shown that JCGT have activating alterations in *AKT1* and *GNAS* that may contribute to the pathogenesis of these tumors.[25]

Sertoli–Leydig cell tumor

Gross

SLCT range from 2 to 35 cm in size. The cut surface is usually yellow-white and solid but can also be solid and cystic or rarely entirely cystic. Hemorrhage and necrosis and may be present.

Microscopic findings

Histologically, the tumors are broadly categorized as well, intermediate, or poorly differentiated based on the proportion of tubular and spindle component present. The tubular component is less represented in intermediate and poorly differentiated tumors. Tumors typically are composed of varying amounts of Sertoli cells and Leydig cells (Fig. 2.8), and the latter may be hard to identify in poorly differentiated tumors.[26] Well-differentiated SLCTs are composed of closely packed hollow or solid tubules separated by fibrous stroma within which clusters of Leydig cells are present. The nuclei of the tubules in well differentiated SLCTs show minimal to no atypia or mitotic activity. Leydig cells are characterized by abundant pink cytoplasm and single small nucleus. Neither heterologous elements nor retiform pattern are identified in well differentiated SLCTs.

SLCTs of intermediate differentiation have a characteristic low power appearance of alternating hyper and hypocellular areas. The cellular areas are composed of short spindle cells with minimal cytoplasm. Admixed Sertoli tubules as well as cords and trabeculae may be present. The Leydig cells may be present either within spindle cell areas or at the periphery of the cellular nodules. The Leydig cells have bland nuclei, no mitotic activity and may rarely contain Reinke crystals.

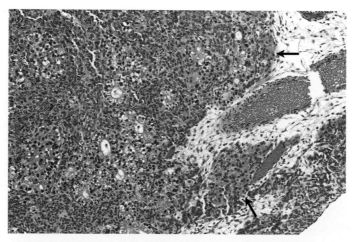

FIG. 2.8 Sertoli–Leydig cell tumor composed of tubules, spindle cells, and aggregates of Leydig cells (*arrows*).

Poorly differentiated SLCTs can be challenging to diagnose as they resemble a high-grade sarcoma, NOS. Typical aforementioned features of SLCT may not be readily identified and additional sampling of the tumor is usually necessary to facilitate the correct diagnosis.

Retiform SLCTs present in younger age group (average 15 years) and patients are less likely to be virilized. The retiform pattern is only associated with intermediate and poorly differentiated SLCTs. Histologically, the tumor cells are arranged in anastomosing, branched/slit-like spaces reminiscent of the normal rete testis.

Heterologous elements are present in approximately 20% of intermediate or poorly differentiated SLCTs. They may be epithelial or mesenchymal. The epithelial-type heterologous elements is more common and composed of glands lined by mucinous epithelium which may be benign, borderline, or carcinoma. Carcinoid tumors have also been described as a heterologous element in SLCTs. The most common mesenchymal-type heterologous elements are immature skeletal muscle (rhabdomyosarcoma) and immature fetal-type cartilage.

Ancillary testing

Immunohistochemical staining of SLCTs is similar to other sex cord/stromal tumors and they are variably positive for inhibin, calretinin and SF-1.

Differential diagnosis

The differential diagnosis of SLCTs is dependent of the degree of differentiation of these tumors. For well-differentiated SLCTs, the two most important differentials to include are sertoliform endometrioid adenocarcinoma and carcinoid tumors.

Diffuse-type AGCT with a prominent corded and trabecular pattern with admixed luteinized stromal cells can mimic SLCTs of intermediate differentiation. Female adnexal tumor of probable Wolffian origin can have some overlapping features with SLCTs but the they lack sertoliform tubules and Leydig cells, and patients do not present with androgenic symptoms.

Molecular alterations

SLCTs are now ascribed to be part of DICER1 syndrome, also known as the pleuropulmonary blastoma familial tumor and dysplasia syndrome, as germline *DICER1* mutations have been identified in these patients.[27] SLCTs with *DICER-1* mutations typically occur in younger women and are either of intermediate or poor differentiation, and have retiform pattern or heterologous elements.[28] On the other hand *FOXL2* mutated SLCTs occur predominantly in postmenopausal women also with intermediate/poor differentiation, but lack retiform and heterologous elements.[28]

Sex cord tumor with annular tubules

Gross

In sporadic cases of sex cord tumors with annular tubules (SCTAT), the tumor size is variable and can range from microscopic to large (up to 20.0 cm). However, in patients with PJS, the tumors are bilateral, small, calcified and usually incidentally detected. The tumors are usually solid but can also have a cystic component and have a yellow white cut surface.

Microscopic findings

The characteristic histologic appearance is the presence of "annular tubules" either simple or complex that encircle the central hyaline basement membrane like material (Fig. 2.9).[29] In the complex type, large islands composed of a network of communicating tubules is present. There is no nuclear atypia and mitoses are usually rare.

Ancillary testing

SCTAT are positive for SF-1, inhibin and calretinin similar to other sex cord/stromal tumors.

Differential diagnosis

The differential diagnosis for SCTAT includes AGCT, Sertoli cell tumor and gonadoblastoma. In AGCT, Call-Exner bodies may mimic the annular tubules of SCTAT, however, the central hyalinized basement membrane material and the ring-shaped tubular pattern seen in the latter are not present in AGCT. Sertoli cell tumor are characterized by individual tubules which is not seen in SCTAT, and they lack the typical annular tubules. Gonadoblastoma can mimic SCTAT due to

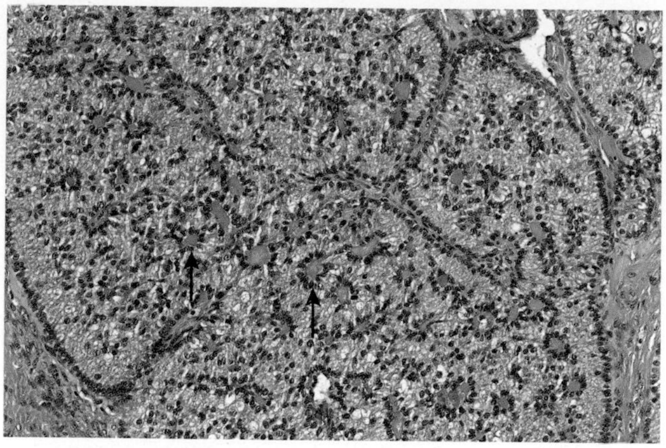

FIG. 2.9 Sex cord tumor with annular tubules (SCTAT) characterized by "annular tubules" that encircle the central hyaline basement membrane-like material (*arrows*).

similar nested pattern, areas of hyalinization and presence of calcification. However, these tumors have both germ cells and sex cord tumor cells and the former are not seen in SCTAT. The germ cells are larger in size and can be highlighted by stains such as OCT4. Furthermore, gonadoblastoma occurs almost exclusively in patients with gonadal dysgenesis.

Molecular alterations

There are only few reports on the molecular genetic alterations of SCTAT. In one study, germline mutations in the *STK11* gene and loss of heterozygosity in the 19p13.3 region were found in the two tested PJS-associated SCTATs.[29] Somatic mutations in the coding region of *STK11* were not identified in the 5 tested sporadic SCTATs.[18]

Diagnosis and workup

Signs and symptoms

The majority of sex cord/stromal tumors are diagnosed in symptomatic patients, and depending on size these symptoms can include distension or abdominal pain referable to mass effect from the tumor itself.[6,7,30] Case reports describe women with advanced or recurrent granulosa cell tumors presenting with acute abdominal pain secondary to hemoperitoneum, but this is a rare occurrence in modern practice.[31,32] Estrogen excess is frequently associated with AGCT of the ovary but can also be seen in other sex cord/stromal tumor subtypes. When present, estrogen production by the tumor can result in abnormal uterine bleeding or other menstrual abnormalities that lead an affected woman to seek medical evaluation, leading to the diagnosis of sex cord/stromal tumor. Similarly, SLCT and pure Leydig cell tumors can produce excess testosterone in 30%–50% of cases,[2] which is often sufficient to enjoin a diagnostic work up as a result of amenorrhea, hirsutism, or frank virilization. A significant minority of sex cord/stromal tumor are never symptomatic and instead are diagnosed incidentally during routine physical examination or imaging studies performed for unrelated indications.[6] It is rare for sex cord/stromal tumor to present with metastatic disease.

Physical exam findings

Pelvic examination reveals a palpable adnexal mass in most cases of sex cord/stromal tumor, which is often firm in character and most often unilateral. In a minority of cases, physical findings associated with hormonal excess are present. In the case of androgen excess, as with SLCT or Leydig cell tumors, the physical findings can range from mild hirsutism to frank virilization including clitoromegaly, deepening of the voice, or other changes in body morphology. As described above, estrogen excess can lead to abnormal uterine bleeding, infertility, or other symptoms that prompt an evaluation eventually leading to the diagnosis of sex cord/stromal tumor.

Differential diagnosis

The preoperative differential diagnosis is often broad in cases where an adnexal mass is ultimately proven to be a sex cord/stromal tumor. In many cases, there is no radiographic evidence of extraovarian spread. Even when the presence of solid

TABLE 2.2 Initial workup of newly diagnosed sex cord/stromal tumor of the ovary.

Physical exam	Complete physical exam with pelvic and rectovaginal examinations
Imaging	Pelvic ultrasound CT MRI pelvis (as indicated, to evaluate pelvic mass)
Laboratories	Inhibin A, Inhibin B, CA125 Total testosterone (if virilization present) Estradiol (if symptoms of estrogen excess present)
Additional testing	Endometrial biopsy or curettage to exclude coexisting uterine malignancy[a]

[a]If abnormal uterine bleeding is present in premenopausal woman or any postmenopausal woman with bleeding or thickened endometrial stripe.

elements on pelvic ultrasound suggests a sex cord/stromal tumor, many of these neoplasms will be benign fibromas or thecomas that can be definitively addressed with removal of the affected ovary. In the premenopausal age group often affected by many types of sex cord/stromal tumor, the differential diagnosis of a complex adnexal mass must include malignant germ cell tumors of the ovary and appropriate serum tumor markers [human chorionic gonadotropin (hCG), alpha-fetoprotein (AFP), lactate dehydrogenase (LDH)] can be obtained preoperatively as indicated. The recommended approach to the initial evaluation of a suspected sex cord/stromal tumor is shown in Table 2.2.

Tumor markers

Except in rare cases where symptoms of hormonal excess prompt an unusually high preoperative index of suspicion, most sex cord/stromal tumor are not diagnosed until pathologic assessment is made following removal of an ovarian mass. Since sex cord/stromal tumor are rare even among women diagnosed with a pelvic mass, the need for measurement of estrogen or testosterone levels during the initial evaluation of a pelvic mass should be guided by the presence of symptoms or clinical findings that indicate an excess of these hormones. For a young woman with a complex ovarian mass on imaging and clinical suspicion for malignancy, consideration should be given for preoperative measurement of epithelial (CA125), germ cell (LDH, hCG, AFP), and sex cord/stromal (inhibin A, inhibin B) ovarian tumor markers.

Elevation in CA125 is not consistently seen with sex cord/stromal tumor[7] and preoperative measurement of serum levels should be performed in the evaluation of an adnexal mass when it is indicated by patient age or radiographic findings suggestive of malignancy. Inhibins A and B are closely related glycoprotein heterodimers produced by granulosa cells in the adult female that together comprise an important feedback signal in the gonadal–hypothalamic–pituitary axis. Of these two hormones, some evidence suggests inhibin B is more sensitive for the detection of granulosa cell tumor but the utility of measuring serum inhibin levels is greatest in the early detection of recurrent disease during surveillance.[33] Anti-Mullerian hormone (AMH) is a glycoprotein normally produced by granulosa cells of preantral and antral follicles of premenopausal women and elevations of AMH can be seen in most cases of AGCT of the ovary and JGCT of the ovary.[34] Although AMH has been shown to have some utility in surveillance for the detection of recurrent disease,[35] it is not routinely measured in the evaluation of an adnexal mass in either premenopausal or postmenopausal women. If intraoperative pathologic evaluation of an adnexal mass is suggestive for granulosa cell tumor, it is recommended that serum inhibins be measured on the day of surgery as a baseline.

Imaging studies

Since diagnostic confirmation or even suspicion for a sex cord/stromal tumor may not be present until after surgical excision and pathologic evaluation have been performed, the choice of preoperative imaging usually includes transvaginal ultrasound or other modalities commonly used to evaluate isolated adnexal masses. Ultrasound findings for sex cord/stromal tumors are variable and can include both solid as cystic elements, as well as areas of internal hemorrhage. In cases where granulosa cell tumors are associated with estrogen excess, a thickened or heterogeneous endometrial stripe can be seen. CT or MRI should be reserved for situations where suspicion for malignancy exists or ultrasound findings are indeterminate.

Diagnostic testing

Estrogen excess from hormonally active sex cord/stromal tumor should be suspected when an adnexal mass is identified in a woman with abnormal uterine bleeding or in a postmenopausal woman with a thickened endometrial stripe on pelvic ultrasound. In these cases, preoperative endometrial biopsy (EMB) is essential since both single-institution and population-based studies indicate that at the time of AGCT of the ovary diagnosis, synchronous endometrial hyperplasia or carcinoma can be found is 25%–30% and 6%–8% of cases, respectively.[36,37] If endometrial hyperplasia or carcinoma is detected preoperatively, hysterectomy can be performed at the time of surgery for management of the adnexal mass along with lymph node evaluation if indicated for endometrial cancer. Except in unusual circumstances where clinically apparent androgen or estrogen excess is present during the initial evaluation of an adnexal mass, it is not necessary in most cases of an isolated adnexal mass to measure hormone levels or perform specialized tumor marker testing preoperatively.

Staging system

Staging for sex cord/stromal tumor utilizes the FIGO staging system for ovarian cancer (Table 2.3). This staging system was last updated in 2014 to incorporate additional subclassification of both early stage and advanced disease. Since most sex cord/stromal tumors are grossly confined to a single ovary at the time of diagnosis (see Section "Prognostic factors"), the majority of these tumors are denoted stage IA.

Prognostic factors

Tumor stage at the time of granulosa cell tumor diagnosis is the most consistent factor linked to prognosis across published studies spanning several decades.[7,11,38] Initial stage is also associated with prognosis in SLCT although more than 95% are stage IA at the time of diagnosis.[2] Given the prognostic importance of tumor stage across subtypes of sex cord/stromal tumor, an area of investigation has been assessment of the utility of surgical staging in these tumor types. Retrospective single-institution studies and population-base epidemiologic data have consistently shown that the rate of lymph node metastases detected in patients with granulosa cell tumor undergoing lymphadenectomy is less than 5%[39–41] and rates of lymph node positivity in apparently early stage SLCT may be even lower.[42] It is important to note that the denominator in most studies designed to estimate the rate of lymph node metastasis is the group of patients who underwent lymphadenectomy. Since the surgeon's decision to perform lymphadenectomy is not independent from clinical factors like tumor size or the presence of gross extraovarian disease, it is likely that published estimates for the rate of lymph node positivity in this disease represent an upper bound and that the true rate could be much lower. Nevertheless, when advanced stage disease or positive lymph nodes are identified, these findings are associated with worse survival outcomes across sex cord/stromal tumor subtypes.[43]

Some retrospective series indicate that tumor size may be an independent prognostic variable for survival outcomes following treatment for sex cord/stromal tumor,[11,44] although other groups have not confirmed this association.[43] In granulosa cell tumor specifically, several clinical and histologic variables such as age at diagnosis, body mass index, tumor mitotic index, or cellular atypia have been inconsistently found to be associated with survival outcomes or recurrence rates,[11,13,14] although none of these factors individually or in combination have been prospectively validated for use in treatment stratification. Tumor rupture, either preoperative or during surgery, increases the FIGO staging of apparently localized disease and there is evidence from retrospective studies that this increases the likelihood of recurrence.[45]

Treatment of primary disease

Initial treatment for sex cord/stromal tumor is primarily determined by the extent of disease at the time of diagnosis (Fig. 2.10). Except in very rare cases where distant metastatic disease is present at the time of diagnosis, primary surgery is the mainstay approach for the treatment of sex cord/stromal tumor. When extraovarian disease is present at the time of surgery, an attempt should be made to remove all grossly visible disease following principles of surgical cytoreduction adapted from the treatment of women with epithelial ovarian cancers. Overall 95% of sex cord/stromal tumors are initially confined to a single ovary which makes it incumbent upon the surgeon to select the most appropriate surgical procedure based upon the age and reproductive goals of the patient. Fertility sparing surgery, including preservation of a contralateral ovary and uterus, is often feasible in the initial treatment of sex cord/stromal tumor and is an important consideration in treatment planning given significant portion of these tumors are diagnosed in premenopausal women.

TABLE 2.3 TNM and FIGO staging for ovary, fallopian tube, and primary peritoneal carcinomas.

T category	FIGO stage	T criteria
		**Primary tumor (T)**
TX		Primary tumor cannot be assessed
T0		No evidence of primary tumor
T1	I	Tumor limited to ovaries (one or both) or fallopian tube(s)
T1a	IA	Tumor limited to one ovary (capsule intact) or fallopian tube, no tumor on ovarian or fallopian tube surface; no malignant cells in ascites or peritoneal washings
T1b	IB	Tumor limited to both ovaries (capsules intact) or fallopian tubes; no tumor on ovarian or fallopian tube surface; no malignant cells in ascites or peritoneal washings
T1c	IC	Tumor limited to one or both ovaries or fallopian tubes, with any of the following:
T1c1	IC1	• Surgical spill
T1c2	IC2	• Capsule ruptured before surgery or tumor on ovarian or fallopian tube surface
T1c3	IC3	• Malignant cells in ascites or peritoneal washings
T2	II	Tumor involves one or both ovaries or fallopian tubes with pelvic extension below pelvic brim or primary peritoneal cancer
T2a	IIA	Extension and/or implants on the uterus and/or fallopian tube(s) and/or ovaries
T2b	IIB	Extension to and/or implants on other pelvic tissues
T3	III	Tumor involves one or both ovaries or fallopian tubes, or primary peritoneal cancer, with microscopically confirmed peritoneal metastasis outside the pelvis and/or metastasis to the retroperitoneal (pelvic and/or paraaortic) lymph nodes
T3a	IIIA2	Microscopic extrapelvic (above the pelvic brim) peritoneal involvement with or without positive retroperitoneal lymph nodes
T3b	IIIB	Macroscopic peritoneal metastasis beyond pelvis 2 cm or less in greatest dimension with or without metastasis to the retroperitoneal lymph nodes
T3c	IIIC	Macroscopic peritoneal metastasis beyond the pelvis more than 2 cm in greatest dimension with or without metastasis to the retroperitoneal lymph nodes (includes extension of tumor to capsule of liver and spleen without parenchymal involvement of either organ)

N category	FIGO stage	N criteria
		**Regional lymph nodes (N)**
NX		Regional lymph nodes cannot be assessed
N0		No regional lymph node metastasis
N0(i+)		Isolated tumor cells in regional lymph node(s) no greater than 0.2 mm
N1	IIIA1	Positive retroperitoneal lymph nodes only (histologically confirmed)
N1a	IIIA1i	Metastasis up to and including 10 mm in greatest dimension
N1b	IIIA1ii	Metastasis more than 10 mm in greatest dimension

M category	FIGO stage	M criteria
		**Distant metastasis (M)**
M0		No distant metastasis
M1	IV	Distant metastasis, including pleural effusion with positive cytology; liver or splenic parenchymal metastasis; metastasis to extraabdominal organs (including inguinal lymph nodes and lymph nodes outside the abdominal cavity); and transmural involvement of intestine
M1a	IVA	Pleural effusion with positive cytology
M1b	IVB	Liver or splenic parenchymal metastases; metastases to extraabdominal organs (including inguinal lymph nodes and lymph nodes outside the abdominal cavity); transmural involvement of intestine

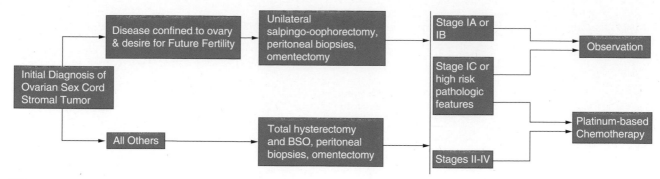

FIG. 2.10   Triage of primary treatment.

A diagnosis of sex cord/stromal tumor is not usually known prior to surgery since preoperative biopsy of a pelvic mass is uncommon. Instead, the most typical situation that prompts surgical evaluation is the presence of a complex adnexal mass, either symptomatic or incidentally detected, for which surgical removal is indicated based upon size or other imaging features.[46] Whenever feasible based upon tumor size and patient factors, removal of an adnexal mass via a minimally invasive laparoscopic approach is preferable since this will minimize surgical morbidity without compromising oncologic outcomes.[47] Spillage of cyst contents should be scrupulously avoided as this increases the FIGO stage and may be associated with an increased risk of recurrence.[45] Regardless of surgical approach, a careful inspection of abdominal contents and peritoneal surfaces is indicated during surgery for an adnexal mass, with biopsies taken of any suspicious areas. If present, ascites should be collected for cytology and otherwise peritoneal washings should be performed.

Low-risk early stage disease

When the tumor is confined to a single ovary and no spillage occurs during surgery, removal of the affected ovary is usually curative for AGCT of the ovary, JGCT of the ovary, or SLCT without high-risk pathologic features (see below). Whenever intraoperative pathology is suggestive of an early stage sex cord/stromal tumor with potentially malignant histology, published guidelines support the performance of surgical staging procedures to assess the extent of disease.[48] For postmenopausal women, complete staging includes total hysterectomy (TAH), bilateral salpingo-oophorectomy (BSO), pelvic washings, peritoneal biopsies, and infra-colic omentectomy. Based on the aforementioned retrospective data demonstrating low rates of lymph node involvement with apparently early stage sex cord/stromal tumor,[39–41] staging lymphadenectomy can be safely omitted although any bulky or suspicious lymph nodes should be biopsied or removed.

Fertility sparing procedures that conserve the uterus and contralateral ovary are associated with excellent outcomes in apparently early stage sex cord/stromal tumor.[49,50] Note that removal of the affected ovary is preferable to cystectomy as retrospective data suggests superior oncologic outcomes with this approach.[49] For women in which a cystectomy has been performed with subsequent identification of a malignant sex cord/stromal tumor on final pathology, these same data suggest that an additional procedure to remove the affected ovary may reduce the risk of recurrence. Specifically, for this cohort of women with early stage granulosa cell tumor, the 5-year disease-free survival (DFS) following unilateral salpingo-oophorectomy (USO) was 84% compared to only 25% for cystectomy.[49] The DFS was 82% for those women who underwent completion USO following initial cystectomy, a favorable outcome more consistent with the group undergoing initial USO. Data on overall survival outcomes and fertility sparing surgery are limited, but suggest the safety of this practice in well-selected women with stage I disease.[51] When uterine conservation is planned and preoperative granulosa cell tumor is suspected, endometrial curettage should also be performed to exclude a coexisting uterine malignancy. Retrospective data support the safety of laparoscopy in the surgical management of apparently early stage granulosa cell tumor with regard to survival outcomes.[47]

Since clinically apparent symptoms of hormonal excess or elevation in tumor markers are not detected preoperatively in most women with sex cord/stromal tumor, a common situation that arises in oncology practice is the referral of women with apparent stage IA sex cord/stromal tumor detected on final pathology following removal of an adnexal mass by a general gynecologist. When one or both ovaries have been removed and no evidence of extraovarian disease or spillage was documented at the time of initial surgery, we recommend initiating surveillance for AGCT of the ovary, JGCT of the ovary and SLCT without high-risk pathologic features rather than performing a second staging surgery due to the low rates of lymph node involvement.[39–41] Also in support of this approach are data suggesting that outcomes are similar when comparing USO with more extensive surgery in the management of apparently early stage granulosa cell tumor.[49] If the surgery was performed by another surgeon and documentation of abdominal survey is incomplete or not available for review, it is essential to perform baseline radiographic assessment to exclude occult extraovarian disease.

High-risk early-stage disease

Certain clinical and pathologic risk factors are associated with a higher risk of sex cord/stromal tumor recurrence and may warrant consideration of adjuvant chemotherapy. Tumor rupture during surgery or the presence of tumor on the ovarian surface or in peritoneal washings all increase the FIGO stage and are features likely associated with an increased risk of recurrence. The MITO-9 group examined whether those women with stage IC granulosa cell tumor derived benefit from adjuvant chemotherapy (carboplatin/paclitaxel or bleomycin/etoposide/cisplatin [BEP]).[52] Of 40 women meeting inclusion criteria for this study, only 23% received adjuvant chemotherapy and there was no statistically significant difference in survival outcomes associated with this practice. National guidelines continue to support adjuvant chemotherapy as an option for stage IC sex cord/stromal tumor[48] but the use of chemotherapy in this setting should be individualized and we encourage a shared decision-making approach in which the areas of uncertainty are clearly explained to the affected individual.

Early-stage, well-differentiated SLCT have little if any risk of recurrence after surgical resection, however those tumors with intermediate differentiation may recur in 11% of cases and poorly differentiated tumors in 59% of cases.[2] Survival also appears to correlate with SLCT grade, with only 62% of women with poorly differentiated tumors alive after 5 years.[30] Similarly, the presence of heterologous (e.g., gastrointestinal (GI)) elements or a retiform pattern have also been linked to a poor prognosis.[2,12] There are no high-quality data to suggest that the use of adjuvant chemotherapy in SLCT with such high-risk pathologic features can effectively reduce the risk of recurrence. Therefore, as with stage IC disease, we recommend individualizing the decision to use adjuvant chemotherapy (carboplatin/paclitaxel or BEP) for early-stage SLCT with high-risk pathologic features.

Metastatic disease

The identification of widespread extraovarian disease at the time of initial sex cord/stromal tumor diagnosis is unusual. For example, one survey of published retrospective series found that stage III–IV disease was present in only 5%–15% of women with newly diagnosed granulosa cell tumor[8] and the rate of advanced stage SLCT is likely even lower.[53] Complete cytoreduction of all visible tumor should be the surgical objective with newly diagnosed advanced stage sex cord/stromal tumor, following principles utilized for the treatment of epithelial ovarian cancer, as both cancer registry data and single institution retrospective series support improved survival outcomes when complete gross resection (CGR) is achieved.[6,54] National guidelines support the use of adjuvant platinum-based chemotherapy for the treatment of advanced stage sex cord/stromal tumor but acknowledge the limited data supporting the efficacy of this practice.[48] Recently published independent analyses of both the Surveillance, Epidemiology, and End Results (SEER) registry and National Cancer Database (NCDB) both failed to find an improvement in DFS associated with the use of adjuvant chemotherapy in the treatment of stage II-IV granulosa cell tumor.[54,55] In contrast, an analysis of NCDB examining a small number of advanced stage nongranulosa cell tumor sex cord/stromal tumor, more than 70% of which were SLCTs, found a survival benefit with the use of adjuvant chemotherapy.[56]

There are no high-quality prospective data to support the superior efficacy of one particular chemotherapy regimen over another for the treatment of sex cord/stromal tumors. Historically, BEP[57] was frequently used to treat advanced stage or high-risk sex cord/stromal tumor but paclitaxel/carboplatin is now our preferred regimen given evidence supporting the efficacy of taxanes in this disease[58,59] and the improved toxicity profile of this combination compared to BEP.

Surveillance for recurrence

As is the case with the more common epithelial ovarian cancer subtypes, the mainstays of posttreatment surveillance for sex cord/stromal tumors include physical examination, careful review of symptoms, and monitoring of serum tumor markers when applicable. Symptoms suggestive of recurrence may be vague or nonspecific but could include new onset of localized or diffuse pain, changes in bowel or bladder habits, weight loss, loss of appetite, bloating, or symptoms of androgenic or estrogenic excess. Periodic physical examination should be performed and must include lymph node surveys as well as abdominal and pelvic examinations. CA125, inhibin A/B, or other serum tumor markers can be measured as part of surveillance and their use should be individualized depending on the tumor subtype and whether an elevation in a specific marker was detected at the time of initial diagnosis. NCCN guidelines dichotomize the recommended frequency of surveillance visits on the basis of initial stage.[48] For sex cord/stromal tumors confined the ovary, surveillance visits should occur every 6–12 months while for high-risk or advanced-stage disease these visits should occur more frequently, typically every 4–6 months. Radiographic assessment should be reserved for situations where physical exam findings, symptoms, or elevated serum tumor markers are suggestive of possible recurrence. Our practice is to use a cross-sectional imaging technique such as CT to evaluated suspected recurrence. Although a previous metaanalysis suggested some utility for the use of PET/CT in evaluating recurrence of epithelial ovarian cancer,[60] the use of this modality should be individualized given higher cost and a lack of data evaluating its use in sex cord/stromal tumor surveillance. Although late recurrences of sex cord/stromal tumor even after 10 years following initial diagnosis, it is still our practice to perform surveillance visits more frequently in the first 2 years and individualize the need for further surveillance after 5 years.

Survival and patterns of failure

Survival outcomes are generally excellent for granulosa cell tumor, with five-year disease-specific survival >95% for stage I disease and 22%–50% for stage III (Table 2.4).[32] These results reflect the indolent, slow growing nature of the disease combined with the high rates of surgical cure when disease is initially confined to the ovary. Well-differentiated (grade 1) SLCT exhibit little, if any, risk of recurrence.[2,30] A retrospective review by the MITO-9 study group demonstrated that while grade 2–3 SLCT as a group had a five-year overall survival rate of 77.8%, the five-year overall survival rate for tumors with stage >I fell to 33.3%.[30] Although granulosa cell tumor can recur five or even 10 years after diagnosis,[61] most SLCT recurrences will occur within the first 5 years.[2,53] The most common sites of sex cord/stromal tumor recurrence are in the abdomen or pelvis.[30,61,62]

Treatment of recurrent disease

There are little data to support definitive recommendations about the management of recurrent sex cord/stromal tumor, and many options are acceptable (Table 2.5). When prospective trials have been completed these have most often included women with all forms of malignant sex cord/stromal tumor or, since it is the most common subtype, only those with granulosa cell tumor. The treatment of rarer forms of sex cord/stromal tumor in the recurrent setting is therefore either based on extrapolation from those trials that have been done or limited retrospective observational studies. When feasible, surgical cytoreduction is attempted in most women with a first recurrence of sex cord/stromal tumor[30,61,62,75] and survival outcomes in the recurrent setting appear superior when complete cytoreduction is achieved.[62] We prefer some form of systemic adjuvant treatment following surgical cytoreduction for women with recurrent sex cord/stromal tumor and will use systemic therapy alone if surgery is not an option. The systemic therapy options outlined below have varied levels of data supporting their use, and there are few prospective published trials examining the comparative effectiveness of various regimens.

Chemotherapy

Due to the longstanding use of BEP in the adjuvant treatment of advanced primary sex cord/stromal tumor,[63] this regimen is also frequently used in the recurrent setting especially for the treatment of younger women or those with an excellent performance status. Newer data on the activity of taxanes[58,59,67] in sex cord/stromal tumor have led to carboplatin/paclitaxel given every 21 days increasingly replacing BEP in our practice and this is an especially reasonable choice for women who are older or frailer, or those who received BEP in the upfront setting and subsequently recurred. More recently an objective response rate of 25% was seen with weekly paclitaxel in a prospective randomized trial examining the addition of bevacizumab to this backbone.[68] A collaborative multicenter prospective randomized trial comparing BEP to carboplatin/paclitaxel for advanced or recurrent sex cord/stromal tumor (GOG-0264) was closed early for futility following

TABLE 2.4 Five- and 10-year survival by stage for granulosa cell tumors.

FIGO stage	5-Year survival (%)	10-Year survival (%)
I	90–100	84–95
II	55–75	50–65
III/IV	22–50	17–33

Reproduced from Schumer ST, Cannistra SA. Granulosa cell tumor of the ovary. *J Clin Oncol.* 2003;21(6):1180–1189.

TABLE 2.5 Therapeutic options for recurrent sex cord/stromal tumors of the ovary

Regimen	Level of support
Bleomycin/etoposide/cisplatin	Single-arm phase II trials[57,63]; case series[64]
Paclitaxel/carboplatin	Case series[65]
Bevacizumab	Single-arm phase II trial[66]
Single-agent paclitaxel	Single-arm phase II trial (every 21 days)[67]; Randomized phase II trial (weekly)[68]
Aromatase inhibitors (anastrozole, letrozole)	Single-arm phase II trial[69]; Case series (see Ref. 70 for summary)
GnRH agonist (leuprolide)	Case series (see Ref. 70 for summary)
Selective estrogen receptor modulator (tamoxifen)	Case series (see Ref. 70 for summary)
Doxorubicin	Case report[71]
Cisplatin/doxorubicin/cyclophosphamide	Single-arm phase II trial[72]
High-dose chemotherapy with hematopoietic progenitor cell support	Case series[73]
Radiation therapy	Case series[74]

a preplanned interim analysis in 2020. It is therefore unlikely that the comparative effectiveness of BEP and carboplatin/paclitaxel will ever be formally evaluated for sex cord/stromal tumors.

Hormonal therapy

Pathologic studies demonstrate that the majority of sex cord/stromal tumor exhibit estrogen or progesterone receptor expression[76] and approaches to the modulation of local or systemic hormone levels serve as an important treatment modality for these diseases. A systematic review of the published evidence for hormonal therapy in granulosa cell tumor identified a pooled overall response rate (ORR) of 71% across a heterogeneous group of treatment regimens, although this is likely an overestimate due to the inherent reporting bias of the retrospective series included in this review.[70] Although the number of evaluable subjects was small, it appeared from this study that aromatase inhibitors (anastrozole and letrozole) exhibited a very high rate of complete and partial response. In contrast, the use of regimens containing gonadotropin releasing hormone agonists (leuprolide) or antagonists (ganirelix acetate and goserelin) was associated with a 30% objective response rate (6 of 18 evaluable subjects) with nearly all responses being among those treated with leuprolide. In contrast to these optimistic results are preliminary results from the PARAGON trial, a phase II study of anastrozole in hormone-receptor positive advanced or recurrent granulosa cell tumor, which found a much lower objective response rate.[69] The overall picture from the available literature is that aromatase inhibitors and leuprolide have some objective evidence for efficacy in the treatment of granulosa cell tumor and are reasonable choices in lieu of salvage chemotherapy, or as maintenance treatment following a response to chemotherapy in the recurrent setting. The use of hormonal agents should also be considered in women with a poor performance status or for whom the quality-of-life impact of chemotherapy may be unacceptable. Additional prospective data will be needed to further clarify the comparative effectiveness of hormonal regimens in sex cord/stromal tumor and whether these regimens could effectively substitute for systemic chemotherapy in some settings.

Angiogenesis inhibitors

Bevacizumab is a humanized monoclonal antibody that acts as an antiangiogenesis agent by inhibiting the action of vascular endothelial growth factor A. Early interest in the use of this agent for treatment of sex cord/stromal tumor led to a small phase II single-arm trial of bevacizumab, which found an ORR of approximately 17%.[66] Importantly, an additional 77% of trial participants had stable disease after a median of 9 cycles of bevacizumab, with a median progression-free survival (PFS) of more than 9 months. More recently the results of the ALIENOR/ENGOT-ov7 were published, which described the results of a randomized trial examining weekly paclitaxel with or without concurrent bevacizumab followed by bevacizumab maintenance.[68] The primary outcome of this study, 6-month PFS, did not significantly differ with the addition of bevacizumab. Thus, although single-agent bevacizumab is a reasonable option for systemic treatment of advanced or recurrent sex cord/stromal tumor in the second line or beyond, more data are needed before the addition of bevacizumab to chemotherapy can be universally recommended.

Radiotherapy

Data supporting the use of external beam radiation in the treatment of sex cord/stromal tumor, either in the adjuvant setting or definitively for oligometastatic disease, are limited to case reports and small single-institution series.[74,77] There are insufficient data to support the routine use of adjuvant pelvic radiation in the treatment of sex cord/stromal tumor, but the directed use of external beam radiation to treat unresectable tumor sites should be individualized on a case-by-case basis.

Special considerations

Some sex cord/stromal tumor subtypes including SLCT and JGCT of the ovary can be diagnosed during adolescence or childhood.[78] Limited small cases series suggest that survival outcomes are excellent when JGCT of the ovary is treated with fertility-sparing surgery in which the uterus and contra-lateral ovary are preserved,[79] potentially even when advanced stage disease is present.[80] Given the extremely rare incidence of sex cord/stromal tumor in this population, we recommend that adolescents and children with a confirmed or suspected diagnosis be treated at referral centers by multidisciplinary teams including pediatric gynecologists and oncologists. JGCT of the ovary have been described in the setting of both Ollier and Maffucci syndromes, related sporadic conditions associated with vascular malformations or enchondromas.[81] When evaluating an adolescent or child with newly diagnosed sex cord/stromal tumor, it is therefore essential to obtain a detailed history and perform a thorough physical examination to identify any evidence for a coexisting pediatric syndrome. Referral to a fertility specialist with experience caring for young women or girls with gynecologic cancers should occur early in the treatment planning process.

Case resolution

This 58 years old first underwent office EMB, which was negative for endometrial adenocarcinoma or hyperplasia. She then underwent primary cytoreductive surgery. Surgery was performed via midline laparotomy incision and included TAH, BSO, and partial mobilization of the liver with complete cytoreduction of all visible disease. Pathology revealed a metastatic AGCT with implants involving the pelvic side wall and liver surface. Uterine pathology was notable for a small focus of complex atypical endometrial hyperplasia. Postoperatively, she received 6 cycles of paclitaxel and carboplatin, given every 21 days, with normalization of inhibin B level and no evidence of disease on posttreatment CT imaging. She tolerated this regimen and remains disease free 5 years following the completion of adjuvant treatment.

References

1. Young RH, Welch WR, Dickersin GR, Scully RE. Ovarian sex cord tumor with annular tubules: review of 74 cases including 27 with Peutz-Jeghers syndrome and four with adenoma malignum of the cervix. *Cancer.* 1982;50(7):1384–1402.
2. Young RH, Scully RE. Ovarian Sertoli-Leydig cell tumors. A clinicopathological analysis of 207 cases. *Am J Surg Pathol.* 1985;9(8):543–569.
3. Torre LA, Trabert B, DeSantis CE, et al. Ovarian cancer statistics, 2018. *CA Cancer J Clin.* 2018;68(4):284–296.
4. *International Classification of Diseases for Oncology.* 2nd ed; 2020.
5. Bryk S, Pukkala E, Martinsen J-IJ-I, et al. Incidence and occupational variation of ovarian granulosa cell tumours in Finland, Iceland, Norway and Sweden during 1953–2012: a longitudinal cohort study. *BJOG Int J Obstet Gynaecol.* 2017;124(1):143–149.
6. Sun HD, Lin H, Jao MS, et al. A long-term follow-up study of 176 cases with adult-type ovarian granulosa cell tumors. *Gynecol Oncol.* 2012;124(2):244–249.
7. Lee IH, Choi CH, Hong DG, et al. Clinicopathologic characteristics of granulosa cell tumors of the ovary: a multicenter retrospective study. *J Gynecol Oncol.* 2011;22(3):188–195. PMCID: PMC3188718.
8. Levin G, Zigron R, Haj-Yahya R, Matan LS, Rottenstreich A. Granulosa cell tumor of ovary: a systematic review of recent evidence. *Eur J Obstet Gynecol Reprod Biol.* 2018;225:57–61.
9. Nasioudis D, Mastroyannis SA, Haggerty AF, Ko EM, Latif NA. Ovarian Sertoli-Leydig and granulosa cell tumor: comparison of epidemiology and survival outcomes. *Arch Gynecol Obstet.* 2020;302(2):481–486. https://doi.org/10.1007/s00404-020-05633-z. Epub 2020 Jun 9. PMID: 32519016.
10. Prat J. Staging classification for cancer of the ovary, fallopian tube, and peritoneum. *Int J Gynecol Obstet.* 2014;124(1):1–5.
11. Miller BE, Barron BA, Wan JY, Delmore JE, Silva EG, Gershenson DM. Prognostic factors in adult granulosa cell tumor of the ovary. *Cancer.* 1997;79(10):1951–1955.

12. Young RH, Scully RE. Ovarian Sertoli-Leydig cell tumors with a retiform pattern: a problem in histopathologic diagnosis. A report of 25 cases. *Am J Surg Pathol.* 1983;7(8):755–771.
13. Stenwig JT, Hazekamp JT, Beecham JB. Granulosa cell tumors of the ovary. A clinicopathological study of 118 cases with long-term follow-up. *Gynecol Oncol.* 1979;7(2):136–152.
14. van Meurs HS, Schuit E, Horlings HM, et al. Development and internal validation of a prognostic model to predict recurrence free survival in patients with adult granulosa cell tumors of the ovary. *Gynecol Oncol.* 2014;134(3):498–504.
15. Heravi-Moussavi A, Anglesio MS, Cheng S-WG, et al. Recurrent somatic DICER1 mutations in nonepithelial ovarian cancers. *N Engl J Med.* 2012;366(3):234–242.
16. Conlon N, Schultheis AM, Piscuoglio S, et al. A survey of DICER1 hotspot mutations in ovarian and testicular sex cord-stromal tumors. *Mod Pathol.* 2015;28(12):1603–1612.
17. Scully RE. Sex cord tumor with annular tubules a distinctive ovarian tumor of the Peutz-Jeghers syndrome. *Cancer.* 1970;25(5):1107–1121.
18. Connolly DC, Katabuchi H, Cliby WA, Cho KR. Somatic mutations in the STK11/LKB1 gene are uncommon in rare gynecological tumor types associated with Peutz-Jegher's syndrome. *Am J Pathol.* 2000;156(1):339–345.
19. Rabban JT, Buza N, Devouassoux-Shisheboran M, Hunstman DG, Kommoss F. Adult granulosa cell tumor. In: WHO Classification of Tumors Editorial Board, ed. *Female Genital Tumors.* World Health Organization Classification of Tumors. Lyon: IARC Press; 2020:105–106.
20. Jamieson S, Butzow R, Andersson N, et al. The FOXL2 C134W mutation is characteristic of adult granulosa cell tumors of the ovary. *Mod Pathol.* 2010;23:1477–1485.
21. Stewart CJR, Amanuel B, De Kock L, et al. Evaluation of molecular analysis in challenging ovarian sex cord-stromal tumours: a review of 50 cases. *Pathology.* 2020;52(6):686–693.
22. Miller K, McCluggage WG. Prognostic factors in ovarian adult granulosa cell tumour. *J Clin Pathol.* 2008;61(8):881–884.
23. Stewart CJR, Ganesa R, Irving JA. Juvenile granulosa cell tumor. In: WHO Classification of Tumors Editorial Board, ed. *Female Genital Tumors.* World Health Organization Classification of Tumors. Lyon: IARC Press; 2020:107–108.
24. Clarke BA, Witkowski L, Ton Nu TN, et al. SMARCA4 (BRG1) protein expression as determined by immunohistochemistry in small-cell carcinoma of the ovary, hypercalcaemic type distinguishes these tumours from their mimics. *Histopathology.* 2016;69(5):727–738.
25. Auguste A, Bessière L, Todeschini AL, et al. Molecular analyses of juvenile granulosa cell tumors bearing *AKT1* mutations provide insights into tumor biology and therapeutic leads. *Hum Mol Genet.* 2015;24(23):6687–6698.
26. Kommoss F, Buza N, Karnezis AN, Shen DH. Sertoli-Leydig cell tumor. In: WHO Classification of Tumors Editorial Board, ed. *Female Genital Tumors.* World Health Organization Classification of Tumors. Lyon: IARC Press; 2020:113–115.
27. de Kock L, Terzic T, McCluggage WG, et al. DICER1 mutations are consistently present in moderately and poorly differentiated Sertoli-Leydig cell tumors. *Am J Surg Pathol.* 2017;41(9):1178–1187.
28. Karnezis AN, Wang Y, Keul K, et al. DICER1 and FOXL2 mutation status correlates with clinicopathologic features in ovarian Sertoli-Leydig cell tumors. *Am J Surg Pathol.* 2019;43(5):628–638.
29. Young RH, Kiyokawa T, Stewart CJR. Sex cord tumor with annular tubules. In: WHO Classification of Tumors Editorial Board, ed. *Female Genital Tumors.* World Health Organization Classification of Tumors. Lyon: IARC Press; 2020:111–112.
30. Sigismondi C, Gadducci A, Lorusso D, et al. Ovarian Sertoli-Leydig cell tumors. A retrospective MITO study. *Gynecol Oncol.* 2012;125(3):673–676.
31. Lee WL, Yuan CC, Lai CR, Wang PH. Hemoperitoneum is an initial presentation of recurrent granulosa cell tumors of the ovary. *Jpn J Clin Oncol.* 1999;29(10):509–512.
32. Schumer ST, Cannistra SA. Granulosa cell tumor of the ovary. *J Clin Oncol.* 2003;21(6):1180–1189.
33. Mom CH, Engelen MJA, Willemse PHB, et al. Granulosa cell tumors of the ovary: the clinical value of serum inhibin A and B levels in a large single center cohort. *Gynecol Oncol.* 2007;105(2):365–372.
34. Lane AH, Lee MM, Fuller AF, Kehas DJ, Donahoe PK, MacLaughlin DT. Diagnostic utility of Mullerian inhibiting substance determination in patients with primary and recurrent granulosa cell tumors. *Gynecol Oncol.* 1999;73(1):51–55.
35. Färkkilä A, Koskela S, Bryk S, et al. The clinical utility of serum anti-Müllerian hormone in the follow-up of ovarian adult-type granulosa cell tumors—a comparative study with inhibin B. *Int J Cancer.* 2015;137(7):1661–1671.
36. Unkila-Kallio L, Tiitinen A, Wahlström T, Lehtovirta P, Leminen A. Reproductive features in women developing ovarian granulosa cell tumour at a fertile age. *Hum Reprod.* 2000;15(3):589–593.
37. Van Meurs HS, Bleeker MCG, Van Der Velden J, Overbeek LIH, Kenter GG, Buist MR. The incidence of endometrial hyperplasia and cancer in 1031 patients with a granulosa cell tumor of the ovary: long-term follow-up in a population-based cohort study. *Int J Gynecol Cancer.* 2013;23(8):1417–1422.
38. Fox H, Agrawal K, Langley FA. A clinicopathologic study of 92 cases of granulosa cell tumor of the ovary with special reference to the factors influencing prognosis. *Cancer.* 1975;35(1):231–241.
39. Brown J, Sood AK, Deavers MT, Milojevic L, Gershenson DM. Patterns of metastasis in sex cord-stromal tumors of the ovary: can routine staging lymphadenectomy be omitted? *Gynecol Oncol.* 2009;113(1):86–90.
40. Kuru O, Boyraz G, Uckan H, et al. Retroperitoneal nodal metastasis in primary adult type granulosa cell tumor of the ovary: can routine lymphadenectomy be omitted? *Eur J Obstet Gynecol Reprod Biol.* 2017;219:70–73.
41. Nasioudis D, Kanninen TT, Holcomb K, Sisti G, Witkin SS. Prevalence of lymph node metastasis and prognostic significance of lymphadenectomy in apparent early-stage malignant ovarian sex cord-stromal tumors. *Gynecol Oncol.* 2017;145(2):243–247.
42. Weng CS, Chen MY, Wang TY, et al. Sertoli-Leydig cell tumors of the ovary: a Taiwanese Gynecologic Oncology Group study. *Taiwan J Obstet Gynecol.* 2013;52(1):66–70.

43. Zhang M, Cheung MK, Shin JY, et al. Prognostic factors responsible for survival in sex cord stromal tumors of the ovary—an analysis of 376 women. *Gynecol Oncol.* 2007;104(2):396–400.

44. Chan JK, Zhang M, Kaleb V, et al. Prognostic factors responsible for survival in sex cord stromal tumors of the ovary—a multivariate analysis. *Gynecol Oncol.* 2005;96(1):204–209.

45. Wilson MK, Fong P, Mesnage S, et al. Stage I granulosa cell tumours: a management conundrum? Results of long-term follow up. *Gynecol Oncol.* 2015;138(2):285–291.

46. American College of Obstetricians and Gynecologists. ACOG Practice Bulletin. Management of adnexal masses. *Obstet Gynecol.* 2007;110(1): 201–214.

47. Bergamini A, Ferrandina G, Candiani M, et al. Laparoscopic surgery in the treatment of stage I adult granulosa cells tumors of the ovary: results from the MITO-9 study. *Eur J Surg Oncol.* 2018;44(6):766–770.

48. National Comprehensive Cancer Network. *Ovarian Cancer (Version 1.2020) [Internet]*; 2020. [cited 2020 Aug 26]. Available from: https://www.nccn.org/professionals/physician_gls/pdf/ovarian.pdf.

49. Bergamini A, Cormio G, Ferrandina G, et al. Conservative surgery in stage I adult type granulosa cells tumors of the ovary: results from the MITO-9 study. *Gynecol Oncol.* 2019;154(2):323–327.

50. Wang D, Cao D, Jia C, et al. Analysis of oncologic and reproductive outcomes after fertility-sparing surgery in apparent stage I adult ovarian granulosa cell tumors. *Gynecol Oncol.* 2018;151(2):275–281.

51. Johansen G, Dahm-Kähler P, Staf C, Flöter Rådestad A, Rodriguez-Wallberg KA. Fertility-sparing surgery for treatment of non-epithelial ovarian cancer: oncological and reproductive outcomes in a prospective nationwide population-based cohort study. *Gynecol Oncol.* 2019; 155(2):287–293.

52. Mangili G, Ottolina J, Cormio G, et al. Adjuvant chemotherapy does not improve disease-free survival in FIGO stage IC ovarian granulosa cell tumors: the MITO-9 study. *Gynecol Oncol.* 2016;143(2):276–280.

53. Bhat RA, Lim YK, Chia YN, Yam KL. Sertoli-Leydig cell tumor of the ovary: analysis of a single institution database. *J Obstet Gynaecol Res.* 2013; 39(1):305–310.

54. Seagle B-L, Ann P, Butler S, Shahabi S. Ovarian granulosa cell tumor: a National Cancer Database study. *Gynecol Oncol.* 2017;146(2): 285–291.

55. Oseledchyk A, Gennarelli RL, Leitao MM, et al. Adjuvant chemotherapy in patients with operable granulosa cell tumors of the ovary: a surveillance, epidemiology, and end results cohort study. *Cancer Med.* 2018;7(6):2280–2287.

56. Nasioudis D, Orfanelli T, Frey MK, Chapman-Davis E, Caputo TA, Witkin SSHK. Role of adjuvant chemotherapy in the management of non-granulosa cell ovarian sex cord-stromal tumors. *J Gynecol Oncol.* 2019;30(2):e19. PMCID: PMC6393626.

57. Gershenson DM, Morris M, Burke TW, Levenback C, Matthews CM, Wharton JT. Treatment of poor-prognosis sex cord-stromal tumors of the ovary with the combination of bleomycin, etoposide, and cisplatin. *Obstet Gynecol.* 1996;87(4):527–531.

58. Brown J, Shvartsman HS, Deavers MT, Burke TW, Munsell MF, Gershenson DM. The activity of taxanes in the treatment of sex cord-stromal ovarian tumors. *J Clin Oncol.* 2004;22(17):3517–3523.

59. Brown J, Shvartsman HS, Deavers MT, et al. The activity of taxanes compared with bleomycin, etoposide, and cisplatin in the treatment of sex cord-stromal ovarian tumors. *Gynecol Oncol.* 2005;97(2):489–496.

60. Limei Z, Yong C, Yan X, Shuai T, Jiangyan X, Zhiqing L. Accuracy of positron emission tomography/computed tomography in the diagnosis and restaging for recurrent ovarian cancer: a meta-analysis. *Int J Gynecol Cancer.* 2013;23(4):598–607.

61. Mangili G, Sigismondi C, Frigerio L, et al. Recurrent granulosa cell tumors (GCTs) of the ovary: a MITO-9 retrospective study. *Gynecol Oncol.* 2013;130(1):38–42.

62. Sehouli J, Drescher FS, Mustea A, et al. Granulosa cell tumor of the ovary: 10 years follow-up data of 65 patients. *Anticancer Res.* 2004;24(2C): 1223–1229.

63. Homesley HD, Bundy BN, Hurteau JA, Roth LM. Bleomycin, etoposide, and cisplatin combination therapy of ovarian granulosa cell tumors and other stromal malignancies: a Gynecologic Oncology Group Study. *Gynecol Oncol.* 1999;72(2):131–137.

64. Van Meurs HS, Buist MR, Westermann AM, Sonke GS, Kenter GG, Van Der Velden J. Effectiveness of chemotherapy in measurable granulosa cell tumors: a retrospective study and review of literature. *Int J Gynecol Cancer.* 2014;24(3):496–505.

65. Zhao D, Zhang Y, Ou Z, Zhang R, Zheng S, Li B. Characteristics and treatment results of recurrence in adult-type granulosa cell tumor of ovary. *J Ovarian Res.* 2020;13(1):1–10.

66. Brown J, Brady WE, Schink J, et al. Efficacy and safety of bevacizumab in recurrent sex cord-stromal ovarian tumors: results of a phase 2 trial of the Gynecologic Oncology Group. *Cancer.* 2014;120(3):344–351.

67. Burton ER, Brady M, Homesley HD, et al. A phase II study of paclitaxel for the treatment of ovarian stromal tumors: an NRG Oncology/Gynecologic Oncology Group Study. *Gynecol Oncol.* 2016;140(1):48–52.

68. Ray-Coquard I, Harter P, Lorusso D, et al. Effect of weekly paclitaxel with or without bevacizumab on progression-free rate among patients with relapsed ovarian sex cord-stromal tumors: the ALIENOR/ENGOT-ov7 randomized clinical trial. *JAMA Oncol.* 2020;1–9.

69. Banerjee SN, Tang M, O'Connell RL, et al. A phase 2 study of anastrozole in patients with oestrogen receptor and/progesterone receptor positive recurrent/metastatic granulosa cell tumors/sex-cord stromal tumors of the ovary: the PARAGON/ANZGOG 0903 trial. *Gynecol Oncol.* 2021; 163(1):72–78.

70. Van Meurs HS, Van Lonkhuijzen LRCW, Limpens J, Van Der Velden J, Buist MR. Hormone therapy in ovarian granulosa cell tumors: a systematic review. *Gynecol Oncol.* 2014;134(1):196–205.

71. Disaia P, Saltz A, Kagan AR, Rich W. A temporary response of recurrent granulosa cell tumor to Adriamycin. *Obstet Gynecol.* 1978;52(3):355–358.

72. Gershenson DM, Copeland LJ, Kavanagh JJ, Stringer CA, Saul PB, Wharton JT. Treatment of metastatic stromal tumors of the ovary with cisplatin, doxorubicin, and cyclophosphamide. *Obstet Gynecol.* 1987;70(5):765–769.

73. De Giorgi U, Nicolas-Virelizier E, Badoglio M, et al. High-dose chemotherapy for adult-type ovarian granulosa cell tumors: a retrospective study of the European Society for Blood and Marrow Transplantation. *Int J Gynecol Cancer.* 2017;27(2):248–251.

74. Wolf JK, Mullen J, Eifel PJ, Burke TW, Levenback C, Gershenson DM. Radiation treatment of advanced or recurrent granulosa cell tumor of the ovary. *Gynecol Oncol.* 1999;73(1):35–41.

75. Meisel JL, Hyman DM, Jotwani A, et al. The role of systemic chemotherapy in the management of granulosa cell tumors. *Gynecol Oncol.* 2015; 136(3):505–511. PMCID: PMC4532352.

76. Farinola MA, Gown AM, Judson K, et al. Estrogen receptor α and progesterone receptor expression in ovarian adult granulosa cell tumors and Sertoli-Leydig cell tumors. *Int J Gynecol Pathol.* 2007;26(4):375–382.

77. Hauspy J, Beiner ME, Harley I, et al. Role of adjuvant radiotherapy in granulosa cell tumors of the ovary. *Int J Radiat Oncol Biol Phys.* 2011;79 (3):770–774.

78. Pommert L, Bradley W. Pediatric gynecologic cancers. *Curr Oncol Rep.* 2017;19(7).

79. Zhao D, Song Y, Zhang Y, Li B. Outcomes of fertility-sparing surgery in ovarian juvenile granulosa cell tumor. *Int J Gynecol Cancer.* 2019;29 (4):787–791.

80. Powell JL, Kotwall CA, Shiro BC. Fertility-sparing surgery for advanced juvenile granulosa cell tumor of the ovary. *J Pediatr Adolesc Gynecol.* 2014;27(4):e89–e92.

81. Young RH, Dickersin GR, Scully RE. Juvenile granulosa cell tumor of the ovary. A clinicopathological analysis of 125 cases. *Am J Surg Pathol.* 1984;8(8):575–596.

Chapter 3

Ovarian carcinosarcoma

Joan R. Tymon-Rosario, M. Herman Chui, and Alessandro D. Santin

Clinical case

A 76-year-old female presents with vague abdominal pain, increased abdominal girth, and early satiety over the past 3 months. On physical exam, she was noted to have abdominal distension, right lower quadrant tenderness on palpation, and a fixed approximately 10 cm adnexal mass. CT of the chest, abdomen, and pelvis with contrast reveals a right-sided 10 cm mass, ascites, carcinomatosis, and no pleural effusions (Fig. 3.1). CA-125 was 305 U/mL, and the patient's health care maintenance was up to date (i.e., pap smear, colonoscopy, and mammography). How do you treat this patient?

Epidemiology

Incidence and mortality

Carcinosarcoma (also known as malignant mixed Müllerian tumor) of the gynecologic tract is a rare and highly aggressive malignancy. Carcinosarcomas are dedifferentiated (metaplastic) carcinomas comprised of both carcinomatous and sarcomatous elements. While the exact mechanism by which these two phenotypes arise within a single tumor remains yet to be elucidated, current molecular evidence with whole-exome sequencing indicates that the epithelioid and spindle-cell components share a single malignant epithelial clonal origin.[1,2]

Ovarian cancer is the most common cause of cancer death in women with gynecologic malignancy and the fifth leading cause of cancer death in the United States. It is projected that there will be approximately 22,000 new cases and 14,000 cancer-related deaths in the United States.[3] Ovarian carcinosarcomas account for 1%–4% of all ovarian malignancies.[4] As such, an estimated 220–880 cases of ovarian carcinosarcoma will be diagnosed in the United States with up to 90% of cases initially presenting with spread to other organs at the time of diagnosis. The median age at diagnosis is 75 years, and patients typically present with advanced stage disease often with a large tumor that has abundant hemorrhage and necrosis.[5] Nevertheless, the prognosis for even localized ovarian carcinosarcoma is also dismal with a high risk of recurrence, both local and distant, occurring within 1 year.[4] Due to the aggressive nature of carcinosarcoma, the survival of women with this disease is worse than the survival of those with other histologic subtypes such as endometrioid and high-grade serous (formerly known as high-grade papillary serous). In fact, women with ovarian carcinosarcoma have a significantly worse five-year, disease-specific survival rate than those with high-grade serous ovarian carcinoma 28.2% vs 38.4% ($P < 0.001$).[6] This difference persists for each FIGO disease stage with 5-year survival consistently being worse for women with ovarian carcinosarcoma when compared to those with high-grade serous ovarian cancer[6] (Table 3.1).

Etiology and risk factors

Ovarian carcinosarcomas are composed of both malignant epithelial and sarcomatous elements. The sarcomatous component may resemble uterine sarcomas (i.e., homologous) such as leiomyosarcoma, endometrial stromal sarcoma, fibrosarcoma, or heterologous differentiation such as rhabdomyosarcoma, chondrosarcoma, liposarcoma, or osteosarcoma. The epithelial component most commonly consist of serous carcinoma whether this may be in a pure or mixed form with other carcinoma types. Molecular studies suggest that carcinosarcomas are predominantly monoclonal in that they arise from the carcinoma component through an epithelial–mesenchymal transition.[1,7–10]

Risk factors for ovarian carcinosarcomas are similar to those of epithelial ovarian carcinoma which include increasing age, early age at menarche or late menopause, and nulliparity. However, demographic factors associated with worse mortality for patient with ovarian carcinosarcoma include increasing age (HR 1.03), African-American race (HR 1.04), and

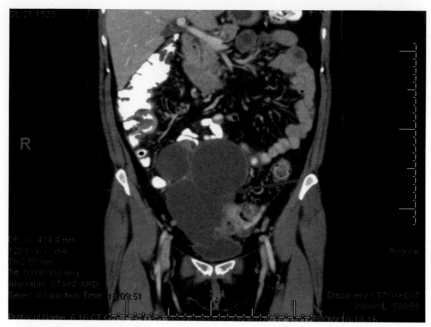

FIG. 3.1 CT scan showing coronal view of large, complex pelvic mass (*arrow*).

TABLE 3.1 Five-year disease-specific survival of ovarian high-grade serous carcinoma versus ovarian carcinosarcoma.

Stage	Papillary serous carcinoma of the ovary		Carcinosarcoma of the ovary		
	Number	5-Year survival	Number	5-Year survival	*P* value
I	793	83.23% (79.94%–86.65%)	105	73.44% (64.92%–83.07%)	*P* = 0.004
II	870	71.80% (68.08%–75.71%)	111	49.47% (39.61%–61.78%)	*P* < 0.001
III	6695	38.98% (37.49%–40.52%)	401	24.26% (19.80%–29.73%)	*P* < 0.001
IV	3643	24.04% (22.30%–25.92%)	249	12.85% (8.54%–19.34%)	*P* < 0.001

Adapted from Rauh-Hain JA, Diver EJ, Clemmer JT, Bradford LS, Clark RM, Growdon WB, et al. Carcinosarcoma of the ovary compared to papillary serous ovarian carcinoma: a SEER analysis. *Gynecol Oncol.* 2013;131:46–51.

unmarried status (HR 0.8 for married status) and have been found to be more commonly associated with ovarian carcinosarcoma.[4,6] Such findings that ovarian carcinosarcoma was more common in unmarried women and that it may be associated with a higher disease-specific mortality warrant further investigation as it perhaps suggests that reproductive history may be more relevant in patients with ovarian carcinosarcoma than those with serous carcinoma.[6]

Pathology

Gross description

Ovarian carcinosarcoma are large (>10 cm) and mostly solid with areas of cystic degeneration, hemorrhage and necrosis. Rarely cartilage and bone maybe grossly identified in tumors with heterologous elements.

Microscopic features

Similar to the more commonly encountered uterine counterpart, ovarian carcinosarcoma is a biphasic tumor composed of high-grade carcinoma and high-grade sarcoma components (Fig. 3.2A). The carcinoma component is usually serous, and less commonly, other histologic subtypes of epithelial ovarian cancer. When derived from a high-grade serous carcinoma, it may be associated with serous tubal intraepithelial carcinoma (STIC) in the fallopian tube.[11] The sarcoma component is classified as homologous when it exhibits a nonspecific spindled appearance, or heterologous, when it exhibits

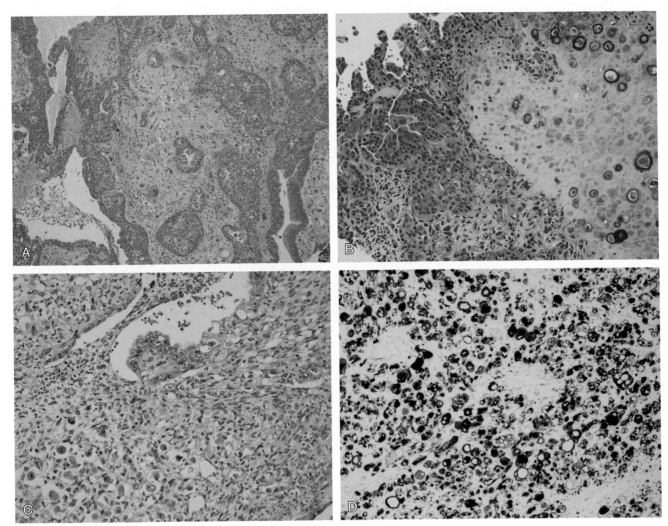

FIG. 3.2 (A) Carcinosarcoma with high-grade carcinoma and sarcoma components. Heterologous elements can include chondrosarcoma (B) and rhabdomyosarcoma (C). (D) Myogenic differentiation in rhabdomyosarcoma is highlighted by desmin immunohistochemical stain.

non-gynecologic tissue differentiation. Rhabdomyosarcoma is the most common heterologous element, though chondrosarcoma, and rarely liposarcoma, osteosarcoma or other sarcoma subtypes may be present (Fig. 3.2B and C). Rarely other components such as yolk sac tumor or primitive neuroectodermal tumor may be present.

Ancillary testing

Immunohistochemical stains may not be necessary for diagnosis, though desmin staining (Fig. 3.2D) may be used to confirm myogenic differentiation, while myogenin or MyoD1 can be more specific to confirm the presence of a rhabdomyosarcoma component. Carcinosarcomas often exhibit an aberrant p53 expression pattern (diffuse staining, or complete absence of staining) in both carcinoma and sarcoma components. A CK7+/CK20−/PAX8+ immunoprofile can confirm Müllerian epithelial origin, when metastasis from another site is under diagnostic consideration.[12]

Pathogenesis and molecular features

Carcinosarcomas are derived from transdifferentiation of high-grade carcinoma through epithelial–mesenchymal transition.[1,13] Most originate as high-grade serous carcinomas, and as such, harbor *TP53* mutations and numerous chromosomal gains and losses. However, the carcinoma component may also be high-grade endometrioid or clear cell carcinoma, or a carcinoma with ambiguous morphologic features.

Differential diagnosis

The differential diagnosis of ovarian carcinosarcoma depends on the histomorphologic features of the particular case in question. Some pure carcinomas are associated with desmoplastic stroma, which can mimic a sarcomatous component. However, in the latter, high-grade nuclear atypia and frequent mitotic figures are present. Immunohistochemical staining showing an aberrant p53 expression pattern in both epithelial and mesenchymal components could serve as confirmation. Sarcomatoid carcinoma can mimic carcinosarcoma; in the former the glandular component merges with the spindle component and the latter usually has diffuse expression of keratin markers. Dedifferentiated carcinoma is another consideration and consists of a low-grade endometrioid carcinoma juxtaposed with discohesive poorly differentiated tumor cells sometimes with rhabdoid morphology. The possibility of metastatic tumor from nongynecologic sites should be excluded. An example is gastric adenocarcinoma (i.e., Krukenberg tumor), which is commonly associated with highly cellular fibromatous stroma, however, predominant signet ring cell morphology is highly unusual in gynecologic primaries. In some carcinosarcomas, the sarcomatous component is predominant, with only focal residual carcinoma, and these cases can occasionally be misclassified as a pure high-grade sarcoma. Carcinosarcoma should be distinguished from other tumors showing multilineage differentiation. These include poorly differentiated Sertoli-Leydig cell tumor with heterologous elements, Müllerian adenosarcoma and immature teratoma. These tumors lack a true high-grade carcinomatous component, though benign or low-grade neoplastic epithelial elements may be present. Pertinent immunohistochemical stains for sex cord and germ cell tumors may be used to facilitate the diagnosis. Ovarian carcinosarcoma should also be distinguished from ovarian metastasis from a uterine primary. In a patient with synchronous endometrial and ovarian tumors, the presence of a large tumor in the uterine cavity would favor an endometrial primary.

Diagnosis and workup

Signs and symptoms

These patients typically present with advanced stage disease with a pelvic mass and peritoneal carcinomatosis. These tumors are typically large at presentation with abundant hemorrhage and necrosis.[4] As with epithelial ovarian carcinoma, the clinical presentation can be either acute or subacute. Those that present in an acute fashion are those with advanced disease whose condition requires urgent evaluation and management (i.e., bowel obstruction, pleural effusion, acute abdominal pain). More often, patients present in a subacute fashion (i.e., vague abdominopelvic pain, bloating, early satiety, gastrointestinal (GI) or genitourinary symptoms) in patients with either early or advanced disease. Women with ovarian cancer frequently report symptoms prior to diagnosis but distinguishing these symptoms from those that normally occur in women remains problematic as they can be confused with other more common GI or genitourinary issues.[14] To date, there is no effective screening modality which has been shown to reduce morbidity or mortality.[15–17] The American College of Obstetricians and Gynecologists (the College) and the Society for Gynecologic Oncology (SGO) both endorse that the best method to diagnose ovarian cancer is for clinicians to have a high index of suspicion in a symptomatic patient.[15,16]

Physical exam findings

As most women present with advanced stage disease, a large pelvic mass that is solid, immobile and with irregular borders is often found on physical examination (Table 3.2). Malignancy-related ascites can result in abdominal distension as a consequence of tumor cell growth in the peritoneal cavity and metastatic spread to the omentum and diaphragm which prevents proper fluid circulation and results in obstruction in the reabsorption of fluid from the peritoneal cavity. Peritoneal

TABLE 3.2 Initial workup of newly diagnosed carcinosarcoma of the ovary.

Physical exam	Complete physical exam with pelvic and rectovaginal examinations
Imaging	Ultrasound CT chest, abdomen, pelvis or PET/CT [a]MRI chest, abdomen, pelvis
Laboratories	CA-125, germline genetic testing

[a]*MRI may be used in those patients where a contrast allergy that precludes use of CT.*

carcinomatosis due to disease spread will also lead to accumulation of ascites due to blockage of draining lymphatic channels and increased vascular permeability.[18] Some patients may present with shortness of breath due to a malignant pleural effusion whereas others may have severe nausea and vomiting due to the extent of their intraabdominal tumor burden obstructing the bowel.

Differential diagnosis

As ovarian carcinosarcomas are rare and highly aggressive malignancies that portend a worse prognosis than their more commonly found epithelial ovarian carcinomas accurate diagnosis is imperative in understanding the usual course of the disease. Typically, the diagnosis will be made on final pathologic review of an ovarian specimen after surgical cytoreduction (see Section "Pathology"). Nonetheless, prior to operative management the differential diagnosis of an adnexal mass must include metastatic disease from endometrial, breast, and some GI malignant neoplasms.[19] As such, one should assure that the patient is up to date with all health care maintenance (i.e., mammogram, colonoscopy).

Tumor markers

CA-125 is the most commonly used biomarker for the evaluation of adnexal masses and as a marker for response to treatment in epithelial ovarian cancer. CA-125 alone has a low sensitivity and low overall specificity for diagnosing malignancy. However, improved survival in women with ovarian carcinosarcoma has been associated with lower CA-125 levels.[20] Therefore, CA-125 may be highly elevated in a subset of ovarian carcinosarcoma and can be used as a marker for response to treatment.

Imaging studies

One of the most important elements in initial evaluation is the finding of an adnexal mass on imaging. Often, this could initially be due to findings on ultrasound which include a mass with solids components, nodules, papillary excrescences, increased Doppler flow, irregularly thick septations and ascites (Fig. 3.3). Once, there is either clinical or radiologic concern for malignancy, imaging studies to assess the extent of disease burden and to evaluate for metastatic disease include computed tomography (CT scan) of the chest, abdomen and pelvis with and without contrast. It must be noted that radiologic staging tends to underestimate the extent of disease, since the majority of clinical stage I tumors have been shown to have lymph node metastasis in up to 60% of cases.[4] If the patient has a contrast allergy that precludes use of CT, magnetic resonance imaging (MRI) may be used instead. There is some data suggesting that positron emission tomography (PET)

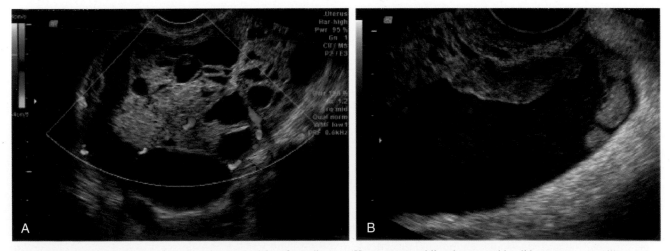

FIG. 3.3 Findings on ultrasound of an adnexal mass suspicious for malignancy. Here you see multilocular mass with solid components, papillary excrescences, increased Doppler flow, increased irregular thick septations on the left (A). On the right, you see fluid in the posterior cul-de-sac which is ascites (B). *(Adapted from Sayasneh et al. The characteristic ultrasound features of specific types of ovarian pathology (review). Published online on: November 18, 2014. https://doi.org/10.3892/ijo.2014.2764. https://www.spandidos-publications.com/10.3892/ijo.2014.2764.)*

alone or combined with CT increases the detection of metastatic ovarian cancer compared with CT alone or MRI; however, further studies of the preoperative use of this imaging modality are needed.[21] Typically, CT scan is the first-line imaging technique performed since it provides adequate anatomic delineation and detection of disease to assist with preoperative staging and surgical planning. The limitation of CT is the inability to use contrast in those with contraindications to contrast agents and the ionizing radiation exposure to the patient. The benefit of PET combined with CT over CT alone in preoperative staging of ovarian cancer has not yet been completely established. It could also potentially improve staging accuracy by improving detection of infra- and supradiaphragmatic metastasis. PET/CT scans may also help in cases of indeterminate lymph node appearance or when there is contraindication to contrast-enhanced CT. However, with PET alone false-positive may result by FDG accumulation in normal tissues (i.e., bowel loops and urinary system), in inflammatory lesions (i.e., diverticulitis) or in atherosclerotic plaques. Nonetheless, the costs of PET/CT are higher than those of ultrasound, CT and MRI.[22] Nevertheless, as part of initial work-up, all women with newly diagnosed disease should undergo either CT scan of the chest, abdomen, and pelvis, PET scan from skull to thigh, or a combined PET/CT scan in order to guide appropriate treatment recommendations.

Diagnostic testing

Diagnosis of ovarian carcinosarcoma is made pathologically with histologic confirmation (biopsy preferred). After assessment by a gynecologic oncologist, if the patient is deemed a surgical candidate primary surgical cytoreduction is performed after which pathological assessment of the tissue provides the diagnosis. If unsure of the feasibility of debulking surgery, laparoscopic evaluation may be performed and if the disease burden is deemed unlikely to be cytoreduced to CGR tissue biopsies can be obtained providing the diagnosis. If the patient is deemed a poor surgical candidate and there is a low likelihood of complete gross cytoreduction, image-guided biopsy can provide histologic confirmation. If biopsy is not feasible, cytopathology from ascites or pleural effusion could allow a diagnosis of malignancy of Müllerian origin but unlikely to provide the diagnosis of carcinosarcoma. Nevertheless, all women with a diagnosis of ovarian, fallopian tube, or peritoneal cancer should have genetic risk evaluation. However, further studies are needed to assess if ovarian carcinosarcoma is an associated hereditary malignancy. Additionally, the tissue used to make the diagnosis of ovarian carcinosarcoma should be assessed for HER2 positivity and sent for somatic testing for the use of potentially targetable treatment. A recent comprehensive analysis of HER2 expression in a large cohort of uterine and ovarian carcinosarcomas demonstrated that up to 13% of tumors (10/80) were positive; however, of the 15 ovarian carcinosarcoma tumors only one ovarian carcinosarcoma was HER2 positive.[23] Additionally, the presence of a germline or somatic BRCA1 or BRCA2 mutation may have treatment implications in maintenance therapy and management of recurrent disease.

Staging system

Ovarian carcinosarcoma is surgically and pathologically staged according to the 2017 eighth edition American Joint Committee on Cancer (AJCC) and the joint 2017 International Federation of Gynecology and Obstetrics (FIGO)/Tumor, Node, Metastasis (TNM) classification system (Table 3.3).

Prognostic factors

Up to 90% of ovarian carcinosarcoma cases present with advanced stage disease with a median overall survival ranging from 7 to 27 months.[4] Overall, the prognosis for ovarian carcinosarcoma is worse than uterine carcinosarcoma (UCS) and high-grade serous carcinoma of similar FIGO stage.[6,24,25] Significant predictors of improved survival for women with ovarian carcinosarcoma include early stage, lower preoperative CA-125 levels (<75 U/mL), and optimal surgical cytoreduction.[20] Improved survival has also been seen in women diagnosed at a younger age and treated with platinum-based chemotherapy regimens.[2] In regards to histopathological prognostic factors, the presence of a $>25\%$ sarcomatous component in the primary tumor was associated with worse survival and serous epithelial components within the tumors adversely affected the survival compared with nonserous components.[26] The significance of the presence of a heterologous mesenchymal component is unclear as some studies suggest it is associated with a poor prognosis while other show that this component has no significant impact on survival.[20,27-29] Molecular markers of ovarian carcinosarcomas such as increased vessel number, increased vascular endothelial growth factor (VEGF) and VEGFR-3 expression have been correlated with poor survival in one study but found not to be statistically significant in another.[30,31] Additionally, the antigen Ki67 which is a nuclear protein associated with cellular proliferation was evaluated in 23 patients with ovarian carcinosarcoma with more than 50% of them showing a high Ki67 labeling index. The 5-year survival rate was 15.9% for the high Ki67 index group

TABLE 3.3 TNM and FIGO staging for ovary, fallopian tube, and primary peritoneal carcinomas.

		Primary tumor (T)
T category	**FIGO stage**	**T criteria**
TX		Primary tumor cannot be assessed
T0		No evidence of primary tumor
T1	I	Tumor limited to ovaries (one or both) or fallopian tube(s)
T1a	IA	Tumor limited to one ovary (capsule intact) or fallopian tube, no tumor on ovarian or fallopian tube surface; no malignant cells in ascites or peritoneal washings
T1b	IB	Tumor limited to both ovaries (capsules intact) or fallopian tubes; no tumor on ovarian or fallopian tube surface; no malignant cells in ascites or peritoneal washings
T1c	IC	Tumor limited to one or both ovaries or fallopian tubes, with any of the following:
T1c1	IC1	• Surgical spill
T1c2	IC2	• Capsule ruptured before surgery or tumor on ovarian or fallopian tube surface
T1c3	IC3	• Malignant cells in ascites or peritoneal washings
T2	II	Tumor involves one or both ovaries or fallopian tubes with pelvic extension below pelvic brim or primary peritoneal cancer
T2a	IIA	Extension and/or implants on the uterus and/or fallopian tube(s) and/or ovaries
T2b	IIB	Extension to and/or implants on other pelvic tissues
T3	III	Tumor involves one or both ovaries or fallopian tubes, or primary peritoneal cancer, with microscopically confirmed peritoneal metastasis outside the pelvis and/or metastasis to the retroperitoneal (pelvic and/or paraaortic) lymph nodes
T3a	IIIA2	Microscopic extrapelvic (above the pelvic brim) peritoneal involvement with or without positive retroperitoneal lymph nodes
T3b	IIIB	Macroscopic peritoneal metastasis beyond pelvis 2 cm or less in greatest dimension with or without metastasis to the retroperitoneal lymph nodes
T3c	IIIC	Macroscopic peritoneal metastasis beyond the pelvis more than 2 cm in greatest dimension with or without metastasis to the retroperitoneal lymph nodes (includes extension of tumor to capsule of liver and spleen without parenchymal involvement of either organ)
		Regional lymph nodes (N)
N category	**FIGO stage**	**N criteria**
NX		Regional lymph nodes cannot be assessed
N0		No regional lymph node metastasis
N0(i+)		Isolated tumor cells in regional lymph node(s) no greater than 0.2 mm
N1	IIIA1	Positive retroperitoneal lymph nodes only (histologically confirmed)
N1a	IIIA1i	Metastasis up to and including 10 mm in greatest dimension
N1b	IIIA1ii	Metastasis more than 10 mm in greatest dimension
		Distant metastasis (M)
M category	**FIGO stage**	**M criteria**
M0		No distant metastasis
M1	IV	Distant metastasis, including pleural effusion with positive cytology; liver or splenic parenchymal metastasis; metastasis to extraabdominal organs (including inguinal lymph nodes and lymph nodes outside the abdominal cavity); and transmural involvement of intestine
M1a	IVA	Pleural effusion with positive cytology
M1b	IVB	Liver or splenic parenchymal metastases; metastases to extraabdominal organs (including inguinal lymph nodes and lymph nodes outside the abdominal cavity); transmural involvement of intestine

and 36.4% for the low index group.[29] In one study of 33 women with uterine and ovarian carcinosarcomas, overexpression of P53 was found in 21 (64%) of patients upon molecular analysis and another smaller study confirmed that P53 overexpression influenced overall survival.[32,33]

Treatment of primary disease
Surgery

Until recently, ovarian carcinosarcoma was considered a sarcoma and treatment was dictated as such. It is now clear that ovarian carcinosarcoma is a metaplastic tumor that derives from the clonal evolution of a poorly differentiated epithelial ovarian cancer and as such, should be treated as a high-risk ovarian carcinoma (Fig. 3.4).[1,4] Due to the aggressive nature of ovarian carcinosarcomas, patients are not candidates for fertility-sparing surgery regardless of age or stage. Surgical staging with pelvic washings, total abdominal hysterectomy, bilateral salpingo-oophorectomy (BSO), omentectomy, pelvic, and paraaortic lymph node dissection is recommended for disease that is limited to the pelvis (i.e., stages I–IIB). Surgical cytoreduction with total abdominal hysterectomy, BSO, omentectomy, pelvic and paraaortic lymph node dissection only for lymph nodes noted to be grossly enlarged, and tumor debulking to no gross residual disease for more advanced stage disease (stage III–IV) and tumor debulking is recommended. Due to the rarity of ovarian carcinosarcomas, the role of cytoreductive surgery has not been prospectively evaluated but several retrospective studies have reported improved outcomes for patients undergoing CGR. In fact, one of the largest studies with a patient cohort of 50 demonstrated a disease-free survival (DFS) for patients with only microscopic disease of 19 months, compared to 10 months for those with less than 1 cm residual disease and only 5 months for those with more than 1 cm ($P = 0.01$).[25] Overall survival in that same study is 47, 18, and 8 months respectively ($P = 0.02$).[25]

Adjuvant chemotherapy

After complete surgical staging, it is recommended that patients with stage I to IV ovarian carcinosarcoma receive adjuvant chemotherapy. As both the carcinomatous and sarcomatous elements arise from a single malignant epithelial precursor and as these tumors tend to behave more like a carcinoma than a sarcoma, treatment regimens for ovarian carcinosarcoma have been based on data extrapolated from other epithelial ovarian histologies with the recommendation to use platinum-based chemotherapy regimens. It is unclear as to whether the platinum should be used alone or in combination. Common

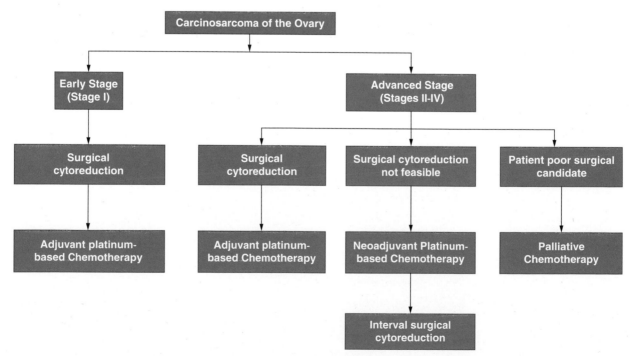

FIG. 3.4 Treatment algorithm for newly diagnosed carcinosarcoma of the ovary.

combination treatments include platinum and paclitaxel and platinum and ifosfamide.[34] However, lower response rates to these agents compared to other histological subtypes have been reported with overall response rates (ORRs) between 25% and 70%.[25,35]

Prospective Gynecologic Oncology Group (GOG) trials demonstrated that doxorubicin is not sufficient and that combination cisplatin with ifosfamide is an active doublet in the treatment of ovarian carcinosarcoma.[36] Another GOG trial of 136 patients, demonstrated that cisplatin is an active single agent in the primary systemic treatment of ovarian carcinosarcoma with a 20% response rate with median PFS and OS of 5.2 and 11.7 months, respectively.[37] In a study of 26 patients with ovarian carcinosarcoma treated with carboplatin and paclitaxel, 16 (55%) had a complete response and 6 (23%) had a partial response. A median OS of 27 months was reported in this study.[34] In one of the largest retrospective series, the ORR to carboplatin and paclitaxel was 62% among 50 women with ovarian carcinosarcoma.[6] The combination of carboplatin and paclitaxel has been compared to other regimens such as ifosfamide and cisplatin. One retrospective study of 29 ovarian carcinosarcoma patients who received adjuvant ifosfamide demonstrated a significantly longer PFS than those who were treated with cisplatin or carboplatin and paclitaxel with 12 months for the carboplatin and paclitaxel group versus not yet reached for the ifosfamide and cisplatin group ($P = 0.005$). This study also demonstrated a favorable 2-year OS of 81% for the ifosfamide and cisplatin group versus 55% for the carboplatin and paclitaxel group ($P = 0.003$).[4,38] Nonetheless, the results have been criticized for potential selection bias in that patients in the ifosfamide and cisplatin group being diagnosed at an earlier stage and having a higher rate of optimal cytoreduction.[4,38] Additionally, the ifosfamide and cisplatin combination was found to be more toxic. Therefore, the choice of paclitaxel versus ifosfamide as the second agent in the doublet regimen depends on tolerability of the patient. Additionally, the recent results from the phase III NRG Oncology clinical trial GOG 261 comparing paclitaxel plus carboplatin to paclitaxel plus ifosfamide in women with stage I-IV carcinosarcoma of the uterus or ovary found that treatment with paclitaxel/carboplatin was not inferior to paclitaxel/ifosfamide based on the primary objective of overall survival (NCT00954174). In fact, paclitaxel/carboplatin was associated with longer progression-free survival (PFS) outcomes when compared with paclitaxel/ifosfamide.

Neoadjuvant chemotherapy

For those patients that are poor surgical candidates or for those whom there is a low likelihood of optimal cytoreduction, neoadjuvant chemotherapy with platinum and paclitaxel is recommended. Interval debulking can be done after 3–4 cycles of platinum-based chemotherapy or after 4–6 cycles based on the clinical judgment of the gynecologic oncologist.

Adjuvant radiation

Given that most ovarian carcinosarcoma cases are advanced stage at presentation, there is little rationale for the use of radiotherapy treatment as adjuvant therapy. However, there may be a role for radiation for isolated recurrences or in a palliative manner. For those patients diagnosed with early stage ovarian carcinosarcoma, the role of radiotherapy remains to be elucidated.[4]

Surveillance for recurrent disease

After treatment, surveillance and follow-up recommendations for epithelial ovarian cancer are also the same as those used for ovarian carcinosarcoma (Table 3.4). As such, office visits with a gynecologic oncologist are recommended every 3–4 months for the first 2 years, every 4–6 months for years 2–3, every 6 months for years 3–5 and then yearly thereafter.[39] At each visit a thorough assessment of symptoms and physical examination, including a pelvic examination, should be done. The role of CA-125 monitoring, should be discussed with the patient. Studies have shown that if initially elevated at the time of diagnosis it can be a good marker of disease status due to the fact that in most cases it is often elevated 2–5 months before clinical detection of relapse.[40] However, a prospective randomized trial of 527 patients demonstrated that for patients treated for recurrent ovarian cancer based on a CA-125 level alone versus clinically evident recurrence that the overall survival outcome did not differ.[41] When a recurrence is suspected based on symptoms, examination or a CA-125 level, a CT scan of the chest, abdomen, and pelvis should be obtained to determine the extent of disease. PET scans can be useful adjuncts when CT scans are indeterminate or for those patients who may be candidates for secondary cytoreductive surgery.[39]

TABLE 3.4 Surveillance recommendations for ovarian carcinosarcoma.

Follow up recommendation intervals

Time from completion of primary therapy	Years 0–2	Years 2–3	Years 3–5	Years >5
Symptom review and examination	3–4 months	4–6 months	6 months	Yearly[a]
Pap test/cytology	Not indicated			
CA-125	Optional			
Radiographic imaging[b]	Insufficient data to support routine use			
Recurrence suspected	CT scans or PET/CT scans			
	CA-125			

[a]May be followed by a gynecologic oncologist or generalist.
[b]May include chest X-ray, PET/CT scans, MRI, ultrasound.
Adapted from Salani, R, Khanna N, Frimer M, Bristow RE, Chen L-M. An updated on post-treatment surveillance and diagnosis of recurrence in women with gynecologic malignancies: Society of Gynecologic Oncology (SGO) recommendations. *Gynecol Oncol.* 2017;146:3–10.

Survival and patterns of failure

The prognosis for ovarian carcinosarcoma is dismal, with an overall 5-year survival rate of less than 30%.[4,6] The prognosis for even localized ovarian carcinosarcoma is also dismal with a high risk of recurrent, both local and distant, occurring within 1 year, with a median overall survival time ranging from 8 to 26 months.[4,25] The overall prognosis for ovarian carcinosarcomas is worse than UCS and other high-grade ovarian carcinomas of a similar stage.[25] In fact, women with ovarian carcinosarcoma have a significantly worse five-year, disease-specific survival rate than those with high-grade serous ovarian carcinoma 28.2% vs 38.4% ($P < 0.001$).[6] Table 3.5 illustrates the 5-year survival rates in women with ovarian carcinosarcoma by stage.[6,42]

Treatment of recurrent disease

As a result of the rarity of ovarian carcinosarcoma, there are no specific trials for women with recurrent disease and thus limited evidence to guide the effective treatment of recurrent disease (Table 3.6). A phase II study of single agent ifosfamide in patients with recurrent ovarian carcinosarcoma showed an ORR of 17.9%.[43] Recently, as noted above results from the phase III NRG Oncology clinical trial GOG 261 that compared carboplatin-paclitaxel to ifosfamide-paclitaxel in women with recurrent stage I–IV carcinosarcoma of the uterus or ovary found that treatment with carboplatin-paclitaxel was not inferior to ifosfamide-paclitaxel based on the primary objective overall survival and carboplatin-paclitaxel was associated with longer PFS outcomes when compared to ifosfamide-paclitaxel (NCT00954174). In the patient cohort with ovarian carcinosarcoma, there was a 30 months median overall survival in the carboplatin-paclitaxel arm vs 25 months in the ifosfamide-paclitaxel arm and 15 months median PFS for the carboplatin-paclitaxel arm and 10 months for the ifosfamide-paclitaxel arm.

TABLE 3.5 Five-year survival rates in women with ovarian carcinosarcoma by FIGO stage.

	5 Year survival
Stage I	73.44% (64.92%–83.07%)
Stage II	49.47% (39.61%–61.78%)
Stage III	24.26% (19.80%–29.73%)
Stage IV	12.85% (8.54%–19.34%)

Adapted from Rauh-Hain JA, Birrer M, del Carmen MG. Carcinosarcoma of the ovary, fallopian tube, and peritoneum: prognostic factors and treatment modalities. *Gynecol Oncol.* 2016;142:248–254.

TABLE 3.6 Therapeutic options for recurrent carcinosarcoma of the ovary.

Regimen	Level of support
Carboplatin/paclitaxel	Phase III trial
Ifosfamide/paclitaxel	Phase III trial
Ifosfamide/mesna	Phase II trial
Cisplatin/ifosfamide	Phase II trial
Carboplatin/gemzar	Extrapolated from treatment of epithelial ovarian cancer
Carboplatin	Extrapolated from treatment of epithelial ovarian cancer
Carboplatin/gemzar/bevacizumab	Extrapolated from treatment of epithelial ovarian cancer
Carboplatin/doxorubicin	Extrapolated from treatment of epithelial ovarian cancer
Bevacizumab	Extrapolated from treatment of epithelial ovarian cancer
PARP Inhibitors	Extrapolated from treatment of epithelial ovarian cancer

In general, similar to the management of high-grade epithelial ovarian carcinoma, treatment of recurrent disease is based on whether it is a platinum sensitive (progression-free interval [PFI] >6 months) recurrence or platinum-resistant (PFI ≤ 6 months) where PFI predicts the expected response rate (RR) and duration of response.[44,45] Treatment for recurrent ovarian cancer should focus on prolongation of life as well as optimization of quality of life. For those with platinum sensitive disease, standard treatment combinations include: carboplatin and paclitaxel; carboplatin and gemcitabine; carboplatin, gemzar, and bevacizumab; and carboplatin and pegylated liposomal doxorubicin (PLD).[44,46] For those with platinum-resistant disease, treatment with single-agent chemotherapy should be employed.[44]

Targeted therapy

Due to the fact that ovarian carcinosarcomas are rare, further research on the genetic and molecular signaling pathways of these biologically aggressive tumors is warranted in order to improve the understanding of these tumors as well as improve their dismal clinical outcomes. Several studies have reported on the genetic landscape of ovarian carcinosarcoma and as such identified potential therapeutic targets. For instance, whole-exome sequencing studies have recently demonstrated mutations or aberrant activation of multiple genes/pathways in carcinosarcomas including *HER2*, PI3K/AKT/mTOR, *EGFR*, and MAPK, genes related to histones and chromatin structure, and genes related to cell-cycle regulation to be attractive contenders for molecularly targeted therapeutic approaches.[47]

HER2 overexpression/amplification has been previously reported in 14%–20% of endometrial carcinosarcomas and a recent phase II clinical trial showed an increase in PFS and overall survival in patients with HER2-positive endometrial serous carcinoma when trastuzumab was used in combination with chemotherapy over chemotherapy alone.[48–51] In addition, in vitro and in vivo studies have also demonstrated antitumor activity of HER2-targeted therapies in ovarian and UCSs.[52–54] Antibody-drug conjugate (ADC) such as Ado-trastuzumab emtansine (T-DM1) utilize a HER2-targeting antibody (i.e., trastuzumab) linked to a toxic payload. In carcinosarcoma patient's preclinical data support the use of T-DMI in carcinosarcomas overexpressing HER2. For instance, Nicoletti et al. demonstrated that T-DM1 was much more active in vivo in reducing tumor formation in carcinosarcoma xenografts overexpressing HER2 with a longer OS compared to trastuzumab.[52] SYD985 is another novel HER2-targeting ADC linking trastuzumab to a highly potent toxin (i.e., duocarmycin) demonstrated excellent preclinical antitumor activity in ovarian carcinosarcoma with both low and high HER2 expression.[53] Neratinib is an irreversible small molecule tyrosine kinase inhibitor (TKI) targeting EGFR (epidermal growth factor receptor) and HER2. Neratinib has been efficacious in the treatment of HER2-amplified carcinosarcoma both in vitro and in vivo.[54]

Another novel target is the *c-Myc* oncogene which is one of the main transcriptional regulators in human cells and plays a critical role in oncogenesis. Amplifications the *c-Myc* gene are one of the most common genetic aberrations in carcinosarcomas. In fact, approximately 50%–78% of carcinosarcomas demonstrate gain of function mutations in *c-Myc*.[1,55] Carcinosarcoma with c-Myc amplification may potentially be targeted using novel BET-inhibitors.[1]

More recently, Sacituzumab-govitecan (SG), which is a new class of ADC targeting the human-trophoblast-cell-surface marker (Trop-2) conjugated with the active metabolite of irinotecan (SN-38), demonstrated activity against biologically aggressive carcinosarcomas. In vitro, Trop-2–positive cell lines showed higher sensitivity to SG when compared to Trop-2 low/negative cell lines. In xenografts, twice-weekly intravenous administration of SG for 3 weeks showed a significant tumor growth inhibition when compared to control, to ADC control and to the naked AB ($P = 0.004$, $P = 0.007$, and $P = 0.0007$, respectively). SG significantly improved overall survival at 90 days when compared to control groups ($P < 0.0001$).[56]

The rate of BRCA1 and BRCA2 germline mutations in women with ovarian carcinosarcoma is currently unknown, but if present could serve evidence for potential benefit of the use of Poly(ADP-ribose) polymerase (PARP) inhibitors. Additionally, as the epithelial component of such biphasic tumors could potentially contain somatic mutations in genes implicated in the HRD pathway (i.e., BRACAness) further studies are warranted to investigate the role of PARP inhibitors in ovarian carcinosarcomas. In conclusion, research should be encouraged to study this rare, yet highly aggressive disease and clinical trials should be broadly opened to include ovarian carcinosarcoma patients.

Case resolution

This 76-year-old patient underwent an exploratory laparotomy, hysterectomy, BSO, omentectomy, and tumor debulking to no gross residual disease. Final pathology revealed stage IIIC ovarian carcinosarcoma. Histologically, the epithelial component of the tumor was of serous histology and the sarcomatous component was heterologous (chondrosarcoma). The tumor also demonstrated HER2/neu overexpression. The patient underwent genetic testing and was found to be germline *BRCA* negative. She was subsequently dispositioned to six cycles of adjuvant carboplatin, paclitaxel, and Herceptin followed by Herceptin maintenance. CA-125 decreased to 24 U/mL after adjuvant platinum-based chemotherapy. Approximately 9 months after completion of her platinum-based chemotherapy, the patient reported worsening abdominal pain and distension. CT scan demonstrated a right upper quadrant nodule, pelvic lymphadenopathy, and moderate ascites consistent with recurrent disease. CA-125 was noted to be increased to 56 U/mL. She underwent another 6 cycles of carboplatin and paclitaxel with improvement in ascites and shrinkage of the right upper quadrant nodule as well as the enlarged pelvic lymph nodes. CA-125 had also decreased to 30 U/mL. After 4 months, the patient returned with abdominal pain and distension where CT scan demonstrated a large abdominal mass, moderate ascites, and bilateral pulmonary nodules consistent with disease recurrence. She was therefore started on dose-dense paclitaxel, but after 7 cycles of treatment, she had progression of disease to which she soon thereafter unfortunately expired as a result of her disease process.

References

1. Zhao S, Bellone S, Lopez S, et al. Mutational landscape of uterine and ovarian carcinosarcomas implicates histone genes in epithelial-mesenchymal transition. *Proc Natl Acad Sci USA.* 2016;113(43):12238–12243.
2. Somarelli JA, Boss MK, Epstein JI, et al. Carcinosarcomas: tumors in transition? *Histol Histopathol.* 2015;30:673.
3. American Cancer Society. *Cancer Facts & Figures 2020.* Atlanta: American Cancer Society; 2020.
4. Berton-Rigaud D, Devouassoux-Shisheboran M, Ledermann JA, et al. Gynecologic Cancer InterGroup (GCIG) consensus review for uterine and ovarian carcinosarcoma. *Int J Gynecol Cancer.* 2014;24:S55–S60.
5. Seidman JD, Kurman RJ. Pathology of ovarian carcinoma. *Hematol Oncol Clin North Am.* 2003;17:909.
6. Rauh-Hain JA, Diver EJ, Clemmer JT, et al. Carcinosarcoma of the ovary compared to papillary serous ovarian carcinoma: a SEER analysis. *Gynecol Oncol.* 2013;131:46–51.
7. Gorai I, Yanagibashi T, Taki A, et al. Uterine carcinosarcoma is derived from a single stem cell: an in vitro study. *Int J Cancer.* 1997;72:821–827.
8. Wada H, Enomoto T, Fujita M, et al. Molecular evidence that most but not all carcinosarcomas of the uterus are combination tumors. *Cancer Res.* 1997;57:5379–5385.
9. Fujii H, Yoshida M, Gong ZX, et al. Frequent genetic heterogeneity in the clonal evolution of gynecological carcinosarcoma and its influence on phenotypic diversity. *Cancer Res.* 2000;60:114–120.
10. McCluggage WG. Uterine carcinosarcomas (malignant mixed Müllerian tumors) are metaplastic carcinomas. *Int J Gynecol Cancer.* 2002;12:687–690.
11. Kurman RJ, Shih IeM. Molecular pathogenesis and extraovarian origin of epithelial ovarian cancer—shifting the paradigm. *Hum Pathol.* 2011;42(7):918–931. https://doi.org/10.1016/j.humpath.2011.03.003. PMID: 21683865; PMCID: PMC3148026.
12. Baker PM, Oliva E. Immunohistochemistry as a tool in the differential diagnosis of ovarian tumors: an update. *Int J Gynecol Pathol.* 2005;24(1):39–55. PMID: 15626916.
13. McConechy MK, Hoang LN, Chui MH, et al. In-depth molecular profiling of the biphasic components of uterine carcinosarcomas. *J Pathol Clin Res.* 2015;1(3):173–185. https://doi.org/10.1002/cjp2.18. PMID: 27499902; PMCID: PMC4939881.

14. Goff BA, Mandel LS, Melancon CH, et al. Frequency of symptoms of ovarian cancer in women presenting to primary care clinics. *JAMA*. 2004; 291(22):2705–2712.

15. Committee Opinion No. 477. The role of the obstetrician-gynecologist in the early detection of epithelial ovarian cancer. *Obstet Gynecol*. 2011;117(3):742–746.

16. Schorge JO, Modesitt SWC, Coleman RL, et al. SGO White Paper on ovarian cancer: etiology, screening and surveillance. *Gynecol Oncol*. 2010; 119(1):7–17.

17. *Screening for Ovarian Cancer, Topic Page*. Rockville, MD: US Department of Health and Human Services; 2004. US Preventive Services Task Force Agency for Healthcare Research and Quality.

18. Runyon BA, Hoefs JC, Morgan TR. Ascitic fluid analysis in malignancy-related ascites. *Hepatology*. 1988;8:1104.

19. Moore RG, Chung M, Granai CO, et al. Incidence of metastasis to the ovaries from nongenital tract primary tumors. *Gynecol Oncol*. 2004;93:87.

20. Sood AK, Sorosky JI, Gelder MS, et al. Primary ovarian sarcoma—analysis of prognostic variables and the role of surgical cytoreduction. *Cancer*. 1998;82:1731–1737.

21. Musto A, Rampin L, Nanni C, et al. Present and future of PET and PET/CT in gynaecologic malignancies. *Eur J Radiol*. 2011;78:12.

22. Fischerova D, Burgetova A. Imaging techniques for the evaluation of ovarian cancer. *Best Pract Res Clin Obstet Gynaecol*. 2014;28(5):697–720.

23. Rottmann D, Snir OL, Wu X, et al. HER2 testing for gynecologic carcinosarcomas: tumor stratification for potential targeted therapy. *Mod Pathol*. 2020;33:118–127.

24. Garg G, Shah J, Kumar S, et al. Ovarian and uterine carcinosarcomas: a comparative analysis of prognostic variables and survival outcomes. *Int J Gynecol Cancer*. 2010;20:888–894.

25. Rauh-Hain JA, Growdon WB, Rodriguez N, et al. Carcinosarcoma of the ovary: a case-control study. *Gynecol Oncol*. 2011;121:477–481.

26. Athavale R, Thomakos N, Godfrey K, et al. The effect of epithelial and stromal tumor components on FIGO stages III and IV ovarian carcinosarcomas treated with primary surgery and chemotherapy. *Int J Gynecol Cancer*. 2007;17:1025–1030.

27. Dictor M. Malignant mixed mesodermal tumor of the ovary: a report of 22 cases. *Obstet Gynecol*. 1985;65:720–724.

28. Muntz HG, Jones MA, Goff BA, et al. Malignant mixed Müllerian tumors of the ovary: experience with surgical cytoreduction and combination chemotherapy. *Cancer*. 1995;76(7):1209–1213.

29. Ariyoshi K, Kawauchi S, Kaku T, Nakano H, Tsuneyoshi M. Prognostic factors in ovarian carcinosarcoma: a clinicopathological and immunohistochemical analysis of 23 cases. *Histopathology*. 2000;37(5):427–436.

30. Nayha V, Stenback F. Angiogenesis and expression of angiogenic agents in uterine and ovarian carcinosarcomas. *APMIS*. 2008;116:107–117.

31. Jensen V, Sorensen FB, Bentzen SM. Proliferative activity (MIB-1 index) is an independent prognostic parameter in patients with high-grade soft tissue sarcomas of subtypes other than malignant fibrous histiocytomas: a retrospective immune-histological study including 216 soft tissue sarcomas. *Histopathology*. 1998;32:536–546.

32. Liu F, Kohler MF, Marks JR, et al. Mutation and overexpression of the P53 tumor suppressor gene frequently occurs in uterine and ovarian sarcomas. *Obstet Gynecol*. 1994;83:118–124.

33. Zorzou MP, Markaki S, Rodolakis A, et al. Clinicopathological features of ovarian carcinosarcomas: a single institution experience. *Gynecol Oncol*. 2005;96(1):136–142.

34. Duska LR, Garett A, Eltabbakh MD, et al. Paclitaxel and platinum chemotherapy for malignant mixed Müllerian tumors of the ovary. *Gynecol Oncol*. 2002;85:459–463.

35. Brown E, Stewart M, Rye T, et al. Carcinosarcoma of the ovary: 19 years of prospective data from a single center. *Cancer*. 2004;100(10):2148–2153.

36. del Carmen MG, Birrer M, Schorge JO. Carcinosarcoma of the ovary: a review of the literature. *Gynecol Oncol*. 2012;125(1):271–277.

37. Tate Thigpen J, Blessing JA, DeGeest K, et al. Cisplatin as initial chemotherapy in ovarian carcinosarcomas: a gynecologic oncology group study. *Gynecol Oncol*. 2004;93:336–339.

38. Rutledge TL, Gold MA, McMeekin DS, et al. Carcinosarcoma of the ovary—a case series. *Gynecol Oncol*. 2006;100(1):128–132.

39. Salani R, Khanna N, Frimer M, Bristow RE, Chen L-M. An updated on post-treatment surveillance and diagnosis of recurrence in women with gynecologic malignancies: Society of Gynecologic Oncology (SGO) recommendations. *Gynecol Oncol*. 2017;146:3–10.

40. Fehm T, Heller F, Krämer S, Jäger W, Gebauer G. Evaluation of CA125, physical and radiological findings in follow-up of ovarian cancer patients. *Anticancer Res*. 2005;25:1551–1554.

41. Rustin GJ, van der Burg ME, On Behalf of MRC and EORTC Collaborators. A randomized trial in ovarian cancer (OC) of early treatment of relapse based on CA125 level alone versus delayed treatment based on conventional clinical indicators (MRC OV05/EORTC 55955 trials). *J Clin Oncol*. 2009;27:18s.

42. Rauh-Hain JA, Birrer M, del Carmen MG. Carcinosarcoma of the ovary, fallopian tube, and peritoneum: prognostic factors and treatment modalities. *Gynecol Oncol*. 2016;142:248–254.

43. Sutton GP, Blessing JA, Homesley HD, Malfetano JH. A phase II trial of ifosfamide and mesna in patients with advanced or recurrent mixed mesodermal tumors of the ovary previously treated with platinum-based chemotherapy: a gynecologic oncology group study. *Gynecol Oncol*. 1994;53(1):24–26.

44. Foley OW, Rauh-Hain JA, del Carmen MG. Recurrent epithelial ovarian cancer: treatment update. *Oncology*. 2013;27(4):288–294.

45. Markman M, Markman J, Webster K, et al. Duration of response to second-line, platinum-based chemo-therapy for ovarian cancer: implications for patient management and clinical trial design. *J Clin Oncol*. 2004;22:3120–3125.

46. Aghajanian C, Blank SV, Goff BA, et al. OCEANS: a randomized, double-blind, placebo-controlled phase III trial of chemotherapy with or without bevacizumab in patients with platinum-sensitive recurrent epithelial ovarian, primary peritoneal, or fallopian tube cancer. *J Clin Oncol*. 2012;30(17): 2039–2045.

47. Han C, Altwerger G, Menderes G, et al. Novel targeted therapies in ovarian and uterine carcinosarcomas. *Discov Med.* 2018;25(140):309–319.

48. Amant F, Vloeberghs V, Woestenborghs H, et al. ERBB-2 gene overexpression and amplification in uterine sarcomas. *Gynecol Oncol.* 2004; 95(3):583–587.

49. Livasy CA, Reading FC, Moore DT, Boggess JF, Lininger RA. EGFR expression and HER2/neu overexpression/amplification in endometrial carcinosarcoma. *Gynecol Oncol.* 2006;100(1):101–106.

50. Fader AN, Roque DM, Siegel E, et al. Randomized phase II trial of carboplatin-paclitaxel versus carboplatin-paclitaxel-trastuzumab in uterine serous carcinomas that overexpress human epidermal growth factor receptor 2/neu. *J Clin Oncol Off J Am Soc Clin Oncol.* 2018;36(20): 2044–2051. https://doi.org/10.1200/JCO.2017.76.5966.

51. Fader AN, Roque DM, Siegel E, et al. Randomized phase II trial of carboplatin-paclitaxel compared with carboplaitn-paclitaxel-trastuzumab in advanced (stage III-IV) or recurrent uterine serous carcinomas that overexpress Her2-/Neu (NCT01367002): updated overall survival analysis. *Clin Cancer Res.* 2020;26(15):3928–3935.

52. Nicoletti R, Lopez S, Bellone S, et al. T-DM1, a novel antibody-drug conjugate, is highly effective against uterine and ovarian carcinosarcomas overexpressing HER2. *Clin Exp Metastas.* 2015;32:29–38.

53. Menderes G, Bonazzoli E, Bellone S, et al. SYD985, a novel duocarmycin-based HER2-targeting antibody-drug conjugate, shows antitumor activity in uterine and ovarian carcinosarcoma with HER2/Neu expression. *Clin Cancer Res.* 2017;23:5836–5845.

54. Schwab CL, English DP, Black J, et al. Neratinib shows efficacy in the treatment of HER2 amplified carcinosarcoma in vitro and in vivo. *Gynecol Oncol.* 2015;139:112–117.

55. Schulten HJ, Gunawan B, Enders C, Donhuijsen K, Emons G, Fuzesi L. Overrepresentation of 8q in carcinosarcomas and endometrial adenocarcinomas. *Am J Clin Pathol.* 2004;122(4):546–551.

56. Lopez S, Perrone E, Bellone S, et al. Preclinical activity of sacituzumab govitecan (IMMU-132) in uterine and ovarian carcinosarcomas. *Oncotarget.* 2020;11(5):560–570.

Chapter 4

Ovarian clear cell carcinoma

Beryl Manning-Geist*, Sushmita Gordhandas*, Preetha Ramalingam, and Oliver Zivanovic

Clinical case

Forty-year-old G1P1 presented to her local emergency department with back pain. A CT scan showed a 14 cm right ovarian cyst, and CA-125 was elevated at 49 U/mL. She underwent a robotic-assisted laparoscopic right salpingo-oophorectomy, with surgical findings of adhesions in the posterior cul-de-sac (Fig. 4.1). Final pathology was consistent with clear cell carcinoma of the ovary with evidence of endometriosis. She subsequently underwent completion staging with total abdominal hysterectomy, left salpingo-oophorectomy, pelvic and paraaortic lymph node dissection, omentectomy, and pelvic washings. Her final stage was FIGO stage IC3, and she was offered chemotherapy with carboplatin and paclitaxel. Is there benefit of adjuvant chemotherapy in stage I ovarian clear cell carcinoma?

Epidemiology
Incidence/mortality

In the United States, it is estimated that there will be 21,410 new diagnoses of ovarian cancer and 13,770 deaths from ovarian cancer. For these women with newly diagnosed ovarian cancer, estimated five-year survival for all stages and histologies is approximately 49%.[1] The most recent average annual age-adjusted incidence of ovarian cancer for all Surveillance, Epidemiology, and End Results (SEER) areas is 10.9 per 100,000 women, and the average age-adjusted mortality rate is 6.7 per 100,000 women .[2]

Ovarian clear cell carcinoma represents 5% to 10% of ovarian cancers in the United States; however, there are known geographical and racial differences in incidence.[3,4] For example, there is a much higher incidence of ovarian clear cell carcinoma in Japan, Taiwan, and Korea, where ovarian clear cell carcinoma represents 15% to 25%, 19%, and 10% of ovarian cancers, respectively.[4] In the United States, Asian/Pacific Islanders have the highest incidence rates of ovarian clear cell carcinoma (1.0 per 100,000 women), which is about twice that of women in other racial groups.[5,6] Environmental and genetic factors likely play a role in development of ovarian clear cell carcinoma but reasons for variation of incidence among racial groups are unclear. Additionally, it is unknown why ovarian clear cell carcinoma is more likely to present in younger women with a median age of 55 years, compared to the more common high-grade serous counterpart, where the median age of presentation is 64 years.[7]

Ovarian clear cell carcinoma is a rare ovarian malignancy; as a result, clinical trials are not powered to make conclusions for ovarian clear cell carcinoma despite known differences in response to treatment. Recommendations for surveillance and treatment of ovarian clear cell carcinoma are nonspecific and follow recommendations for the most common histology of ovarian cancer, high-grade serous. In this chapter we will highlight the known distinct features of ovarian clear cell carcinoma and treatment recommendations.

Etiology/risk factors

Similar to endometrioid ovarian carcinoma, ovarian clear cell carcinoma is often associated with or arises from endometriosis.[8] Women with endometriosis have a significantly elevated age-adjusted incidence rate ratio for ovarian clear cell carcinoma (2.29, 95% CI, 1.24–4.20).[9] A metaanalysis combining data from 13 ovarian cancer case–control studies found that self-reported endometriosis significantly increased the risk of ovarian clear cell carcinoma (OR 3.05, 95% CI, 2.4–3.8).[10]

---

*These authors contributed equally to this work.

Diagnosis and Treatment of Rare Gynecologic Cancers. https://doi.org/10.1016/B978-0-323-82938-0.00004-5

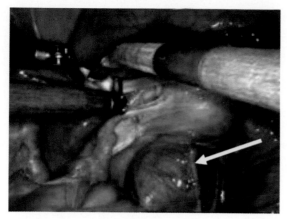

FIG. 4.1 Right adnexal mass (*yellow arrow*). Final diagnosis was clear cell carcinoma of the ovary.

On final pathology, endometriosis is identified in up to 51% of ovarian clear cell carcinoma cases.[11] The association of endometriosis is further supported by the protective nature of tubal ligation against the development of ovarian clear cell carcinoma.[12] The Ovarian Cancer Cohort Consortium found that tubal ligation and hysterectomy were associated with a significantly reduced risk of ovarian clear cell carcinoma (RR 0.35, 95% CI, 0.18–0.69; RR 0.57, 95% CI, 0.36–0.88, respectively).[13] Theoretically, occlusion of the tubes or hysterectomy could prevent retrograde menstruation and subsequent development of endometriosis. However, the effect of endometriosis may confound these results. Most women undergo tubal ligation after childbearing is complete and women with endometriosis have higher rates of infertility. The group who did not undergo tubal ligation may have a disproportionate number of patients with endometriosis.

Endometriosis with cytologic atypia or complex hyperplasia (atypical endometriosis) is the most likely precursor to clear cell ovarian cancers.[14] Studies have found that similar gene mutations are detected in ovarian clear cell carcinoma and adjacent atypical endometriosis.[15] Chronic inflammation associated with endometriosis has also been identified as a potential risk factor for development of cancers, involving the intensive release of cytokines and infiltration of immune cells.[16]

In addition to endometriosis, patients with germline mutations associated with *BRCA1/2* or Lynch syndrome also have an increased risk of ovarian clear cell carcinoma. In a study of 1119 *BRCA1/2* associated ovarian cancers, 2% were of clear cell histology.[17] In Lynch syndrome, a Swedish/Danish cancer registry found that ovarian cancer subtypes differed from the sporadic population, with 35% endometrioid and 17% clear cell histology.[18] Therefore, as in all epithelial ovarian cancers, women with ovarian clear cell carcinoma should be recommended to undergo genetic testing.

Pathology

Gross

The gross appearance of ovarian clear cell carcinoma is variable with cut surface being entirely solid, entirely cystic or solid and cystic. The entirely cystic tumors are grossly not distinguishable from other benign ovarian cysts.

Microscopic findings

Histologically ovarian clear cell carcinomas are heterogeneous with papillary (Fig. 4.2), tubulocystic, and solid patterns. The papillae of ovarian clear cell carcinomas are lined by cells with clear cytoplasm that have characteristic hobnail appearance, lining a hyalinized fibrovascular core.[19] The tubulocystic pattern (Fig. 4.3) is composed of numerous dilated cysts with markedly flattened epithelium that may impart a "benign" appearance on low power examination. However, on high power review, the prominent cytologic atypia is usually apparent. In ovarian clear cell carcinoma, the nuclei are variably atypical and usually round without significant pleomorphism, though bizarre cells may be seen in a subset of cases. Prominent "cherry-red" nucleoli, though not specific, are typically seen in ovarian clear cell carcinomas. While majority of ovarian clear cell carcinomas have typical cytoplasmic clearing, in some cases the cells have eosinophilic cytoplasm, and can mimic endometrioid or serous carcinoma. The mitotic activity is usually low. Ovarian clear cell carcinoma has been shown to have significant interobserver variability, even among gynecologic pathology experts, as both endometrioid adenocarcinoma and high-grade serous carcinoma can have prominent clear cell changes.[20]

Ancillary testing

The currently available immunohistochemical (IHC) stains used to establish a diagnosis of ovarian clear cell carcinoma, are unfortunately neither sensitive nor specific, limiting their utility. The tumors are positive for PAX-8, hepatocyte nuclear factor 1 beta (HNF-1B) (Fig. 4.4), napsin A (Fig. 4.5), and α-methylacyl-coenzyme A racemase (AMACR, p504S), while negative for WT-1.[21] Estrogen and progesterone receptors (ER and PR) are typically negative in ovarian clear cell

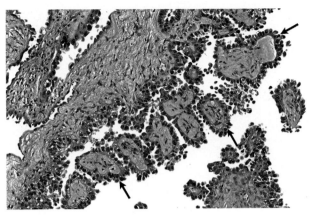

FIG. 4.2 Ovarian clear cell carcinoma showing papillary pattern with hyalinized fibrovascular cores (*asterisks*) and hobnailing (*black arrows*).

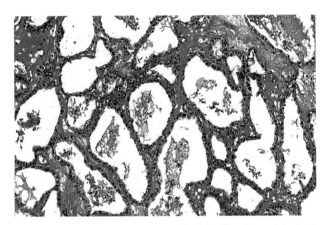

FIG. 4.3 Ovarian clear cell carcinoma showing tubulocystic pattern characterized by dilated cysts/glands that are lined by flattened epithelium with cytoplasmic clearing.

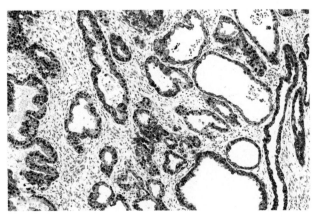

FIG. 4.4 Ovarian clear cell carcinoma showing diffuse strong nuclear staining for HNF-1B.

carcinomas; however, focal and or diffuse weak staining can be seen in a subset of tumors. HNF-1B, frequently used to confirm ovarian clear cell carcinoma is highly sensitive but not specific, as it can be expressed in both endometrioid and serous carcinomas. Conversely, AMACR and napsin-A are more specific for a diagnosis of ovarian clear cell carcinoma but their low sensitivity results in them not being helpful in many cases.

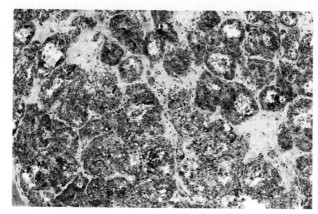

FIG. 4.5 Ovarian clear cell carcinoma showing granular cytoplasmic staining for napsin-A.

Differential diagnosis

The differential diagnosis of clear cell carcinoma is quite vast and encompasses epithelial, germ cell and sex cord tumors, as well as metastatic tumors with clear cytoplasm. As mentioned earlier both endometrioid carcinoma and serous carcinoma can mimic ovarian clear cell carcinoma. IHC stains can show overlapping expression among ovarian clear cell carcinomas, serous carcinoma and endometrioid carcinoma, making a definite diagnosis challenging in some cases. This is further compounded by the lack of sensitivity and specificity of the available immunomarkers used to confirm a diagnosis of clear cell carcinoma. In typical cases endometrioid carcinoma and serous carcinoma will have hormone receptor expression with absent staining for HNF-1B, and napsin-A. p53 staining has limited utility in distinguishing serous carcinoma from clear cell carcinoma in isolation, as the former can rarely show wild-type staining and the latter can show p53 overexpression. An important differential is yolk sac tumor (YST), which can have histologic features that are virtually indistinguishable from clear cell carcinoma. Young age of presentation, elevated serum alpha-fetoprotein (AFP) and presence of Schiller-Duval bodies would favor YST. YSTs are positive for SALL-4, and AFP while negative for CK7, while ovarian clear cell carcinomas will show the opposite staining pattern. The solid variant of clear cell carcinoma can mimic steroid cell tumor and metastatic renal cell carcinoma. Steroid cell tumors and ovarian clear cell carcinomas have completely different immunoprofiles that will facilitate the correct diagnosis. Metastatic clear cell renal cell carcinoma (RCC) can be more challenging due to overlapping immunomarker expression such as PAX-8, napsin-A, and HNF-1B. Presence of a renal mass and positivity for RCC-specific markers will help in making the correct diagnosis.

Molecular findings

In ovarian clear cell carcinoma, the most common molecular genetic alterations are somatic inactivating mutations of AT-rich interactive domain 1A *(ARID1A)*, activating mutations of phosphatidylinositol-4,5-bisphosphate 3-kinase, catalytic subunit alpha *(PIK3CA),* and deletion of phosphatase and tensin homolog *(PTEN).*[22] *ARID1A* mutations are present in approximately 50% of ovarian clear cell carcinomas, but there are also reports of its presence in the adjacent foci of atypical endometriosis.[23] This finding suggests that *ARID1A* mutations represent an early molecular event in ovarian clear cell carcinomas, and that endometriosis may be a precursor lesion for these tumors.[24]

Diagnosis and workup

Differential diagnosis

Diagnosis of ovarian clear cell carcinoma is difficult due to the diversity of clinical presentation, nonspecific symptoms and endometriosis-associated symptoms. In contrast to the more common high-grade serous ovarian cancer, patients with ovarian clear cell carcinoma often present with unilateral, sometimes large adnexal masses and more commonly present with earlier stage disease. The differential diagnosis for an adnexal mass is quite large, including but not limited to ectopic pregnancy, physiologic/ functional cysts, polycystic ovaries, serous/mucinous cystadenomas, germ cell tumors, sex cord stromal tumors, peritoneal inclusion cysts, fibroids, endometriosis, tubo-ovarian abscess, appendiceal/diverticular abscess, colon cancer, and/or metastasis from a different primary. The workup for an adnexal mass must keep this broad differential diagnosis in mind.

Signs and symptoms

Ovarian clear cell carcinoma typically presents as a pelvic mass, often large pelvic mass. In early-stage ovarian clear cell carcinoma, initial presentation is often an asymptomatic adnexal mass discovered incidentally during workup for another condition. Some may present with pelvic pain and pressure due to a growing, typically unilateral, adnexal tumor. Clinical presentation of patients with advanced ovarian cancer varies, and symptoms are often nonspecific, such as fatigue, loss of appetite, early satiety, nausea, and anorexia, and may overlap with symptoms of concurrent endometriosis. Symptoms in advanced-stage ovarian clear cell carcinoma may be due to ascites, pleural effusions and peritoneal carcinomatosis. Because symptoms overlap with more common disorders (e.g., endometriosis, menopause, constipation, irritable bowel syndrome) diagnosis may be delayed.[5]

Ovarian clear cell carcinoma tumors range up to 30 cm in diameter, with a mean of 13 to 15 cm.[25] As the mass grows, it may cause bulk symptoms. Urinary complaints are common including urinary urgency and frequency.[26] As these tumors expand posteriorly, they can compress the colon, leading to constipation and pain. Pelvic and abdominal symptoms include bloating, and diffuse, dull, constant abdominal pain. Adnexal masses may also present with acute onset abdominal pain, which may be associated with rupture, torsion, or bowel obstruction.

Deep venous thrombosis (DVT) may develop due to the hypercoagulability associated with advanced cancer, or the tumor pressing on the pelvic veins.[27] Of the epithelial ovarian cancers, ovarian clear cell carcinoma are most commonly associated with DVT which occur in up to 42% of cases.[28] Ovarian clear cell carcinoma expresses high levels of tissue factor, a transmembrane protein that is associated with hypercoagulability.[29] Complaints of lower extremity swelling/pain, shortness of breath, and pleuritic chest pain must be evaluated thoroughly due to elevated risk of DVT and pulmonary embolism. Hypercalcemia is observed at a higher frequency in ovarian clear cell carcinoma compared to other ovarian cancers due to production of parathyroid hormone-related protein.[30]

There is no evidence that screening for symptoms aids in recognizing ovarian cancers at earlier stage or improves detection with use of CA-125 or ultrasound.[31,32] Early referral to a gynecologic oncologist for patients with symptomatic, persistent or growing adnexal masses, ascites, or evidence of abdominal/ distant metastases is imperative.[33]

Physical exam findings

Physical exam findings are similar for benign and malignant adnexal masses. It is nearly impossible to identify a malignant mass based on clinical exam alone. A comprehensive exam is essential, including evaluation of extremities, lungs, supra-clavicular nodes, and breasts. Lower extremity edema, tenderness, or a palpable cord is suggestive of a DVT. Abdominal exam should include palpation and percussion. If the tumor produces a large amount of ascites, the abdominal cavity may be distended, causing increased abdominal circumference and marked discomfort. Ascites can also cause dyspnea, as the lower lungs are compressed by abdominal distension.

On pelvic exam, a bimanual and rectovaginal exam should be performed. Visually, a cystocele may indicate the presence of ascites. During pelvic exam, the clinician should note the size, borders, mobility, and location of the mass. Invasive cancers are typically large, fixed, and have irregular borders. Exam may also reveal involvement of the parametrium or nodularity of the rectovaginal septum, also known as a Blumer's shelf.

Tumor markers

The most studied tumor marker associated with epithelial ovarian cancer is CA-125. Pretreatment CA-125 levels are elevated in the majority of patients with ovarian clear cell carcinoma, but levels do not predict clinical outcome. A retrospective case–control study of 375 patients with ovarian clear cell carcinoma, found that pretreatment CA-125 levels were not associated with relapse-free survival (RFS) or overall survival. Pretreatment CA-125 is normal in 30% of early-stage and 13% of advanced-stage ovarian clear cell carcinoma.[34,35] The majority of ovarian clear cell carcinomas are diagnosed at early stage so elevated CA-125 levels are not a reliable marker of malignancy in these patients (Table 4.1).

For advanced-stage ovarian cancers, CA-125 values are highest for patients with serous histology with a median of 2000 U/mL; patients with clear cell histology have lower CA-125 values with a median of 154 U/mL (normal <35 U/mL).[35,36] CA-125 normalization after initiation of chemotherapy is correlated with overall survival and is likely a surrogate for inherent chemosensitivity.[34] A retrospective review of seven previously reported GOG phase three trials

TABLE 4.1 Basic workup for ovarian clear cell carcinoma.

		Early-stage	Advanced-stage
Imaging	Pelvic ultrasound: detect and characterize adnexal mass	Papillary surface excrescences, areas of necrosis, internal solid elements	Suspicious adnexal mass and ascites, upper abdominal disease
	CT scan: assess extent of disease, assist with surgical planning		
Tumor markers	CA-125	Elevated in 70%	Elevated in 87%
Diagnostic tests	Pathologic tissue diagnosis required: – Surgical resection: confirm whether malignancy is present, proceed with staging and cytoreduction – Biopsy: for pathologic tissue diagnosis in patients who cannot tolerate surgical cytoreduction, or for those with distant metastases or disease that is unlikely to be optimally cytoreduced		

in patients with stage III/IV ovarian clear cell carcinoma found that changes in CA-125 at the end of treatment compared to baseline can serve as an indicator of progression-free survival (PFS) and overall survival.[35]

It should be noted that elevated CA-125 levels may be false positives. For example, other gynecologic conditions that cause peritoneal or pelvic inflammation can elevate CA-125 levels, including endometriosis. Meanwhile, conditions that lead to ascites, such as cirrhosis or heart failure may also elevate the CA-125. Overall, tumor markers can be useful in monitoring treatment and surveillance of ovarian clear cell carcinoma, but clinical history remains integral to diagnosis.

Imaging

Imaging findings associated with epithelial ovarian cancer include partially solid and cystic components to the mass, irregularity of borders, and fixed location. The three main imaging modalities used for ovarian clear cell carcinoma are ultrasound, CT scan, and MRI. Imaging findings particular to ovarian clear cell carcinoma include unilocular or large cysts with solid protrusions into the cavity.[37] Due to association with endometriosis, large endometriomas with solid components are highly suspicious for ovarian clear cell carcinoma. On CT scan, ovarian clear cell carcinoma margins are typically smooth, solid protrusions are rounded and few in number with high-attenuated cystic or necrotic portions.[38] On T1-weighted MRI images, signal intensity varies from low to very high.[37] Imaging can help identify patients in whom aggressive initial surgical cytoreduction may not be the most beneficial primary treatment option, as they have a lower chance of optimal cytoreduction. Preoperative imaging can also identify disease in unresectable locations.

Diagnostic tests

The diagnosis of ovarian clear cell carcinoma requires pathologic tissue diagnosis. Patients with early-stage disease benefit from removal of the adnexal mass intact, although data are conflicting on whether intraoperative mass rupture truly worsens prognosis.[39] Therefore, imaging-guided biopsy of the ovary should not be performed when the patient is a good candidate for surgical exploration. The goal of surgery is to confirm whether malignancy is present and if so, proceed with staging and cytoreduction. In patients who are unable to tolerate aggressive surgical cytoreduction or with extensive/unresectable disease, image guided biopsy, paracentesis, or thoracentesis may be used to establish a tissue diagnosis.

Staging system

Ovarian clear cell carcinoma is diagnosed at an earlier stage than serous carcinoma, with 57% to 81% of patients presenting at stage I, and 19% to 22% at stage II.[7] Epithelial ovarian cancers are surgically and pathologically staged according to the 2017 eighth edition American Joint Committee on Cancer (AJCC) and the joint 2017 International Federation of Gynecology and Obstetrics (FIGO)/Tumor, Node, Metastasis (TNM) classification system (Table 4.2). The standard staging procedure for epithelial ovarian cancer includes total extra-fascial hysterectomy and bilateral salpingo-oophorectomy (BSO) with pelvic and paraaortic lymph node dissection if there is no gross evidence of intraperitoneal disease.

TABLE 4.2 TNM and FIGO staging for ovary, fallopian tube, and primary peritoneal carcinomas.

Primary tumor (T)		
T category	**FIGO stage**	**T criteria**
TX		Primary tumor cannot be assessed
T0		No evidence of primary tumor
T1	I	Tumor limited to ovaries (one or both) or fallopian tube(s)
T1a	IA	Tumor limited to one ovary (capsule intact) or fallopian tube, no tumor on ovarian or fallopian tube surface; no malignant cells in ascites or peritoneal washings
T1b	IB	Tumor limited to both ovaries (capsules intact) or fallopian tubes; no tumor on ovarian or fallopian tube surface; no malignant cells in ascites or peritoneal washings
T1c	IC	Tumor limited to one or both ovaries or fallopian tubes, with any of the following:
T1c1	IC1	• Surgical spill
T1c2	IC2	• Capsule ruptured before surgery or tumor on ovarian or fallopian tube surface
T1c3	IC3	• Malignant cells in ascites or peritoneal washings
T2	II	Tumor involves one or both ovaries or fallopian tubes with pelvic extension below pelvic brim or primary peritoneal cancer
T2a	IIA	Extension and/or implants on the uterus and/or fallopian tube(s) and/or ovaries
T2b	IIB	Extension to and/or implants on other pelvic tissues
T3	III	Tumor involves one or both ovaries or fallopian tubes, or primary peritoneal cancer, with microscopically confirmed peritoneal metastasis outside the pelvis and/or metastasis to the retroperitoneal (pelvic and/or paraaortic) lymph nodes
T3a	IIIA2	Microscopic extrapelvic (above the pelvic brim) peritoneal involvement with or without positive retroperitoneal lymph nodes
T3b	IIIB	Macroscopic peritoneal metastasis beyond pelvis 2 cm or less in greatest dimension with or without metastasis to the retroperitoneal lymph nodes
T3c	IIIC	Macroscopic peritoneal metastasis beyond the pelvis more than 2 cm in greatest dimension with or without metastasis to the retroperitoneal lymph nodes (includes extension of tumor to capsule of liver and spleen without parenchymal involvement of either organ)

Regional lymph nodes (N)		
N category	**FIGO stage**	**N criteria**
NX		Regional lymph nodes cannot be assessed
N0		No regional lymph node metastasis
N0(i+)		Isolated tumor cells in regional lymph node(s) no greater than 0.2 mm
N1	IIIA1	Positive retroperitoneal lymph nodes only (histologically confirmed)
N1a	IIIA1i	Metastasis up to and including 10 mm in greatest dimension
N1b	IIIA1ii	Metastasis more than 10 mm in greatest dimension

Distant metastasis (M)		
M category	**FIGO stage**	**M criteria**
M0		No distant metastasis
M1	IV	Distant metastasis, including pleural effusion with positive cytology; liver or splenic parenchymal metastasis; metastasis to extraabdominal organs (including inguinal lymph nodes and lymph nodes outside the abdominal cavity); and transmural involvement of intestine
M1a	IVA	Pleural effusion with positive cytology
M1b	IVB	Liver or splenic parenchymal metastases; metastases to extraabdominal organs (including inguinal lymph nodes and lymph nodes outside the abdominal cavity); transmural involvement of intestine

Pelvic washings are collected, and omentectomy is performed. Further cytoreduction is dependent on each individual clinical situation.

For patients who underwent comprehensive staging for clinical stage I ovarian clear cell carcinoma (disease grossly confined to the ovary) the rate of lymph node metastasis is 4.8%. In cases with ovarian surface involvement, 37.5% had lymph node metastasis.[40] This brings to question the yield of detecting nodal metastasis in ovarian clear cell carcinoma cases lacking ovarian surface involvement. Takano et al. found that peritoneal cytology (pelvic washings) status was an independent prognostic factor for PFS but not overall survival, and that completion of surgical staging procedures was not a prognostic factor.[41] Eight percent of all stages of ovarian clear cell carcinomas are bilateral, only 4% of stage I cases are bilateral.[25]

Prognostic factors

Ovarian clear cell carcinoma typically presents at an early-stage (stage I or II) and has a relatively good prognosis. Patients with stage I ovarian clear cell carcinoma have 5-year PFS of 85.3% compared to 86.4% for women with serous carcinoma, 92.7% for endometrioid, and 93.1% for mucinous disease. Patients with stage II disease have 5-year PFS of 60.3% compared to 66.4% for women with serous carcinoma, 81.9% for endometrioid, and 61.3% for mucinous histologies.[7] In a review of 9531 patients participating in 12 prospective randomized Gynecologic Oncology Group (GOG) studies, PFS was significantly better in stage I and II ovarian clear cell carcinoma when compared with serous ovarian carcinoma (PFS HR 0.69, 95% CI, 0.50–0.96) but PFS and OS were significantly worse in advanced-stage ovarian clear cell carcinoma (OS HR 1.66, 95% CI, 1.43–1.91).[42]

When diagnosed at an advanced stage, ovarian clear cell carcinoma has a worse prognosis than serous or endometrioid ovarian cancer.[7] For patients with stage III ovarian clear cell carcinoma, 5-year OS is 31.5% compared to 35.0% for patients with serous carcinoma, 50.6% for women with endometrioid carcinoma, and 34.5% for those with mucinous histology. Meanwhile, 5-year OS is 17.5% for patients with stage IV ovarian clear cell carcinoma compared to 22.2% for patients with stage IV serous carcinoma, 34.6% for women with endometrioid carcinoma, and 17.5% for those with mucinous histology.[7] In a study of oncologic outcomes in ovarian clear cell carcinoma, 68% and 94% of deaths occurred within 12 and 24 of recurrence, respectively. In comparison, 41% and 73% of deaths occurred within 12 and 24 months of serous ovarian cancer recurrence, respectively.[43] Poorer oncologic outcomes for advanced-stage ovarian clear cell carcinoma have been confirmed in SEER database studies as well as meta-analyses.[44,45]

The incidence of vascular thrombotic events, such as DVT and pulmonary embolism, is high in patients with ovarian clear cell carcinoma (27%–42%) and is considered an independent poor prognostic factor.[27,28] Studies on prognosis in endometriosis-associated ovarian clear cell carcinoma are mixed, but overall suggest no difference in survival after controlling for variables such as stage of disease.[46] It is unclear if MMRd, MSI, TMB, PDL-1 IHC, or hormone receptor status is associated with survival.

Treatment of primary disease

Surgery

Early-stage disease

Staging surgery is a fundamental aspect of ovarian clear cell carcinoma care, as it both prognosticates and guides treatment decisions in early-stage disease (Fig. 4.6). In cases of presumed early-stage disease, surgery should also include a lymphadenectomy, as risk of lymph node metastases in ovarian clear cell carcinoma is 5% to 15%. While lymphadenectomy has not been associated with improved survival in advanced stages, it has been associated with significantly improved disease-specific survival in patients with pT1 or pT2 disease in several large, retrospective cohorts including the Multicenter Italian Trials in Ovarian Cancer (MITO 9) study.[47–49]

In patients desiring fertility preservation with apparent early-stage disease, full peritoneal staging (including washings, inspection of the cavity, and biopsies if necessary) accompanied by unilateral salpingo-oophorectomy (USO), omentectomy, and lymph node dissection should be considered.[50] While laparotomy is generally favored for advanced-stage disease, minimally invasive surgery may be considered in early-stage ovarian cancer.[51,52] A systematic review comparing 1450 patients undergoing laparoscopy and 1615 undergoing laparotomy demonstrated no difference in survival outcomes between route of surgery.[52] Patients undergoing laparoscopy had a significantly lower estimated blood loss, shorter length of stay, fewer postoperative complications, and shorter time to chemotherapy compared to patients who underwent an open approach.[52] A subsequent National Cancer Database (NCDB) analysis of 1096 patients (including 195 patients with ovarian

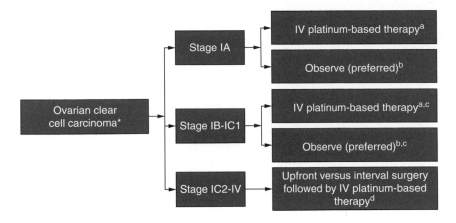

^a**Primary Systemic Therapy Regimens for Stage I Disease**

Preferred Regimens	Other Recommended Regimens	Useful in Certain Circumstances
• Paclitaxel/carboplatin (3-6 cycles)	• Carboplatin/liposomal doxorubicin • Docetaxel/carboplatin	• Single-agent carboplatin (if unable to tolerate doublet, such as elderly or with comorbidities)

^bSurgical staging including washings, pelvic/para-aortic lymph node dissection, omentectomy, and peritoneal biopsies as well as hysterectomy/bilateral salpingo-oophorectomy (unless planning fertility preservation)
^cESMO guidelines offer observation for stages IB-IC1 disease; NCCN guidelines recommend 3-6 cycles IV platinum-based chemotherapy for stages IB-IC1 disease; based on available data, little proven benefit to chemotherapy.

^d**Primary Systemic Therapy Regimens for Stage II-IV Disease**

Preferred Regimen	Other Recommended Regimens	Useful in Certain Circumstances
• Paclitaxel/carboplatin (6 cycles)	• Paclitaxel weekly/carboplatin weekly • Paclitaxel weekly/carboplatin q3 weeks • Carboplatin/docetaxel • Carboplatin/liposomal doxorubicin	• IP/IV paclitaxel/cisplatin (for optimally debulked stage II-III disease)

*In all cases, recommend panel genetic testing and consideration of MMR IHC.

FIG. 4.6 Treatment algorithm for patients with ovarian clear cell carcinoma.

clear cell carcinoma) demonstrated no survival benefit to laparotomy compared with laparoscopic staging after propensity score matching.[53] Given these data, it is reasonable to offer a minimally invasive approach to women with presumed early-stage disease, although it should be noted that this has been independently associated with an almost 20% relative increase in capsule rupture among all epithelial ovarian cancer patients.[54]

In patients desiring fertility, preservation of the contralateral ovary and uterus may be considered in select cases after careful patient counseling as this is a deviation from the standard of care. Data informing the decision to offer fertility-sparing surgery are limited, but evidence thus far suggests that this approach is relatively safe. An NCDB Analysis of 33 women with stage IA and 24 women with stage IC ovarian clear cell carcinoma undergoing fertility preservation demonstrated no difference in survival between patients undergoing fertility sparing surgery versus those undergoing radical cytoreduction.[55] A systematic review of 132 patients with stage IA-IC ovarian clear cell carcinoma undergoing fertility sparing surgery demonstrated a relapse rate of 15.2%, a median of 18 months from surgery. Of patients with available staging and recurrence data, 5 (12.5%) of 40 patients with IA disease recurred, 6 (21.4%) of 28 patients with stage IC1 recurred, and 5 (38.5%) of 13 patients with IC2/3 disease recurred. Sites of relapse included local sites including retroperitoneal lymph nodes, the remaining ovary, the pelvis as well as distant sites including the lung, the brain, and perihepatic soft tissue.[55]

Surgery for advanced stage ovarian clear cell carcinoma

In advanced-stage disease, surgery should include an exploratory laparotomy, pelvic washings, hysterectomy, BSO, omentectomy, and removal of all gross visible disease including upper abdominal tumor. As in all epithelial ovarian cancers, complete gross resection (CGR) confers maximum overall survival compared to optimal or suboptimal residual disease

$(P < 0.001)$.[56] In fact, the survival curves for optimal residual disease and suboptimal residual disease after cytoreductive surgery for ovarian clear cell carcinoma are relatively similar. Thus, all efforts should be made to remove all visible tumor at time of debulking surgery.

Because ovarian clear cell carcinoma thought to be less responsive to platinum-based chemotherapy regimens when compared to high-grade serous counterpart, there may be a risk that patients will have refractory disease and lose the opportunity to derive surgical benefit. In certain instances, however, such as in patients with stage IVB disease, extremely poor functional status, or thromboembolic disease, neoadjuvant chemotherapy followed by interval debulking surgery (NACT-IDS) should be considered. Data are limited on the efficacy of NACT-IDS in ovarian clear cell carcinoma: the two largest randomized controlled trials comparing NACT-IDS to primary debulking surgery (EORTC-55971 and CHORUS) included only 10 (out of 670) and 17 (out of 550) ovarian clear cell carcinoma patients among the study populations, respectively.[57]

Systemic treatment of ovarian clear cell carcinoma

Although ovarian clear cell carcinoma appears to be less chemosensitive than other epithelial ovarian histologic subtypes, treatment guidelines recommend an approach paralleling high-grade serous carcinoma.[56] Current National Comprehensive Cancer Network (NCCN) guidelines recommend systemic therapy for all patients with stage IB, IC, and II–IV disease, while patients with stage IA cancer should be offered IV platinum-based chemotherapy versus observation[50] (Fig. 4.6). The European Society for Medical Oncology (ESMO) guidelines differ from NCCN guidelines in offering either adjuvant chemotherapy or observation in patients with completely staged IA, IB, or IC1 ovarian clear cell carcinoma.

Chemotherapy

The optimal first-line treatment regimen for clear cell carcinoma is a carboplatin/paclitaxel doublet (paclitaxel 175 mg/m^2 IV followed by carboplatin AUC 5–6 IV day 1 q3 weeks), which can be dose-reduced if required by patient comorbidities such as kidney dysfunction or poor performance status. Special attention should be paid to dose-reduction of carboplatin based on renal function.[58] It is estimated that the response rate of ovarian clear cell carcinoma to this platinum doublet is 22% to 79%.[8,59]

Special considerations

Early-stage disease

The largest debate surrounding treatment in ovarian clear cell carcinoma is in early-stage disease, and data informing adjuvant treatment guidelines in this setting are limited by the relative rarity of this disease. The two largest randomized trials addressing this issue are the ICON1 trial, which included 36 ovarian clear cell carcinoma patients randomized to observation and 31 ovarian clear cell carcinoma patients randomized to adjuvant chemotherapy and ACTION trial, which included 26 ovarian clear cell carcinoma patients randomized to observation and 37 ovarian clear cell carcinoma patients randomized to adjuvant chemotherapy.[60,61] Although these studies were not powered to offer an ovarian clear cell carcinoma-specific subgroup analysis, ICON1 performed a subgroup analysis of high-risk patients, including those with stage IB/IC grade 2/3 or any stage I grade 3 or clear cell histology. The greatest benefit of adjuvant chemotherapy was observed in this high-risk subgroup, with a PFS and OS HR of 0.48 (95% CI, 0.31–0.73) and 0.52 (95% CI, 0.33–0.81) at 10 years, respectively.[62]

Large, retrospective cohort studies can also offer additional guidance on the association between adjuvant chemotherapy and survival in patients with early-stage ovarian clear cell carcinoma. A SEER database review of 1995 patients with stage I ovarian clear cell carcinoma found no OS survival benefit associated with adjuvant chemotherapy when analyzed by stage.[63] For patients with stage IA/B disease, 5-year OS was 87% with chemotherapy versus 84% without chemotherapy ($P = 0.308$). For patients with stage IC disease, 5-year OS was 83% with chemotherapy versus 80% without ($P = 0.620$). Given the above findings, it is recommended that chemotherapy be offered to all patients with stage IC2 and above ovarian clear cell carcinoma.

Society guidelines differ with regards to patients with stages IA, IB, and IC1 disease. Although data are limited, it should be noted that patients upstaged to IC1 by intraoperative capsule rupture carry a similar prognosis to patients with stage IA disease.[64,65] A retrospective study of 93 patients with stage IC1 ovarian clear cell carcinoma found no survival benefit to adjuvant chemotherapy in this subgroup.[66] However, patients with preoperative capsule rupture (positive washings) demonstrate a less favorable prognosis: in one study, patients with IC disease and negative washings ($n = 74$) had a 86% 5-year PFS while patients with IC disease and positive washings ($n = 33$) had a 41% 5-year PFS.[67]

In early-stage ovarian clear cell carcinoma, the number of cycles of adjuvant therapy is also a point of contention. GOG-157 compared 3 to 6 cycles of a carboplatin/paclitaxel doublet in early-stage epithelial ovarian carcinoma and found a nonsignificant decreased risk of recurrence with additional cycles (HR 0.76, 95% CI, 0.51–1.13).[68] A subgroup analysis of GOG-157 explored survival differences in 3 versus 6 cycles of carboplatin/paclitaxel based on histologic subtype. Among 130 patients with ovarian clear cell carcinoma, there was no difference in PFS (HR 0.90, 95% CI, 0.43–1.91) among those receiving 3 versus 6 cycles of chemotherapy.[69] A subsequent retrospective multiinstitutional study of 210 patients confirmed these findings, demonstrating no difference in PFS or OS in stage IA-II ovarian clear cell carcinoma patients receiving 3 versus 6 cycles of chemotherapy.[70] Ultimately, the number of cycles of therapy to pursue should be tailored to individual patients, taking into consideration toxicities of adjuvant treatment.

Role of radiation

There are limited studies examining the role of primary radiation in early-stage ovarian clear cell carcinoma. The largest available study by Hoskins et al. reported on 241 patients with stage I and II ovarian clear cell carcinoma treated with 6 abdominopelvic radiation versus observation after 3 to 6 cycles of adjuvant carboplatin/paclitaxel. This study found no benefit associated with radiation for patients with stage IA–IC1 disease, while patients with IC2/3 disease undergoing abdominopelvic radiation had a 20% improvement in PFS at 5 years (RR 0.54, 95% CI, 0.33–0.95).[67] A follow-up study compared 153 patients with stage IC2/3-II ovarian clear cell carcinoma treated with adjuvant chemotherapy versus chemoradiotherapy (chemoRT) (i.e., whole abdominal radiotherapy (WAR)/ pelvic nodal radiotherapy).[71] Receipt of chemoRT ($n = 90$) was associated with improvement in PFS and disease-specific survival compared to chemotherapy alone ($n = 63$) (HR 0.57, 95% CI, 0.34–0.94; HR 0.46, 95% CI, 0.24–0.89, respectively). Several smaller studies have also demonstrated a survival advantage of adjuvant radiation. In a 2007 study comparing 16 patients with stage IC-III ovarian clear cell carcinoma treated with WAR to a historical cohort of 12 patients who underwent cyclophosphamide/ adriamycin/cisplatin (CAP), authors noted a 5-year PFS of 81.2% versus 25.0% ($P = 0.006$) and OS of 81.8% versus 33.3% in the WAR versus historical cohort ($P = 0.031$).[72] However, it should be noted that survival rates of the historical controls were lower than expected. Another prospective study that included 11 ovarian clear cell carcinoma patients showed improvement in patient outcomes after combining chemotherapy with WAR.[73]

Of note, one large retrospective study of 163 patients with stage I or II ovarian clear cell carcinoma failed to demonstrate a survival benefit associated with radiation therapy.[74] This study reported that patients receiving radiation ($n = 44$) had no survival advantage compared to patients who did not ($n = 119$): 10-year PFS was 65% with radiation versus 59% without radiation, and 10-year OS was 70% in both groups. Similar to the Hoskins study, these authors investigated the benefit of radiation in a "high-risk" subgroup that included patients with stages IC2/3 or II disease versus "low-risk" patients with stage IA, IB, and IC1 disease. In the high-risk subgroup, 9 (45%) of 20 patients receiving radiation recurred, while 13 (33%) of 39 women in the nonradiation group recurred. Radiation was not associated with improved PFS (HR 1.07, 95% CI, 0.47–2.43) or OS (HR 0.81, 95% CI, 0.28–2.33). It is unclear if endometriosis-associated ovarian clear cell carcinoma responds different to radiation treatment than nonendometriosis associated ovarian clear cell carcinoma.

Endometriosis-associated ovarian clear cell carcinoma

Endometriosis is predicted to affect 3% to 10% of reproductive-aged women and confers an approximately 3 times increased risk of ovarian clear cell carcinoma.[10,75] Estimates suggest that 0.5% to 1.0% of endometriosis cases are complicated by neoplasia.[76] In most cases, endometriosis is observed adjacent to or in continuity with ovarian clear cell carcinoma, suggesting that malignant transformation occurs, particularly in cases of ovarian endometriosis.[77] This hypothesis is further supported by the observed spectrum of atypia in endometriosis, which can be subtyped into benign ectopic endometrial glands and atypical endometriosis.

The genetic underpinnings of this malignant transformation have begun to be elucidated, with *ARID1A* mutations identified in approximately 53% of ovarian clear cell carcinoma.[15] *ARID1A* encodes the BAF250a protein, which acts as an accessory subunit in the chromatin remodeling pathway. Other commonly observed mutations are seen in important oncogenes, such as *KRAS* and *PI3K*, that are part of the MAPK and PI3K pathways.[78] Similarly, mutations in the tumor suppressor gene *PTEN* are observed in approximately 21% of ovarian clear cell carcinoma.[79] While these observational studies are important, it should be noted that whole-exome sequencing has identified many of these mutations, including *ARID1A, PIK3CA, KRAS,* and *PP2R1A,* in benign infiltrating endometriotic lesions without concurrent cancer, suggesting that there are additional drivers necessary for malignant transformation.[80]

There is debate surrounding whether endometriosis-associated ovarian clear cell carcinoma carries a poorer prognosis.[67,81,82] This debate is further complicated by the difficulty in classifying tumors as arising in endometriosis, because ovarian clear cell carcinoma may overgrow and replace endometriosis in an unknown portion of cases. Further, the demonstration of histologic continuity between endometriosis and cancer may be limited by sampling bias. A large meta-analysis of ovarian cancer (all histologies) in women with endometriosis demonstrated improved survival in women with endometriosis; however, authors noted these patients were more likely to have stage I–II and grade 1 disease.[83,84] Another meta-analysis specific to ovarian clear cell carcinoma demonstrated no difference in PFS or OS in 331 patients with endometriosis-associated ovarian clear cell carcinoma versus 412 patients with nonendometriosis associated ovarian clear cell carcinoma (HR 1.15, 95% CI, 0.80–1.67 and HR 0.86, 95% CI, 0.63–1.17, respectively).[85] Single-site studies have also echoed these conclusions, finding no survival difference in patients with a diagnosis of endometriosis, while only a few smaller, single-site studies have associated improved survival with endometriosis.[86–88] In several studies, the reported improvement in survival associated with endometriosis disappears after controlling for stage, suggesting that these smaller scale studies may be confounded by the lower stage of diagnosis in patients with endometriosis.[82,89,90]

Surveillance for recurrence

Surveillance intervals

Although routine follow-up of epithelial ovarian cancer patients has not been shown to improve outcomes, both NCCN and ESMO advocate for routine follow-up while emphasizing cost-effectiveness (Table 4.3).[50,91–93]

Patient visit and physical exam

In approximately 50% of epithelial ovarian cancer patients, symptoms are the earliest harbinger of recurrence. For these reasons, both NCCN and ESMO emphasize a thorough history, as well as a physical exam, during routine follow-up appointments.

Laboratory testing and imaging

While NCCN guidelines for epithelial ovarian cancer recommend imaging and CA-125 as clinically indicated, CA-125 is less reliable in ovarian clear cell carcinoma and may not elevate with recurrence. Prospective randomized data also suggest that treatment of recurrent ovarian cancer based on CA-125 values alone does not improve overall survival.[94] For these reasons, caution is advised in using CA-125 to guide treatment decisions, confirm relapse, or monitor treatment response in ovarian clear cell carcinoma.

In cases such as ovarian clear cell carcinoma when tumor markers are unreliable or there is a high risk of recurrence, the NCCN states that surveillance imaging may be indicated.[50] In the majority of cases, imaging includes a CT scan with oral and IV contrast. CT scans have a sensitivity of 40% to 93% and specificity of 50% to 98% for detecting recurrent ovarian cancer. In comparison, MRI has a sensitivity of 62% to 91% and specificity of 40% to 100%. CT scans are more cost-effective, making them the primary imaging modality for surveillance.[94] PET-CT should only be used in exceptional circumstances and ovarian clear cell carcinoma may be less FDG avid than other histologies.[93]

TABLE 4.3 Surveillance for patients with ovarian clear cell carcinoma.

	Years 0–2	Year 3–5	Year 5 and beyond
NCCN-proposed surveillance interval	Every 2–4 months	Every 3–6 months	Annual visits
ESMO-proposed surveillance interval	Every 3–4 months	Every 6 months	As individually decided upon

Survival and patterns of failure

Early disease (stage IA to IIA)

The literature on recurrence in patients with early-stage ovarian clear cell carcinoma shows that the median time to recurrence for stage I disease is 138.5 months and 33.4 months for stage II disease.[46] Median overall survival is 112.4 months for patients with stage II disease. The majority of patients who recur will do so in the pelvis. Other sites of recurrence may include the abdomen, retroperitoneal lymph nodes, or more rarely distant sites, such as the chest or the brain.[95] While this distribution mimics other epithelial ovarian cancers, it should be noted that patients with ovarian clear cell carcinoma are more likely to have nodal recurrences. In fact, patients with ovarian clear cell carcinoma may have isolated nodal recurrences in up to 18% of cases, compared to only 4.2% of serous ovarian cancer patients.[74,96]

In most cases, patients with early-stage ovarian clear cell carcinoma have multisite recurrence, and less than 20% of patients have single-site recurrent disease.[96] Evidence suggests that patients with single-site and nodal recurrences may have improved 5-year postrecurrence survival compared to those with multisite recurrence (54.4 and 30.1 months vs 13.7 months, respectively).[96]

Advanced disease (stage IIB to IV)

Patients with advanced-stage ovarian clear cell carcinoma have poor disease-free and overall survival compared to patients with other epithelial ovarian cancer histologies. Median recurrence-free and overall survival is 19.3 months and 48.7 months, respectively, for patients with stage III ovarian clear cell carcinoma and 9.7 months and 18.3 months, respectively, for patients with stage IV ovarian clear cell carcinoma.[7] Recurrence patterns in advanced-stage disease parallel those of early-stage disease, although available data indicate that greater than 90% of patients with advanced-stage disease will recur in multiple sites.[96]

Treatment of recurrent disease

"Standard" or commonly used regimens: Platinum-sensitive disease

Patients with recurrent ovarian clear cell carcinoma have significantly poorer survival compared to patients with recurrent serous carcinoma—a study of platinum and paclitaxel in platinum-sensitive recurrent EOC demonstrated a response rate of just 9% in patients with ovarian clear cell carcinoma.[43] For this reason, all patients with recurrent ovarian clear cell carcinoma should consider clinical trials, as there are multiple ongoing studies evaluating targeted therapies, as reviewed below.

For patients with platinum-sensitive disease, the NCCN recommends carboplatin/gemcitabine; carboplatin/pegylated liposomal doxorubicin (PLD); carboplatin/paclitaxel; or cisplatin/gemcitabine. Each agent may be combined with bevacizumab 10 to 15 mg/m^2 IV q2–3 weeks, as discussed below. Similar to trials on platinum-resistant disease, treatment responses of ovarian clear cell carcinoma to these regimens are difficult to estimate due to the rarity of the disease (see Table 4.4).

"Standard" or commonly used regimens: Platinum-resistant disease

In cases of platinum-refractory or resistant recurrence, clinical trial or supportive care is recommended, although acceptable cytotoxic therapies include cyclophosphamide/bevacizumab, docetaxel, etoposide, gemcitabine, liposomal doxorubicin +/− bevacizumab, paclitaxel (weekly) +/− bevacizumab, or topotecan +/− bevacizumab.[50] It should be noted that the trials supporting these recommended regimens included few ovarian clear cell carcinoma patients, as outlined in Table 4.5.

Surgery

For patients with platinum-sensitive recurrent ovarian clear cell carcinoma, secondary cytoreduction may be considered in cases deemed to be resectable. When secondary cytoreduction is pursued, effort should be made to resect all recurrent tumor

TABLE 4.4 Commonly used treatments for recurrent, platinum sensitive ovarian carcinoma.

Regimen*	Total patients included	Ovarian clear cell carcinoma patients included	Outcome (all patients)	ORR (ovarian clear cell carcinoma)
Carboplatin AUC 5 IV D1 + PLD 30 mg/m^2 IV D1 + bevacizumab 10 mg/kg D1 and D15 q4 weeks followed by bevacizumab 15 mg/kg q3 weeks vs carboplatin AUC4 IV D1 + gemcitabine 800–1000 mg/m^2 IV D1 and D8 + bevacizumab 15 mg/kg D1 q3 weeks[126]	345 vs 337	NR	PFS 13.3 vs 11.6 months ($P = 0.012$) and OS 31.9 vs 27.8 months ($P = 0.032$)	NR
Carboplatin AUC 5 (minimum) IV vs cisplatin 50 mg/m^2 plus 135–185 mg/m^2 IV paclitaxel D1 q3 weeks vs conventional treatment (3–6 cycles)[127]	392	NR	1-year PFS 13 vs 10 months ($P = 0.0004$) and 2-year OS 29 vs 24 months ($P = 0.02$)	NR
Gemcitabine 800–1000 mg/m^2 IV D1 and D8 and carboplatin AUC 4 IV D1 q3 weeks[128]	40	NR	Median PFS 9.6 months	NR

NR, not reported.
*Suggested dose ranges.

TABLE 4.5 Commonly used treatments for recurrent platinum-resistant ovarian clear cell carcinoma.

Regimen*	Total patients included	Ovarian clear cell carcinoma patients included	ORR (all patients)	ORR (ovarian clear cell carcinoma)
Bevacizumab 10 mg/kg IV q14d and cyclophosphamide 50 mg oral qday[129]	66	3	42.4%	66.7%
Docetaxel 75–100 mg/m^2 IV ×1 h q21d[130]	61	4	22.4%	NR
Etoposide 30–50 mg/m^2/d oral x21d q4 weeks[131]	53	5	26.8%	NR
Gemcitabine 800–1000 mg/m^2 IV D1 and D8 q21d vs Pegylated liposomal doxorubicin 30–50 mg/m^2 IV D1 q28d[132]	195 (99 vs 96)	NR	6.1% vs 8.3%	NR
Pegylated liposomal doxorubicin 40 mg/m^2 IV D1 q28d +/− bevacizumab 10 mg/kg IV q2 weeks[133]	126	NR	7.8% vs 13.7% (with bevacizumab)	NR
Paclitaxel 80 mg/m^2 IV D1, D8, D15 q4 weeks +/− bevacizumab 10–15 mg/kg IV q2 weeks[134]	70	NR	48% vs 63% (with bevacizumab)	NR
Topotecan 2–4 mg/m^2 IV D1, D8, D15 q4 weeks +/− bevacizumab 10–15 mg/kg IV q3 weeks[133]	120	NR	0.0% vs 17.0% (with bevacizumab)	NR

NR, not reported.
*Suggested dose ranges.

to confer maximum survival benefit.[97] Following secondary cytoreduction, platinum-based chemotherapy, clinical trial, or supportive care may be considered.[50] Surgery for platinum resistant ovarian clear cell carcinoma is generally not recommended.

Radiation

There are no randomized trials available comparing radiation and chemotherapy in the treatment of recurrent ovarian clear cell carcinoma. The largest retrospective study comparing these two regimens included 47 women with recurrent disease. Treatment benefit was loosely defined as if "all disease resolved," there was "lesser degree of disease resolution," or there was "stable disease." While outcomes were not stratified by first, second, and third-line, among 105 treatment cycles, benefit was seen in 24% of patients receiving chemotherapy, 64% receiving radiation, and 100% of patients receiving both chemotherapy and radiation therapy.[98]

Applying treatments from similar tumors at other sites

Ovarian clear cell carcinoma shares features with renal clear cell carcinoma. Genomic studies have found several mutational similarities between the diseases, including alterations in the chromatin remodeling SWI-SNF and PIK3/AKT/mTOR pathways, and a shared hypoxia-like mRNA expression signature. Both ovarian clear cell carcinoma and renal clear cell carcinoma exhibit upregulation of angiogenesis pathways, and many currently approved anti-VEGF therapies for renal clear cell carcinoma are being studied in ovarian clear cell carcinoma.[99] NiCCC (ENGOT-GYN1), a randomized phase II study of nintedanib in recurrent clear cell carcinoma of the ovary or endometrium is currently recruiting.[100]

Potential therapeutic targets/molecular testing/mutations

Kuo et al. published on a series of 97 ovarian clear cell carcinoma that were sequenced for potentially actionable genetic alterations, including in *KRAS, BRAF, PIK3CA, TP53, PTEN,* and *CTNNB1*.[101] They reported a mutation rate of 33% in *PIK3CA* and only 15% in *TP53*, which is present in approximately 96% of high-grade serous ovarian cancers. A subsequent preclinical study of a dual PI3K/mTOR inhibitor led to G1 phase arrest and apoptosis in ovarian clear cell carcinoma cell lines as well as inhibition of tumor growth in mice.[102] Unfortunately, there has not yet been widespread translation of this work into the clinical setting. Table 4.6 presents mutation rates in clear cell and high-grade serous ovarian cancers from Memorial Sloan Kettering-Integrated Mutation Profiling of Actionable Cancer Targets (MSK-IMPACT), a hybridization capture-based next-generation panel that is capable of detecting all protein-coding mutations in 341 cancer-associated genes.[103–106]

PARP

The only landmark trial on poly(ADP-ribose) polymerase inhibitors (PARPi) that included clear cell histology was Study 10.[107] Only one ovarian clear cell carcinoma was included in the phase II study evaluating oral rucaparib in patients with platinum-sensitive ovarian cancer with a germline *BRCA1/2* mutation. The patient with ovarian clear cell carcinoma achieved a partial response. Investigators have associated *PTEN* mutations, and PI3K inhibition with homologous

TABLE 4.6 Gene mutation rates per MSK-IMPACT.

Gene	Mutation rate in ovarian cancers	
	Clear cell (*n* = 138)	High-grade serous (*n* = 1438)
PIK3CA	48.6%	4.9%
TP53	13.8%	94.2%
KRAS	13.0%	1.1%
PTEN	8.7%	0.9%
CTNNB1	5.8%	0.5%
BRAF	4.3%	0.9%

MSK-IMPACT, Memorial Sloan Kettering-Integrated Mutation Profiling of Actionable Cancer Targets.[103–106]

recombination deficiency (HRD), and possible susceptibility to PARPi.[108,109] Overall, data on PARPi efficacy are lacking and difficult to extrapolate to this clinical setting.

VEGF

Several trials have evaluated the role of VEGF inhibitors, including bevacizumab, sorafenib, sosunitinib, cabozantinib, and ENMD-2076, in newly diagnosed or persistent/recurrent ovarian clear cell carcinoma (Table 4.7). Unfortunately, reported response rates have been low. A subgroup analysis of newly diagnosed ovarian clear cell carcinoma receiving carboplatin/ paclitaxel alone versus carboplatin/ paclitaxel /bevacizumab as part of ICON7 demonstrated no improvement in OS (HR 1.09, 95% CI, 0.64–1.88).[110] An additional randomized phase II trial compared topotecan plus oral sorafenib versus topotecan with placebo in patients with platinum-resistant ovarian cancer. The trial included 172 total patients, 36 patients with nonserous histology, and reported a median PFS with sorafenib of 6.7 months versus 4.4 months with placebo (HR 0.60, 95% CI, 0.48–0.83).[111]

Phase II trials of sunitinib, cabozantinib, and ENMD-2076 have found minimal response in ovarian clear cell carcinoma in the recurrent setting. In GOG-254, a phase II trial of orally administered sunitinib, there was a response rate of 6.7% in patients with one or two prior lines of therapy.[112] NRG-GY001, a phase II study of single agent cabozantinib in persistent or recurrent ovarian clear cell carcinoma found minimal activity in the second- and third-line treatment of ovarian clear cell carcinoma.[113] Oral ENMD-2076 (a multitarget kinase selective against Aurora A and VEGF) in patients with recurrent ovarian clear cell carcinoma who received prior platinum-based chemotherapy had a 22% overall 6-month PFS, not meeting preset threshold for efficacy (40%).[114]

mTOR

GOG-268 evaluated temsirolimus (mTOR inhibitor) in combination with carboplatin/paclitaxel versus carboplatin/ paclitaxel alone in patients with newly diagnosed stage III or IV ovarian clear cell carcinoma as first-line therapy (Table 4.8). This trial reported no statistically significant increase in PFS compared with historical control.[115]

PD-L1

In a phase II study looking at nivolumab in 20 patients with advanced or relapsed, platinum-resistant ovarian cancer, only two patients had clear cell histology and only one exhibited a complete response.[116] The phase 1b JAVELIN Solid Tumor Trial examining avelumab in recurrent/refractory ovarian cancer included two patients with ovarian clear cell carcinoma, both of whom had a partial response.[117] Several trials incorporating PD-L1 inhibitors for treatment of persistent or recurrent ovarian clear cell carcinoma are ongoing.

TABLE 4.7 Clinical trials using molecular targeted therapies for treatment of recurrent or persistent ovarian clear cell carcinoma.

Study	ClinicalTrials.gov identifier	Study drug	Target	Trial phase	Outcomes		
					n	ORR	Median PFS (months)
GOG-254	NCT00979992	Sunitinib	PDGFRs and VEGFRs	II	667	6.7%	2.7
NRG-GY001	NCT02315430	Cabozantinib	MET, RET, VEGFR2, and AXL	II	13	0%	3.6
ENMD-2076-OCC	NCT01914510	ENMD-2076	AURKA, VEGFRs, FGFRs, Flt3, and c-kit	II	40	5%	3.7

AURKA, aurora kinase A; *FGFR*, fibroblast growth factor receptor; *Flt3*, FMS-like tyrosine kinase; *MET*, MET proto-oncogene, receptor tyrosine kinase; *ORR*, overall response rate; *PDGFR*, platelet-derived growth factor receptor; *PFS*, progression-free survival; *RET*, RET proto-oncogene, receptor tyrosine kinase; *VEGFR*, vascular endothelial growth factor receptor.

TABLE 4.8 Clinical trials using molecular targeted therapies for newly diagnosed ovarian clear cell carcinoma.

Study	ClinicalTrials.gov identifier	Regimen	Target	Phase	n	Outcome
ICON7	NCT00483782	Carboplatin, paclitaxel and bevacizumab vs standard therapy	VEGFRs	III	82 vs 77	OS HR: 0.99 (95% CI, 0.85–1.14) PFS HR: 0.93 (95% CI, 0.83–1.05)
GOG-268	NCT01196429	Paclitaxel, carboplatin, and temsirolimus ➔ temsirolimus maintenance	mTOR	II	90	No statistically significant increase in PFS vs historical controls

HR, hazard ratio; *mTOR*, mammalian target of rapamycin; *OS*, overall survival; *PFS*, progression-free survival; *VEGFR*, vascular endothelial growth factor receptor.

Mismatch repair protein deficiency/microsatellite instability

Data are limited on the prevalence of MMR deficiency and microsatellite instability (MSI) in patients with ovarian clear cell carcinoma; however, it is well known that ovarian cancer patients with Lynch Syndrome have a disproportionate likelihood of having nonserous histologies, including mixed types (33%), endometrioid (25%), and clear cell (12%).[118] One of the largest studies on MSI in 42 ovarian clear cell carcinoma tumors demonstrated a 14.3% rate of MSI-high disease.[119] Another study of 30 ovarian clear cell carcinoma tumors reported 10% with MMR protein expression loss and MSI-high tumors.[120] Other studies have demonstrated lower rates of deficient MMR: a study that included 33 women with ovarian clear cell carcinoma found that only 3.0% of patients had MMR loss of expression on IHC.

In patients with MSI-high, mismatch repair deficient (MMR-D), or high tumor mutational burden solid tumors with progression following prior treatment, disease-agnostic immunotherapies, such as PD-L1 inhibitors, may be considered. Isolated case reports have reported responses to avelumab in heavily pretreated ovarian clear cell carcinoma.[121] Further, studies of MSI-high ovarian clear cell carcinoma demonstrate high rates of CD3+ and CD8+ tumor-infiltrating lymphocytes (TILs), suggesting a potential therapeutic benefit of PD-L1 inhibitors in these patients.[120]

ER/PR

A multiinstitutional study of 155 cases of ovarian clear cell carcinoma demonstrated ER or PR positivity in only 5 of 137 cases (3.6%) with available IHC.[122] It is postulated that there are low rates of ER positivity in ovarian clear cell carcinoma because loss of ER expression is required for ovarian clear cell carcinoma lesion progression from endometriosis.[123] Due to the relative rarity of ER positivity in ovarian clear cell carcinoma, the role of hormonal blockade in the rare cases of ER+ ovarian clear cell carcinoma is unknown. Hormonal blockade is emerging as a treatment strategy for endometrioid ovarian cancers or renal clear cell carcinomas, which have much higher rates of ER positivity.[124,125]

Case resolution

The patient received six cycles of adjuvant carboplatin and paclitaxel. Twenty-seven months after completing chemotherapy, she was diagnosed with an isolated recurrence in a right inguinal lymph node. At the time of her recurrence, CA-125 was 12 U/mL. She underwent excision of the enlarged node, and pathology was consistent with metastatic clear cell carcinoma. Following surgery, she received 5040 cGy radiotherapy to the right groin with cisplatin sensitization. Ten months after her first recurrence, an abdominal wall mass biopsy showed recurrent clear cell carcinoma. The abdominal wall mass was resected and she was started on letrozole. She is now 36 months out from her tertiary cytoreduction and is currently being monitored with CT scans every 6 months. Her most recent imaging demonstrated no evidence of disease.

References

1. Siegel RL, Miller KD, Fuchs HE, Jemal A. Cancer statistics, 2021. *CA Cancer J Clin.* 2021;71(1):7–33.
2. Siegel RL, Miller KD, Jemal A. Cancer statistics, 2020. *CA Cancer J Clin.* 2020;70(1):7–30.
3. Banks E. *The Epidemiology of Ovarian Cancer. Ovarian Cancer.* Humana Press; 2001:3–11.

4. Iida Y, Okamoto A, Hollis RL, Gourley C, Herrington CS. Clear cell carcinoma of the ovary: a clinical and molecular perspective. *Int J Gynecol Cancer.* 2020. https://doi.org/10.1136/ijgc-2020-001656.

5. Torre LA, Trabert B, Desantis CE, et al. Ovarian cancer statistics, 2018. *CA Cancer J Clin.* 2018;68(4):284–296.

6. Fuh KC, Java JJ, Chan JK, et al. Differences in presentation and survival of Asians compared to Caucasians with ovarian cancer: an NRG oncology/ GOG ancillary study of 7914 patients. *Gynecol Oncol.* 2019;154(2):420–425.

7. Chan JK, Teoh D, Hu JM, Shin JY, Osann K, Kapp DS. Do clear cell ovarian carcinomas have poorer prognosis compared to other epithelial cell types? A study of 1411 clear cell ovarian cancers. *Gynecol Oncol.* 2008;109(3):370–376.

8. del Carmen MG, Birrer M, Schorge JO. Clear cell carcinoma of the ovary: a review of the literature. *Gynecol Oncol.* 2012;126(3):481–490.

9. Hermens M, Van Altena AM, Nieboer TE, et al. Incidence of endometrioid and clear-cell ovarian cancer in histological proven endometriosis: the ENOCA population-based cohort study. *Am J Obstet Gynecol.* 2020;223(1). 107.e1–.e11.

10. Pearce CL, Templeman C, Rossing MA, et al. Association between endometriosis and risk of histological subtypes of ovarian cancer: a pooled analysis of case-control studies. *Lancet Oncol.* 2012;13(4):385–394.

11. Stamp JP, Gilks CB, Wesseling M, et al. BAF250a expression in atypical endometriosis and endometriosis-associated ovarian Cancer. *Int J Gynecol Cancer.* 2016;26(5):825.

12. Hankinson SE. Tubal ligation, hysterectomy, and risk of ovarian cancer. *J Am Med Assoc.* 1993;270(23):2813.

13. Wentzensen N, Poole EM, Trabert B, et al. Ovarian cancer risk factors by histologic subtype: an analysis from the ovarian cancer cohort consortium. *J Clin Oncol.* 2016;34(24):2888–2898.

14. Vercellini P, Somigliana E, Buggio L, Bolis G, Fedele L. Endometriosis and ovarian cancer. *Lancet Oncol.* 2012;13(5). e188–e9.

15. Wiegand KC, Shah SP, Al-Agha OM, et al. ARID1A mutations in endometriosis-associated ovarian carcinomas. *N Engl J Med.* 2010;363 (16):1532–1543.

16. Schildkraut JM, Moorman PG, Halabi S, Calingaert B, Marks JR, Berchuck A. Analgesic drug use and risk of ovarian Cancer. *Epidemiology.* 2006; 17(1):104–107.

17. Candido-Dos-Reis FJ, Song H, Goode EL, et al. Germline mutation in BRCA1 or BRCA2 and ten-year survival for women diagnosed with epithelial ovarian cancer. *Clin Cancer Res.* 2015;21(3):652–657.

18. Ketabi Z, Bartuma K, Bernstein I, et al. Ovarian cancer linked to lynch syndrome typically presents as early-onset, non-serous epithelial tumors. *Gynecol Oncol.* 2011;121(3):462–465.

19. Kobel M, Bennett JA, Cheung AN, et al. Clear cell carcinoma of the ovary. In: WHO Classification of Tumors Editorial Board, ed. *Female Genital Tumors.* World Health Organization Classification of Tumors. *Lyon: IARC Press.* 2020;65–67.

20. Han G, Gilks CB, Leung S, et al. Mixed ovarian epithelial carcinomas with clear cell and serous components are variants of high-grade serous carcinoma: an interobserver correlative and immunohistochemical study of 32 cases. *Am J Surg Pathol.* 2008;32(7):955–964.

21. Fadare O, Zhao C, Khabele D, et al. Comparative analysis of Napsin A, alpha-methylacyl-coenzyme A racemase (AMACR, P504S), and hepatocyte nuclear factor 1 beta as diagnostic markers of ovarian clear cell carcinoma: an immunohistochemical study of 279 ovarian tumours. *Pathology.* 2015;47(2):105–111.

22. Mabuchi S, Sugiyama T, Kimura T. Clear cell carcinoma of the ovary: molecular insights and future therapeutic perspectives. *J Gynecol Oncol.* 2016;27(3): e31.

23. Jones S, Wang TL, Shih IM, et al. Frequent mutations of chromatin remodeling gene ARID1A in ovarian clear cell carcinoma. *Science.* 2010;330 (6001):228–231.

24. Yamamoto S, Tsuda H, Takano M, et al. Loss of ARID1A protein expression occurs as an early event in ovarian clear-cell carcinoma development and frequently coexists with PIK3CA mutations. *Mod Pathol.* 2012;25(4):615–624.

25. Kurman RJ, Hedrick Ellenson L, Ronnett BM. *Blaustein's Pathology of the Female Genital Tract.* Cham: Springer International Publishing AG; 2019.

26. Goff BA, Mandel LS, Drescher CW, et al. Development of an ovarian cancer symptom index. *Cancer.* 2007;109(2):221–227.

27. Matsuura Y, Robertson G, Marsden DE, Kim S-N, Gebski V, Hacker NF. Thromboembolic complications in patients with clear cell carcinoma of the ovary. *Gynecol Oncol.* 2007;104(2):406–410.

28. Duska LR, Garrett L, Henretta M, Ferriss JS, Lee L, Horowitz N. When 'never-events' occur despite adherence to clinical guidelines: the case of venous thromboembolism in clear cell cancer of the ovary compared with other epithelial histologic subtypes. *Gynecol Oncol.* 2010;116 (3):374–377.

29. Uno K, Homma S, Satoh T, et al. Tissue factor expression as a possible determinant of thromboembolism in ovarian cancer. *Br J Cancer.* 2007; 96(2):290–295.

30. Sugiyama T, Kamura T, Kigawa J, et al. Clinical characteristics of clear cell carcinoma of the ovary. *Cancer.* 2000;88(11):2584–2589.

31. Lim AWW, Mesher D, Gentry-Maharaj A, et al. Predictive value of symptoms for ovarian Cancer: comparison of symptoms reported by questionnaire, interview, and general practitioner notes. *J Natl Cancer Inst.* 2012;104(2):114–124.

32. Pavlik EJ, Saunders BA, Doran S, et al. The search for meaning-symptoms and transvaginal sonography screening for ovarian cancer. *Cancer.* 2009;115(16):3689–3698.

33. Committee Opinion No. 716. The role of the obstetrician-gynecologist in the early detection of epithelial ovarian Cancer in women at average risk. *Obstet Gynecol.* 2017;130(3). e146–e9.

34. Bai H, Sha G, Xiao M, et al. The prognostic value of pretreatment CA-125 levels and CA-125 normalization in ovarian clear cell carcinoma: a two-academic-institute study. *Oncotarget.* 2016;7(13):15566–15576.

35. Tian C, Markman M, Zaino R, et al. CA-125 change after chemotherapy in prediction of treatment outcome among advanced mucinous and clear cell epithelial ovarian cancers: a gynecologic oncology group study. *Cancer.* 2009;115(7):1395–1403.

36. Morales-Vásquez F, Pedernera E, Reynaga-Obregón J, et al. High levels of pretreatment CA125 are associated to improved survival in high grade serous ovarian carcinoma. *J Ovarian Res.* 2016;9(1).

37. Jung SE, Lee JM, Rha SE, Byun JY, Jung JI, Hahn ST. CT and MR imaging of ovarian tumors with emphasis on differential diagnosis. *Radiographics.* 2002;22(6):1305–1325.

38. Choi HJ, Lee JH, Seok Lee J, et al. CT findings of clear cell carcinoma of the ovary. *J Comput Assist Tomogr.* 2006;30(6):875–879.

39. Shu CA, Zhou Q, Jotwani AR, et al. Ovarian clear cell carcinoma, outcomes by stage: the MSK experience. *Gynecol Oncol.* 2015;139(2):236–241.

40. Mueller JJ, Holzapfel M, Han CH, et al. Staging lymphadenectomy in patients with clear cell carcinoma of the ovary. *Int J Gynecol Cancer.* 2016;26(1):120–124.

41. Takano M, Tsuda H, Sugiyama T. Clear cell carcinoma of the ovary: is there a role of histology-specific treatment? *J Exp Clin Cancer Res.* 2012;31 (1):53.

42. Oliver KE, Brady WE, Birrer M, et al. An evaluation of progression free survival and overall survival of ovarian cancer patients with clear cell carcinoma versus serous carcinoma treated with platinum therapy: an NRG oncology/gynecologic oncology group experience. *Gynecol Oncol.* 2017;147(2):243–249.

43. Kajiyama H, Shibata K, Mizuno M, et al. Postrecurrent oncologic outcome of patients with ovarian clear cell carcinoma. *Int J Gynecol Cancer.* 2012;22(5):801–806.

44. Lee Y-Y, Kim T-J, Kim M-J, et al. Prognosis of ovarian clear cell carcinoma compared to other histological subtypes: a meta-analysis. *Gynecol Oncol.* 2011;122(3):541–547.

45. Liu H, Xu Y, Ji J, Dong R, Qiu H, Dai X. Prognosis of ovarian clear cell cancer compared with other epithelial cancer types: A population-based analysis. *Oncol Lett.* 2020;19(3):1947–1957.

46. Lee HY, Hong JH, Byun JH, et al. Clinical characteristics of clear cell ovarian cancer: a retrospective multicenter experience of 308 patients in South Korea. *Cancer Res Treat.* 2020;52(1):277–283.

47. Kajiyama H, Suzuki S, Yoshikawa N, Tamauchi S, Shibata K, Kikkawa F. The impact of systematic retroperitoneal lymphadenectomy on long-term oncologic outcome of women with advanced ovarian clear-cell carcinoma. *J Gynecol Oncol.* 2020;31(4), e47.

48. Suzuki S, Kajiyama H, Shibata K, et al. Is there any association between retroperitoneal lymphadenectomy and survival benefit in ovarian clear cell carcinoma patients? *Ann Oncol.* 2008;19(7):1284–1287.

49. Magazzino F, Katsaros D, Ottaiano A, et al. Surgical and medical treatment of clear cell ovarian cancer: results from the multicenter Italian trials in ovarian cancer (MITO) 9 retrospective study. *Int J Gynecol Cancer.* 2011;21(6):1063–1070.

50. Armstrong DK, Alvarez RD, Bakkum-Gamez JN, et al. NCCN guidelines insights: ovarian cancer, version 1.2019. *J Natl Compr Canc Netw.* 2019;17(8):896–909.

51. Chi DS, Abu-Rustum NR, Sonoda Y, et al. The safety and efficacy of laparoscopic surgical staging of apparent stage I ovarian and fallopian tube cancers. *Am J Obstet Gynecol.* 2005;192(5):1614–1619.

52. Bogani G, Borghi C, Leone Roberti Maggiore U, et al. Minimally invasive surgical staging in early-stage ovarian carcinoma: a systematic review and meta-analysis. *J Minim Invasive Gynecol.* 2017;24(4):552–562.

53. Melamed A, Keating NL, Clemmer JT, et al. Laparoscopic staging for apparent stage I epithelial ovarian cancer. *Am J Obstet Gynecol.* 2017;216(1). 50 e1–e12.

54. Matsuo K, Huang Y, Matsuzaki S, et al. Minimally invasive surgery and risk of capsule rupture for women with early-stage ovarian Cancer. *JAMA Oncol.* 2020;6(7):1110–1113.

55. Nasioudis D, Mulugeta-Gordon L, McMinn E, Frey MK, Chapman-Davis E, Holcomb K. Fertility sparing surgery for patients with FIGO stage I clear cell ovarian carcinoma: a database analysis and systematic review of the literature. *Int J Gynecol Cancer.* 2020;30(9):1372–1377.

56. Melamed A, Manning-Geist B, Bregar AJ, et al. Associations between residual disease and survival in epithelial ovarian cancer by histologic type. *Gynecol Oncol.* 2017;147(2):250–256.

57. Vergote I, Trope CG, Amant F, et al. Neoadjuvant chemotherapy or primary surgery in stage IIIC or IV ovarian cancer. *N Engl J Med.* 2010;363(10):943–953.

58. Calvert AH, Newell DR, Gumbrell LA, et al. Carboplatin dosage: prospective evaluation of a simple formula based on renal function. *J Clin Oncol.* 1989;7(11):1748–1756.

59. Utsunomiya H, Akahira J, Tanno S, et al. Paclitaxel-platinum combination chemotherapy for advanced or recurrent ovarian clear cell adenocarcinoma: a multicenter trial. *Int J Gynecol Cancer.* 2006;16(1):52–56.

60. Trimbos JB, Vergote I, Bolis G, et al. Impact of adjuvant chemotherapy and surgical staging in early-stage ovarian carcinoma: European Organisation for Research and Treatment of Cancer-adjuvant ChemoTherapy in ovarian neoplasm trial. *J Natl Cancer Inst.* 2003;95(2):113–125.

61. Colombo N, Guthrie D, Chiari S, et al. International collaborative ovarian neoplasm trial 1: a randomized trial of adjuvant chemotherapy in women with early-stage ovarian cancer. *J Natl Cancer Inst.* 2003;95(2):125–132.

62. Collinson F, Qian W, Fossati R, et al. Optimal treatment of early-stage ovarian cancer. *Ann Oncol.* 2014;25(6):1165–1171.

63. Oseledchyk A, Leitao Jr MM, Konner J, et al. Adjuvant chemotherapy in patients with stage I endometrioid or clear cell ovarian cancer in the platinum era: a surveillance, epidemiology, and end results cohort study, 2000-2013. *Ann Oncol.* 2017;28(12):2985–2993.

64. Higashi M, Kajiyama H, Shibata K, et al. Survival impact of capsule rupture in stage I clear cell carcinoma of the ovary in comparison with other histological types. *Gynecol Oncol.* 2011;123(3):474–478.

65. Kajiyama H, Mizuno M, Shibata K, et al. A recurrence-predicting prognostic factor for patients with ovarian clear-cell adenocarcinoma at reproductive age. *Int J Clin Oncol.* 2014;19(5):921–927.

66. Mizuno M, Kajiyama H, Shibata K, et al. Adjuvant chemotherapy for stage i ovarian clear cell carcinoma: is it necessary for stage IA? *Int J Gynecol Cancer.* 2012;22(7):1143–1149.

67. Hoskins PJ, Lc N, Gilks B, et al. Low-stage ovarian clear cell carcinoma: population-based outcomes in British Columbia, Canada, with evidence for a survival benefit as a result of irradiation. *J Clin Oncol.* 2012;30(14):1656–1662.

68. Bell J, Brady MF, Young RC, et al. Randomized phase III trial of three versus six cycles of adjuvant carboplatin and paclitaxel in early stage epithelial ovarian carcinoma: a gynecologic oncology group study. *Gynecol Oncol.* 2006;102(3):432–439.

69. Chan JK, Tian C, Fleming GF, et al. The potential benefit of 6 vs. 3 cycles of chemotherapy in subsets of women with early-stage high-risk epithelial ovarian cancer: an exploratory analysis of a gynecologic oncology group study. *Gynecol Oncol.* 2010;116(3):301–306.

70. Prendergast EN, Holzapfel M, Mueller JJ, et al. Three versus six cycles of adjuvant platinum-based chemotherapy in early stage clear cell ovarian carcinoma - a multi-institutional cohort. *Gynecol Oncol.* 2017;144(2):274–278.

71. Roy S, Hoskins P, Tinker A, Brar H, Bowering G, Bahl G. Adjuvant treatment of early ovarian clear cell carcinoma: a population-based study of whole abdominal versus pelvic nodal radiotherapy. *J Natl Compr Canc Netw.* 2020;1–9.

72. Nagai Y, Inamine M, Hirakawa M, et al. Postoperative whole abdominal radiotherapy in clear cell adenocarcinoma of the ovary. *Gynecol Oncol.* 2007;107(3):469–473.

73. Dinniwell R, Lock M, Pintilie M, et al. Consolidative abdominopelvic radiotherapy after surgery and carboplatin/paclitaxel chemotherapy for epithelial ovarian cancer. *Int J Radiat Oncol Biol Phys.* 2005;62(1):104–110.

74. Hogen L, Thomas G, Bernardini M, et al. The effect of adjuvant radiation on survival in early stage clear cell ovarian carcinoma. *Gynecol Oncol.* 2016;143(2):258–263.

75. Eskenazi B, Warner ML. Epidemiology of endometriosis. *Obstet Gynecol Clin North Am.* 1997;24(2):235–258.

76. Matias-Guiu X, Stewart CJR. Endometriosis-associated ovarian neoplasia. *Pathology.* 2018;50(2):190–204.

77. Stern RC, Dash R, Bentley RC, Snyder MJ, Haney AF, Robboy SJ. Malignancy in endometriosis: frequency and comparison of ovarian and extra-ovarian types. *Int J Gynecol Pathol.* 2001;20(2):133–139.

78. Grandi G, Toss A, Cortesi L, Botticelli L, Volpe A, Cagnacci A. The association between endometriomas and ovarian cancer: preventive effect of inhibiting ovulation and menstruation during reproductive life. *Biomed Res Int.* 2015;2015:751571.

79. Sato N, Tsunoda H, Nishida M, et al. Loss of heterozygosity on 10q23.3 and mutation of the tumor suppressor gene PTEN in benign endometrial cyst of the ovary: possible sequence progression from benign endometrial cyst to endometrioid carcinoma and clear cell carcinoma of the ovary. *Cancer Res.* 2000;60(24):7052–7056.

80. Anglesio MS, Papadopoulos N, Ayhan A, et al. Cancer-associated mutations in endometriosis without cancer. *New Engl J Med.* 2017;376(19):1835–1848.

81. Behbakht K, Randall TC, Benjamin I, Morgan MA, King S, Rubin SC. Clinical characteristics of clear cell carcinoma of the ovary. *Gynecol Oncol.* 1998;70(2):255–258.

82. Zhao T, Lu Y. Endometriosis does not confer improved prognosis in ovarian clear cell carcinoma. *Bjog-Int J Obstet Gy.* 2018;125:15–16.

83. Kim HS, Kim TH, Chung HH, Song YS. Risk and prognosis of ovarian cancer in women with endometriosis: a meta-analysis. *Br J Cancer.* 2014;110(7):1878–1890.

84. Orezzoli JP, Russell AH, Oliva E, Del Carmen MG, Eichhorn J, Fuller AF. Prognostic implication of endometriosis in clear cell carcinoma of the ovary. *Gynecol Oncol.* 2008;110(3):336–344.

85. Kim HS, Kim MA, Lee M, et al. Effect of endometriosis on the prognosis of ovarian clear cell carcinoma: a two-center cohort study and Meta-analysis. *Ann Surg Oncol.* 2015;22(8):2738–2745.

86. Komiyama S, Aoki D, Tominaga E, Susumu N, Udagawa Y, Nozawa S. Prognosis of Japanese patients with ovarian clear cell carcinoma associated with pelvic endometriosis: clinicopathologic evaluation. *Gynecol Oncol.* 1999;72(3):342–346.

87. Cuff J, Longacre TA. Endometriosis does not confer improved prognosis in ovarian carcinoma of uniform cell type. *Am J Surg Pathol.* 2012;36(5):688–695.

88. Schnack TH, Hogdall E, Thomsen LN, Hogdall C. Demographic, clinical, and prognostic factors of ovarian clear cell adenocarcinomas according to endometriosis status. *Int J Gynecol Cancer.* 2017;27(9):1804–1812.

89. Bai H, Cao D, Yuan F, et al. Prognostic value of endometriosis in patients with stage I ovarian clear cell carcinoma: experiences at three academic institutions. *Gynecol Oncol.* 2016;143(3):526–531.

90. Ye S, Yang J, You Y, et al. Comparative study of ovarian clear cell carcinoma with and without endometriosis in People's Republic of China. *Fertil Steril.* 2014;102(6):1656–1662.

91. Geurts SM, van Altena AM, de Vegt F, et al. No supportive evidence for clinical benefit of routine follow-up in ovarian cancer: a Dutch multicenter study. *Int J Gynecol Cancer.* 2011;21(4):647–653.

92. Clarke T, Galaal K, Bryant A, Naik R. Evaluation of follow-up strategies for patients with epithelial ovarian cancer following completion of primary treatment. *Cochrane Database Syst Rev.* 2014;9, CD006119.

93. Colombo N, Sessa C, Bois AD, et al. ESMO-ESGO consensus conference recommendations on ovarian cancer: pathology and molecular biology, early and advanced stages, borderline tumours and recurrent disease. *Int J Gynecol Cancer.* 2019;29(4):728–760.

94. Salani R, Khanna N, Frimer M, Bristow RE, Chen LM. An update on post-treatment surveillance and diagnosis of recurrence in women with gynecologic malignancies: Society of Gynecologic Oncology (SGO) recommendations. *Gynecol Oncol.* 2017;146(1):3–10.

95. Macrie BD, Strauss JB, Helenowski IB, et al. Patterns of recurrence and role of pelvic radiotherapy in ovarian clear cell adenocarcinoma. *Int J Gynecol Cancer.* 2014;24(9):1597–1602.

96. Hogen L, Vicus D, Ferguson SE, et al. Patterns of recurrence and impact on survival in patients with clear cell ovarian carcinoma. *Int J Gynecol Cancer.* 2019;29(7):1164–1169.

97. Kajiyama H, Suzuki S, Yoshikawa N, et al. Oncologic outcomes after secondary surgery in recurrent clear-cell carcinoma of the ovary. *Int J Gynecol Cancer.* 2019;29(5):910–915.

98. Al-Barrak J, Santos JL, Tinker A, et al. Exploring palliative treatment outcomes in women with advanced or recurrent ovarian clear cell carcinoma. *Gynecol Oncol.* 2011;122(1):107–110.

99. Ji JX, Wang YK, Cochrane DR, Huntsman DG. Clear cell carcinomas of the ovary and kidney: clarity through genomics. *J Pathol.* 2018;244 (5):550–564.

100. Glasspool RM, McNeish IA, Paul J, et al. NiCCC (ENGOT-GYN1): A randomized phase II study of nintedanib (BIBF1120) compared to chemotherapy in patients with recurrent clear-cell carcinoma of the ovary or endometrium. *J Clin Oncol.* 2016;34(15_suppl). TPS5603-TPS.

101. Kuo KT, Mao TL, Jones S, et al. Frequent activating mutations of PIK3CA in ovarian clear cell carcinoma. *Am J Pathol.* 2009;174 (5):1597–1601.

102. Oishi T, Itamochi H, Kudoh A, et al. The PI3K/mTOR dual inhibitor NVP-BEZ235 reduces the growth of ovarian clear cell carcinoma. *Oncol Rep.* 2014;32(2):553–558.

103. Zehir A, Benayed R, Shah RH, et al. Mutational landscape of metastatic cancer revealed from prospective clinical sequencing of 10,000 patients. *Nat Med.* 2017;23(6):703–713.

104. Cerami E, Gao J, Dogrusoz U, et al. The cBio Cancer genomics portal: an open platform for exploring multidimensional Cancer genomics data: figure 1. *Cancer Discov.* 2012;2(5):401–404.

105. Cheng DT, Mitchell TN, Zehir A, et al. Memorial Sloan Kettering-integrated mutation profiling of actionable Cancer targets (MSK-IMPACT). *J Mol Diagn.* 2015;17(3):251–264.

106. Gao J, Aksoy BA, Dogrusoz U, et al. Integrative analysis of complex cancer genomics and clinical profiles using the cBioPortal. *Sci Signal.* 2013;6(269). pl1–pl.

107. Kristeleit R, Shapiro GI, Burris HA, et al. A phase I-II study of the Oral PARP inhibitor Rucaparib in patients with germline BRCA1/2-mutated ovarian carcinoma or other solid tumors. *Clin Cancer Res.* 2017;23(15):4095–4106.

108. Ibrahim YH, García-García C, Serra V, et al. PI3K inhibition impairs BRCA1/2 expression and sensitizes BRCA-proficient triple-negative breast Cancer to PARP inhibition. *Cancer Discov.* 2012;2(11):1036–1047.

109. Saal LH, Gruvberger-Saal SK, Persson C, et al. Recurrent gross mutations of the PTEN tumor suppressor gene in breast cancers with deficient DSB repair. *Nat Genet.* 2008;40(1):102–107.

110. Oza AM, Cook AD, Pfisterer J, et al. Standard chemotherapy with or without bevacizumab for women with newly diagnosed ovarian cancer (ICON7): overall survival results of a phase 3 randomised trial. *Lancet Oncol.* 2015;16(8):928–936.

111. Chekerov R, Hilpert F, Mahner S, et al. Sorafenib plus topotecan versus placebo plus topotecan for platinum-resistant ovarian cancer (TRIAS): a multicentre, randomised, double-blind, placebo-controlled, phase 2 trial. *Lancet Oncol.* 2018;19(9):1247–1258.

112. Chan JK, Brady W, Monk BJ, et al. A phase II evaluation of sunitinib in the treatment of persistent or recurrent clear cell ovarian cancer: an NRG oncology/gynecologic oncology group study (GOG-254). *Gynecol Oncol.* 2018;150(2):247–252.

113. Konstantinopoulos PA, Brady WE, Farley J, Armstrong A, Uyar DS, Gershenson DM. Phase II study of single-agent cabozantinib in patients with recurrent clear cell ovarian, primary peritoneal or fallopian tube cancer (NRG-GY001). *Gynecol Oncol.* 2018;150(1):9–13.

114. Lheureux S, Tinker AV, Clarke BA, et al. A clinical and molecular Phase II trial of oral ENMD-2076 in ovarian clear cell carcinoma (OCCC): A study of the Princess Margaret Phase II Consortium. *Clin Cancer Res.* 2018. clincanres.1244.

115. Farley JH, Brady WE, Fujiwara K, et al. A phase II evaluation of temsirolimus in combination with carboplatin and paclitaxel followed by temsirolimus consolidation as first-line therapy in the treatment of stage III–IV clear cell carcinoma of the ovary. *J Clin Oncol.* 2016;34 (15_suppl):5531.

116. Hamanishi J, Mandai M, Ikeda T, et al. Safety and antitumor activity of anti–PD-1 antibody, Nivolumab, in patients with platinum-resistant ovarian Cancer. *J Clin Oncol.* 2015;33(34):4015–4022.

117. Disis ML, Taylor MH, Kelly K, et al. Efficacy and safety of avelumab for patients with recurrent or refractory ovarian Cancer. *JAMA Oncol.* 2019; 5(3):393.

118. Helder-Woolderink JM, Blok EA, Vasen HF, Hollema H, Mourits MJ, De Bock GH. Ovarian cancer in lynch syndrome; a systematic review. *Eur J Cancer.* 2016;55:65–73.

119. Cai KQ, Albarracin C, Rosen D, et al. Microsatellite instability and alteration of the expression of hMLH1 and hMSH2 in ovarian clear cell carcinoma. *Hum Pathol.* 2004;35(5):552–559.

120. Howitt BE, Strickland KC, Sholl LM, et al. Clear cell ovarian cancers with microsatellite instability: a unique subset of ovarian cancers with increased tumor-infiltrating lymphocytes and PD-1/PD-L1 expression. *Onco Targets Ther.* 2017;6(2), e1277308.

121. Hamanishi J, Mandai M, Ikeda T, et al. Safety and antitumor activity of anti-PD-1 antibody, Nivolumab, in patients with platinum-resistant ovarian Cancer. *J Clin Oncol.* 2015;33(34):4015–4022.

122. DeLair D, Oliva E, Kobel M, Macias A, Gilks CB, Soslow RA. Morphologic spectrum of immunohistochemically characterized clear cell carcinoma of the ovary: a study of 155 cases. *Am J Surg Pathol.* 2011;35(1):36–44.

123. Soslow RA. Histologic subtypes of ovarian carcinoma: an overview. *Int J Gynecol Pathol.* 2008;27(2):161–174.

124. Czarnecka AM, Niedzwiedzka M, Porta C, Szczylik C. Hormone signaling pathways as treatment targets in renal cell cancer (review). *Int J Oncol.* 2016;48(6):2221–2235.

125. Rambau P, Kelemen LE, Steed H, Quan ML, Ghatage P, Kobel M. Association of hormone receptor expression with survival in ovarian endometrioid carcinoma: biological validation and clinical implications. *Int J Mol Sci.* 2017;18(3).

126. Pfisterer J, Shannon CM, Baumann K, et al. Bevacizumab and platinum-based combinations for recurrent ovarian cancer: a randomised, open-label, phase 3 trial. *Lancet Oncol.* 2020;21(5):699–709.

127. Parmar MK, Ledermann JA, Colombo N, et al. Paclitaxel plus platinum-based chemotherapy versus conventional platinum-based chemotherapy in women with relapsed ovarian cancer: the ICON4/AGO-OVAR-2.2 trial. *Lancet.* 2003;361(9375):2099–2106.

128. Kose MF, Sufliarsky J, Beslija S, et al. A phase II study of gemcitabine plus carboplatin in platinum-sensitive, recurrent ovarian carcinoma. *Gynecol Oncol.* 2005;96(2):374–380.

129. Barber EL, Zsiros E, Lurain JR, Rademaker A, Schink JC, Neubauer NL. The combination of intravenous bevacizumab and metronomic oral cyclophosphamide is an effective regimen for platinum-resistant recurrent ovarian cancer. *J Gynecol Oncol.* 2013;24(3):258–264.

130. Rose PG, Blessing JA, Ball HG, et al. A phase II study of docetaxel in paclitaxel-resistant ovarian and peritoneal carcinoma: a gynecologic oncology group study. *Gynecol Oncol.* 2003;88(2):130–135.

131. Rose PG, Blessing JA, Soper JT, Barter JF. Prolonged oral etoposide in recurrent or advanced leiomyosarcoma of the uterus: a gynecologic oncology group study. *Gynecol Oncol.* 1998;70(2):267–271.

132. Mutch DG, Orlando M, Goss T, et al. Randomized phase III trial of gemcitabine compared with pegylated liposomal doxorubicin in patients with platinum-resistant ovarian cancer. *J Clin Oncol.* 2007;25(19):2811–2818.

133. Poveda AM, Selle F, Hilpert F, et al. Bevacizumab combined with weekly paclitaxel, Pegylated liposomal doxorubicin, or Topotecan in platinum-resistant recurrent ovarian Cancer: analysis by chemotherapy cohort of the randomized phase III AURELIA trial. *J Clin Oncol.* 2015;33(32): 3836–3838.

134. O'Malley DM, Richardson DL, Rheaume PS, et al. Addition of bevacizumab to weekly paclitaxel significantly improves progression-free survival in heavily pretreated recurrent epithelial ovarian cancer. *Gynecol Oncol.* 2011;121(2):269–272.

Chapter 5

Mucinous ovarian carcinomas

Sarah H. Kim, Roisin E. O'Cearbhaill, Preetha Ramalingam, and Jennifer J. Mueller

Clinical case

A 34-year-old female presents with worsening abdominal distension. She is found to have a 22 cm solid and cystic pelvic mass likely arising from the right ovary on MRI, and no evidence of metastatic disease (Fig. 5.1). CA-125 is within normal range for a premenopausal female at 36 (ULN 46 U/mL), hCG and prolactin levels are normal, and CEA is elevated to 15 (ULN 5 ng/mL). The patient undergoes surgical removal of the mass, right tube and ovary via laparotomy. The mass is removed intact with no evidence of intraoperative rupture. On histopathological evaluation, the tumor is determined to be a primary mucinous ovarian carcinoma with expansile-type pattern of invasion. She desires fertility preservation.

How do you approach the management of this patient?

Epidemiology

Incidence/mortality

Mucinous carcinomas of the ovary are a rare subtype of epithelial ovarian carcinomas, accounting for less than 3% of all epithelial ovarian cancers (Table 5.1).[1–4] Historical studies cite the frequency of primary mucinous ovarian carcinoma ranging from 6% to 25%; however, after excluding tumors of low malignant potential or borderline tumors, and metastatic tumors to the ovary, largely from the GI tract, the true incidence of these tumors is much lower.[5] Therefore, out of the 21,750 new cases of ovarian cancer estimated to be diagnosed in the United States, approximately 650 of these cases will be mucinous ovarian carcinomas.[6] The rarity of these tumors is reflected in the low percentage of primary mucinous ovarian carcinomas represented in clinical trials. In fact, mucinous ovarian carcinomas represented 2–4% of enrolled patients in landmark GOG trials that helped establish current platinum-based treatment paradigms in epithelial ovarian cancer.[7–9]

Over 80% of mucinous ovarian carcinomas are diagnosed at an early stage, with disease confined to the ovary. The clinical presentation will typically be a young woman reporting pelvic pain or discomfort in the setting of a large (10–15 cm) unilateral ovarian mass.[10,11] This contrasts with patients who are diagnosed with the more common type of epithelial ovarian cancer, high-grade serous ovarian carcinoma, which tends to present with advanced-stage disease due to the later onset of symptoms.[4,12] Another feature distinguishing mucinous tumors from the high-grade serous subtype is that they are diagnosed more frequently in younger women, at a median age of 53 years, with 26% diagnosed in women younger than 44 years.[2,12,13] In contrast, patients with high-grade serous ovarian carcinoma have a median age at diagnosis of 61 years, with less than 7% being younger than 44 years (Table 5.2).[12,13]

Women diagnosed with mucinous ovarian carcinoma have an overall better prognosis than those diagnosed with high-grade serous ovarian carcinoma. This is due to the fact that the majority of mucinous ovarian carcinomas are stage I at the time of diagnosis, in contrast to high-grade serous ovarian carcinomas, where stage I disease is rarely diagnosed (83% vs 4%).[2] While early-stage mucinous ovarian carcinomas are associated with a 5-year overall survival exceeding 90%, patients with advanced-stage mucinous carcinomas tend to fare worse than their high-grade serous counterparts, with a median overall survival of less than 15 months.[11,12,14–18] This is largely due to the relative resistance of mucinous ovarian carcinomas to platinum-based chemotherapy regimens[19–21] (Table 5.2).

Etiology/risk factors

It is now commonly believed that the majority of high-grade serous ovarian carcinomas or tubal carcinomas originate in the fimbriae of the tube and then exfoliate onto the surface of the adjacent ovary.[22] In contrast, mucinous ovarian carcinoma

Diagnosis and Treatment of Rare Gynecologic Cancers. https://doi.org/10.1016/B978-0-323-82938-0.00005-7

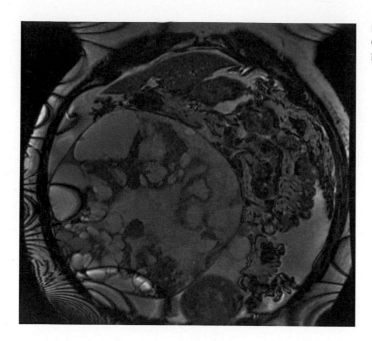

FIG. 5.1 Preoperative MRI (coronal section) demonstrating a large complex mass likely arising from the right ovary in a patient with primary mucinous ovarian carcinoma.

TABLE 5.1 Subtypes of epithelial ovarian cancer.

Subtype	Frequency[a]
High-grade serous	70%
Low-grade serous	10%
Endometrioid	10%
Clear cell	5%
Mucinous	3%
Other (Brenner, undifferentiated)	2%

[a]*Frequencies for women in North American and Europe, frequencies differ in Asia.*
From Stephanie Lheureux, Marsela Braunstein, Amit M. Oza. Epithelial ovarian cancer: evolution of management in the era of precision medicine. *CA Cancer J Clin.* 2019;69(4):280–304.

appears to develop as a continuum, arising from benign epithelium, progressing to a mucinous borderline tumor before developing into an invasive malignancy.[11,22–24] This is supported by the observation that invasive mucinous carcinomas often coexist with benign mucinous cystadenomas and/or borderline tumors within the same ovarian mass.[25] Mucinous carcinomas can also arise from mature cystic teratomas or Brenner tumors.[24] Histologically, the distinction between these different mucinous entities can be subtle, making an accurate pathologic diagnosis challenging.[26–28]

Unlike high-grade serous ovarian carcinomas, for which nulliparity, early menarche, late menopause and germline *BRCA1* or *BRCA2* mutations are established risk factors, smoking is the only known risk factor associated with mucinous ovarian carcinomas (Table 5.2).[29] In a systematic review, current or prior history of smoking was associated with an increased risk for mucinous ovarian carcinoma (RR 2.1, 95% CI 1.7–2.1) but not the other epithelial subtypes of ovarian cancer.[30] Current and former smokers also have worse cancer-specific survival compared with nonsmokers, with a hazard ratio of 1.9 (95% CI 1.01–3.65).[31]

Genetic sequencing can help distinguish mucinous ovarian carcinomas from other epithelial subtypes and from extra-ovarian primaries. The vast majority of mucinous ovarian carcinomas harbor *KRAS* mutations (45%–71%), compared with

TABLE 5.2 Epidemiological, clinical, pathologic and genetic factors of mucinous ovarian carcinomas as compared with high-grade serous ovarian carcinomas.

	Mucinous carcinoma	High-grade serous carcinoma
Median age at diagnosis (years)	53	61
<44 years at diagnosis (%)	26	7
Risk factors	Smoking	Germline *BRCA* mutations, nulliparity, early menarche, late menopause
Rate of bilaterality (%)	<20	>50
Stage I at diagnosis (%)	65–83	<5
Rate of lymph node metastasis for stage I disease (%)	0 (Expansile) up to 30 (infiltrative)	10
Serum tumor markers	CEA or CA 19-9	CA-125
Rate of response to platinum-based chemotherapy (%)	12.5–38.5	67.6–70
Overall survival		
Stage I, at 5 years (%)	>90	>80
Advanced stage (months)	14.8	45.2

Data presented in this table are from Peres LC, et al. Invasive epithelial ovarian cancer survival by histotype and disease stage. *J Natl Cancer Inst.* 2019;111 (1):60–68; Torre LA, et al. Ovarian cancer statistics, 2018. *CA Cancer J Clin.* 2018;68(4):284–296; Hess V, et al. Mucinous epithelial ovarian cancer: a separate entity requiring specific treatment. *J Clin Oncol.* 2004;22(6):1040–4; Morice P, Gouy S, Leary A. Mucinous ovarian carcinoma. *N Engl J Med.* 2019;380 (13):1256–1266; Seidman JD, Kurman RJ, Ronnett BM. Primary and metastatic mucinous adenocarcinomas in the ovaries: incidence in routine practice with a new approach to improve intraoperative diagnosis. *Am J Surg Pathol.* 2003;27(7):985–93; Jordan SJ, et al. Risk factors for benign, borderline and invasive mucinous ovarian tumors: epidemiological evidence of a neoplastic continuum? *Gynecol Oncol.* 2007;107(2):223–30 and Schiavone MB, et al. Natural history and outcome of mucinous carcinoma of the ovary. *Am J Obstet Gynecol.* 2011;205(5):480 e1-8.

only 10% of endometrioid ovarian carcinomas, 5% of high-grade serous ovarian carcinomas, and 0% of clear cell carcinomas.[32–37] Notably, the same *KRAS* mutations have been found in the associated benign and borderline lesions, suggesting that this mutation is a founder event.[32,34,36] While *TP53* mutations are characteristic of high-grade serous ovarian carcinomas (>96%), 56%–75% of mucinous ovarian carcinomas harbor these alterations.[34,35,37,38] Additionally, amplification of *ERBB2* (HER2) is also seen in 18%–35% of cases.[39] Mutations in *ERBB2* (HER2) and *TP53* are only observed in the carcinoma component, suggesting that these alterations occur (develop) later in the process of malignant transformation.[32,34]

Pathology

Gross

Majority of primary ovarian mucinous carcinomas are grossly large unilateral masses. This appearance is different from metastatic tumors involving the ovary, which are frequently bilateral; and the ovaries are small and multinodular with a bosselated surface. While the aforementioned appearance is typical, on occasion large unilateral tumors may represent metastasis from the gastrointestinal (GI) tract or pancreas rather than ovarian primaries; therefore, careful histologic evaluation is necessary.

Microscopic findings

Histologically primary ovarian mucinous carcinomas usually show a heterogeneous appearance with areas of cystadenoma, borderline tumor, and carcinoma. The majority of mucinous carcinomas are of intestinal type with the lining epithelium containing goblet cells. Mucinous ovarian carcinomas show two patterns of invasion, i.e., expansile type and infiltrative type. In the expansile pattern the glands are back to back with minimal or no intervening stroma, and this area should measure at least 5 mm in one dimension; importantly there is no stromal invasion or desmoplastic reaction around the glands (Fig. 5.2). Infiltrative invasion is characterized by haphazard glands surrounded by desmoplastic stroma, measuring at least 5 mm in one linear dimension (Fig. 5.3). If the infiltrative pattern of invasion is focal and measures <5 mm, in a

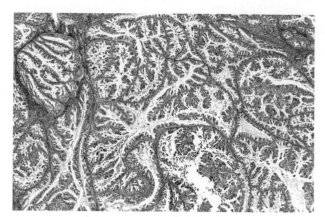

FIG. 5.2 Mucinous carcinoma with expansile pattern of invasion showing back to back glands with minimal or no intervening stroma.

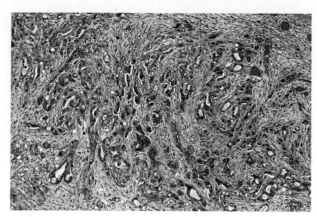

FIG. 5.3 Mucinous carcinoma with infiltrative invasion characterized by haphazard glands surrounded by desmoplastic stroma.

background of a mucinous borderline tumor, the term microinvasive carcinoma is used. The size criteria are based on the WHO Classification of Tumors of the Female Reproductive Organs.[40] Of note, intestinal-type mucinous carcinomas may arise in a background of an ovarian teratoma and mimic metastasis due to extensive pseudomyxoma ovarii/peritonei.[41]

A subset of mucinous carcinomas have mural nodules which may be composed of anaplastic carcinoma, or sarcoma. These two components have histologic overlap but the anaplastic carcinoma is diffusely positive for keratin markers, while negative in sarcoma. The presence of anaplastic carcinoma and sarcoma may be associated with an adverse outcome but some studies have not shown this to be the case in stage IA tumors; however, experience is limited. Sarcoma-like mural nodule, on the other hand, is a reactive proliferation composed of mitotically active spindle cells with numerous osteoclast-like giant cells, and as such is a benign proliferation that does not alter the outcome.

Ancillary testing

Primary ovarian mucinous tumors are usually positive for CK7 (diffuse) (Fig. 5.4). CK20 (Fig. 5.5), PAX-8 and ER show variable staining ranging from negative to focal or patchy staining but are not usually diffuse and strong.[42] Markers of intestinal differentiation such as SATB2 are negative in the surface epithelial tumors, but can be positive in mucinous tumors arising in a background of teratoma.[28] Distinction from metastasis can be challenging on histologic evaluation hence, doing a panel of immunostains is prudent.

Differential diagnosis

The differential diagnosis for ovarian mucinous carcinoma is quite diverse. Among other ovarian primaries, endometrioid carcinoma and clear cell carcinoma can show extensive mucinous differentiation and may be classified as mucinous

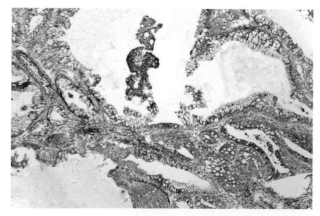

FIG. 5.4 Mucinous carcinoma showing diffuse staining for CK7.

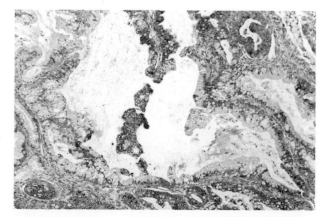

FIG. 5.5 Mucinous carcinoma showing variable staining for CK20.

carcinoma. Diffuse strong expression of ER and PR favors endometrioid carcinoma over mucinous carcinoma. Expression of HNF-1B and napsin-A would support clear cell carcinoma. Distinguishing metastatic mucinous ovarian carcinoma from a primary ovarian mucinous carcinoma can be particularly challenging. Histologic features such as dirty necrosis are typical of metastatic colonic adenocarcinoma, and the presence of pseudomyxoma ovarii/peritonei is almost always associated with an appendiceal primary. But in many cases there are overlapping histologic features and immunohistochemical (IHC) stains are necessary to make the correct diagnosis. The two most important markers are CK7 and CK20, the former being diffusely positive in ovarian mucinous carcinomas and the latter in tumors of the lower GI tract. However, right-sided colonic adenocarcinomas that are microsatellite unstable may be diffusely CK7 positive and negative for CK20, and most ovarian mucinous carcinomas can show focal CK20 staining; these factors must be considered when interpreting the stains. CDX2 is often positive in ovarian mucinous carcinomas which limits its utility in this differential. Other metastatic tumors that are morphologically virtually indistinguishable from ovarian mucinous carcinomas are tumors of the pancreatico-biliary tract and some cervical carcinomas. Pancreaticobiliary tract tumors show loss of DPC4 in about 50% of cases and this marker may facilitate the diagnosis as other markers are not specific in this differential. Unlike primary ovarian mucinous carcinomas, HPV-associated cervical carcinoma will be diffusely positive for p16 and show positivity for high risk HPV by in-situ hybridization. Despite the use of immunomarkers, in a subset of cases, distinguishing primary from metastatic tumors is not possible, and correlation with clinical and radiologic findings is necessary to determine the primary site of origin.

Molecular alterations

The most common molecular alterations in ovarian mucinous carcinoma, besides copy number loss, are mutations in *CDKN2A, KRAS,* and *TP53* genes.[42] *HER2* gene amplification has been reported in approximately 25% of cases.

Diagnosis and workup

Differential diagnosis

It is challenging to accurately diagnose mucinous ovarian carcinomas. Ovarian metastases from extraovarian primary cancers account for the majority of mucinous carcinomas involving the ovary. In 2011, Zaino et al. published a landmark paper revealing that, in a prospective GOG trial, the vast majority of diagnosed primary mucinous ovarian carcinomas were, in fact, metastases from other sites.[18] Less than a quarter (23%) of mucinous carcinomas involving the ovary will be primary ovarian cancers. The most common primary origin of these carcinomas will belong to the GI tract (45%), followed by pancreas (20%), cervix (13%), breast (8%), and uterus (3%).[5] Given this, expert gynecologic pathology review is essential and additional clinical evaluation is needed to rule out metastases from nonovarian primaries. This includes upper endoscopy, colonoscopy, mammogram, computed tomography (CT) and/or positron emission tomography (PET) and serum tumors markers.[43] This work-up should be completed in patients diagnosed with mucinous ovarian carcinomas, given the high frequency with which an extraovarian primary will be diagnosed.

A validated algorithm that uses size and laterality of the tumor can help confirm the diagnosis of primary versus metastatic mucinous tumors. Unilateral tumors greater than 10 cm in diameter have been shown to be an ovarian primary in over 80% of patients, while 88% of unilateral masses smaller than 10 cm and 94% of bilateral masses will be metastases (Fig. 5.6).[5] Primary mucinous ovarian carcinomas are greater in size, with a mean of 16–20 cm (range 5–48 cm) compared with metastatic mucinous carcinomas, which are 11–12 cm on average (range 2–24 cm).[5,25] Given the broad differential diagnosis of these tumors, which includes GI malignancies, in addition to upper endoscopy and colonoscopy patients should undergo careful inspection of the peritoneal cavity, including the small and large bowel, by a gynecologic oncologist (Fig. 5.7).

The origin of mucinous tumors, whether primary to the ovary or originating elsewhere, can be difficult to determine by histologic examination alone. Measuring the size and laterality of the tumor is helpful. Additional features that favor an ovarian primary include the following: the coexistence of borderline and/or benign mucinous component or teratoma, Brenner tumor, mural nodules or an expansile (confluent) pattern. Features that favor metastatic adenocarcinoma include the following: ovarian surface involvement, vascular invasion, hilar involvement, extensive infiltrative pattern, signet-ring cells, prominent desmoplastic response, small clusters of tumor cells within corpora lutea or albicantia, numerous pools of mucin dissecting the ovarian stroma, or a nodular pattern of invasion.[44,45] (Table 5.5).

IHC markers can help narrow the diagnosis. While immunostaining with PAX8 is typical for tumors of gynecologic origin, PAX8 staining is usually focal and weak in primary mucinous ovarian carcinomas.[26,27,46,47] Meanwhile, colorectal tumors tend to express SATB2, although mucinous tumors arising from mature teratomas can also stain diffusely positive

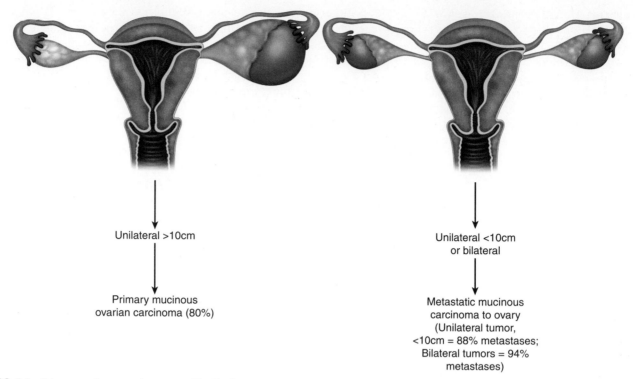

FIG. 5.6 Primary mucinous ovarian cancer will typically present as large, unilateral mass and metastatic disease to the ovary as smaller, bilateral masses.

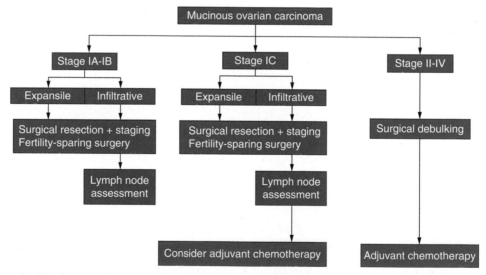

FIG. 5.7 Treatment algorithm for newly diagnosed primary mucinous ovarian cancer.

for SATB2.[24,28] Additionally, primary mucinous ovarian carcinomas stain positive for CK7 and CK20, while colorectal primaries tend only to express CK20, and breast primaries are usually CK7 positive and CK20 negative.[27] Unlike endometrioid tumors of gynecologic origin and primary breast cancers, mucinous ovarian carcinomas do not express estrogen or progesterone receptors (ERs or PRs).[27,46] HPV in situ hybridization and p16 immunostaining can be helpful in diagnosing a cervical primary, as p16 staining is usually negative in primary mucinous ovarian carcinomas.[24,27] While the application of massively parallel sequencing is not yet widely available in the clinical setting, some have advocated a targeted gene panel with select IHC to narrow the differential diagnosis.[35]

TABLE 5.3 Initial work-up of newly diagnosed mucinous carcinoma of the ovary.	
Physical exam	Complete physical exam with pelvic and rectovaginal examination Consider breast examination if indicated
Imaging	CT chest/abdomen/pelvis with contrast MRI pelvis if indicated PET CT (optional) Obtain endoscopy and colonoscopy pre or post operatively If breast etiology suspected, obtain mammogram as clinically indicated
Tumor markers	CEA, CA 19-9, CA-125

Signs and symptoms

In the case of primary mucinous ovarian carcinomas, the tumors tend to be large and unilateral.[44,48] Most patients present with pelvic pain or discomfort, prompting medical evaluation.[49] Patients with advanced-stage disease often have omental caking and peritoneal spread of disease in the pelvis and upper abdomen, and report increasing abdominal girth, bloating, early satiety and weight loss symptoms, similar to those experienced by patients with high-grade serous ovarian carcinomas.[50–52]

Physical exam findings

In the majority of patients with primary mucinous ovarian carcinomas, abdominal and pelvic examination will reveal a large abdominopelvic mass. Laterality cannot always be determined based on examination alone, given the large size of these tumors. A thorough physical exam, including a pelvic exam to rule out a cervical or uterine mass, and a rectovaginal exam, should be performed to help determine extent of disease and to assess for a rectal primary. A breast examination should be considered if clinically indicated, as metastatic breast cancer can present with ovarian metastases (Table 5.3).

Tumor markers

Approximately a third of all ovarian cancers will have elevated carcinoembryonic antigen (CEA) levels; however, CEA is more likely to be elevated in mucinous ovarian carcinomas specifically.[53–55] CEA is an oncofetal antigen that is found in embryonic and fetal tissue and disappears almost completely after birth; however, small amounts may persist in the adult colon.[53] CEA may also be elevated in colon and pancreatic cancer and benign diseases involving the liver, lung and GI tract.[53] CA-125, while elevated in 85% of high-grade serous carcinomas, is only elevated in 12% of mucinous ovarian carcinomas, with a mean CA-125 of 44.2 U/mL compared with 235 U/mL for high-grade serous carcinomas.[56,57] Given the specificity for mucinous carcinomas, CEA is a more useful marker preoperatively and throughout the patient's post-operative or treatment course. Carbohydrate antigen 19-9 (CA 19-9) is also more likely to be elevated in mucinous ovarian carcinomas and may help distinguish benign mucinous neoplasms from invasive carcinoma.[58]

Imaging studies

CT scan of the chest, abdomen and pelvis with contrast is helpful in the primary work-up of a suspicious adnexal mass, to evaluate the lesion and radiologic extent of disease. While transvaginal ultrasound may be obtained as part of the initial evaluation of pelvic pain or when an adnexal mass is palpated on pelvic examination, ultrasound is insufficient to capture the entire size of these lesions and will not rule out the possibility of metastatic disease. MRI may be used to further characterize the tumor and its relationship with key structures of the pelvis (Fig. 5.1); however, CT remains the preferred imaging modality. PET scans can be considered if nonovarian metastatic mucinous carcinoma is suspected; however, we do not routinely obtain PET scans in our practice.

Diagnostic testing

In addition to obtaining a detailed clinical history, a complete physical examination including a pelvic exam and rectovaginal exam should be performed. Imaging for pelvic masses typically begins with transvaginal ultrasound, given the wide availability of this modality. However, if there is suspicion for malignancy, a CT scan, preferably of the chest, abdomen and pelvis, should be obtained to assess for metastatic disease and resectability. Relevant tumor markers, including CA-125, CEA and CA 19-9, should be obtained (Table 5.3). While a primary mucinous ovarian carcinoma may be suspected based on clinical presentation and imaging findings, the diagnosis is made on pathological evaluation following surgical resection. Given the large size of these tumors, it may be difficult to provide a diagnosis of invasive carcinoma on frozen section, making it a challenge to counsel a patient on management until the final pathology is clarified. Furthermore, distinguishing a primary mucinous ovarian carcinoma from metastatic mucinous ovarian carcinoma adds another layer of complexity, given the morphologic similarity of these tumors.[26–28] In addition to endoscopic studies to rule out a GI primary, including upper endoscopy and colonoscopy, IHC studies can help narrow the diagnosis (see Sections "Pathology" and "Differential diagnosis").[27,47]

Staging system

Mucinous ovarian carcinomas are staged according to the International Federation of Gynecology and Obstetrics (FIGO) ovarian cancer staging system (Table 5.4). Surgical staging of mucinous ovarian carcinomas follows epithelial ovarian cancer guidelines and includes removal of the uterus, cervix, both tubes and ovaries, and obtaining peritoneal cytology, multiple peritoneal biopsies, and an omental biopsy or omentectomy. For patients desiring fertility preservation, the unaffected contralateral ovary and uterus may be retained if disease is confined to a single ovary; however, staging with or without lymphadenectomy should still be performed.[43] The current staging guidelines include comprehensive lymphadenectomy; however, given the rarity of occult nodal involvement ($<$2%) in mucinous ovarian carcinomas, lymph node sampling can be omitted.[10,50–52,59] While many institutions grade mucinous ovarian carcinomas according to the FIGO system, it is important to note that there is no standardized grading system for primary mucinous ovarian carcinomas.

TABLE 5.4 TNM and FIGO staging for ovary, fallopian tube, and primary peritoneal carcinomas.

T category	FIGO stage	T criteria
		Primary tumor (T)
TX		Primary tumor cannot be assessed
T0		No evidence of primary tumor
T1	I	Tumor limited to ovaries (one or both) or fallopian tube(s)
T1a	IA	Tumor limited to one ovary (capsule intact) or fallopian tube, no tumor on ovarian or fallopian tube surface; no malignant cells in ascites or peritoneal washings
T1b	IB	Tumor limited to both ovaries (capsules intact) or fallopian tubes; no tumor on ovarian or fallopian tube surface; no malignant cells in ascites or peritoneal washings
T1c	IC	Tumor limited to one or both ovaries or fallopian tubes, with any of the following:
T1c1	IC1	• Surgical spill
T1c2	IC2	• Capsule ruptured before surgery or tumor on ovarian or fallopian tube surface
T1c3	IC3	• Malignant cells in ascites or peritoneal washings
T2	II	Tumor involves one or both ovaries or fallopian tubes with pelvic extension below pelvic brim or primary peritoneal cancer
T2a	IIA	Extension and/or implants on the uterus and/or fallopian tube(s) and/or ovaries
T2b	IIB	Extension to and/or implants on other pelvic tissues
T3	III	Tumor involves one or both ovaries or fallopian tubes, or primary peritoneal cancer, with microscopically confirmed peritoneal metastasis outside the pelvis and/or metastasis to the retroperitoneal (pelvic and/or paraaortic) lymph nodes
T3a	IIIA2	Microscopic extrapelvic (above the pelvic brim) peritoneal involvement with or without positive retroperitoneal lymph nodes

TABLE 5.4 TNM and FIGO staging for ovary, fallopian tube, and primary peritoneal carcinomas—cont'd

Primary tumor (T)		
T category	**FIGO stage**	**T criteria**
T3b	IIIB	Macroscopic peritoneal metastasis beyond pelvis 2 cm or less in greatest dimension with or without metastasis to the retroperitoneal lymph nodes
T3c	IIIC	Macroscopic peritoneal metastasis beyond the pelvis more than 2 cm in greatest dimension with or without metastasis to the retroperitoneal lymph nodes (includes extension of tumor to capsule of liver and spleen without parenchymal involvement of either organ)
Regional lymph nodes (N)		
N category	**FIGO stage**	**N criteria**
NX		Regional lymph nodes cannot be assessed
N0		No regional lymph node metastasis
N0(i+)		Isolated tumor cells in regional lymph node(s) no greater than 0.2 mm
N1	IIIA1	Positive retroperitoneal lymph nodes only (histologically confirmed)
N1a	IIIA1i	Metastasis up to and including 10 mm in greatest dimension
N1b	IIIA1ii	Metastasis more than 10 mm in greatest dimension
Distant metastasis (M)		
M category	**FIGO stage**	**M criteria**
M0		No distant metastasis
M1	IV	Distant metastasis, including pleural effusion with positive cytology; liver or splenic parenchymal metastasis; metastasis to extraabdominal organs (including inguinal lymph nodes and lymph nodes outside the abdominal cavity); and transmural involvement of intestine
M1a	IVA	Pleural effusion with positive cytology
M1b	IVB	Liver or splenic parenchymal metastases; metastases to extraabdominal organs (including inguinal lymph nodes and lymph nodes outside the abdominal cavity); transmural involvement of intestine

TABLE 5.5 Characteristics favoring primary mucinous ovarian cancer versus metastatic mucinous carcinoma involving the ovary.

Primary mucinous ovarian cancer	Metastatic mucinous cancer to ovary
Unilateral	Bilateral
>10 cm	<10 cm
Intact ovarian capsule	Ovarian surface involvement
Absence of vascular invasion, hilar involvement and extensive infiltration	Presence of vascular invasion, hilar involvement and extensive infiltration
IHC Markers: +CK7, +CK20	IHC Markers: Colorectal primary: -CK7, +CK20 Breast primary: +CK7, −CK20 Cervical primary: +p16 Endometrial primary: +ER, +PR

Data presented in this table from Lee KR, Young RH. The distinction between primary and metastatic mucinous carcinomas of the ovary: gross and histologic findings in 50 cases. *Am J Surg Pathol*. 2003;27(3):281–92; Hart WR. Mucinous tumors of the ovary: a review. *Int J Gynecol Pathol*. 2005;24(1):4–25 and McCluggage WG, Wilkinson N. Metastatic neoplasms involving the ovary: a review with an emphasis on morphological and immunohistochemical features. *Histopathology*. 2005;47(3):231–47.

The vast majority (greater than 80%) of patients with mucinous ovarian carcinomas are stage I at the time of diagnosis. This is in contrast to high-grade serous ovarian carcinomas, less than 5% of which are confined to the ovary at diagnosis (Table 5.2).[2]

Invasive mucinous ovarian carcinomas are characterized by two different patterns of invasion: expansile/confluent and infiltrative/destructive (see Section "Pathology").[24] There are reports of an increased rate of occult nodal metastases with an infiltrative pattern of invasion (17%–30%), and in these cases, lymph node sampling should be considered along with peritoneal staging. Pattern of invasion is not typically available at the time of frozen section diagnosis, and these considerations are often based on final pathology.[60,61] The risk of upstaging increases with an infiltrative pattern of invasion. This should be discussed with patients, along with the risks associated with staging lymphadenectomy.

Prognostic factors

The majority of primary mucinous ovarian carcinomas are stage I at the time of diagnosis and are associated with a favorable prognosis. According to a SEER database analysis of different epithelial ovarian cancer histotypes from 2004 to 2014, the 5-year survival rate for mucinous ovarian carcinomas is 91% for stage I, 76% for stage II, and 17% for stage III/IV disease.[12] Given that the majority of patients are diagnosed with stage I disease, women with mucinous ovarian carcinoma overall have a better prognosis than those with high-grade serous ovarian carcinoma, who are rarely diagnosed at stage I (overall survival of 70 months vs 34 months).[62] However, women with advanced-stage mucinous ovarian carcinoma fare worse than those with metastatic high-grade serous ovarian carcinoma due to the relative resistance of mucinous ovarian carcinomas to platinum-based chemotherapy (Table 5.2).[14]

Histologic subtype has important prognostic implications. Mucinous carcinomas with expansile invasion have a more favorable prognosis than those with infiltrative invasion.[25,49,61] Over 95% of women with expansile subtype of mucinous ovarian carcinomas present with stage I disease, supporting the low metastatic potential of these tumors. In contrast, women with infiltrative mucinous ovarian carcinomas are more likely to present with advanced disease at the time of diagnosis (>25%).[61] Overall, the infiltrative subtype is associated with higher risk of relapse, metastatic potential, lymph node involvement and worse overall survival.[61] The rate of occult lymph node involvement in patients who appear to have ovary-confined disease in infiltrative versus expansile subtype carcinomas is 17%–30% vs 0% in the published literature.[60]

Treatment of primary disease

Early-stage disease

For early-stage disease, defined as disease confined to one ovary, initial management is surgery. Fertility-sparing surgery with unilateral salpingo-oophorectomy (USO), with preservation of the contralateral ovary and uterus, can be considered in motivated patients with apparent ovary-confined disease.[43] For patients selected for fertility preservation surgical staging treatment (with and without lymphadenectomy), the 5-year progression-free survival (PFS) is reported to range from 73% to 80% for patients with stage I-II disease, with overall lower recurrence rates than patients with stage I serous carcinomas (6% vs 20%).[63–65] We recommend discussing fertility preserving options with all motivated patients under 45 years of age. For patients desiring fertility, we recommend referral to a reproductive endocrinologist to discuss fertility preservation, including oocyte cryopreservation as clinically indicated. In all patients with suspected early-stage disease, surgical staging with thorough inspection of the peritoneal cavity, including the small and large bowel and pancreas, and peritoneal biopsies should be done to rule out a nonovarian primary or occult higher stage disease. Previously, routine appendectomy was recommended at the time of surgical resection of mucinous ovarian carcinomas. An appendectomy is now indicated only if the appendix appears abnormal; otherwise, documenting a normal-appearing appendix in the operative report is appropriate.[43] Care should be taken to remove the mass intact and avoid any intraoperative spillage, which will upstage a patient to stage IC, increasing risk of recurrence. If it is anticipated that the tumor will exceed the size of a specimen retrieval bag or is at higher risk of capsular rupture, then open surgery is the preferred option. Minimally invasive surgery with the aid of specimen retrieval bags can be considered in select cases. Pelvic and paraaortic lymphadenectomy should only be considered in the setting of infiltrative patterns of invasion, given the higher rates of lymph node involvement in these cases (17%–30%)[60,61] (Fig. 5.2). If mucinous ovarian carcinoma is incidentally diagnosed on postoperative pathology, and the original surgery was performed by a gynecologic oncologist, we recommend second look surgery with lymph node evaluation only for infiltrative subtype. This is recommended even if postoperative imaging is negative for metastatic disease, given the high rates of lymph node metastases for infiltrative subtype. For patients found to have expansile subtype with no evidence of metastatic disease on postoperative imaging, and in whom the original surgery was performed by a gynecologic oncologist, we do not recommend a second look surgery; these patients can be observed. Data regarding the use of adjuvant chemotherapy for early-stage mucinous ovarian carcinoma is limited. This is due to the inherent challenges in studying rare tumors. Per the NCCN guidelines, chemotherapy is recommended for stage II and above, and can be considered for those with stage IC disease.[43] In two large randomized trials (ICON1 and ACTION) that helped establish guidelines regarding adjuvant chemotherapy for early-stage epithelial ovarian cancer, only 20% of the patients had primary mucinous ovarian carcinoma. Both trials showed improved recurrence-free survival (RFS) in those patients with early-stage mucinous ovarian carcinoma who received chemotherapy versus those who were observed; however, no difference in overall survival was seen.[66–68] A recent large national database analysis study reviewing over 4800 patients from 2004 to 2014 found that approximately 30% of patients with stage I mucinous ovarian carcinoma received adjuvant chemotherapy, with the vast majority treated with a multiagent regimen (>92%). Factors associated with receiving chemotherapy were the following: stage IC disease, tumor size $\geq$10 cm, higher histologic grade, or lymph node dissection performed. Importantly, there was no difference in overall survival between those patients who received adjuvant chemotherapy and those who did not (85.6% vs 85.1%).[69] Given the limited and mainly retrospective data available to guide management, there is no clear consensus regarding adjuvant chemotherapy for stage IC patients. It is reasonable to consider chemotherapy for patients with adverse prognostic features such as infiltrative pattern of invasion or incomplete surgical staging (Fig. 5.2).[70–72]

Metastatic disease

Women with advanced-stage mucinous ovarian carcinoma have a worse prognosis than those with other subtypes of epithelial ovarian cancer.[14] While studies assessing the efficacy of surgical management for advanced-stage disease are limited, optimal debulking surgery remains the gold standard in the upfront management of patients with stage III or IV mucinous ovarian carcinomas, who are determined to have resectable disease[73,74] (Fig. 5.2). Complete gross resection (CGR) of metastatic disease is especially important, given the lower response rates to chemotherapy seen in mucinous ovarian carcinomas.[3,14,16,74,75] Following surgical debulking, adjuvant chemotherapy with intravenous carboplatin (AUC 5–6) and paclitaxel (175 mg/m^2) every 3 weeks for a total of 6 cycles is recommended, although these recommendations stem from clinical trials in which accrual of primary mucinous ovarian carcinomas was exceedingly low (see Sections "Epidemiology," "Incidence/mortality") (Fig. 5.2).[7–9] Due to the low accrual on clinical trials that evaluated carboplatin and paclitaxel, and as mucinous ovarian cancer, unlike high-grade serous ovarian cancer, does not seem to respond to these drugs, some have advocated for chemotherapy regimens similar to those utilized for GI mucinous malignancies (see below).

There is a growing consensus in recent years that mucinous ovarian carcinomas are genetically, biologically and clinically distinct entities that should be studied separately from other epithelial subtypes of ovarian cancer.[76] Despite the low percentage of patients with true primary mucinous ovarian carcinomas enrolled in clinical trials, multiple randomized controlled trials have demonstrated decreased PFS and overall survival in advanced-stage disease compared with high-grade serous ovarian cancer.[7–9,77] The poorer prognosis in the setting of metastatic disease is attributed to lower response rates to platinum-based chemotherapy regimens, with studies citing rates of 12.5%–38.5% vs 67.6%–70% in mucinous tumors and high-grade serous ovarian carcinomas, respectively.[3,16] The relative resistance to platinum-based chemotherapy is likely due, in part, to a lack of *BRCA* mutations or homologous recombination deficiency (HRD) signatures in these tumors. Therefore, patients with mucinous ovarian carcinoma are also unlikely to benefit from treatment with PARP inhibition.[78]

Mucinous ovarian carcinomas are genetically heterogeneous and have a genetic profile distinct from that of high-grade serous ovarian carcinomas. Mucinous ovarian carcinomas are characterized by a high frequency of mutations or alterations in *KRAS* (45%–65%), *c-MYC* (65%), *PI3KCA* (13%), *BRAF* (23%), *ERBB2* (23%), *CDKN2A* (60%), and *TP53* (52%–57%). The genetic and morphologic similarities of mucinous ovarian carcinomas to adenocarcinomas of the GI tract have led some to rationalize the use of GI-type chemotherapy regimens.[10,35]

Studies have evaluated the efficacy of GI chemotherapy regimens compared to those used in a gynecologic treatment paradigm with carboplatin and paclitaxel.[79,80] Researchers have compared the use of FOLFOX (IV oxaliplatin 85 mg/m^2 and IV leucovorin 400 mg/m^2 and 5-FU 400 mg/m^2 IV bolus followed by 5-FU 2400 mg/m^2 infusion over 48 h.) with IV carboplatin and paclitaxel, and observed similar response rates of approximately 30%.[16,81–83] The GOG 241 attempted to compare the efficacy of a GI regimen (capecitabine-oxaliplatin (CapeOX)) with or without bevacizumab to carboplatin and paclitaxel with or without bevacizumab. The study was closed prematurely due to low accrual; however, of the data collected, there were no significant differences in response rates to the four treatment regimens (15.4% vs 25% in the capecitabine-oxaliplatin $\pm$ bevacizumab and carboplatin/paclitaxel $\pm$ bevacizumab arms, respectively). There was also no significant benefit to adding bevacizumab to either regimen. However, the data was insufficient to draw any conclusions.[84] The rarity of true primary mucinous ovarian carcinomas makes prospective clinical trials challenging, as highlighted in the early termination of an international randomized study (GOG 241) due to slow accrual.[84] Investigators at Memorial Sloan Kettering Cancer Center published their experience of 62 surgically treated patients with mucinous ovarian carcinoma and report oncologic outcomes in patients receiving either a gynecologic- (GYN-) or GI-type adjuvant chemotherapy regimen (FOLFOX or CapeOX). The 3-year PFS was 90.9% vs 53.3%, and 3-year overall survival was 90.9% versus 76.2% for the GYN and GI chemotherapy regimens, respectively. The authors of this study noted that patients receiving a GI regimen had more advanced-stage disease, and the number of patients who received the GI regimen was small ($n = 9$); therefore, conclusions regarding chemotherapy regimens should be made with caution.[21] In a retrospective review from MD Anderson Cancer Center and Johns Hopkins University examining GI versus GYN regimens in patients with mucinous ovarian carcinoma, GI-type chemotherapy was associated with improved overall survival (HR 0.2, 95% CI 0.1–0.8) compared with GYN-type chemotherapy. Of note, patients receiving GI-type chemotherapy were more likely to have received concomitant bevacizumab.[19] Considering the results from these small but key studies, it is reasonable to consider either a GI- or GYN-type chemotherapy regimen; however, current practice is now leaning toward GI regimens. This is largely based upon the molecular profile of mucinous ovarian carcinoma, which overlaps most closely with that of GI malignancies. Clinicians can consider adding bevacizumab, as this has been associated with extended survival in retrospective reports.[19]

In recent years, hyperthermic intraperitoneal chemotherapy (HIPEC) has been explored as a treatment option for patients with stage III epithelial ovarian cancer undergoing surgical debulking.[85] Only 3 patients with mucinous ovarian carcinoma were enrolled in the pivotal Van Driel Phase III randomized controlled trial of cisplatin HIPEC at interval debulking surgery for stage III epithelial ovarian cancer.[86] A recent multicenter international working group published a retrospective cohort of over 200 patients treated with cytoreductive surgery plus HIPEC in rare subtypes of ovarian cancer, including 80 patients with mucinous ovarian carcinoma. In this cohort, various HIPEC regimens were used; the majority of patients were treated with cisplatin, mitomycin C, or oxaliplatin. Patients with mucinous ovarian carcinoma experienced the longest disease- survival and overall survival benefit, particularly with complete resection of visible disease at time of surgery, though median survivals were not reached.[87] This remains an area of active investigation, and prospective surgical trials are needed to better delineate the role of HIPEC in advanced mucinous ovarian carcinoma.

Surveillance for recurrent disease

Regardless of stage, following primary treatment, the NCCN guidelines recommend surveillance visits every 2–4 months for the first 2 years, every 3–6 months for 3 years, and annually after 5 years, with physical exam including pelvic exam, and tumor markers (CA125, CEA, CA19-9) if these were elevated upon diagnosis. Imaging, preferably with CT of the chest, abdomen and pelvis with contrast, is performed as clinically indicated.[43] For patients with a contralateral ovary and/or uterus in situ, there are no consensus-based guidelines regarding imaging of the remaining ovary. In our practice, we use ultrasound and tumor markers for surveillance of patients that have undergone fertility-sparing surgery, given the low cost and minimally invasive nature of these tests. Imaging, such as a CT of the chest, abdomen and pelvis, should be performed as clinically indicated. Clinicians should continue to use imaging as indicated by the patient's symptoms and physical exam findings.

Survival and patterns of failure

Recurrences tend to occur within 3 years of diagnosis. The most common site of recurrence is the peritoneum (64% of all recurrent cases).[88] Recurrent mucinous ovarian carcinoma has low response rates to chemotherapy compared with recurrent nonmucinous ovarian carcinomas (see Section "Treatment of recurrent disease").[20] Upon diagnosis of recurrent disease, patients with mucinous ovarian carcinoma have a worse PFS (4.5 vs 8 months) and overall survival (17.9 vs 28.8 months) compared with patients with nonmucinous ovarian carcinomas.[20]

Treatment of recurrent disease

Due to the rarity of mucinous ovarian carcinomas, there is a paucity of high-quality data to guide the management of recurrent disease. The general approach and treatment regimens are extrapolated from data for high-grade serous ovarian carcinomas and GI carcinomas (Table 5.6). In patients who are considered to be appropriate surgical candidates, secondary cytoreductive surgery with the goal of CGR should be considered, especially given the relative resistance of this disease to both GYN- and GI-based chemotherapy regimens.[78,88,89] HIPEC at the time of secondary cytoreductive surgery for

TABLE 5.6 Chemotherapy regimens for recurrent mucinous ovarian carcinoma.

Carboplatin (AUC 5–6 on day 1 every 21 days) + paclitaxel (175 mg/m^2 on day 1 or 80 mg/m^2 on days 1, 8 and 15 every 21 days) ± bevacizumab (15 mg/kg on day 1 every 21 days)

Carboplatin (AUC 5–6 on day 1 every 21 days) + albumin-bound paclitaxel (175 mg/m^2 on day 1 or 80 mg/m^2 on days 1, 8, and 15 every 21 days) (for confirmed taxane hypersensitivity)

Carboplatin (AUC 4 on day 1 every 21 days) + gemcitabine (1000 mg/m^2 on days 1 and 8 every 21 days) ± bevacizumab (15 mg/kg on day 1 every 21 days)

Carboplatin (AUC 5 on day 1 every 28 days) + liposomal doxorubicin (30 mg/m^2 on day 1 every 28 days) ± bevacizumab (10 mg/kg on days 1 and 15 every 28 days)

Cisplatin (50–75 mg/m^2 every 21 days)

Carboplatin (AUC 5–6 on day 1 every 21 days) + docetaxel (60–75 mg/m^2 on day 1 every 21 days)

Carboplatin (AUC 4–6 on day 1 every 21 days)

Paclitaxel (60–80 mg/m^2 on days 1, 8 and 15 every 28 days) or albumin-bound paclitaxel (80 mg/m^2 on days 1, 8 and 15 every 28 days) ± bevacizumab (10 mg/kg on days 1 and 15 every 28 days)

Doxorubicin (60 mg/m^2 on day 1 every 21 days)

Irinotecan (60–90 mg/m^2 on days 1 and 8 every 21 days)

Pemetrexed (375 or 500 mg/m^2 on day 1 every 21 days)

Topotecan (1.25 mg/m^2 on days 1 and 5 every 21 days) ± bevacizumab (15 mg/kg on day 1 every 21 days)

Alternative regimen (weekly): Topotecan (3–4 mg/m^2 on days 1, 8 and 15 every 28 days) ± bevacizumab (10 mg/kg on days 1 and 15 every 28 days)

Vinorelbine (20–30 mg/m^2 on days 1 and 8 every 21 days)

Specific regimens to consider for mucinous ovarian carcinoma

5-FU (400 mg/m^2 on day 1, 2400 mg/m^2 infusion over 48 h on day 1) + leucovorin (400 mg/m^2 on day 1) + oxaliplatin (85 mg/m^2 on day 1) ± bevacizumab (5 mg/kg on day 1) every 14 days

Capecitabine (850–1000 mg/m^2 twice daily on days 1–14) + oxaliplatin (130 mg/m^2 on day 1) ± bevacizumab (7.5 mg/kg on day 1) every 21 days

Data presented in this table adapted from National Comprehensive Cancer Network. Ovarian cancer (version 1.2019). 2020, November 27, 2020; Available from: http://www.nccn.org/professionals/physician_gls/pdf/ovarian.pdf.

recurrent mucinous ovarian carcinoma, as in the primary setting, is an intriguing but understudied practice, and should be considered investigational at this time.[90,91]

Given the lack of consensus on the appropriate second-line chemotherapy for recurrent mucinous ovarian carcinoma, multiple retrospective analyses have published on a wide range of regimens used in this setting.[20,78,92] In Pignata et al., single-agent platinum was used more frequently than a platinum doublet (42.1 vs 31.6%). Nonplatinum chemotherapy was employed in less than a third of cases (26.3%). In this series, recurrent mucinous ovarian carcinomas were less likely to respond to chemotherapy than recurrent high-grade serous ovarian carcinomas (36% vs 63% responding, $P = 0.04$).[20] In a Phase II prospective study, Ueda et al. demonstrated that a regimen of docetaxel and irinotecan may be considered in patients with recurrent platinum-refractory or resistant mucinous ovarian carcinoma (15% response rate).[92] Of note, in the largest known cohort of mucinous ovarian carcinomas studied as part of a multicenter international collaboration, 16 different therapeutic regimens were prescribed across 23 cases of recurrent disease. This highlights the lack of true consensus for the management of this rare subtype of epithelial ovarian cancer.[78]

HER2 amplified tumors may benefit from HER2-directed therapies.[93,94] Additionally, mutations in the PI3-kinase pathway occur most frequently with a *KRAS* mutation, and are potentially targetable with MEK and PI3K inhibitors.[95] Microsatellite instability (MSI) is detected in up to 20% of mucinous ovarian carcinomas, and these tumors may respond to immune-checkpoint inhibitors such as pembrolizumab.[96–98] Potential targetable genetic alterations based on available therapeutics, or those that are currently under investigation in other cancer types, are listed in Table 5.7.

TABLE 5.7 Potential non-FDA approved targeted therapies in mucinous ovarian cancer.

Genetic alteration	Potential therapy
ERBB2 (HER2) amplification/mutation	Anti-Her2 monoclonal antibody therapies, Anti-Her2 tyrosine kinase inhibitors
KRAS, NRAS mutations	RAS/RAF inhibitors, MEK inhibitors
EGFR amplification/mutation	EGFR inhibitors
FGFR2 mutation	FGFR2 tyrosine kinase inhibitor
PIK3CA/PTEN mutations	PI3-kinase tyrosine kinase inhibitor, AKT inhibitor
BRAF mutation	BRAF inhibitors
TP53 mutation	Mutant p53 reactivators
ARID1A mutation	BET, EZH2 and ATR inhibitors
RNF43 mutation	FZD and PORCN inhibitors
Src alteration	Src tyrosine kinase
Mismatch repair deficiency	Immune checkpoint inhibitors
HRD	Platinums, PARP inhibitors
ER positivity	Antiestrogens, CDK4/6 inhibitors

Special considerations

Primary mucinous ovarian carcinoma is a clinically, biologically and genetically distinct entity. Given the diminishing likelihood of prospective study, as demonstrated by the recent premature closure of GOG 241, many questions remain regarding the management of this rare disease. These issues must be creatively addressed with tumor registries and institutional collaborations that allow for accurate and uniform data capture. A large, cooperative database with central pathology review would provide a foundation from which researchers can study multiple unanswered questions: which patients will benefit from adjuvant chemotherapy in early-stage disease, the most effective chemotherapy regimens, the role of HIPEC at time of surgical debulking, the role of lymph node assessment in apparent early-stage disease, and use of molecular data to determine eligibility for targeted therapeutics and clinical trials (Table 5.5).

Case resolution

USO, sparing the contralateral ovary and tube and the uterus, is a reasonable approach in patients desiring fertility preservation. Preoperatively, the patient should be referred to a reproductive endocrinologist to discuss fertility preservation options, including oocyte cryopreservation. At the time of surgery, it is important that the patient undergo staging with cytology, peritoneal biopsies, and omental biopsy or omentectomy. Care should be taken to rule out a GI primary with inspection of the small and large bowel, appendix and pancreas. An upper endoscopy and colonoscopy should be performed postoperatively, if not already performed perioperatively. If the patient is found to have infiltrative pattern of invasion, a pelvic and paraaortic lymph node assessment should be strongly considered, given the high rate of nodal involvement reported in clinically apparent stage I infiltrative pattern mucinous ovarian carcinoma (17%–30% vs <2% in expansile type). Following fertility-sparing surgery, patients should undergo active surveillance, which includes physical exam with pelvic exam at regular intervals per the NCCN guidelines (see Section "Surveillance for recurrent disease"). Tumor markers should be trended if initially elevated upon diagnosis, and imaging with transvaginal ultrasound or CT should be performed as clinically indicated.

References

1. Heinzelmann-Schwarz VA, et al. A distinct molecular profile associated with mucinous epithelial ovarian cancer. *Br J Cancer*. 2006;94(6):904–913.
2. Seidman JD, et al. The histologic type and stage distribution of ovarian carcinomas of surface epithelial origin. *Int J Gynecol Pathol*. 2004;23(1):41–44.
3. Shimada M, et al. Clinicopathological characteristics of mucinous adenocarcinoma of the ovary. *Gynecol Oncol*. 2009;113(3):331–334.

4. Torre LA, et al. Ovarian cancer statistics, 2018. *CA Cancer J Clin.* 2018;68(4):284–296.
5. Seidman JD, Kurman RJ, Ronnett BM. Primary and metastatic mucinous adenocarcinomas in the ovaries: incidence in routine practice with a new approach to improve intraoperative diagnosis. *Am J Surg Pathol.* 2003;27(7):985–993.
6. SEER. *Surveillance, Epidemiology, and End Results Program (seer.cancer.gov) Cancer Stats Facts: Ovarian Cancer*; 2020. https://seer.cancer.gov/statfacts/html/ovary.html. [cited 2020 11.22].
7. Bookman MA, et al. Evaluation of new platinum-based treatment regimens in advanced-stage ovarian cancer: a Phase III Trial of the Gynecologic Cancer Intergroup. *J Clin Oncol.* 2009;27(9):1419–1425.
8. McGuire WP, et al. Cyclophosphamide and cisplatin compared with paclitaxel and cisplatin in patients with stage III and stage IV ovarian cancer. *N Engl J Med.* 1996;334(1):1–6.
9. Muggia FM, et al. Phase III randomized study of cisplatin versus paclitaxel versus cisplatin and paclitaxel in patients with suboptimal stage III or IV ovarian cancer: a gynecologic oncology group study. *J Clin Oncol.* 2000;18(1):106–115.
10. Morice P, Gouy S, Leary A. Mucinous ovarian carcinoma. *N Engl J Med.* 2019;380(13):1256–1266.
11. Prat J, D'Angelo E, Espinosa I. Ovarian carcinomas: at least five different diseases with distinct histological features and molecular genetics. *Hum Pathol.* 2018;80:11–27.
12. Peres LC, et al. Invasive epithelial ovarian cancer survival by histotype and disease stage. *J Natl Cancer Inst.* 2019;111(1):60–68.
13. Schiavone MB, et al. Natural history and outcome of mucinous carcinoma of the ovary. *Am J Obstet Gynecol.* 2011;205(5). 480 e1-8.
14. Hess V, et al. Mucinous epithelial ovarian cancer: a separate entity requiring specific treatment. *J Clin Oncol.* 2004;22(6):1040–1044.
15. Mackay HJ, et al. Prognostic relevance of uncommon ovarian histology in women with stage III/IV epithelial ovarian cancer. *Int J Gynecol Cancer.* 2010;20(6):945–952.
16. Pectasides D, et al. Advanced stage mucinous epithelial ovarian cancer: the Hellenic Cooperative Oncology Group experience. *Gynecol Oncol.* 2005;97(2):436–441.
17. Simons M, et al. Survival of patients with mucinous ovarian carcinoma and ovarian metastases: a population-based cancer registry study. *Int J Gynecol Cancer.* 2015;25(7):1208–1215.
18. Zaino RJ, et al. Advanced stage mucinous adenocarcinoma of the ovary is both rare and highly lethal: a Gynecologic Oncology Group study. *Cancer.* 2011;117(3):554–562.
19. Kurnit KC, et al. Effects of gastrointestinal-type chemotherapy in women with ovarian mucinous carcinoma. *Obstet Gynecol.* 2019;134(6):1253–1259.
20. Pignata S, et al. Activity of chemotherapy in mucinous ovarian cancer with a recurrence free interval of more than 6 months: results from the SOCRATES retrospective study. *BMC Cancer.* 2008;8:252.
21. Schlappe BA, et al. A descriptive report of outcomes of primary mucinous ovarian cancer patients receiving either an adjuvant gynecologic or gastrointestinal chemotherapy regimen. *Int J Gynecol Cancer.* 2019.
22. Kurman RJ, Shih Ie M. The origin and pathogenesis of epithelial ovarian cancer: a proposed unifying theory. *Am J Surg Pathol.* 2010;34(3):433–443.
23. Jordan SJ, et al. Risk factors for benign, borderline and invasive mucinous ovarian tumors: epidemiological evidence of a neoplastic continuum? *Gynecol Oncol.* 2007;107(2):223–230.
24. World Health Organization. *WHO classification of tumours: female genital tumours.* vol. 4. 5th ed. World Health Organization; 2020:632.
25. Lee KR, Scully RE. Mucinous tumors of the ovary: a clinicopathologic study of 196 borderline tumors (of intestinal type) and carcinomas, including an evaluation of 11 cases with 'pseudomyxoma peritonei'. *Am J Surg Pathol.* 2000;24(11):1447–1464.
26. de Waal YR, et al. Secondary ovarian malignancies: frequency, origin, and characteristics. *Int J Gynecol Cancer.* 2009;19(7):1160–1165.
27. McCluggage WG, Wilkinson N. Metastatic neoplasms involving the ovary: a review with an emphasis on morphological and immunohistochemical features. *Histopathology.* 2005;47(3):231–247.
28. Strickland S, et al. Immunohistochemistry in the diagnosis of mucinous neoplasms involving the ovary: the added value of SATB2 and biomarker discovery through protein expression database mining. *Int J Gynecol Pathol.* 2016;35(3):191–208.
29. Wentzensen N, et al. Ovarian cancer risk factors by histologic subtype: an analysis from the ovarian cancer cohort consortium. *J Clin Oncol.* 2016;34(24):2888–2898.
30. Jordan SJ, et al. Does smoking increase risk of ovarian cancer? A systematic review. *Gynecol Oncol.* 2006;103(3):1122–1129.
31. Praestegaard C, et al. Cigarette smoking is associated with adverse survival among women with ovarian cancer: results from a pooled analysis of 19 studies. *Int J Cancer.* 2017;140(11):2422–2435.
32. Chang KL, et al. The status of Her2 amplification and Kras mutations in mucinous ovarian carcinoma. *Hum Genomics.* 2016;10(1):40.
33. Gemignani ML, et al. Role of KRAS and BRAF gene mutations in mucinous ovarian carcinoma. *Gynecol Oncol.* 2003;90(2):378–381.
34. Mackenzie R, et al. Targeted deep sequencing of mucinous ovarian tumors reveals multiple overlapping RAS-pathway activating mutations in borderline and cancerous neoplasms. *BMC Cancer.* 2015;15:415.
35. Mueller JJ, et al. Massively parallel sequencing analysis of mucinous ovarian carcinomas: genomic profiling and differential diagnoses. *Gynecol Oncol.* 2018;150(1):127–135.
36. Pieretti M, et al. Heterogeneity of ovarian cancer: relationships among histological group, stage of disease, tumor markers, patient characteristics, and survival. *Cancer Invest.* 2002;20(1):11–23.
37. Ryland GL, et al. Mutational landscape of mucinous ovarian carcinoma and its neoplastic precursors. *Genome Med.* 2015;7(1):87.
38. The Cancer Genome Atlas Research Network. Integrated genomic analyses of ovarian carcinoma. *Nature.* 2011;474(7353):609–615.
39. Chao WR, et al. Assessing the HER2 status in mucinous epithelial ovarian cancer on the basis of the 2013 ASCO/CAP guideline update. *Am J Surg Pathol.* 2014;38(9):1227–1234.
40. Vang R, Khunamornpong S, Kobel M, et al. Mucinous carcinoma of the ovary. In: WHO Classification of Tumors Editorial Board, ed. *Female Genital Tumors.* World Health Organization Classification of Tumors. Lyon: IARC Press; 2020:53–54.

41. Ronnett BM, Seidman JD. Mucinous tumors arising in ovarian mature cystic teratomas: relationship to the clinical syndrome of pseudomyxoma peritonei. *Am J Surg Pathol.* 2003;27(5):650–657.

42. Cheasley D, Wakefield MJ, Ryland GL, et al. The molecular origin and taxonomy of mucinous ovarian carcinoma. *Nat Commun.* 2019;10:3935.

43. National Comprehensive Cancer Network. *Ovarian cancer (version 1.2019)*; 2020. November 27, 2020; Available from: http://www.nccn.org/professionals/physician_gls/pdf/ovarian.pdf.

44. Hart WR. Mucinous tumors of the ovary: a review. *Int J Gynecol Pathol.* 2005;24(1):4–25.

45. Lee KR, Young RH. The distinction between primary and metastatic mucinous carcinomas of the ovary: gross and histologic findings in 50 cases. *Am J Surg Pathol.* 2003;27(3):281–292.

46. Madore J, et al. Characterization of the molecular differences between ovarian endometrioid carcinoma and ovarian serous carcinoma. *J Pathol.* 2010;220(3):392–400.

47. McCluggage WG. Immunohistochemistry in the distinction between primary and metastatic ovarian mucinous neoplasms. *J Clin Pathol.* 2012;65 (7):596–600.

48. Hart WR, Norris HJ. Borderline and malignant mucinous tumors of the ovary. Histologic criteria and clinical behavior. *Cancer.* 1973;31 (5):1031–1045.

49. Riopel MA, Ronnett BM, Kurman RJ. Evaluation of diagnostic criteria and behavior of ovarian intestinal-type mucinous tumors: atypical proliferative (borderline) tumors and intraepithelial, microinvasive, invasive, and metastatic carcinomas. *Am J Surg Pathol.* 1999;23(6):617–635.

50. Cho YH, et al. Is complete surgical staging necessary in patients with stage I mucinous epithelial ovarian tumors? *Gynecol Oncol.* 2006;103(3):878–882.

51. Roger N, et al. Should pelvic and Para-aortic lymphadenectomy be different depending on histological subtype in epithelial ovarian cancer? *Ann Surg Oncol.* 2008;15(1):333–338.

52. Schmeler KM, et al. Prevalence of lymph node metastasis in primary mucinous carcinoma of the ovary. *Obstet Gynecol.* 2010;116(2 pt. 1):269–273.

53. Barakat RR, Markman M, Randall ME. *Principles and Practice of Gynecologic Oncology.* 5th ed. Philadelphia: Lippincott Wiliams & Wilkins; 2009:1072.

54. Tholander B, et al. Pretreatment serum levels of CA-125, carcinoembryonic antigen, tissue polypeptide antigen, and placental alkaline phosphatase, in patients with ovarian carcinoma, borderline tumors, or benign adnexal masses: relevance for differential diagnosis. *Gynecol Oncol.* 1990;39(1):16–25.

55. Tuxen MK, Soletormos G, Dombernowsky P. Tumor markers in the management of patients with ovarian cancer. *Cancer Treat Rev.* 1995;21(3):215–245.

56. Badgwell D, Bast Jr RC. Early detection of ovarian cancer. *Dis Markers.* 2007;23(5–6):397–410.

57. Choi JH, et al. Preoperative serum levels of cancer antigen 125 and carcinoembryonic antigen ratio can improve differentiation between mucinous ovarian carcinoma and other epithelial ovarian carcinomas. *Obstet Gynecol Sci.* 2018;61(3):344–351.

58. Cho HY, Kyung MS. Serum CA19-9 as a predictor of malignancy in primary ovarian mucinous tumors: a matched case-control study. *Med Sci Monit.* 2014;20:1334–1339.

59. Hoogendam JP, et al. Surgical lymph node assessment in mucinous ovarian carcinoma staging: a systematic review and meta-analysis. *BJOG.* 2017;124(3):370–378.

60. Gouy S, et al. Staging surgery in early-stage ovarian mucinous tumors according to expansile and infiltrative types. *Gynecol Oncol Rep.* 2017;22:21–25.

61. Muyldermans K, et al. Primary invasive mucinous ovarian carcinoma of the intestinal type: importance of the expansile versus infiltrative type in predicting recurrence and lymph node metastases. *Eur J Cancer.* 2013;49(7):1600–1608.

62. Ji J, et al. Survival in ovarian cancer patients by histology and family history. *Acta Oncol.* 2008;47(6):1133–1139.

63. Bentivegna E, et al. Long-term follow-up of patients with an isolated ovarian recurrence after conservative treatment of epithelial ovarian cancer: review of the results of an international multicenter study comprising 545 patients. *Fertil Steril.* 2015;104(5):1319–1324.

64. Lee JY, et al. Safety of fertility-sparing surgery in primary mucinous carcinoma of the ovary. *Cancer Res Treat.* 2015;47(2):290–297.

65. Mueller JJ, et al. International study of primary mucinous ovarian carcinomas managed at tertiary medical Centers. *Int J Gynecol Cancer.* 2018;28 (5):915–924.

66. Colombo N, et al. International *Collaborative Ovarian Neoplasm* trial 1: a randomized trial of adjuvant chemotherapy in women with early-stage ovarian cancer. *J Natl Cancer Inst.* 2003;95(2):125–132.

67. Ledermann JA, et al. Gynecologic Cancer InterGroup (GCIG) consensus review for mucinous ovarian carcinoma. *Int J Gynecol Cancer.* 2014;24(9 suppl. 3):S14–S19.

68. Trimbos JB, et al. International Collaborative Ovarian Neoplasm trial 1 and Adjuvant ChemoTherapy In Ovarian Neoplasm trial: two parallel randomized phase III trials of adjuvant chemotherapy in patients with early-stage ovarian carcinoma. *J Natl Cancer Inst.* 2003;95(2):105–112.

69. Nasioudis D, et al. Adjuvant chemotherapy is not associated with a survival benefit for patients with early stage mucinous ovarian carcinoma. *Gynecol Oncol.* 2019;154(2):302–307.

70. Colombo N, et al. ESMO-ESGO consensus conference recommendations on ovarian cancer: pathology and molecular biology, early and advanced stages, borderline tumours and recurrent disease. *Int J Gynecol Cancer.* 2019.

71. Kajiyama H, et al. Survival impact of capsule status in stage I ovarian mucinous carcinoma-a mulicentric retrospective study. *Eur J Obstet Gynecol Reprod Biol.* 2019;234:131–136.

72. Matsuo K, et al. Effectiveness of postoperative chemotherapy for stage IC mucinous ovarian cancer. *Gynecol Oncol.* 2019;154(3):505–515.

73. du Bois A, et al. Role of surgical outcome as prognostic factor in advanced epithelial ovarian cancer: a combined exploratory analysis of 3 prospectively randomized phase 3 multicenter trials: by the Arbeitsgemeinschaft Gynaekologische Onkologie Studiengruppe Ovarialkarzinom (AGO-OVAR) and the Groupe d'Investigateurs Nationaux Pour les Etudes des Cancers de l'Ovaire (GINECO). *Cancer.* 2009;115(6):1234–1244.

74. Karabuk E, et al. Comparison of advanced stage mucinous epithelial ovarian cancer and serous epithelial ovarian cancer with regard to chemosensitivity and survival outcome: a matched case-control study. *J Gynecol Oncol.* 2013;24(2):160–166.

75. Pisano C, et al. Activity of chemotherapy in mucinous epithelial ovarian cancer: a retrospective study. *Anticancer Res.* 2005;25(5):3501–3505.

76. Frumovitz M, et al. Unmasking the complexities of mucinous ovarian carcinoma. *Gynecol Oncol.* 2010;117(3):491–496.

77. Winter 3rd WE, et al. Prognostic factors for stage III epithelial ovarian cancer: a Gynecologic Oncology Group Study. *J Clin Oncol.* 2007;25 (24):3621–3627.

78. Gorringe KL, et al. Therapeutic options for mucinous ovarian carcinoma. *Gynecol Oncol.* 2020;156(3):552–560.

79. Sato S, et al. Combination chemotherapy of oxaliplatin and 5-fluorouracil may be an effective regimen for mucinous adenocarcinoma of the ovary: a potential treatment strategy. *Cancer Sci.* 2009;100(3):546–551.

80. Xu W, et al. Mucinous ovarian cancer: a therapeutic review. *Crit Rev Oncol Hematol.* 2016;102:26–36.

81. Lee HJ, et al. Feasibility of Oxaliplatin, Leucovorin, and 5-fluorouracil (FOLFOX-4) chemotherapy in heavily Pretreated patients with recurrent epithelial ovarian cancer. *Cancer Res Treat.* 2013;45(1):40–47.

82. Rosa DD, et al. Oxaliplatin/5fluorouracil-based chemotherapy was active and well tolerated in heavily pretreated patients with ovarian carcinoma. *Arch Gynecol Obstet.* 2008;278(5):457–462.

83. Sundar S, et al. Phase II trial of oxaliplatin and 5-fluorouracil/leucovorin combination in epithelial ovarian carcinoma relapsing within 2 years of platinum-based therapy. *Gynecol Oncol.* 2004;94(2):502–508.

84. Gore M, et al. An international, phase III randomized trial in patients with mucinous epithelial ovarian cancer (mEOC/GOG 0241) with long-term follow-up: and experience of conducting a clinical trial in a rare gynecological tumor. *Gynecol Oncol.* 2019;153(3):541–548.

85. Cowan RA, et al. Current status and future prospects of hyperthermic intraoperative intraperitoneal chemotherapy (HIPEC) clinical trials in ovarian cancer. *Int J Hyperthermia.* 2017;33(5):548–553.

86. van Driel WJ, et al. Hyperthermic intraperitoneal chemotherapy in ovarian cancer. *N Engl J Med.* 2018;378(3):230–240.

87. Mercier F, et al. Peritoneal Carcinomatosis of rare ovarian origin treated by cytoreductive surgery and hyperthermic intraperitoneal chemotherapy: a multi-institutional cohort from PSOGI and BIG-RENAPE. *Ann Surg Oncol.* 2018;25(6):1668–1675.

88. Massad LS, et al. Clinical outcomes among women with mucinous adenocarcinoma of the ovary. *Gynecol Obstet Invest.* 2016;81(5):411–415.

89. Cheng X, et al. The role of secondary cytoreductive surgery for recurrent mucinous epithelial ovarian cancer (mEOC). *Eur J Surg Oncol.* 2009;35 (10):1105–1108.

90. Babaier A, Ghatage P. Mucinous cancer of the ovary: overview and current status. *Diagnostics (Basel).* 2020;10(1).

91. Nasioudis D, et al. Advanced stage primary mucinous ovarian carcinoma. Where do we stand? *Arch Gynecol Obstet.* 2020;301(4):1047–1054.

92. Ueda Y, et al. A phase II study of combination chemotherapy using docetaxel and irinotecan for TC-refractory or TC-resistant ovarian carcinomas (GOGO-OV2 study) and for primary clear or mucinous ovarian carcinomas (GOGO-OV3 Study). *Eur J Obstet Gynecol Reprod Biol* 2013;170 (1):259–263.

93. Jain A, Ryan PD, Seiden MV. Metastatic mucinous ovarian cancer and treatment decisions based on histology and molecular markers rather than the primary location. *J Natl Compr Canc Netw.* 2012;10(9):1076–1080.

94. McAlpine JN, et al. HER2 overexpression and amplification is present in a subset of ovarian mucinous carcinomas and can be targeted with trastuzumab therapy. *BMC Cancer.* 2009;9:433.

95. Spreafico A, et al. Genotype-matched treatment for patients with advanced type I epithelial ovarian cancer (EOC). *Gynecol Oncol.* 2017;144(2):250–255.

96. Murphy MA, Wentzensen N. Frequency of mismatch repair deficiency in ovarian cancer: a systematic review. This article is a US Government work and, as such, is in the public domain of the United States of America. *Int J Cancer.* 2011;129(8):1914–1922.

97. Pal T, et al. Systematic review and meta-analysis of ovarian cancers: estimation of microsatellite-high frequency and characterization of mismatch repair deficient tumor histology. *Clin Cancer Res.* 2008;14(21):6847–6854.

98. Segev Y, et al. Risk factors for ovarian cancers with and without microsatellite instability. *Int J Gynecol Cancer.* 2013;23(6):1010–1015.

Chapter 6

Low-grade serous ovarian cancer

Rachel N. Grisham and Preetha Ramalingam

Clinical case

A 36-year-old, G1P1, previously healthy woman presents with left sided pelvic pain. She presents to her PCP who performs a CBC and comprehensive panel that are unrevealing, abdominal exam shows bloating without point tenderness. She has a history of normal menses. She has no family history of cancer, and her both parents are alive and healthy. She is referred to her gynecologist who performs a transvaginal pelvic ultrasound which reveals bilateral multilocular ovarian cysts with mural nodularity, papillary projections and solid components. She is sent for a contrast CT scan of abdomen and pelvis which shows left ovarian mass consistent with an ovarian neoplasm, mild abdominopelvic peritoneal disease and small slightly complex right ovarian cyst (Fig. 6.1). Dedicated chest CT shows clear lungs with no signs of metastatic disease to the chest. Blood tests show CA-125 of 125 U/mL.

She is seen in consultation by a gynecologic oncologist who recommends surgical staging. The patient is seen by reproductive endocrinology prior to surgery. She does not plan to have further children and decides to not attempt harvesting of oocytes prior to surgery. At time of surgery an open laparotomy is performed with TAH/BSO, omentectomy, washings, and resection of all gross disease. She is found to have involvement of the ovaries, left fallopian tube, uterine serosa, omentum, and abdominal and pelvic peritoneal disease, consistent with stage IIIc ovarian cancer. Pathology examination shows serous adenocarcinoma, arising in serous borderline disease with micropapillary features. The invasive component is p53 wild-type, ER+, PR-, WT-1, and PAX-8 positive, consistent with low-grade serous ovarian cancer.

The patient undergoes germline and somatic testing and is found to have no BRCA mutation but a somatic *KRAS* mutation. She is treated postoperatively with 6 cycles of carboplatin and paclitaxel chemotherapy followed by letrozole maintenance therapy. She is routinely followed with blood work and exam every 3 months and CT scan of chest, abdomen, and pelvis every 6 months. Three years into maintenance therapy she is found to have recurrent disease with an isolated peritoneal implant. She undergoes secondary debulking surgery with her gynecologic oncologist. Postoperatively she is treated with 6 cycles of carboplatin and gemcitabine, which she tolerates well, but at end of treatment repeat CT imaging shows recurrence of disease with multiple peritoneal nodules and supradiaphragmatic nodes. Biopsy confirms recurrent low-grade serous ovarian cancer. At this time, what systemic therapies would you consider and how may molecular testing help in your decision making?

Epidemiology

Incidence/mortality

Low-grade serous ovarian cancer is a rare form of epithelial ovarian, fallopian tube or primary peritoneal cancer, accounting for approximately 5%–7% of cases of epithelial ovarian cancer. Like the most common form of ovarian cancer, high-grade serous ovarian cancer (which accounts for ~70% of cases), low-grade serous ovarian cancer is typically diagnosed at an advanced stage. Patients with low-grade serous ovarian cancer tend to have a more protracted disease course with a median survival of approximately 10 years; however, patients have limited responses to systemic therapy with most ultimately succumbing to their cancer. A retrospective study by Bodurka et al. reviewed the data from 290 patients with stage III serous ovarian cancer treated with surgery and chemotherapy on GOG 158; blinded pathology review was performed by a panel of 6 gynecologic pathologists to regrade the tumors using the 2-tier (low-grade vs. high-grade) histologic classification system. Patients with low-grade serous ovarian cancer had a significantly longer PFS (45 vs 19.8 months respectively; $P = 0.01$) and women with high-grade serous ovarian cancer demonstrated a significantly higher risk of death

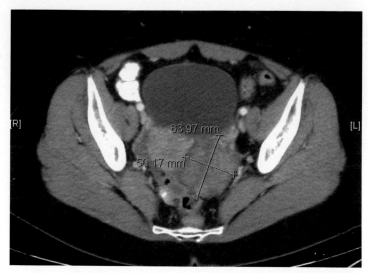

FIG. 6.1 CT of abdomen and pelvis showing left ovarian mass in a 36 year old woman with newly diagnosed stage IIIc low-grade serous ovarian cancer.

vs those with low-grade serous (HR, 2.43; 95% CI, 1.17–5.04; $P = 0.02$).[1] Patients with low-grade serous ovarian cancer also have a younger median age of diagnosis than those with high-grade serous ovarian cancer, with patients commonly diagnosed in their 20s or 30s[2] (Table 6.1).

Etiology/risk factors

Unlike high-grade serous ovarian cancer, the incidence of *BRCA* mutations in patients with low-grade serous ovarian cancer approaches that of the general population. There is not a known hereditary or environmental predisposition for development of this disease. The primary risk factor for development of invasive low-grade serous ovarian cancer is a personal history of its precursor lesion, serous borderline disease. Benign ovarian cystadenoma can progress in a step wise fashion to serous borderline tumor (SBT), SBT with micropapillary features, and ultimately invasive low-grade serous ovarian cancer (Fig. 6.2). A comprehensive population study performed by Vang et al. involved the entire female population of Denmark and included all patients diagnosed with a SBT between 1978 and 2002 or with low-grade serous ovarian cancer between 1997 and 2002. In total 1042 cases of serous borderline disease were included; subsequent development of carcinoma occurred in 4% of patients, of which 93% were low-grade and 7% were high-grade serous carcinoma. Median time to development of subsequent invasive cancer was 10 years, with a range up to 25 years.[3] Presence of a somatic *V600E BRAF* mutation in patients with serous borderline disease may predict for improved prognosis and decreased likelihood of progression.[4,5] In a retrospective study by Grisham et al. of 75 tumors of serous borderline or low-grade serous ovarian

TABLE 6.1 Key characteristics of low-grade vs high-grade serous ovarian cancer.

Clinical/molecular features	Low-grade serous	High-grade serous
Median age at diagnosis	40–50 years	50–60 years
Molecular genetics	Mutant: RAS, BRAF Wild type: p53	Mutant: p53, BRCA Wild type: BRAF, RAS
Response rate to neoadjuvant chemotherapy	4%–23%	80%–90%
Response rates to chemotherapy in the recurrent setting	2%–25%	12%–57%
Median PFS/OS for patients with Stage III optimally debulked disease treated on GOG 158 (blinded pathology review)	$n = 21$ PFS: 45 months OS: 126.2 months	$n = 220$ PFS: 19.8 months OS: 53.8 months

References: Grisham, RN. *Oncology.* 2016;7:650–2. *J Natl Cancer Inst.* 2014;106(4):1–8; Bodurka et al. *Cancer.* 2012;118:3087–94; Schmeler et al. *Gynecol Oncol.* 2008;108:510–4; Grabowski et al. *Gynecol Oncol.* 2016;140(3):457–462. Gershenson et al. *Gynecol Oncol.* 2009;114(1):48–52. Pujade-Lauraine et al. *J Clin Oncol.* 2014;32(13):1302–8. Aghajanian et al. *J Clin Oncol* 2012;30(17):2039–45.

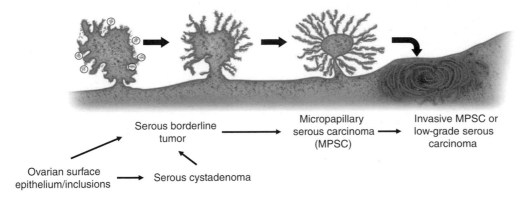

Serous borderline tumor → Micropapillary serous carcinoma (MPSC) → Invasive MPSC or low-grade serous carcinoma

Ovarian surface epithelium/inclusions → Serous cystadenoma → Serous borderline tumor

FIG. 6.2 Development of low-grade serous carcinoma in step wise fashion from.

cancer histology, 57 tumors harbored either a *KRAS* (*n* = 17) or *BRAF V600E* (*n* = 26) mutation.[6] The presence of *BRAF V600E* mutation was associated significantly with early disease stage (stage I/II; $P < 0.001$) and serous borderline histology ($P = 0.002$). While patients with serous borderline disease are at increased risk of developing low-grade serous ovarian cancer, systemic therapy is reserved for those with confirmed invasive disease.

Pathology

Serous borderline tumors

Gross findings

SBTs can range in size from 1 to 35 cm (mean size: 11.0 cm). The tumors may be purely intracystic, purely surface tumors or involve both cyst wall and the ovarian surface. The tumor grossly is composed of papillary excrescences and the papillae are typically soft, edematous and have a tan-yellow appearance. The cyst contents are mostly serous-type fluid, but can also be mucinous. In some cases, the gross appearance is that of cystadenofibroma and the borderline component is only identified microscopically; therefore, sampling of these areas is important even in the absence of the characteristic papillary excrescences.

Histologic features

Microscopically SBTs demonstrate complex arborizing papillae with hierarchical tufting (Fig. 6.3). By definition there is no evidence of stromal invasion in these tumors, though SBT can be present in the background of low-grade serous carcinoma (LGSC) (Fig. 6.3). The lining epithelium can be either low cuboidal or stratified, and ciliated cells are identified at least focally. Cells with abundant eosinophilic cytoplasm can be seen in a subset of SBTs. Cytologic atypia is mild to moderate, and marked atypia is not a feature of SBTs. Per the WHO criteria, at least 10% of the tumor must show epithelial proliferation to be considered SBT;[7] however, in a few cases, even patients with small foci of SBT can recur. Hence, our practice has been to call these tumors "focal" SBTs if the epithelial proliferation is less than 10%.

A subset (5%–15%) of SBTs have a micropapillary pattern (SBT-MP). Histologically, these tumors are characterized by large edematous papillae from which emanate slender papillae devoid of fibrovascular cores that are 5 times as long as they are wide, and has been likened to a Medusa head appearance (Fig. 6.4). This pattern must measure ≥ 5.0 mm to meet criteria for a diagnosis of SBT-MP. A subset of SBT-MP can show cribriform architecture, which is thought to result from fusion of the micropapillae. Of note, the term noninvasive LGSC is not accepted for these tumors in the WHO classification of Tumors of Female Reproductive Organs, and is not used at our institution.

Autoimplants may present either on the surface or between papillae. Histologically, they are composed of plaque-like lesions with features of a desmoplastic noninvasive implant. They are not shown to be associated with adverse outcome.

Another important feature in SBT is the presence of microinvasion. This is defined as the presence of small papillae or single tumor cells with surrounding clear spaces or "halos" measuring <5 mm in one linear dimension, per the WHO criteria. At our institution we use a cut-off of 3 mm. While microinvasion has not been consistently associated with adverse outcome, multiple foci should prompt additional sampling to exclude microscopic foci of LGSC.

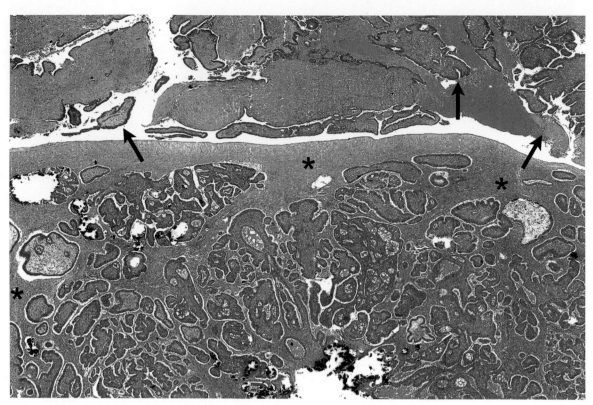

FIG. 6.3 Low grade serous carcinoma (*asterisks*) in a background of serous borderline tumor (*arrows*) which demonstrates complex arborizing papillary with hierarchical tufting and cell detachment.

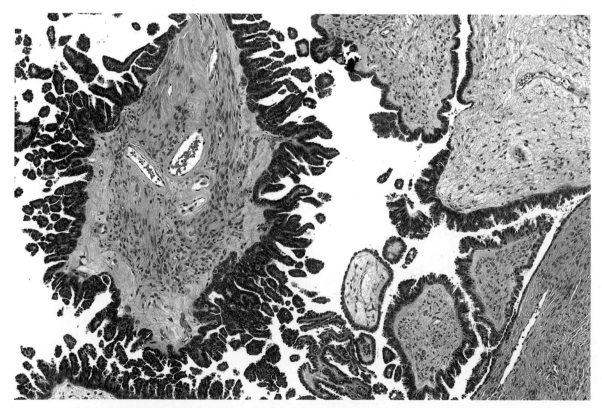

FIG. 6.4 Serous borderline tumor with micropapillary pattern characterized by a large edematous papilla from which emanate slender papillae devoid of fibrovascular cores that are 5 times as long as they are wide.

Peritoneal implants associated with SBT are either noninvasive or invasive. Noninvasive implants are divided into epithelial implants and desmoplastic implants, and are collectively called implants. Invasive implants are now considered to be synonymous with LGSC. Epithelial implants are composed of papillary proliferations within cystically lined spaces that are present within the invagination of the omental fat. Desmoplastic implants are characterized by loose spindle cells within which glands, papillae and single cells are embedded, but overall has to be a stroma rich proliferation. When small biopsies are taken without surrounding adipose tissue, distinguishing noninvasive from invasive implants may be difficult, and the implants may be considered indeterminate.

Ancillary testing

SBTs are positive for PAX-8, WT-1, ER, and PR. They typically show patchy staining for p16 and wild-type staining for p53.

Differential diagnosis

The differential diagnosis for SBTs includes high-grade serous carcinoma with a "borderline-like" architectural pattern, but the latter is identified by the presence of marked cytologic atypia. The diagnosis can be further supported by p53 stain which is only overexpressed in high-grade serous carcinoma. Ovarian clear cell carcinoma is another differential, as a subset of SBTs can show cytoplasmic clearing. Presence of solid, and tubulocystic patterns, hobnailing, and marked cytologic atypia would support a diagnosis of ovarian clear cell carcinoma. If needed immunostains such as WT-1 for SBTs, and napsin-A and HNF-1B for ovarian clear cell carcinoma may be considered.

Serous carcinoma

Gross findings

LGSCs are frequently bilateral and the presence of extensive calcification can give it a gritty appearance. The tumors can be cystic with papillary excrescences, especially if arising in a background of SBT, or solid and cystic. The average size of the tumors is about 8.0 cm.

Histologic features

Histologically, LGSC is characterized by small papillae surrounded by clear spaces/halos that haphazardly infiltrate the stroma (Fig. 6.3). Usually there are numerous psammoma bodies admixed with the tumor cells. Frequently an associated SBT is present. Per the 2020 WHO Classification of Female Genital Tumors, the foci of invasion must measure at least 5 mm in one linear dimension to meet criteria for LGSC, and smaller foci are designated as microinvasion.[8] We use a 3 mm cut off for distinguishing microinvasion from LGSC. From a cytologic point of view LGSC can show mild to moderate nuclear atypia and small nucleoli. Mitotic activity is usually <12/10 hpfs in these tumors.

Ancillary testing

LGSCs are positive for PAX-8, WT-1 (Fig. 6.5), ER and PR. They typically show patchy staining for p16 and wild-type staining for p53 (Fig. 6.6).

Differential diagnosis

Distinguishing LGSC from high-grade serous carcinoma is dependent on the presence of marked nuclear pleomorphism and >12 mitoses/10 hpfs in the latter. Some LGSCs, especially post therapy, can have nuclear pleomorphism and may be difficult to distinguish from high-grade serous carcinoma. In such cases immunostains such as p16, p53 and Ki-67 may be used to differentiate the two tumors. Though uncommon, a few patients with LGSC can have admixed high-grade areas or can recur as high-grade serous carcinoma, hence careful examination of the entire sampled tumor is necessary. Another important differential for LGSC is malignant mesothelioma, which it can mimic histologically. While some stains such as WT1 are positive in both tumors, there are several markers that are discriminatory between these two tumors, that when employed will facilitate the correct diagnosis.

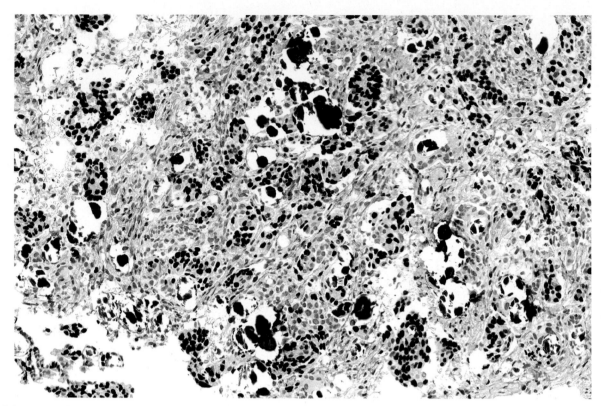

FIG. 6.5 Low-grade serous carcinoma in a peritoneal biopsy showing positive staining for WT1.

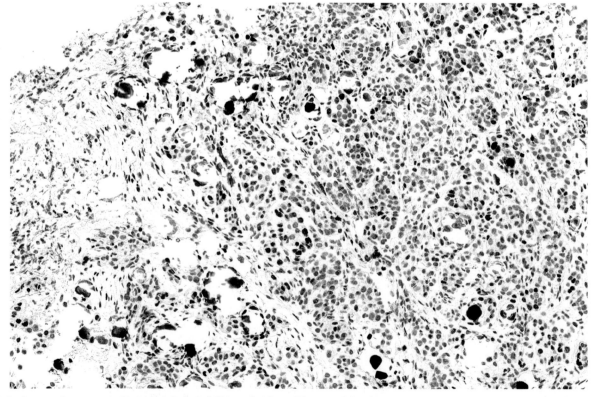

FIG. 6.6 Low-grade serous carcinoma in a peritoneal biopsy showing wild-type staining for p53.

Genetic studies

LGSC typically has fewer mutations than most other solid tumors.[9] The most frequent mutations in LGSC are *KRAS* and *BRAF*, in about 35% and 33% of cases, respectively.[10,11] Of note, *KRAS* mutations at codons 12 and 13 and *BRAF* mutations at codon 599 are mutually exclusive in a given tumor.[11]

Diagnosis and workup
Differential diagnosis

In young women presenting with an ovarian mass low-grade serous ovarian cancer is one of several different histologies that should be considered, including malignant sex cord-stromal tumors and malignant germ cell tumors, in addition to benign etiologies such as dermoid and serous borderline disease. Tumor markers including inhibin, beta-human chorionic gonadotropin (β-hCG) and alpha-fetoprotein (AFP), which are not typically elevated in cases of low-grade serous ovarian cancer, can help steer one toward these other rare histologies.

Signs and symptoms

Similar to other histologies of epithelial ovarian cancer, patients with low-grade serous ovarian cancer often do not present with symptoms until they have developed advanced stage disease. In addition, since patients may present at a younger age, ovarian cancer is generally not considered in the initial differential diagnosis. Possible symptoms include pelvic pain, abdominal bloating, early satiety, and change in bowel function.

Physical exam findings

While patients may present with palpable ascites, physical exam at time of initial diagnosis may be unrevealing. Patients may have weight loss and/or abdominal distention on exam. Pelvic exam may reveal adnexal tenderness or an adnexal mass.

Tumor markers

While CA-125 is the tumor marker most commonly elevated in low-grade serous ovarian cancer, levels may not reach that seen in high-grade serous ovarian cancer. In a *post-hoc* analysis of GOG-182 it was found that significantly fewer patients with grade 1 (low-grade serous ovarian cancer) had pretreatment CA-125 values above the normal range (85%) vs those with high-grade disease (93%).[12] Median pretreatment CA-125 was 119 for those with grade 1 serous ovarian cancer (low-grade), vs 247 for those with grade 2–3 (high-grade).

Imaging

At time of diagnosis patients generally have a contrasted CT scan of abdomen and pelvis performed (Table 6.2). Chest imaging should be performed prior to surgical staging as well, with a minimum of a PA and Lateral chest X-ray to rule out supra-diaphragmatic disease. It is difficult to distinguish between premalignant serous borderline disease and invasive low-grade serous ovarian cancer based on imaging alone. However, the presence of bilateral ovarian masses ($P = 0.03$), the presence of peritoneal disease ($P = 0.002$), and higher solid tumor volumes ($P = 0.002$) of ovarian masses were all associated with low-grade serous ovarian cancer vs borderline disease in a retrospective study of 59 women with serous borderline disease or low-grade serous ovarian cancer.[13] Low-grade serous ovarian cancer also frequently has intratumor calcifications see on CT imaging and may display increased calcifications in response to treatment.

Diagnostic tests

A diagnosis of low-grade serous ovarian cancer is most frequently made at time of explorative surgery. Patients are often taken to the operating room for a suspicious pelvic mass or for carcinomatosis. When imaging shows radiologic abnormalities limited to the ovaries only, patients should have intact removal of the mass without spillage and subsequent upstaging of disease. A percutaneous biopsy should never be performed in this scenario. When patients have widely metastatic disease eon imaging and are either poor surgical candidates or perceived

TABLE 6.2 Diagnostic tests/work-up at time of diagnosis of low-grade serous ovarian cancer.

Imaging	Contrasted CT of abdomen and pelvis and chest imaging with PA and lateral chest X-ray or chest CT
Tumor marker	CA-125
Genetic testing	BRCA (germline) and tumor somatic testing to look for BRCA and MAPK alterations
Counseling	In those patients of child bearing age with suspected early stage disease, discussion should be had regarding potential for oocyte retrieval prior to surgery and/or fertility sparing surgery Genetic counseling for those patients with confirmed deleterious germline mutation
Surgical consultation	All patients with suspected ovarian cancer should meet with a gynecologic oncologist prior to surgical intervention

to have undebulkable disease, a percutaneous biopsy may be considered for diagnostic purposes to guide systemic therapies.

Staging system

Epithelial ovarian cancers, including low-grade serous tumors, are surgically and pathologically staged according to the 2017 eighth edition American Joint Committee on Cancer (AJCC) and the joint 2017 International Federation of Gynecology and Obstetrics (FIGO)/Tumor, Node, Metastasis (TNM) classification system (Table 6.3). The standard staging procedure for epithelial ovarian cancer includes total extra-fascial hysterectomy and bilateral salpingo-oophorectomy (BSO) with pelvic and paraaortic lymph node dissection if there is no gross evidence of intraperitoneal disease. Pelvic washings are collected, and omentectomy is performed. Further cytoreduction is dependent on each individual clinical situation.

Prognostic factors

Patients with serous borderline disease with micropapillary features are more likely to progress to invasive low-grade serous ovarian cancer than those without micropapillary features. In a study of 52 invasive low-grade serous ovarian tumors by Ahn et al., 95% of the low-grade serous ovarian tumors exhibited a micropapillary and/or complex papillary pattern of invasion. Therefore, some pathologists label SBT with a micropapillary pattern as noninvasive low-grade serous cancer, even in the absence of destructive stromal invasion.[14] Immunohistochemistry and somatic tumor testing many help to both aide in determination of treatment options for recurrent disease and help with prognostication.[15] Presence of a somatic *V600E BRAF* mutation in patients with serous borderline disease may be associated with improved prognosis and decreased likelihood of progression.[4,5] In a study by Chui et al., mutational analysis of the *KRAS* and *BRAF* genes was performed on 201 SBTs following centralized pathology review. The *BRAF* mutated tumors were less likely to exhibit micropapillary features ($P < 0.0001$) and were more frequently stage I ($P = 0.0023$).[16] While presence of a *KRAS* or *BRAF* mutation in the tumor of patients with low-grade serous ovarian cancer is prognostic of better outcomes, it may also predict for better response rates to treatment with MEK inhibitors. In a study of 79 cases of low-grade serous ovarian cancer with tumor tissue available for Sanger sequencing analysis, the 21 patients with presence of *KRAS* or *BRAF* mutation had a significantly better overall survival than those with wild-type *KRAS* or *BRAF* ($n = 58$) [106.7 months (95% CI, 50.6–162.9) vs 66.8 months (95% CI, 43.6–90)], respectively ($P = 0.018$).[17] A *post hoc* analysis performed by Grisham et al. on archival tumor tissues submitted at time of study entry to the MILO/ENGOT-ov11 Phase III study of binimetinib vs physicians choice of chemotherapy showed that those patients harboring a *KRAS* mutation in their tumor had 3.4 times the odds of responding to treatment with the MEK inhibitor binimetinib vs those without a KRAS mutation (95% CI, 1.57–7.67; $P = 0.002$).[18]

Treatment of primary disease

At time of diagnosis all patients should be referred to a gynecologic oncologist for surgical staging (Fig. 6.7). Fertility-sparing surgery with unilateral salpingo-oophorectomy (USO) or BSO can be considered in patients with early stage disease desiring future fertility. Patients being considered for fertility sparing surgery should have disease grossly limited to one

TABLE 6.3 TNM and FIGO staging for ovary, fallopian tube, and primary peritoneal carcinomas.

T category	FIGO stage	T criteria
		Primary tumor (T)
TX		Primary tumor cannot be assessed
T0		No evidence of primary tumor
T1	I	Tumor limited to ovaries (one or both) or fallopian tube(s)
T1a	IA	Tumor limited to one ovary (capsule intact) or fallopian tube, no tumor on ovarian or fallopian tube surface; no malignant cells in ascites or peritoneal washings
T1b	IB	Tumor limited to both ovaries (capsules intact) or fallopian tubes; no tumor on ovarian or fallopian tube surface; no malignant cells in ascites or peritoneal washings
T1c	IC	Tumor limited to one or both ovaries or fallopian tubes, with any of the following:
T1c1	IC1	• Surgical spill
T1c2	IC2	• Capsule ruptured before surgery or tumor on ovarian or fallopian tube surface
T1c3	IC3	• Malignant cells in ascites or peritoneal washings
T2	II	Tumor involves one or both ovaries or fallopian tubes with pelvic extension below pelvic brim or primary peritoneal cancer
T2a	IIA	Extension and/or implants on the uterus and/or fallopian tube(s) and/or ovaries
T2b	IIB	Extension to and/or implants on other pelvic tissues
T3	III	Tumor involves one or both ovaries or fallopian tubes, or primary peritoneal cancer, with microscopically confirmed peritoneal metastasis outside the pelvis and/or metastasis to the retroperitoneal (pelvic and/or paraaortic) lymph nodes
T3a	IIIA2	Microscopic extrapelvic (above the pelvic brim) peritoneal involvement with or without positive retroperitoneal lymph nodes
T3b	IIIB	Macroscopic peritoneal metastasis beyond pelvis 2 cm or less in greatest dimension with or without metastasis to the retroperitoneal lymph nodes
T3c	IIIC	Macroscopic peritoneal metastasis beyond the pelvis more than 2 cm in greatest dimension with or without metastasis to the retroperitoneal lymph nodes (includes extension of tumor to capsule of liver and spleen without parenchymal involvement of either organ)

N category	FIGO stage	N criteria
		Regional lymph nodes (N)
NX		Regional lymph nodes cannot be assessed
N0		No regional lymph node metastasis
N0(i+)		Isolated tumor cells in regional lymph node(s) no greater than 0.2 mm
N1	IIIA1	Positive retroperitoneal lymph nodes only (histologically confirmed)
N1a	IIIA1i	Metastasis up to and including 10 mm in greatest dimension
N1b	IIIA1ii	Metastasis more than 10 mm in greatest dimension

M category	FIGO stage	M criteria
		Distant metastasis (M)
M0		No distant metastasis
M1	IV	Distant metastasis, including pleural effusion with positive cytology; liver or splenic parenchymal metastasis; metastasis to extraabdominal organs (including inguinal lymph nodes and lymph nodes outside the abdominal cavity); and transmural involvement of intestine
M1a	IVA	Pleural effusion with positive cytology
M1b	IVB	Liver or splenic parenchymal metastases; metastases to extraabdominal organs (including inguinal lymph nodes and lymph nodes outside the abdominal cavity); transmural involvement of intestine

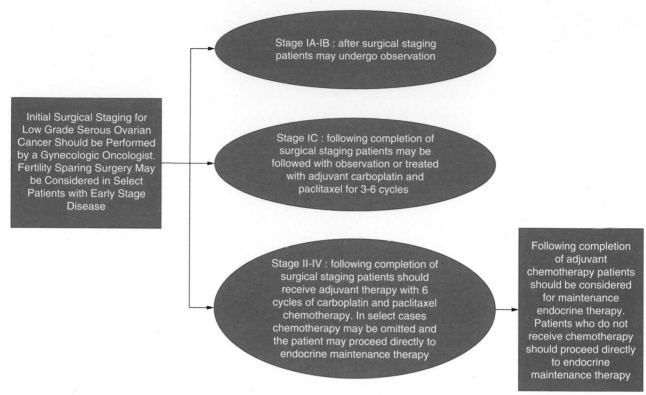

FIG. 6.7   Treatment algorithm for newly diagnosed low-grade serous ovarian cancer.

ovary and should be referred to a reproductive endocrinologist for consideration of preoperative oocyte retrieval. Patients with advanced disease should under complete surgical staging with total hysterectomy (TAH), BSO, omentectomy lymph node dissection, washings, and attempted removal of all gross disease via either and open or minimally invasive approach.

Following completion of surgical staging for those patients with Stage Ia or Ib disease, observation alone is recommended. For those patients with Stage Ic disease observation or 3 cycles of adjuvant chemotherapy may be considered. For those patients receiving adjuvant chemotherapy the standard regimen is chemotherapy with carboplatin (at an AUC of 5–6) administered in conjunction with paclitaxel 175 mg/m^2 in a 3 week cycle. For those patients with stage II-IV disease 6 cycles of adjuvant carboplatin/paclitaxel chemotherapy are recommended with consideration for maintenance endocrine therapy (most commonly with an aromatase inhibitor, i.e., letrozole 2.5 mg daily) following completion of chemotherapy. There is not currently a standard of care as to how long aromatase inhibitor therapy is continued following completion of upfront chemotherapy; however if well tolerated and there is no evidence of disease progression, it is generally continued for 5–10 years after completion of chemotherapy. The recommendation for use of aromatase inhibitor maintenance following completion of adjuvant chemotherapy is based upon a retrospective study performed by Gershenson and colleagues examining their patients with stage II-IV low-grade serous ovarian cancer treated at MD Anderson Cancer Center between 1981 and 2013. All patients examined were treated with primary cytoreductive surgery followed by platinum based-chemotherapy. At completion of chemotherapy patients were either followed with observation or endocrine maintenance therapy, as per their attending physician's discretion. Median PFS for patients followed with observation following chemotherapy was 26.4 months compared with 64.9 months for those receiving endocrine maintenance therapy after completion of chemotherapy ($P < 0.001$); however, there was not a statistically significant difference observed in overall survival between the two groups (102.7 vs 115.7 months, respectively).[19] Multiple retrospective studies have shown that response rates to cytotoxic chemotherapy in the frontline setting are lower in low-grade serous ovarian cancer then in high-grade serous ovarian cancer. Grabowski and colleagues examined 5114 patients treated on 4 randomized phase III trials with first-line platinum based chemotherapy in women with metastatic epithelial ovarian cancer, response rates to chemotherapy in those patients with suboptimal debulking were reported, and found a response rate of 23.1% in the patients with low-grade serous ovarian cancer vs 90.1% in those with high-grade serous ovarian cancer.[20] In select patients, particularly those at higher risk of chemotherapy associated complications, or those who decline chemotherapy, hormonal maintenance therapy alone (without adjuvant chemotherapy) may be considered. The addition of bevacizumab 15 mg/kg in combination with upfront carboplatin/paclitaxel chemotherapy, followed by 15 months of bevacizumab maintenance at completion of chemotherapy, may also be considered for patients with advanced disease, particularly those with high-risk features of suboptimal debulking or stage IV disease; however, for patients without high-risk features, bevacizumab is often omitted in favor of aromatase inhibitor maintenance.

Surveillance for recurrence

Following completion of surgery and adjuvant chemotherapy (if chemotherapy is delivered) all patients should continue in active follow-up with monitoring for recurrence of disease. All patients should have follow-up visits every 2–4 months for 2 years and then every 3–6 months for 3 years, and then at least annually after 5 years. Patients require long term follow-up as late recurrences can occur after 5 years of remission. At each follow-up visit a physical exam, review of systems, and ca-125 blood test (if elevated at time of diagnosis) should be performed. Serial imaging with contrasted CT of abdomen and pelvis and chest imaging with CT or X-ray should be done as clinically indicated, and we recommend completed every 6 months for those patients with advanced disease at time of diagnosis, spacing out to annually after at least 3 years of follow-up. Patients being maintained on aromatase inhibitor maintenance therapy should have a bone density performed prior to start of treatment and annually thereafter, with osteoporosis treated as clinically appropriate.

Survival and patterns of failure

Similar to high-grade serous ovarian cancer, the majority of patents with low-grade serous ovarian cancer will initially present with advanced stage disease and ultimately develop recurrent disease. For those patients who develop recurrent disease it is generally considered to be a chronic (incurable) condition. Given the relatively chemoresistant nature of low-grade serous ovarian cancer, it is important that patients with low-grade serous ovarian cancer continue to follow with a gynecologic oncologist for consideration of future debulking surgery. Patients may have multiple resections of recurrent disease over the course of their life and should be considered for secondary, and in some cases even later line debulking surgery as clinically appropriate. A randomized phase III study of secondary cytoreduction followed by chemotherapy vs chemotherapy alone in platinum-sensitive relapsed ovarian cancer (SOC-1) allowed enrollment of all patients with epithelial ovarian cancer and found a significantly longer median progression-free survival (PFS) of 17.4 months (95% CI, 15–19.8) in the surgery group vs 11.9 months in the no surgery group (HR 0.58; 95% CI, 0.45–0.74; $P < 0.0001$); however, the majority of patients enrolled to the study had serous grade 2 or 3 disease (303/357), and data is not available regarding outcomes in patients with low-grade serous ovarian cancer in particular.[21] In a retrospective study of 41 women with recurrent low-grade serous ovarian cancer, those who achieved a complete gross resection (CGR) of disease had a significantly better PFS (60.3 months vs 10.7 months) and OS (93.6 months vs 45.8 months) from the time of secondary surgery when compared with those patients who had gross residual disease following surgery.[22]

Treatment of recurrent disease
"Standard" or commonly used regimens

As is the case with high-grade serous ovarian cancer, at time of recurrence patients are classified as platinum sensitive or platinum resistant based upon the time between completion of last platinum based chemotherapy and diagnosis of recurrent disease (Table 6.4). For those patients with platinum sensitive disease (>6 months since completion of last platinum based chemotherapy) it is appropriate to treat with a platinum based doublet again. Platinum based doublets can include carboplatin in combination with paclitaxel, carboplatin in combination with gemcitabine, or carboplatin in combination with pegylated liposomal doxorubicin (PLD), all either alone or in combination with bevacizumab followed by bevacizumab maintenance. For those patients with platinum resistant disease (recurrence <6 months since completion of last platinum based therapy) PLD or weekly paclitaxel, alone or in combination with bevacizumab are early line options. Bevacizumab has been observed to have activity in patients with recurrent low-grade serous ovarian cancer either alone or in combination with chemotherapy in multiple retrospective studies.[23,24]

Unlike in high-grade serous ovarian cancer, endocrine therapy is frequently used in the treatment of recurrent low-grade serous ovarian cancer, especially for those patients with low volume or indolent disease where disease stability is sought. The majority of low-grade serous ovarian cancer cases are hormone receptor positive (87%

TABLE 6.4 Common options for systemic treatment of low-grade serous ovarian cancer.

Chemotherapy	
	Platinum sensitive regimens:
	– Carboplatin (AUC of 4) in combination with gemcitabine (1000 mg/m^2) ± bevacizumab 15 mg/kg
	– Carboplatin (AUC of 5) in combination with liposomal doxorubicin 30 mg/m^2 ± bevacizumab 15 mg/kg
	– Carboplatin (AUC of 5) in combination with paclitaxel (175 mg/m^2) ± bevacizumab 15 mg/kg
	Platinum resistant regimens:
	– Doxil 40 mg/m^2 ± bevacizumab 10 mg/kg
	– Weekly Paclitaxel 80 mg/m^2 ± bevacizumab 10 mg/kg
	– Topotecan 1.25 mg/m^2 daily × 5 days ± bevacizumab 15 mg/kg
	– Pemetrexed 375 mg/m^2
	– Vinorelbine 30 mg/m^2
	– Gemcitabine 1000 mg/m^2
	– Oral etoposide 50 mg/m^2
Biologic	
	Bevacizumab 15 mg/kg
Endocrine	
	Letrozole 2.5 mg
	Anastrozole 1 mg
	Exemestane 25 mg
	Fulvestrant 500 mg
	Tamoxifen 20 mg
	Leuprolide acetate
Targeted therapy	
	Trametinib 2 mg
	Binimetinib 45mg BID

ER positive; 58% PR positive).[25] In a single-institution study of 64 patients with recurrent low-grade serous ovarian cancer treated with 89 endocrine regimens over time the objective response rate to endocrine therapy was 9% and 61.8% of patients experienced stable disease.[26] The most common hormonal agents used for treatment in this study were anastrozole, fulvestrant, letrozole, leuprolide, and megace. In the phase II/III study of trametinib vs physicians' choice of therapy in patients with recurrent low-grade serous ovarian cancer, patients treated in the control arm were allowed to receive chemotherapy or endocrine therapy with letrozole or tamoxifen. While 0/27 patients treated with tamoxifen achieved an objective response the response rate to letrozole was 13.6% (6/44). Therefore, letrozole is generally the preferred regimen for endocrine therapy of this disease.[27] Potential Therapeutic Targets/Molecular testing/mutations.

Low-grade serous ovarian cancer has a distinct molecular profile from high-grade serous ovarian cancer. In high-grade serous ovarian cancer p53 mutations are ubiquitous and alterations affecting the MAP Kinase (mitogen-activated protein kinase) pathway are quite rare, while in low-grade serous ovarian cancer patient's tumors are generally p53 wildtype.[28] The genomic alterations found in tumors of patients with low-grade serous ovarian cancer are most frequently those affecting the MAP Kinase pathway. The most common somatic mutation identified is a *KRAS* mutation, which is found in 33% of patients with recurrent disease; other MAP Kinase pathway alterations identified in this population include *NRAS* (8%), *RAF1* (2%), *NF1* (5%), and *BRAFV600E* (6%) mutations.[11,18,29,30] This, in combination with the comparatively lower response rates to chemotherapy vs high-grade serous ovarian cancer, has led to considerable interest in the development of targeted therapies for treatment of recurrent low-grade serous ovarian cancer.

The first prospective clinical trial to examine the use of single agent MEK inhibitors for recurrent low-grade serous ovarian cancer was a single arm study (GOG 0239) that treated women with recurrent measurable low-grade serous ovarian cancer with selumetinib (AZD6244) until time of progression or intolerable toxicity. The study showed a promising objective response rate of 15%. No correlation was found between presence of *KRAS* or *BRAF* mutation and response to therapy; however, sufficient DNA was available for analysis in only 34 (65%) of the 52 of evaluable patients.[31]

Since that time, two randomized phase 3 studies have been performed comparing single agent MEK inhibitors to standard of care therapy in patients with recurrent measurable low-grade serous ovarian cancer. The GOG 0281 phase II/III study of the MEK inhibitor trametinib vs physician's choice of chemotherapy or endocrine therapy in patients with recurrent disease and unlimited prior lines of chemotherapy found a significant difference in median PFS with trametinib (13 months) vs physician's choice of chemotherapy (7.2 months; HR = 0.48; $P < 0.001$). The overall response rate (ORR) was 26 and 6.2% for trametinib and physician's choice, respectively ($P < 0.0001$).[27] The MILO/ENGOT-ov11 study was a phase III study of the MEK inhibitor binimetinib vs physician's choice of chemotherapy in patients with recurrent low-grade serous ovarian. Unlike GOG 0281, the MILO/EBGOT-ov11 study limited patients to a maximum of three prior lines of chemotherapy. Although the study was discontinued early based on an interim analysis revealing that the PFS hazard ratio crossed the predefined futility boundary, an updated analysis indicated a median PFS of 10.4 months for binimetinib vs 11.5 months for physician's choice (HR = 1.15; $P = 0.748$), and an ORR of 24% in both arms of the study. Notably, for patients treated with binimetinib, the ORR and median PFS in the *KRAS* mutant group (ORR = 44%; median PFS = 17.7 months) were significantly better than in the *KRAS* wild-type group (ORR = 19%; median PFS = 10.8 months) ($P = 0.006$)[32] indicating that patients with somatic *KRAS* mutations may be most likely to respond to MEK inhibitor treatment. Trametinib and binimetinib are NCCN compendium listed for treatment of recurrent low-grade serous ovarian cancer and multiple clinical trials are ongoing with MEK inhibitor combinations, seeking to build upon the response rate seen with single agent therapy and to define the molecular subgroup of patients most likely to benefit from targeted therapy.

There is a paucity of data regarding the use of PARP inhibitors in low-grade serous ovarian cancer. However, given that low-grade serous ovarian cancer is less sensitive to platinum based chemotherapy in the upfront and recurrent setting, and rarely associated with BRCA mutations, we generally favor the use of endocrine maintenance or bevacizumab maintenance over the use of PARP inhibitor maintenance for these patients.

Immunotherapy targets

Immunotherapy is currently not a standard of care therapy for low-grade serous ovarian cancer and should not be administered outside of a clinical trial unless the patient meets one of the molecular solid tumor criteria for treatment with immunotherapy in the recurrent setting (MMR deficient, MSI-high, or TMB high).

Case resolution

At this time the patient has platinum resistant recurrent low-grade serous ovarian cancer. Options for therapy include chemotherapy with or without bevacizumab, biologic therapy with bevacizumab alone, endocrine therapy, or targeted therapy. As noted in the history, her initial molecular testing showed a *KRAS* mutation, which may predicted for improved response rate to targeted therapy with a MEK inhibitor based on the MILO/ENGOT-ov11 study. While multiple options are available, treatment either on a clinical trial with targeted therapy or initiation of standard of care therapy with trametinib 2 mg by mouth daily or binimetinib 45mg PO BID would be good options.

References

1. Bodurka DC, et al. Reclassification of serous ovarian carcinoma by a 2-tier system: a gynecologic oncology group study. *Cancer*. 2012;118 (12):3087–3094.
2. Grisham RN. Low-grade serous carcinoma of the ovary. *Oncology (Williston Park)*. 2016;30(7):650–652.
3. Vang R, et al. Long-term behavior of serous borderline tumors subdivided into atypical proliferative tumors and noninvasive low-grade carcinomas: a population-based clinicopathologic study of 942 cases. *Am J Surg Pathol*. 2017;41(6):725–737.
4. Grisham RN, et al. BRAF mutation is associated with early stage disease and improved outcome in patients with low-grade serous ovarian cancer. *Cancer*. 2012.
5. Wong KK, et al. BRAF mutation is rare in advanced-stage low-grade ovarian serous carcinomas. *Am J Pathol*. 2010;177(4):1611–1617.

6. Grisham RN, et al. BRAF mutation is associated with early stage disease and improved outcome in patients with low-grade serous ovarian cancer. *Cancer.* 2013;119(3):548–554.

7. Vang R, Davidson B, Kong CS, et al. Serous borderline tumor of the ovary. In: WHO Classification of Tumors Editorial Board, ed. *Female Genital Tumors.* World Health Organization Classification of Tumors. Lyon: IARC Press; 2020:38–42.

8. Longacre TA, Davidson B, Folkins AK, et al. Low grade serous carcinoma of the ovary. In: WHO Classification of Tumors Editorial Board, ed. *Female Genital Tumors.* World Health Organization Classification of Tumors. Lyon: IARC Press; 2020:43–44.

9. Jones S, Wang T-L, Kurman RJ, et al. Low-grade serous carcinomas of the ovary contain very few point mutations. *J Pathol.* 2012;226(3):413–420.

10. Sieben NL, Macropoulos P, Roemen GM, et al. In ovarian neoplasms, BRAF, but not KRAS, mutations are restricted to low-grade serous tumours. *J Pathol.* 2004;202(3):336–340.

11. Singer G, Oldt 3rd R, Cohen Y, et al. Mutations in BRAF and KRAS characterize the development of low-grade ovarian serous carcinoma. *J Natl Cancer Inst.* 2003;95(6):484–486.

12. Fader AN, et al. The prognostic significance of pre- and post-treatment CA-125 in grade 1 serous ovarian carcinoma: a gynecologic oncology group study. *Gynecol Oncol.* 2014;132(3):560–565.

13. Nougaret S, et al. CT features of ovarian tumors: defining key differences between serous borderline tumors and low-grade serous carcinomas. *AJR Am J Roentgenol.* 2018;210(4):918–926.

14. Ahn G, et al. Low-grade serous carcinoma of the ovary: clinicopathologic analysis of 52 invasive cases and identification of a possible noninvasive intermediate lesion. *Am J Surg Pathol.* 2016;40(9):1165–1176.

15. Turashvili G, et al. BRAF(V)(600E) mutations and immunohistochemical expression of VE1 protein in low-grade serous neoplasms of the ovary. *Histopathology.* 2018.

16. Chui MH, et al. BRAF(V600E)-mutated ovarian serous borderline tumors are at relatively low risk for progression to serous carcinoma. *Oncotarget.* 2019;10(64):6870–6878.

17. Gershenson DM, Sun CC, Wong KK. Impact of mutational status on survival in low-grade serous carcinoma of the ovary or peritoneum. *Br J Cancer.* 2015;113(9):1254–1258.

18. Grisham RN, Banerjee SN, Drill EN, et al. Molecular results and potential biomarkers identified from MILO/ENGOT-ov11 phase 3 study of binimetinib versus physicians choice of chemotherapy (PCC) in recurrent low-grade serous ovarian cancer (LGSOC). *J Clin Oncol.* 2021;39 [suppl 15; abstr 5519].

19. Gershenson DM, et al. Hormonal maintenance therapy for women with low-grade serous cancer of the ovary or peritoneum. *J Clin Oncol.* 2017; 35(10):1103–1111.

20. Grabowski JP, et al. Operability and chemotherapy responsiveness in advanced low-grade serous ovarian cancer. An analysis of the AGO study group metadatabase. *Gynecol Oncol.* 2016;140(3):457–462.

21. Shi T, et al. Secondary cytoreduction followed by chemotherapy versus chemotherapy alone in platinum-sensitive relapsed ovarian cancer (SOC-1): a multicentre, open-label, randomised, phase 3 trial. *Lancet Oncol.* 2021;22(4):439–449.

22. Crane EK, et al. The role of secondary cytoreduction in low-grade serous ovarian cancer or peritoneal cancer. *Gynecol Oncol.* 2015;136(1):25–29.

23. Grisham RN, et al. Bevacizumab shows activity in patients with low-grade serous ovarian and primary peritoneal cancer. *Int J Gynecol Cancer.* 2014;24(6):1010–1014.

24. Dalton HJ, et al. Activity of bevacizumab-containing regimens in recurrent low-grade serous ovarian or peritoneal cancer: a single institution experience. *Gynecol Oncol.* 2017;145(1):37–40.

25. Sieh W, et al. Hormone-receptor expression and ovarian cancer survival: an ovarian tumor tissue analysis consortium study. *Lancet Oncol.* 2013; 14(9):853–862.

26. Gershenson DM, et al. Hormonal therapy for recurrent low-grade serous carcinoma of the ovary or peritoneum. *Gynecol Oncol.* 2012;125(3):661–666.

27. Gershenson DM, Miller A, Brady W, et al. A randomized phase II/III study to assess the efficacy of trametinib in patients with recurrent or progressive low-grade serous ovarian or peritoneal cancer. *Ann Oncol.* 2019;30(suppl. 5):v851–v934. https://doi.org/10.1093/annonc/mdz394.2019.

28. Vang R, Shih Ie M, Kurman RJ. Ovarian low-grade and high-grade serous carcinoma: pathogenesis, clinicopathologic and molecular biologic features, and diagnostic problems. *Adv Anat Pathol.* 2009;16(5):267–282.

29. Grisham RN, et al. Extreme outlier analysis identifies occult mitogen-activated protein kinase pathway mutations in patients with low-grade serous ovarian cancer. *J Clin Oncol.* 2015;33(34):4099–4105.

30. Kelemen L, et al. BRAF polymorphisms and the risk of ovarian cancer of low malignant potential. *Gynecol Oncol.* 2005;97(3):807–812.

31. Farley J, et al. Selumetinib in women with recurrent low-grade serous carcinoma of the ovary or peritoneum: an open-label, single-arm, phase 2 study. *Lancet Oncol.* 2012.

32. Monk BJ, et al. MILO/ENGOT-ov11: binimetinib versus physician's choice chemotherapy in recurrent or persistent low-grade serous carcinomas of the ovary, fallopian tube, or primary peritoneum. *J Clin Oncol.* 2020;, JCO2001164.

Chapter 7

Small cell carcinoma of the ovary, hypercalcemic type

Douglas A. Levine, Donato Callegaro Filho, Elizabeth Kertowidjojo, and M. Herman Chui

Clinical case

A 22-year-old G0 female presents with a newly diagnosed small cell carcinoma of the ovary, hypercalcemic type (SCCOHT). She reported pelvic pain and her physical exam was within normal limits. Pelvic sonography identified a 5 cm complex cystic mass in the left ovary with increased vascularity in multiple nodules (Fig. 7.1). She was thought to have an endometrioma and was taken to the operating room by a gynecologist where she had a left ovarian cystectomy performed. Intraoperative findings did not identify any evidence of disseminated disease. There was cyst rupture during the procedure, and preoperative tumor markers were not sent. Final pathology identified SCCOHT, and the patient underwent completion left oophorectomy with comprehensive minimally invasive surgical staging by a gynecologic oncologist. She was diagnosed with FIGO stage IIIA SCCOHT with disease found in the residual ovary and one aortocaval node, but all other specimens were negative. She is in excellent health and has her contralateral ovary *in situ*. The patient desires fertility-sparing treatment for her disease. How do you treat this patient?

Epidemiology

Incidence and mortality

SCCOHT unfortunately shares a similar name with small cell neuroendocrine carcinoma of the ovary (sometimes termed pulmonary type), and these two exceedingly rare histologies are often confused. The molecular basis of these two malignancies is distinct, and the cells of origin, though unknown at present, are likely different. This chapter will focus on SCCOHT. SCCOHT is a very rare and aggressive malignancy usually identified in teenage girls and young women. The mean age at diagnosis is 24 years and most cases occur before age 40.[1] The long-term survival for advanced stage cases is extremely dismal; however, more recent reports suggest some anecdotal success with targeted therapeutics, as discussed below. The true incidence of SCCOHT is unknown due to historical difficulty with making a definitive diagnosis and a myriad of histologic mimics, such as poorly differentiated sex cord stromal tumors and various tumors that are metastatic to the ovary.[2] Based on informal discussions with various global experts who have access to registry data, a very rough estimate of SCCOHT incidence of 0.1% of all ovarian cancer cases are SCCOHT, which would translate to ~22 cases per year in the United States. The true incidence is unknown; however, as definitive diagnoses are becoming more robust, this estimate may become more precise over the next decade. The ensure the most accurate diagnosis, histologic assessments should be routinely coupled with protein or DNA analyses as discussed below. The largest collective case series to date collated 293 patients to analyze clinical, pathologic, and genetic features.[3] The overall survival for all patients with available data was 39%, and few patients recurred after 5 years as may be expected for an aggressive malignancy. Stage for stage, SCCOHT has a worse prognosis than most ovarian cancers. The collective review reports a five-year survival of 55% for stage I patients, 30 to 40% for stage II and III, and no long-term survival for patients diagnosed at stage IV (Fig. 7.2). The actual survival for patients with available data was 39% and few patients recurred after 5 years as may be expected for an aggressive malignancy.

Etiology and risk factors

The etiology of SCCOHT remains mostly a mystery at this point. A number of laboratories are conducting complex studies to try and identify the cell of origin. The tumor has many molecular and morphologic similarities to malignant rhabdoid

Diagnosis and Treatment of Rare Gynecologic Cancers. https://doi.org/10.1016/B978-0-323-82938-0.00007-0

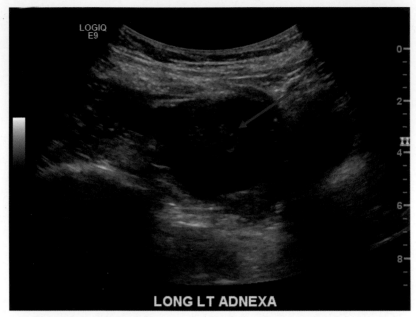

FIG. 7.1 Ultrasound view of complex mass on left ovary. Arrow showing solid component.

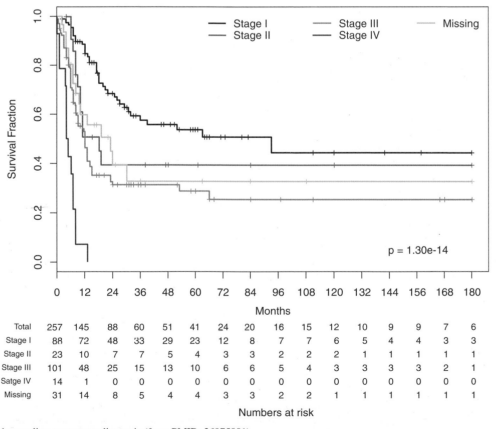

FIG. 7.2 Survival according to stage at diagnosis (from PMID: 26975901).

tumors suggesting a mesenchymal origin, but details are far from clear.[4] The only well-defined risk factor for SCCOHT is genetic predisposition due to inherited germline mutation in *SMARCA4*. These germline mutations should certainly be suspected in any family member with more than one case of SCCOHT, which unfortunately has been reported several times in addition to other known cases that have not been published.[5] The exact frequency of *SMARCA4* germline mutations in SCCOHT is estimated to be between 10% and 40% and the penetrance is presently unknown though inheritance patterns are generally paternal.[3,6] This wide range of estimates is due to ascertainment bias where some cases are collected from genetic testing clinics and others originate from oncologic practices. All patients with SCCOHT should have germline genetic testing for *SMARCA4*. If the proband is unavailable for testing, at-risk first-degree family members should have genetic counseling and consider testing. *SMARCA4* is a member of the SWI/SNF chromatin-remodeling complexes and has defined roles in transcriptional regulation, DNA-damage repair, and immune surveillance.[7]

Pathology

Gross

Tumors are unilateral, large (mean 15 cm), soft and fleshy, gray-tan, and predominantly solid, but may have a cystic component, and often with areas of hemorrhage and necrosis. The external surface is smooth or nodular. Familial cases may be bilateral.

Histopathologic features

SCCOHT is typically characterized by small monomorphic undifferentiated cells with high nuclear-cytoplasmic ratio and brisk mitotic activity (Fig. 7.3A). The tumor cells are arranged in solid sheets, nests, cords, or trabeculae with little intervening stroma. Follicle-like spaces filled with eosinophilic or basophilic secretions are a characteristic histologic feature (Fig. 7.3B). Areas of geographic necrosis and vascular invasion are frequent findings. Approximately half of these tumors exhibit varying proportions of large cells with abundant eosinophilic cytoplasm and are designated as the "large cell variant of small cell carcinoma."[8] The tumor cells have eccentrically placed nuclei and along with the abundant eosinophilic cytoplasm impart a rhabdoid appearance. Mucinous cysts and glands may be present in a subset of cases. Rarely the mucinous component may be malignant.

Immunohistochemistry

SCCOHT are variably positive for epithelial markers, including cytokeratins (CAM5.2, AE1/AE3), EMA, and Claudin-4 (CLDN4). WT1, CD10, and calretinin can be positive, and tumors may exhibit diffuse overexpression of p53. Negative immunoreactivity is seen with inhibin, CD99, TTF1, and desmin. BRG1 (SMARCA4) shows loss of expression and is diagnostic of this tumor; it is lost in greater than 95% of SCCOHT and is almost always intact in other tumors in the differential diagnosis[2] (Fig. 7.3C).

Differential diagnosis

The differential diagnosis includes granulosa cell tumor, particularly the juvenile type. In juvenile granulosa cell tumor (JGCT), small cells are not typically present, and the lining of follicles tends to be smoother with more cellular cohesion compared to SCCOHT, in which the follicle-like spaces tend to be irregular with cellular discohesion. Adult granulosa cell tumors exhibit characteristic nuclear grooves, not seen in SCCOHT. Other small round blue cell tumors that enter into the differential diagnosis include lymphoma, melanoma, rhabdomyosarcoma (embryonal-type), and desmoplastic small round cell tumor. Usually, these can be excluded by careful immunohistochemical workup, as they show distinct immunomarker profiles. In particular, loss of BRG1 (SMARCA4) expression has been shown to be a sensitive and specific marker for SCCOHT.[2]

Molecular features

SCCOHTs are characterized by pathognomonic inactivating somatic or germline mutations in *SMARCA4* gene (encoding protein BRG1), implicated in the SWI/SNF chromatin remodeling complex.[6] *SMARCA4* acts as a tumor suppressor gene requiring loss of both alleles to result in development of SCCOHT. Consideration of removal of the uninvolved ovary and testing of close family members should be considered in patients with germline mutations.[9] Despite frequently showing p53 overexpression by immunohistochemistry, *TP53* mutation is extremely rare in this tumor type. SCCOHT is typically diploid and exhibits low mutational burden.

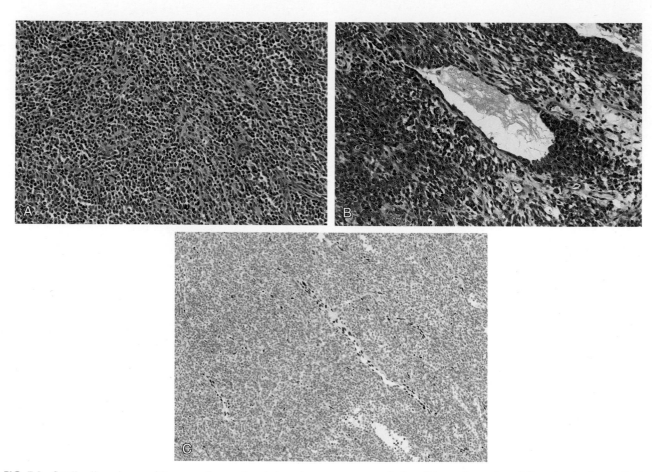

FIG. 7.3 Small cell carcinoma of the ovary, hypercalcemic type, is a tumor composed of small hyperchromatic undifferentiated cells (A). Foci of follicle-like spaces filled with eosinophilic and or basophilic secretions are frequently identified (B). Immunohistochemical staining shows loss of BRG1 (SMARCA4) in the tumor cells (C).

Diagnosis and workup

Signs and symptoms

Women with SCCOHT may present with various symptoms associated with a pelvic mass or advanced ovarian cancer. These commonly would include pelvic pain, frequent urination, bloating, early satiety, nausea, and menstrual irregularities. Increased abdominal girth may be a sign associated with a large abdomino-pelvic mass or large volume ascites.

Physical exam findings

For most women with small ovarian masses, physical exam findings may be within normal limits. A pelvic mass may be appreciated on pelvic exam if the mass is of sufficient size to be differentiated from surrounding soft tissues. Abdominal exam may identify a palpable abdominal mass in women with sizable omental disease, or other related findings. Imaging features are likely to be more useful during the initial evaluation of symptoms than physical findings.

Differential diagnosis

Differential diagnosis for SCCOHT can be wide. There are numerous histologic mimics of SCCOHT discussed previously (see Section "Pathology").[2] Based on the extreme rarity of this tumor, initial clinical symptoms, and radiographic presentation, it can be very challenging for a reasonable practitioner to include SCCOHT in a preoperative differential diagnosis. Thus, most cases are encountered incidentally and only diagnosed at the time of permanent histologic sectioning. This lack of preoperative suspicion also hampers research efforts that often rely on newly diagnosed, untreated specimens for tissue banking and creation of patient-derived xenograft models.

Tumor markers

There are no clear serum tumor markers for women with SCCOHT. CA125 is often elevated due to involvement of the ovary and/or peritoneum. The increased expression can be variable, but when elevated preoperatively it can be a useful surveillance tool for recurrent disease. Other routine tumor markers such as CEA, CA19–9, inhibin, AFP, LDH, and hCG can be useful in the preoperative differential diagnosis. In some situations, these tumor markers may be elevated, but this would also open the differential to other types of ovarian tumors.

Hypercalcemia is found in up to 60% of cases. Common symptoms of hypercalcemia include dehydration, nausea, vomiting, constipation as well as neurologic symptoms such as confusion, lethargy, and fatigue. Serum calcium levels should be monitored at diagnosis and certainly in the recurrent setting.

Imaging studies

Many women with SCCOHT present with a pelvic mass. Often a pelvis sonogram is ordered based on symptomatology or findings at the time of pelvic exam. If a suspicious pelvic mass is identified, a CT scan of the abdomen and pelvis with oral and nonionic intravenous contrast should be performed. A chest CT should be added if extra-pelvic disease is identified. Common sites for metastatic disease outside the pelvis include the omentum, peritoneum, lymph nodes, and the liver. An MRI of the pelvis can be helpful to further characterize the morphology of a pelvic mass and identify invasion into surrounding structures.

Diagnostic testing

The definitive diagnosis if SCCOHT is made with tissue evaluation. Surgical resection, excisional biopsy, and incisional biopsy are all reasonable approaches to diagnose SCCOHT. Due to the rarity of this entity as well as the presence of histologic mimics, a correct diagnosis of SCCOHT can be quite challenging. In 2014, three independent research groups identified universal *SMARCA4* mutations in SCCOHT.[6,10,11] Robust antibodies exist for SMARCA4 protein. DNA sequencing or immunohistochemistry protein evaluation should be performed on all suspected cases of SCCOHT. If a mutation or loss of protein expression is not identified in the tumor cells, a diagnosis of SCCOHT should be strongly reconsidered. SMARCA2 protein is also, and uniquely, lost in SCCOHT, which can help with evaluating the differential diagnosis.[12] SMARCA4 is the most useful biomarker for confirming the diagnosis of SCCOHT.

Staging system

Staging for SCCOHT utilizes the FIGO staging system for ovarian cancer (Table 7.1). Unlike prior versions of the FIGO staging system for ovarian cancer, the 2014 version considers both microscopic disease outside of the pelvis and lymph node spread in a similar category.[13] The Tumor, Node, Metastasis (TNM) staging system (Table 7.1) may also be used to describe extent of disease but this is employed less often among gynecologic oncologists.

Prognostic factors

Clinical stage at diagnosis is the most important prognostic factor.[3] Five-year survival is 55% for stage I patients, 30% to 40% for stage II and III, and no long-term survival for patients diagnosed at stage IV (Fig. 7.2). Other reported prognostic factors include age at diagnosis and treatment modality. Patients diagnosed after age 40 appeared to have a worse outcome with a HR for death of 2.1 from multivariate analyses compared with patients less than 20 years old ($P = 0.04$). This may be a reflection of underlying disease biology or the inability to tolerate aggressive treatment regimens. Some oncologists recommend high-dose chemotherapy (HDC) with autologous stem cell rescue for patients who are in complete clinical remission after completion of initial adjuvant therapy. In a retrospective review, this treatment seemed to result in more favorable outcomes for a small subset of patients with stage II–IV disease. All multimodal therapies had improved outcomes compared to surgery alone with HR ranging from 0.14 for surgery and chemotherapy to 0.03 for surgery combined with chemotherapy, radiation therapy, and stem cell rescue. Though promising, these results are limited by sample size, retrospective survival bias, and selection bias.[14] The presence of hypercalcemia did not have an effect on prognosis.

Treatment of primary disease

There is no evidence-based consensus for the optimal treatment of SCCOHT. The available data are mainly composed of published case reports or retrospective series. A multimodal approach including nonconservative debulking surgery, multiagent chemotherapy and radiotherapy is proposed (Fig. 7.4).

TABLE 7.1 TNM and FIGO staging for ovary, fallopian tube, and primary peritoneal carcinomas.

Primary tumor (T)		
T category	**FIGO stage**	**T criteria**
TX		Primary tumor cannot be assessed
T0		No evidence of primary tumor
T1	I	Tumor limited to ovaries (one or both) or fallopian tube(s)
T1a	IA	Tumor limited to one ovary (capsule intact) or fallopian tube, no tumor on ovarian or fallopian tube surface; no malignant cells in ascites or peritoneal washings
T1b	IB	Tumor limited to both ovaries (capsules intact) or fallopian tubes; no tumor on ovarian or fallopian tube surface; no malignant cells in ascites or peritoneal washings
T1c	IC	Tumor limited to one or both ovaries or fallopian tubes, with any of the following:
T1c1	IC1	• Surgical spill
T1c2	IC2	• Capsule ruptured before surgery or tumor on ovarian or fallopian tube surface
T1c3	IC3	• Malignant cells in ascites or peritoneal washings
T2	II	Tumor involves one or both ovaries or fallopian tubes with pelvic extension below pelvic brim or primary peritoneal cancer
T2a	IIA	Extension and/or implants on the uterus and/or fallopian tube(s) and/or ovaries
T2b	IIB	Extension to and/or implants on other pelvic tissues
T3	III	Tumor involves one or both ovaries or fallopian tubes, or primary peritoneal cancer, with microscopically confirmed peritoneal metastasis outside the pelvis and/or metastasis to the retroperitoneal (pelvic and/or paraaortic) lymph nodes
T3a	IIIA2	Microscopic extrapelvic (above the pelvic brim) peritoneal involvement with or without positive retroperitoneal lymph nodes
T3b	IIIB	Macroscopic peritoneal metastasis beyond pelvis 2 cm or less in greatest dimension with or without metastasis to the retroperitoneal lymph nodes
T3c	IIIC	Macroscopic peritoneal metastasis beyond the pelvis more than 2 cm in greatest dimension with or without metastasis to the retroperitoneal lymph nodes (includes extension of tumor to capsule of liver and spleen without parenchymal involvement of either organ)

Regional lymph nodes (N)		
N category	**FIGO stage**	**N criteria**
NX		Regional lymph nodes cannot be assessed
N0		No regional lymph node metastasis
N0(i+)		Isolated tumor cells in regional lymph node(s) no greater than 0.2 mm
N1	IIIA1	Positive retroperitoneal lymph nodes only (histologically confirmed)
N1a	IIIA1i	Metastasis up to and including 10 mm in greatest dimension
N1b	IIIA1ii	Metastasis more than 10 mm in greatest dimension

Distant metastasis (M)		
M category	**FIGO stage**	**M criteria**
M0		No distant metastasis
M1	IV	Distant metastasis, including pleural effusion with positive cytology; liver or splenic parenchymal metastasis; metastasis to extraabdominal organs (including inguinal lymph nodes and lymph nodes outside the abdominal cavity); and transmural involvement of intestine
M1a	IVA	Pleural effusion with positive cytology
M1b	IVB	Liver or splenic parenchymal metastases; metastases to extraabdominal organs (including inguinal lymph nodes and lymph nodes outside the abdominal cavity); transmural involvement of intestine

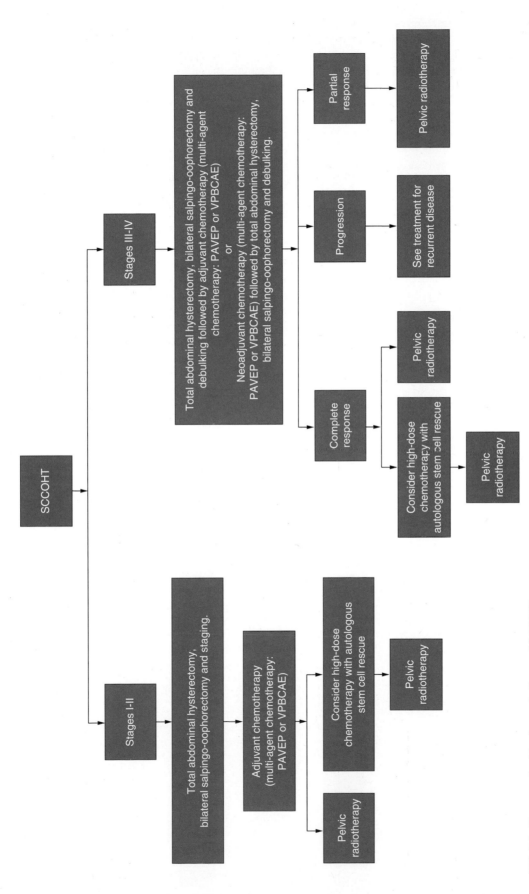

FIG. 7.4 Treatment algorithm for newly diagnosed SCCOHT.

Surgical resection is considered the main therapeutic modality, especially for early stage disease. For selected patients with more advance disease where primary debulking surgery is not considered to be achievable, the use of neoadjuvant chemotherapy may be considered on an individual basis. Fertility-sparing surgery followed by adjuvant therapy is debated since most of women are in the reproductive age group and the majority presents with unilateral ovarian involvement at diagnosis.[8,15,16] However, nonfertility conserving debulking surgery initially or after three to six cycles of chemotherapy is suggested, even for stage IA tumors. The more radical approach is based on the poor prognosis of the disease; trend toward better results with bilateral salpingo-oophorectomy (BSO)[8]; potential infertility with multiagent chemotherapy and/or radiotherapy; the frequent recurrence at the contralateral ovary and the relationship between germline mutations of *SMARCA4* and familial cases with bilateral involvement of the ovary.[5,17] There is one reported case of pregnancy following fertility-sparing surgery.[18] For these reasons, BSO at staging surgery should be strongly considered for all patients when there is already a definitive diagnosis, which is often not available at the time of initial surgical intervention.

SCCOHTs are particularly chemosensitive at the outset. In the majority of cases, platinum-based regimens are the treatment choice extrapolated on studies of small cell lung cancer, epithelial and nonepithelial ovarian cancer (Table 7.2).[19] Retrospective data suggest an overall survival superiority for cisplatin and etoposide compared to paclitaxel and carboplatin.[20] The recent advance on the molecular genetics and a better understanding of the pathogenesis would guide optimal management, although the rarity of SCCOHT limits prospective clinical trials. Multiagent including vinblastine, cisplatin, cyclophosphamide, bleomycin, doxorubicin, and etoposide (VPCBAE) chemotherapy may be justified by those finding, and retrospective data suggests to be more effective than a platinum doublet.[19,21–23]

HDC for patients who achieved a complete response, after surgery and/or chemotherapy with autologous hematopoietic stem-cell transplantation (AHSCT) rescue has been associated in prospective studies with better survival.[3] The French group has reported the two-year survival rate of 49% and 40% from two prospective studies.[14,24]

TABLE 7.2 Recommendations for newly diagnosed small cell carcinoma of the ovary, hypercalcemic type.

Surgical modality:

Early stage: Nonconservative debulking surgery initially: total hysterectomy, bilateral oophorectomy, omentectomy, pelvic and lumbar-aortic lymph node dissection and peritoneal biopsies.

Advanced stage: Nonconservative debulking surgery initially or after three to six cycles of chemotherapy: total hysterectomy, bilateral oophorectomy and debulking.

Treatment regimens:

(1) Clinical trial, if available.

(2) High-dose chemotherapy with autologous stem cell rescue: Four to six cycles of chemotherapy (PAVEP) with granulocyte colony-stimulating factor. In case of a complete remission, high-dose chemotherapy with CARBOPEC or ICE and stem-cell support +/− pelvic radiotherapy.
   - PAVEP regimen: Cisplatin (80–100 mg/m²); doxorubicin (40 mg/m²), etoposide (75 mg/m² days 1–3), cyclophosphamide (300 mg/m² days 1–3). Granulocyte colony-stimulating factor (G-CSF): filgrastim 5 mcg/kg/day days 7–12. Repeat every 3 weeks for four to six cycles.
   - CARBOPEC or ICE regimen: high-dose consolidation chemotherapy. CARBOPEC: carboplatin (400 mg/m²/day days 1–4), etoposide (450 mg/m²/day days 1–4), and cyclophosphamide (1600 mg/m²/day days 1–4). ICE: ifosfamide (5 g/m² with equivalent dose of MESNA given over 24 h by continuous infusion on day 2), carboplatin (area under the curve (AUC) of 5 with a maximum of 800 mg on day 2) and etoposide (100 mg/m²/day on days 1 to 3). Followed by autologous hematopoietic stem-cell transplantation (AHSCT).
   - Stem cells were collected after the third or fourth cycle of PAVEP supported by G-CSF (filgrastim or lenograstim), 5 Lg/kg/day, from day 6 until apheresis. The concentration of CD34+ cells required for the administration of high-dose therapy was at least 3 · 106 cells/kg of body weight. In case of harvest failure, a new attempt at stem-cell mobilization using a double G-CSF dose >5 days from steady state was proposed to the patient after the next course of PAVEP or alone.

(3) VPBCAE regimen: Six cycles of chemotherapy with granulocyte colony-stimulating factor, +/− pelvic radiotherapy.
   - Vinblastine 6 mg/m², cisplatin 90 mg/m², cyclophosphamide 1.000 mg/m², bleomycin 15 units/m², doxorubicin 45 mg/m² and etoposide 200 mg/m². Granulocyte colony-stimulating factor (G-CSF): pegfilgrastim 6 mg days every 3 weeks.

(4) BEP regimen: Four cycles of chemotherapy, +/− pelvic radiotherapy.
   - Bleomycin 20–30 units per dose, etoposide 100 mg/m² per day, on days 1–5 plus cisplatin 20 mg/m², per day on days 1–5, every 21 days.

(5) For those with poor performance status:
   - Refer for palliative care assessment.
   - Paclitaxel/carboplatin: Paclitaxel 175 mg/m² and carboplatin AUC = 5 or 6; repeat every 21 days for 6 cycles.
   - Etoposide/ cisplatin: cisplatin 20 mg/m² per day, on days 1–5 and etoposide 100 mg/m² per day, on days 1–5 every 21 days.

The role of radiotherapy in the treatment of SCCOHT is largely unknown, but there is limited information to suggest a potential benefit more relevant when compared to other types of ovarian cancers and similarly to what is seen in malignant rhabdoid tumors.[8,19,20,25,26] This may be a reasonable consideration when disease is confined to a single radiation portal, but some practitioners advocate pelvic radiotherapy for all patients to reduce the likelihood of pelvic recurrence.

Treatment of recurrent disease

The tumors at recurrence tend to be poorly responsive to chemotherapy and prolonged remissions are rarely achieved with second-line regimen usually used in small cell carcinoma of the lung (Table 7.3).[8,24] However, there are a few reports of rare patients who have survived after multimodality treatment that included surgery, chemotherapy and radiotherapy for recurrent disease.[8,27] Some chemotherapy regimens have been reported including the combination of cyclophosphamide, doxorubicin and vincristine; paclitaxel and carboplatin including dose-dense regimes; and topotecan monotherapy. The use of antiangiogenic in combination with chemotherapy (bevacizumab and paclitaxel), was reported in a second line swimmer plot with a case of complete response (Fig. 7.5). The other two patients who received paclitaxel and bevacizumab had prolonged partial responses of 10 and 15 months.[14]

TABLE 7.3 Recommendations for recurrent small cell carcinoma of the ovary, hypercalcemic type.

Surgical modality:
Palliative surgical procedures may be appropriate in select patients.
Debulking surgery (selective cases only).

Treatment regimens:
(1) Clinical trial, if available.
(2) PD-1/PD-L1 blockade for PD-L1 positive tumors, regardless of low-mutational burden tumors.
  - Nivolumab 240 mg every 2 weeks.
  - Pembrolizumab 200 mg every 3 weeks.
(3) Chemotherapy regimens (dosage according to epithelial ovarian cancer and small cell lung cancer)
  - Cyclophosphamide, doxorubicin and vincristine
  - Paclitaxel and carboplatin
  - Dose dense paclitaxel and carboplatin
  - Paclitaxel and bevacizumab
  - Topotecan
(4) Radiotherapy in selected cases.
(5) For those with poor performance status:
  - Refer for palliative care assessment.

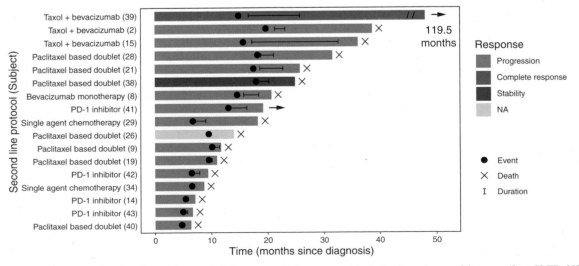

FIG. 7.5 Swimmer plot of the duration of response to second-line treatments for women with small cell carcinoma of the ovary (from PMID: 32723678).

Although SCCOHT are low–mutational burden tumors, their immunogenic microenvironment resembles the landscape of tumors that respond well to treatment with PD-1/PD-L1 blockade.[28] Protein studies have demonstrated PD-L1 expression with strong associated T-cell infiltration. PD-L1 expression was detected in both tumor and stromal cells, with macrophages being the most abundant PD-L1–positive cells in some tumors. Transcriptional profiling revealed increased expression of genes related to Th1 and cytotoxic cell function in PD-L1–high tumors, suggesting that PD-L1 acts as a pathway of adaptive immune resistance in SCCOHT. However, in one study only 1 of 4 patients who received a PD-1 inhibitor had a response and this partial response was short lived nonetheless.[12]

Phase I trials should be considered for all patients if available and patients that remains with good performance status.

Case resolution

This 22-year-old patient diagnosed with FIGO stage IIIA SCCOHT had been counseled for completion surgery with hysterectomy and contralateral oophorectomy but wanted to pursue fertility-sparing surgery. She was then treated with the six-drug chemotherapy regimen VPBCAE. HDC with autologous stem cell rescue was discussed, but based on uncertain selection bias, she chose to undergo a period of observation with CT scans every 3 months for the first two years, followed by six-month CT scans after that until she is disease free for 5 years. Pelvic radiotherapy was not given for consolidation since she had extra-pelvic disease at the time of diagnosis. Germline genetic testing for SMARCA4 was performed and found to be negative. If she does recur, current treatment options would likely include immune checkpoint blockade or combination chemotherapy with paclitaxel and bevacizumab. In the future, she would receive second line therapy based on emerging data in the published peer-reviewed literature, clinical trial, or have consultation with a member of the recently formed International SCCOHT Consortium (ISC).

References

1. Patibandla JR, Fehniger JE, Levine DA, Jelinic P. Small cell cancers of the female genital tract: molecular and clinical aspects. *Gynecol Oncol.* 2018;149(2):420–427.
2. Conlon N, Silva A, Guerra E, et al. Loss of SMARCA4 expression is both sensitive and specific for the diagnosis of small cell carcinoma of ovary, hypercalcemic type. *Am J Surg Pathol.* 2016;40(3):395–403.
3. Witkowski L, Goudie C, Ramos P, et al. The influence of clinical and genetic factors on patient outcome in small cell carcinoma of the ovary, hypercalcemic type. *Gynecol Oncol.* 2016;141(3):454–460.
4. Foulkes WD, Clarke BA, Hasselblatt M, Majewski J, Albrecht S, McCluggage WG. No small surprise - small cell carcinoma of the ovary, hypercalcaemic type, is a malignant rhabdoid tumour. *J Pathol.* 2014;233(3):209–214.
5. Witkowski L, Donini N, Byler-Dann R, et al. The hereditary nature of small cell carcinoma of the ovary, hypercalcemic type: two new familial cases. *Fam Cancer.* 2017;16(3):395–399.
6. Jelinic P, Mueller JJ, Olvera N, et al. Recurrent SMARCA4 mutations in small cell carcinoma of the ovary. *Nat Genet.* 2014;46(5):424–426.
7. Mittal P, Roberts CWM. The SWI/SNF complex in cancer - biology, biomarkers and therapy. *Nat Rev Clin Oncol.* 2020;17(7):435–448.
8. Young RH, Oliva E, Scully RE. Small cell carcinoma of the ovary, hypercalcemic type. A clinicopathological analysis of 150 cases. *Am J Surg Pathol.* 1994;18(11):1102–1116.
9. Berchuck A, Witkowski L, Hasselblatt M, Foulkes WD. Prophylactic oophorectomy for hereditary small cell carcinoma of the ovary, hypercalcemic type. *Gynecol Oncol Rep.* 2015;12:20–22.
10. Witkowski L, Carrot-Zhang J, Albrecht S, et al. Germline and somatic SMARCA4 mutations characterize small cell carcinoma of the ovary, hypercalcemic type. *Nat Genet.* 2014;46(5):438–443.
11. Ramos P, Karnezis AN, Craig DW, et al. Small cell carcinoma of the ovary, hypercalcemic type, displays frequent inactivating germline and somatic mutations in SMARCA4. *Nat Genet.* 2014;46(5):427–429.
12. Jelinic P, Schlappe BA, Conlon N, et al. Concomitant loss of SMARCA2 and SMARCA4 expression in small cell carcinoma of the ovary, hypercalcemic type. *Mod Pathol.* 2016;29(1):60–66.
13. Mutch DG, Prat J. 2014 FIGO staging for ovarian, fallopian tube and peritoneal cancer. *Gynecol Oncol.* 2014;133(3):401–404.
14. Blanc-Durand F, Lefeuvre-Plesse C, Ray-Coquard I, et al. Dose-intensive regimen treatment for small-cell carcinoma of the ovary of hypercalcemic type (SCCOHT). *Gynecol Oncol.* 2020;159(1):129–135.
15. Woopen H, Sehouli J, Pietzner K, Darb-Esfahani S, Braicu EI, Fotopoulou C. Clinical experience of young patients with small cell ovarian carcinoma of the hypercalcemic type (OSCCHT). *Eur J Obstet Gynecol Reprod Biol.* 2012;165(2):313–317.
16. Dykgraaf RH, de Jong D, van Veen M, Ewing-Graham PC, Helmerhorst TJ, van der Burg ME. Clinical management of ovarian small-cell carcinoma of the hypercalcemic type: a proposal for conservative surgery in an advanced stage of disease. *Int J Gynecol Cancer.* 2009;19(3):348–353.
17. Lavrut PM, Le Loarer F, Normand C, et al. Small cell carcinoma of the ovary, hypercalcemic type: report of a bilateral case in a teenager associated with SMARCA4 germline mutation. *Pediatr Dev Pathol.* 2016;19(1):56–60.
18. Phoolcharoen N, Woodard T, James D, et al. Successful pregnancy following chemotherapy in a survivor of small cell carcinoma of the ovary, hypercalcemic type (SCCOHT): a case report and review of literature. *Gynecol Oncol Rep.* 2020;32:100576.

19. Callegaro-Filho D, Gershenson DM, Nick AM, et al. Small cell carcinoma of the ovary-hypercalcemic type (SCCOHT): a review of 47 cases. *Gynecol Oncol.* 2016;140(1):53–57.
20. Harrison ML, Hoskins P, du Bois A, et al. Small cell of the ovary, hypercalcemic type—analysis of combined experience and recommendation for management. A GCIG study. *Gynecol Oncol.* 2006;100(2):233–238.
21. Wallbillich JJ, Nick AM, Ramirez PT, Watkins JL, Euscher ED, Schmeler KM. Vinblastine, cisplatin, cyclophosphamide, bleomycin, doxorubicin, and etoposide (VPCBAE) in the management of three patients with small-cell carcinoma of the ovary. *Gynecol Oncol Case Rep.* 2012;2(2):58–60.
22. Tewari K, Brewer C, Cappuccini F, Macri C, Rogers LW, Berman ML. Advanced-stage small cell carcinoma of the ovary in pregnancy: long-term survival after surgical debulking and multiagent chemotherapy. *Gynecol Oncol.* 1997;66(3):531–534.
23. Senekjian EK, Weiser PA, Talerman A, Herbst AL. Vinblastine, cisplatin, cyclophosphamide, bleomycin, doxorubicin, and etoposide in the treatment of small cell carcinoma of the ovary. *Cancer.* 1989;64(6):1183–1187.
24. Pautier P, Ribrag V, Duvillard P, et al. Results of a prospective dose-intensive regimen in 27 patients with small cell carcinoma of the ovary of the hypercalcemic type. *Ann Oncol.* 2007;18(12):1985–1989.
25. Sultan I, Qaddoumi I, Rodriguez-Galindo C, Nassan AA, Ghandour K, Al-Hussaini M. Age, stage, and radiotherapy, but not primary tumor site, affects the outcome of patients with malignant rhabdoid tumors. *Pediatr Blood Cancer.* 2010;54(1):35–40.
26. Dickersin GR, Kline IW, Scully RE. Small cell carcinoma of the ovary with hypercalcemia: a report of eleven cases. *Cancer.* 1982;49(1):188–197.
27. Callegaro-Filho D, Burke TW, Eifel PJ, Ramirez PT, Euscher EE, Schmeler KM. Radiotherapy for recurrent small cell carcinoma of the ovary: a case report and review of the literature. *Gynecol Oncol Rep.* 2015;11:23–25.
28. Jelinic P, Ricca J, Van Oudenhove E, et al. Immune-active microenvironment in small cell carcinoma of the ovary, hypercalcemic type: rationale for immune checkpoint blockade. *J Natl Cancer Inst.* 2018;110(7):787–790.

Chapter 8

Other rare ovarian cancers: Transitional cell carcinoma, malignant Brenner tumor, endometrioid carcinoma, mesothelioma, squamous cell carcinoma, sarcoma

Sahana Somasegar, Elizabeth Kertowidjojo, M. Herman Chui, Preetha Ramalingam, Ying Liu, and Emeline Aviki

Introduction

Ovarian cancer encompasses a wide variety of tumors, all with different clinical patterns, histologies, and molecular features. Ovarian cancer is typically classified as epithelial (serous, mucinous, endometrioid, clear cell, carcinosarcoma, and mixed) vs nonepithelial (germ cell and sex cord stromal cell). Epithelial ovarian cancers, which comprise 90% to 95% of all ovarian cancer cases, are more common than nonepithelial ovarian cancer. However, there are a group of ultrarare subtypes such as transitional cell carcinoma, endometrioid carcinoma, neuroendocrine tumors (NETs), mesothelioma, squamous cell carcinoma, and ovarian sarcomas. Most of the literature for these subtypes comes from case reports, small case series, and population database resources whose data sources lack the details necessary to make any specific treatment recommendations. In this chapter, we will review these ultrarare subtypes of ovarian malignancies and make recommendations for treatment based on the current literature as well as drawing from similar histologic subtypes from other primary tumor sites.

Transitional cell carcinoma

Transitional cell carcinoma of the ovary is a rare histological type of epithelial ovarian cancer that was first described in 1987 by Austin and Norris[1] (Table 8.1). Similar to other transitional cell tumors such as Brenner tumors of the ovary, transitional cell carcinomas of the ovary contain urothelial-like tissue that closely resembles transitional cell carcinoma of the bladder.[2-5] Unlike Brenner tumors, however, they lack the dense stromal calcifications and epithelial-type histologic patterns.[5] In fact, molecular and immunohistochemical studies have further distinguished transitional cell carcinoma of the ovary from Brenner tumors by showing a resemblance to high-grade serous carcinomas.[6] Molecular and genetic analysis also demonstrated that ovarian transitional cell carcinomas follow a tumorigenic pathway like that of high-grade serous tumors with frequent TP53 mutations.[6] In the light of new evidence, in the new WHO classification system released in 2014, transitional cell carcinoma of the ovary is no longer considered a separate entity but a variant of high-grade serous (or rarely endometrioid) ovarian carcinoma.

Very few studies have examined the clinical significance of ovarian transitional cell carcinomas. Given the rarity of this tumor, the true incidence of the disease is unknown, but studies have reported incidences ranging from 1% to 2% of cases of ovarian cancer.[6,7] The clinical presentation is like that of other epithelial ovarian cancers, including symptoms such as abdominal pain, bloating, back pain, and urinary or bowel symptoms.[5] Given the close resemblance to transitional cell carcinomas of the bladder, the differential diagnosis includes metastatic urothelial carcinoma of the urinary tract. Often, it is very difficult to discern the origin of transitional cell carcinomas based on conventional histological stains alone.[2,5,8] While Brenner tumors of the ovary and transitional cell carcinomas of urothelial origin express certain cytokeratins and uroplakins, ovarian transitional cell carcinomas usually do not.[2,5,8] Therefore, in some cases, immunohistochemistry may be helpful in distinguishing transitional cell carcinomas of ovarian origin from those of urothelial origin. The lack of expression of urothelial markers also supports the idea that transitional cell carcinomas of the ovary originate from Mullerian epithelium rather than being a urothelial neoplasm.

TABLE 8.1 Frequency of epithelial ovarian cancer subtypes.

Subtype	Frequency[a]
High-grade serous	70%
Low-grade serous	10%
Clear cell	5%
Endometrioid	10%
Mucinous	3%
Other (Transitional, undifferentiated)	2%

[a]*Frequencies for women in North American and Europe, frequencies differ in Asia.*
From Stephanie Lheureux, Marsela Braunstein, Amit M. Oza. Epithelial ovarian cancer: Evolution of management in the era of precision medicine. CA Cancer J Clin. 69 (4) (2019) 280–304.

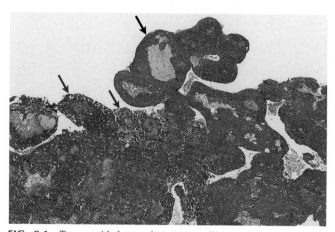

FIG. 8.1 Tumor with large edematous papillae resembling urothelial mucosa (*black arrow*). Areas of more typical high-grade serous carcinoma with micropapillae (*red arrows*).

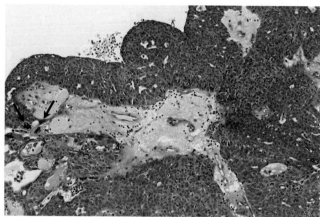

FIG. 8.2 High power images showing multilayered epithelium with punched out spaces and cells with marked pleomorphism (*black arrows*).

The gross appearance of the tumor is similar to high-grade serous carcinoma, with no specific distinguishing features. Tumors are large and can be solid and cystic with areas of hemorrhage and necrosis.

As mentioned earlier, the 2014 WHO Classification of Female Genital Tumors transitional cell carcinoma was considered a variant of high-grade serous carcinoma. The 2020 WHO Classification of Female Genital Tumors further highlights that high grade serous carcinoma with homologous recombination-deficiency frequently display solid, endometrial-like and transitional patterns.[9] Tumors with transitional pattern are characterized by large papillae lined by multilayered/stratified epithelium, resembling urothelial mucosa (Fig. 8.1). Microcysts or punched out spaces are typically seen with the epithelium (Fig. 8.2). The nuclei are high-grade with significant pleomorphism. Most cases, upon adequate sampling, show

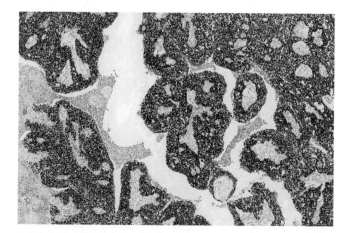

FIG. 8.3 Transitional cell carcinoma showing diffuse positivity for WT-1 in the tumor cells.

areas of more typical high-grade serous carcinoma with papillary, cribriform, slit-like, and glandular patterns. Transitional cell carcinoma and high-grade serous carcinoma share similar immunophenotype. Both tumors are positive for PAX-8, WT-1 (Fig. 8.3), and hormone receptors.

The most important differential diagnoses are metastatic urothelial carcinoma to the ovary and malignant Brenner tumor (MBT). Clinical history of bladder cancer is essential to exclude metastatic urothelial carcinoma. Histologically, the two tumors are very similar; however, the presence of more typical areas of high-grade serous carcinoma would support an ovarian primary. Immunohistochemically, unlike ovarian transitional cell carcinoma, urothelial carcinomas are positive for CK20, GATA3, and uroplakin (~50% of cases), while negative for WT-1 and hormone receptors. PAX-8 can be positive in both tumors.

MBTs usually have infiltrating nests of tumor cells with urothelial-like appearance. The hallmark of the diagnosis is the presence of benign or borderline Brenner tumor, and sometimes extensive sampling is necessary to find these components.[10] MBTs are usually negative for WT-1 and hormone receptors, though the latter may be weakly expressed. The expression of markers of urothelial differentiation such as GATA3 is not well studied currently, limiting its use.

The molecular profile of transitional cell carcinomas is not well-studied due to the lack of consistency in reporting and accurately diagnosing these tumors. A recent study has shown that proteins associated with cell death, apoptosis and necrosis were highly expressed in transitional cell carcinomas (defined as tumors having >50% of said morphology).[11] Conversely, proteins with reduced expression included those associated with DNA homologous recombination, cell mitosis, proliferation and survival, and cell cycle progression pathways. Proteomic analysis revealed three biomarkers including Claudin-4 (CLDN4), ubiquitin carboxyl-terminal esterase L1 (UCHL1), and minichromosome maintenance protein 7 (MCM7) that were enriched in transitional cell carcinoma over high-grade serous carcinoma, but were not able to distinguish the two tumors with 100% sensitivity and specificity. Additional studies are necessary to confirm these differences and determine their clinical significance.

Like epithelial ovarian cancers, ovarian transitional cell carcinomas are staged according to International Federation of Gynecology and Obstetrics (FIGO) staging (Table 8.2). As there have been so few reported cases of these tumors, there is not much data on overall prognosis and survival. Kommoss et al. found that ovarian transitional cell carcinomas had a significantly better prognosis as compared to all other types of ovarian carcinomas after standardized chemotherapy (5-year survival was 57% as compared to 31% for patients with ovarian carcinomas of other types, $P = 0.03$).[4] In addition, the authors found that even among patients with postoperative residual tumor <1 cm, there was still a trend toward better survival.[4] It has also been suggested by other researchers that ovarian transitional cell carcinomas are more chemosensitive than epithelial ovarian cancers and this may explain the better prognosis compared to other more common serous carcinomas. Guseh et al. found that patients with these tumors are less likely to demonstrate resistance to platinum chemotherapy and have improved overall survival when compared to patients with papillary serous ovarian cancer.[5] The authors suggested that a propensity for micronodular rather than macronodular extraovarian spread and better surgical resectability due to lesser degree of diffuse infiltrative growth may also be factors contributing to the overall improved survival and prognosis.[5]

Patients with transitional cell carcinoma of the ovary appear to benefit from optimal surgical resection, followed by adjuvant platinum-based chemotherapy.[4,5] Given the scarcity of reported cases, there are no current recommendations for surveillance and treatment of recurrence. Because transitional cell carcinomas of the ovary follow a similar tumorigenic pathway to high-grade serous ovarian cancer and have been shown to be associated with better prognosis after following a similar treatment paradigm, surveillance for recurrence and treatment of recurrent disease should be the same as that for epithelial ovarian cancers (Fig. 8.4).

Malignant Brenner tumors

MBTs are a rare subtype of epithelial ovarian cancer. Originally identified by Fritz Brenner in 1907, Brenner tumors of the ovary represent <1% of all ovarian neoplasms.[6] These tumors can be benign, borderline, or malignant. The vast majority of Brenner tumors will be benign or borderline with only 5% malignant.[12] The median age for diagnosis in women with MBTs is 65 years old (range 34–95).[13] This age at diagnosis is older than other epithelial ovarian cancers. For example, the median age at diagnosis for serous ovarian cancer is 60 years old, 58 years old for endometrioid, 55 for clear cell, and 52 for mucinous ovarian cancer.[14] There are no known risk factors for developing these tumors.

MBTs resemble ovarian transitional cell carcinomas and careful pathologic review should be performed to distinguish the two. These two entities were first differentiated in 1987 by Austin and Norris.[1] Although they share similar histologic features, MBTs are generally felt to be low-grade malignancies while transitional cell carcinomas are considered more aggressive high-grade tumors. For diagnosis, MBTs require the presence of both benign and malignant epithelial components with destructive stromal invasion. As described above, in contrast, transitional cell carcinomas resemble urothelial carcinomas and are marked by the absence of any Brenner tumor component.[15]

Tumors are usually unilateral but can occasionally be bilateral with a median size of 10 cm (Fig. 8.5).[13] They may be completely solid or cystic with mural nodules. MBT, by definition, is composed of a frankly malignant component, akin to high-grade papillary urothelial carcinoma, with associated benign or borderline areas (Fig. 8.6). The malignant component

TABLE 8.2 TNM and FIGO staging for ovary, fallopian tube, and primary peritoneal carcinomas.

Primary tumor (T)		
T category	**FIGO stage**	**T criteria**
TX		Primary tumor cannot be assessed
T0		No evidence of primary tumor
T1	I	Tumor limited to ovaries (one or both) or fallopian tube(s)
T1a	IA	Tumor limited to one ovary (capsule intact) or fallopian tube, no tumor on ovarian or fallopian tube surface; no malignant cells in ascites or peritoneal washings
T1b	IB	Tumor limited to both ovaries (capsules intact) or fallopian tubes; no tumor on ovarian or fallopian tube surface; no malignant cells in ascites or peritoneal washings
T1c	IC	Tumor limited to one or both ovaries or fallopian tubes, with any of the following:
T1c1	IC1	• Surgical spill
T1c2	IC2	• Capsule ruptured before surgery or tumor on ovarian or fallopian tube surface
T1c3	IC3	• Malignant cells in ascites or peritoneal washings
T2	II	Tumor involves one or both ovaries or fallopian tubes with pelvic extension below pelvic brim or primary peritoneal cancer
T2a	IIA	Extension and/or implants on the uterus and/or fallopian tube(s) and/or ovaries
T2b	IIB	Extension to and/or implants on other pelvic tissues
T3	III	Tumor involves one or both ovaries or fallopian tubes, or primary peritoneal cancer, with microscopically confirmed peritoneal metastasis outside the pelvis and/or metastasis to the retroperitoneal (pelvic and/or paraaortic) lymph nodes
T3a	IIIA2	Microscopic extrapelvic (above the pelvic brim) peritoneal involvement with or without positive retroperitoneal lymph nodes
T3b	IIIB	Macroscopic peritoneal metastasis beyond pelvis 2 cm or less in greatest dimension with or without metastasis to the retroperitoneal lymph nodes
T3c	IIIC	Macroscopic peritoneal metastasis beyond the pelvis more than 2 cm in greatest dimension with or without metastasis to the retroperitoneal lymph nodes (includes extension of tumor to capsule of liver and spleen without parenchymal involvement of either organ)
Regional lymph nodes (N)		
N category	**FIGO stage**	**N criteria**
NX		Regional lymph nodes cannot be assessed
N0		No regional lymph node metastasis
N0(i+)		Isolated tumor cells in regional lymph node(s) no greater than 0.2 mm
N1	IIIA1	Positive retroperitoneal lymph nodes only (histologically confirmed)
N1a	IIIA1i	Metastasis up to and including 10 mm in greatest dimension
N1b	IIIA1ii	Metastasis more than 10 mm in greatest dimension
Distant metastasis (M)		
M category	**FIGO stage**	**M criteria**
M0		No distant metastasis
M1	IV	Distant metastasis, including pleural effusion with positive cytology; liver or splenic parenchymal metastasis; metastasis to extraabdominal organs (including inguinal lymph nodes and lymph nodes outside the abdominal cavity); and transmural involvement of intestine
M1a	IVA	Pleural effusion with positive cytology
M1b	IVB	Liver or splenic parenchymal metastases; metastases to extraabdominal organs (including inguinal lymph nodes and lymph nodes outside the abdominal cavity); transmural involvement of intestine

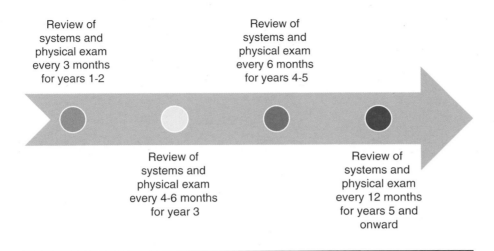

FIG. 8.4 Society of Gynecologic Oncology. Society of gynecologic oncology guidelines for epithelial ovarian cancer surveillance.

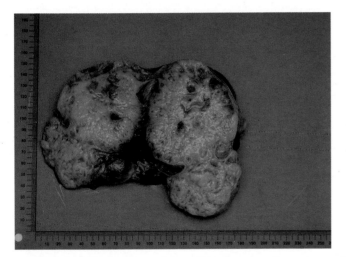

FIG. 8.5 Gross image shows a large, solid and cystic yellow mass with hemorrhagic areas.

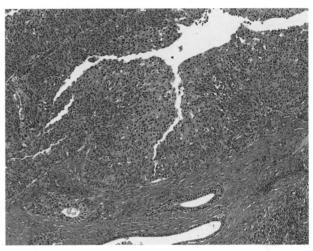

FIG. 8.6 The morphologic features are akin to high-grade papillary urothelial carcinoma with papillary architecture and marked cytologic atypia.

comprises of nests of tumor cells with transitional type epithelium that invade the ovarian stroma (Fig. 8.7). The tumor nests can be haphazard with angulated and infiltrative pattern or have a solid growth pattern. The tumor cells usually show nuclear pleomorphism and mitotic activity. Foci of squamous or glandular differentiation may be present. Areas of necrosis are common. In the absence of a benign or borderline component an alternative diagnosis should be considered. In rare cases a coexisting mucinous adenocarcinoma may be present.

Brenner tumors are positive for cytokeratin, EMA, PAX-8, p63, and GATA-3 while negative for ER, PR, and WT-1. Immunohistochemistry for p53 shows a wild-type pattern of staining.[16] Most exhibit a CK7-positive and CK20-negative profile.

MBT arises from benign and borderline Brenner tumors (Fig. 8.8). Repeated *PIK3CA* mutations and *MDM2* amplification have been reported. In contrast, no mutations have been observed in the *TP53* gene or the *TERT* promoter region, which is frequently seen in urothelial carcinoma.[17,18]

The diagnosis of MBT is made only in the presence of benign or borderline Brenner tumor. Tumors lacking a benign Brenner component (previously designated as transitional cell carcinoma) are now regarded as high-grade serous carcinoma with transitional-like features.[6] High-grade serous carcinoma displays a greater degree of cytologic atypia and nuclear pleomorphism with staining for WT-1 and aberrant p53 expression (overexpression or null-type pattern).

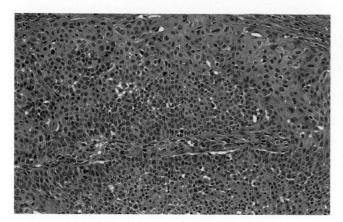

FIG. 8.7 Areas of solid and invasive growth are often present.

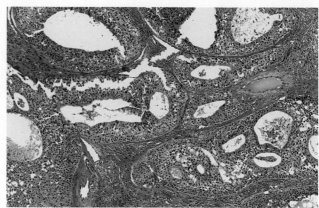

FIG. 8.8 By definition, an associated benign or borderline Brenner tumor must be present.

Metastatic urothelial carcinomas from the urinary tract are usually associated with a deeply invasive and clinically evident primary tumor. Metastatic disease involving the ovary is usually bilateral and in the form of multiple small nodules with ovarian surface involvement. Urothelial carcinomas are positive for CK7 and CK20 while MBTs are generally negative for CK20.

Women with MBTs may present with abdominal distension or pelvic discomfort although many will be asymptomatic with diagnosis made incidentally after removal of the ovary for other reasons. Although these tumors do not produce or secrete hormones, women may experience dysfunctional uterine bleeding or postmenopausal bleeding.[19] The etiology for bleeding symptoms is unknown. Less than 10% of women with MBT will have ascites at diagnosis and its presence should make the clinician consider other types of epithelial ovarian cancers. That said, if ascites is present and paracentesis reveals squamous cells, there is a higher likelihood that the patient has a MBT.[12]

As with other ovarian neoplasms, CA-125 is the tumor marker most commonly assessed. In one large population-based study, CA-125 was elevated in 70% of women with MBT in whom it was drawn; however, the level of CA-125 level did not seem to correlate with tumor burden.[13] Other studies have reported only 30% to 40% of patients with MBTs as having an elevated CA-125.[20] One report of 2 cases showed that CA 72–4 may be elevated in women with MBT although this is not a commonly used tumor marker.[21]

Imaging work-up should include either a CT scan or MRI. PET scan is unlikely to add useful information beyond CT scan or MRI. Although median tumor size is 10 cm, a large proportion of patients will have small tumors (< 2 cm).[22] Larger tumors will have both solid and cystic components with amorphous calcifications seen in the solid component.[22] In contrast to many other types of epithelial ovarian cancers, MBTs are unlikely to show evidence of hemorrhage or necrosis on imaging.

Staging for MBTs is the same as those for other epithelial ovarian cancers (Table 8.2). Women with MBT tend to present with unilateral ovarian masses (84%).[13] Fifty-five percent will be stage I at diagnosis, while 14% will have stage II disease, 18% stage III, and 12% stage IV (Table 8.3). Histologically, 13% will be grade 1 tumors, 30% grade 2, and 57% will have grade 3 disease.[13]

As the majority of women will present with unilateral, stage I disease, the overall prognosis is quite good (Table 8.3). For these women, 5-year disease-specific survival (DSS) is 95% with 5 year overall survival 69%. The median overall survival for women with stage I disease is 91 months compared to 49 months for those with extra-ovarian disease at

TABLE 8.3 Stage at diagnosis and survival for women with malignant Brenner tumor.

Stage	Stage at diagnosis	5 year DSS	5 year OS
I	55%	95%	69%
II	14%	52%	42%
III	18%	62%	62%
IV	12%	37%	29%

DSS—disease-specific survival; OS—overall survival.
Adapted from: D. Nasioudis, G. Sisti, K. Holcomb, T. Kanninen, S.S. Witkin. Malignant Brenner tumors of the ovary; a population-based analysis. Gynecol Oncol. 142(1) (2016) 44–49. doi: https:/doi.org/10.1016/j.ygyno.2016.04.538. Epub 2016 May 11. PMID: 27130406.

diagnosis.[13] Women with low-grade tumors (grade 1 or 2) also have improved DSS compared to those with high-grade (grade 3) neoplasms (94% vs 44%). However, this does not translate to a difference in overall survival although that may just be due to small sample sizes in these studies.[13]

Surgical resection with an attempt at complete cytoreduction is the mainstay of initial treatment for women with MBT. The role of lymphadenectomy (LAD) as part of the initial cytoreductive surgery is unknown. Only 5% of women will have metastatic disease to the lymph nodes and there does not appear to be a survival advantage for those women who underwent LAD compared to those who did not.[13] In addition, there is a low likelihood of nodal disease even when imaging suggests possible metastasis. In one study, 6 out of 10 patients with MBT had preoperative imaging suggestive of nodal disease; however, none of these patients had findings of metastatic disease on pathologic examination of surgical specimens.[19] We recommend resection of suspicious nodes on preoperative imaging or on intraoperative assessment of the retroperitoneum.

Adjuvant chemotherapy with 6 cycles of platinum/taxane regimen should be administered to all patients with stage II-IV disease. In addition, postoperative chemotherapy should be given to women with stage IC disease. For women with stages IA–IB disease, there are limited data on which to base the decision for observation or chemotherapy. In one study, three patients with stage IA/IB were observed. Two women were without recurrence at 47 months (one with stage IA, the other with stage IB) while 1 woman with stage IB disease recurred at 12 months.[23] In another study, 4 women with stage IA disease were observed after surgery. None had recurred at a median follow-up of 75 months. A fifth patient with stage IA disease received postoperative chemotherpay and was without recurrence at 8 months.[20] In one last report of 4 women with stage IA or IB disease, 2 received adjuvant chemotherapy and were without disease at 60 months, one was observed and without disease at 126 months, and one was lost to follow-up.[19] Based on these limited data, we would recommend observation for all women with stage IA MBTs (all grades) and for those with stage IB, grade 1 or 2 disease. For women with stage IB, grade 3 disease, we would recommend adjuvant chemotherapy with a platinum and taxane regimen.

As mentioned, the overall prognosis for women with stage I disease is excellent (5-year DSS 95%) while those with stage II–IV disease have a 5-year DSS of 51% (Table 8.3). Median time to recurrence is 11 months.[12] The most common sites of recurrence are the peritoneal cavity and lung with reports of recurrences in the dura, the skin, and bone.[15]

Treatment for recurrence typically mimics those for other epithelial ovarian cancers with similar agents for platinum-sensitive and platinum-resistant recurrences. Chemotherapy for recurrences is unlikely to be curative; however, there have been reports of long-term survivals even in women with distant recurrences.[20] The role of secondary cytoreductive surgery and radiation are unknown and should be considered on an individualized basis. One patient had a pelvic recurrence after upfront therapy that included bevacizumab maintenance. She underwent secondary cytoreductive surgery followed by pelvic irradiation and was without recurrence at 24 months after treatment.[12] Another patient with recurrence had a good response to radiation followed by cyclophosphamide and doxorubicin.[24]

MBTs are microsatellite stable with low tumor mutational burden so the role of single agent immunotherapy may be limited. These tumors have been shown to have alterations in FGFR3 in 45% of cases.[25] Anti-FGFR inhibitors such as erdafitinib and pemigatinib in recurrent MBTs that harbor these alterations may be considered.

Endometrioid carcinoma

Endometrioid ovarian carcinoma is an ultrarare subtype of epithelial ovary cancer. The first cases of endometrioid ovarian carcinoma were described by Dr. John A. Sampson in 1925, when he described cases that were frequently associated with endometriosis and closely resembling the most common carcinoma of the uterine corpus.[26] Over the subsequent few decades, additional cases were described in individual case reports and small case series.

Endometrioid ovarian carcinoma can be associated with Lynch syndrome, an autosomal dominant syndrome in which a germline mutation in the DNA mismatch repair mechanisms results in an increased risk of carcinogenesis in various organs.[27–29] It is estimated that patients with Lynch syndrome have a 10% lifetime risk of developing endometrioid ovarian carcinoma, with some variation depending on mutation type.[27–30] In North American and European populations, the endometrioid subtype accounts for approximately 10% of all epithelial ovarian cancer (Table 8.1).[31] A family history in a first-degree relative has been associated with an increased risk of endometrioid ovarian carcinoma with relative risks ranging from 2.81 to 3.81.[32] These tumors are thought to be primarily derived from progenitor cells in endometriosis that differentiate toward a secretory cell lineage, and 11% to 30% of patients also have a concurrent endometrioid carcinoma in the uterus.[33,34] The concurrent presence of ovarian cancer with endometrial cancer, also known as synchronous endometrial and ovarian cancer is not a rare clinical entity and occurs in approximately 3% of endometrial cancers.[35,36] When it comes to grading, grades I and II endometrioid ovarian carcinomas represent approximately 84% to 95% of all cases, and grade III cancers represent the remaining 5% to 16% of cases.[33,37,38]

Tumors are usually unilateral and large with a smooth surface. They are variably cystic and solid and may be associated with an endometriotic cyst. Similar to endometrial endometrioid carcinoma, the ovarian counterpart shows a wide spectrum of morphologic patterns. Well-differentiated adenocarcinomas show back-to-back glandular, cribriform, and/or villo-glandular growth. Higher-grade tumors show areas of solid growth. In general, the cytologic features are concordant with the architectural grade of the tumor. Squamous, morular, and mucinous metaplasia, as well as secretory change, are often present. Some tumors may also display sex cord-like features or corded and hyalinized morphology.

Endometrioid carcinomas express cytokeratins (with a CK7-positive, CK20-negative profile), EMA, PAX-8, ER, and PR. They are usually negative for WT-1 (positive in ~10%) and napsin-A (positive in ~8%).[39] The vast majority display a wild-type pattern of p53 staining.

Most ovarian endometrioid carcinomas originate in a background of endometriosis. The molecular alterations are analogous to that of endometrial endometrioid carcinoma, including the WNT/β-catenin signaling pathway (*CTNNB1* mutations, 53%), the PI3K pathway (*PIK3CA*), the MAPK pathway (*KRAS*, 33%), and the SWI/SNF complex (*ARID1A*, 30%).[40,41] Molecular subtyping, analogous to that of endometrial endometrioid carcinoma as defined by The Cancer Genome Atlas (TCGA), has been proposed for ovarian endometrioid carcinoma.

Metastatic disease can mimic primary ovarian endometrioid carcinoma, particularly colorectal adenocarcinoma, endometrial endometrioid adenocarcinoma, and endocervical adenocarcinoma. Bilaterality, nodularity, and surface involvement are factors that favor metastases. On the other hand, presence of associated endometriosis, adenofibroma, or borderline tumor supports an ovarian primary. Colorectal adenocarcinoma is characterized by a "garland" pattern of glands lined by cytologically malignant columnar cells surrounding central areas of dirty necrosis. In contrast to endometrioid carcinoma, the majority of colorectal carcinomas display a CK7-negative, CK20-positive profile. SATB2, a marker of colorectal carcinoma, is negative. However, endometrioid carcinoma may show positive staining for CDX2 (typically positive in colorectal carcinomas), particularly in areas of mucinous and squamous differentiation. p16 staining is usually patchy in endometrioid carcinomas and diffuse in endocervical primaries, with the caveat being that a subset of high-grade endometrioid carcinomas may show diffuse staining. Detection of high-risk HPV subtypes indicates a metastasis from the endocervix. Lastly, distinction between synchronous endometrial and ovarian endometrioid tumor *versus* metastatic disease can be difficult. Morphologic features and immunohistochemical profile may be similar at the two sites. A low-grade, low-stage endometrial tumor, in conjunction with an ovarian endometrioid carcinoma that arises in a background of endometriosis would favor synchronous primaries. On the other hand, a deeply invasive tumor with bilateral ovarian tumors and surface involvement would favor metastasis. Immunohistochemistry for mismatch repair proteins, ARID1A, and PTEN may be helpful if the two sites show contrasting staining pattern. Recent molecular studies have shown that the majority of synchronous ovarian and endometrial endometrioid carcinomas are clonally related.[42,43]

There is also morphologic overlap between ovarian endometrioid carcinoma with other ovarian primary tumors. High-grade serous carcinomas, particularly those with a solid, pseudo-endometrioid, and transitional (SET) pattern, may mimic endometrioid carcinoma. Immunohistochemistry for WT-1 and p53 are helpful in differentiating the two entities. Cytoplasmic clearing due to secretory change or squamous differentiation in endometrioid carcinoma may mimic clear cell carcinoma. Furthermore, clear cell carcinoma is also associated with endometriosis. Immunohistochemistry for ER, PR, and napsin-A is helpful in this differential. Lastly, sex cord-like features in endometrioid carcinoma may be confused with a sex cord stromal tumor. Areas of conventional endometrioid morphology, particularly the presence of squamous metaplasia, an adenofibromatous component, and the presence of endometriosis are helpful in favoring endometrioid carcinoma. Sex cord stromal tumors often stain with cytokeratin; however, they are almost always negative for EMA and positive for sex cord markers such as SF-1, inhibin and calretinin.

The clinical presentation is similar to that of other epithelial ovarian cancers, including vague symptoms such as abdominal pain, bloating, back pain, and urinary or bowel symptoms. The cancer antigen 125 (CA-125) level at initial presentation is found to vary widely but is most commonly modestly elevated.[38] The differential diagnosis is broad and includes endometrioid adenofibroma, borderline ovarian tumor, dedifferentiated endometrioid carcinoma, high-grade serous carcinoma, clear cell carcinoma, carcinosarcoma, sex-cord stromal tumors, metastatic adenocarcinoma from extragenital sites, glandular yolk sac tumor (YST), and metastatic endometrioid carcinoma from the uterus.[44]

For endometrioid ovarian carcinoma, the WHO classification recommends the same FIGO staging that is applicable for epithelial ovarian cancers (Table 8.2). In cases where synchronous endometrial and ovarian cancers are found, a recent study using next generation sequencing suggests that sporadic synchronous endometrioid endometrial and ovarian cancers are clonally related and likely represent disseminated disease from one site to the other.[43] Therefore, in cases of synchronous endometrial and ovarian cancer, FIGO staging that is applicable for uterine cancer is recommended (Table 8.4). Data from the Surveillance, Epidemiology, and End Results (SEER) showed that the 1-year, 5-year, and 10-year overall survival for localized OEC are 96.9%, 87.1%, and 72.5%, respectively.[45] Stage has been shown to be a significant prognostic factor in endometrioid ovarian carcinoma. Other positive prognostic factors include ER expression (HR = 0.18) and PR expression (HR = 0.22).[46] Lymphovascular invasion, p16-block positivity (HR = 1.88), BAF250a loss, nuclear beta-catenin expression (HR = 2.25), and aberrant p53 expression (HR = 3.41) have been found to be negative prognostic factors.[47-49] Given

TABLE 8.4 FIGO staging system for endometrial cancer.

FIGO stage	Description
I	Tumor confined to the corpus uteri, including endocervical glandular involvement
IA	Tumor limited to the endometrium or invading less than half the myometrium
IB	Tumor invading one half or more of the myometrium
II	Tumor invading the stromal connective tissue of the cervix but not extending beyond the uterus. Does NOT include endocervical glandular involvement.
III	Tumor involving serosa, adnexa, vagina, or parametrium
IIIA	Tumor involving the serosa and/or adnexa (direct extension or metastasis)
IIIB	Vaginal involvement (direct extension or metastasis) or parametrial involvement
IIIC1	Regional lymph node metastasis to pelvic lymph nodes
IIIC2	Regional lymph node metastasis to paraaortic lymph nodes, with or without positive pelvic lymph nodes
IVA	Tumor invading the bladder mucosa and/or bowel mucosa
IVB	Distance metastasis (includes metastasis to inguinal lymph nodes, intraperitoneal disease, lung, liver, or bone).

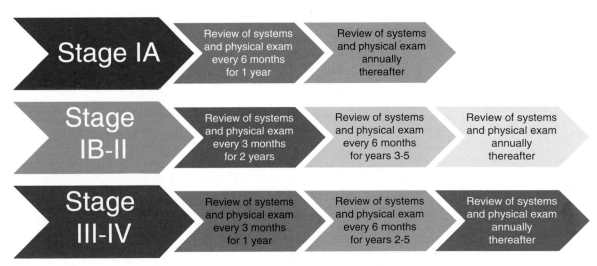

FIG. 8.9 Society of Gynecologic Oncology guidelines for endometrial cancer surveillance.

the association with Lynch Syndrome and frequent presence of high microsatellite insufficiency (MSI-H) and mismatch repair deficiency (MMR-D), it is reasonable to perform immunohistochemistry for mismatch repair proteins or assess for MSI in these tumors, particularly given implications for effectiveness of checkpoint inhibitors.[50,51] In fact, Liu et al. found that in 74 cases of ovarian endometrioid carcinomas, 20% of the tumors were microsatellite instability (MSI) high, with at least 2 of 4 microsatellite markers (BAT25, BAT26, D5S346, and D17S250) showing instability.[50]

Like epithelial ovarian cancers, optimal surgical resection followed by adjuvant platinum-based chemotherapy is the current standard of care for endometrioid ovarian carcinoma. Storey et al. found that after receiving platinum-based chemotherapy, histological type was an independent predictor of survival favoring endometrioid adenocarcinoma along with debulking status and FIGO stage.[52] The authors found that survival is better for patients with endometrioid tumors than for patients with serous adenocarcinoma, even with stage III disease or poorly differentiated tumors.[52] Given limited cases and data, there are no current recommendations for surveillance and treatment of recurrence. When endometrioid ovarian carcinomas are diagnosed in the absence of a synchronous uterine cancer, surveillance for recurrence and any subsequent treatments should resemble that of other epithelial cancers. However, in the setting of synchronous ovarian and uterine endometrioid tumors surveillance for recurrence and treatment of recurrent disease should be like that of endometrial cancer (Fig. 8.9).

Neuroendocrine tumors

Neuroendocrine tumors (NETs) are well-differentiated neoplasms that are derived from enterochromaffin cells.[53] They are classically found throughout the gastrointestinal (GI) and bronchopulmonary systems and can also occur in other locations in patients with multiple endocrine neoplasia type 1 (MEN1).[53] MEN1 is an autosomal dominant condition, caused by a germline mutation in the *MEN1* gene, leading to the growth of tumors of the parathyroid glands, anterior pituitary, and pancreas.[54] While the majority of MEN1 syndrome-associated NETs originate from the foregut, those that originate from the ovary can be seen in rare cases in patients with and without MEN1. Ovarian NETs are rare, comprising 0.1% of all ovarian neoplasms.[53–55] Very few cases of primary ovarian NETs have been reported in the literature. In the limited existing data, the average age of diagnosis is 50.8 years with a range of 16 to 83 years.[56]

Although most patients have some of the same vague signs or symptoms as seen in patients with epithelial ovarian cancer at diagnosis, approximately 30% patients are diagnosed incidentally.[54] For patients who do present with signs and symptoms, the most common ones are a palpable abdominal mass, abdominal pain, diarrhea, flushing, and weight loss.[54] Isolated primary ovarian NETs are rare, and in a study of 329 patients with ovarian NETs, 57.4% were found to be associated with a teratoma.[56] However, in patients with MEN1, it is exceedingly rare for ovarian NETs to be associated with teratomas.[56]

Since MEN1 can be associated with NETs of other origins, diagnosis of primary ovarian NET can be challenging. Once an ovarian NET is diagnosed, thorough attempts should be made to identify an alternate origin of the tumor, given the rarity of these tumors. It is especially important to rule out a primary pancreatic NET as the treatment approach is unique for cases of primary pancreatic disease.[54] When an ovarian NET is diagnosed, initial evaluation should include lab studies, imaging studies, and investigation of alternate primary sites *via* esophagogastroduodenoscopy, colonoscopy, CT imaging, MRI imaging, and/or somatostatin receptor-based diagnostic imaging (In-111 pentetreotide imaging or OctreoScan or ^{68}Ga-DOTATATE positron emission tomography (PET) imaging).[54]

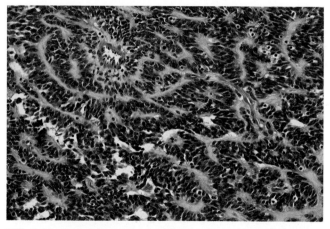

FIG. 8.10 Some cases show a corded, trabecular growth pattern with pseudo-rosette formation.

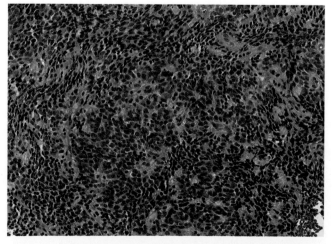

FIG. 8.11 Small cell carcinoma, comprised of small hyperchromatic cells with nuclear molding.

Grossly the tumors are solid and cystic, yellow to gray homogeneous masses that range in size from small to quite large. If associated with a mature teratoma, the tumor may form a nodule in the wall of the cyst. Necrosis and hemorrhage are rare in well-differentiated NETs but are often seen in neuroendocrine carcinomas. Well-differentiated NETs (carcinoids) are composed of monotonous round, cuboidal, or columnar cells with stippled "salt-and-pepper" chromatin and infrequent mitotic figures. Carcinoids can be classified based on their histology into the following categories: insular, trabecular, strumal, mucinous, and mixed types. Insular carcinoid is the most common subtype[57] and is histologically similar to its intestinal counterpart with islands of cells separated by a hyalinized or fibrous stroma. Trabecular carcinoid is similar to foregut and hindgut carcinoid and is composed of columnar cells in cords, ribbons, or trabeculae.[58] Strumal carcinoid contains both carcinoid and mature thyroid tissue (struma).[59] The carcinoid component may display an insular, trabecular, or mixed insular-trabecular pattern and may colonize thyroid follicles. Finally, mucinous carcinoid is the least common of the subtypes and resembles goblet cell carcinoids of the appendix[60] with round or tubular glands lined by columnar neuroendocrine cells admixed with goblet cells. Malignant transformation (carcinoma ex-goblet cell carcinoid) can occur.

High-grade neuroendocrine carcinomas of the ovary include small cell carcinoma (to be distinguished from small cell carcinoma of the ovary, hypercalcemic type (SCCOHT)) and large cell neuroendocrine carcinoma. These tumors show solid sheet-like, corded or nested growth (Fig. 8.10) and exhibit extensive necrosis and brisk mitoses. Small cell carcinoma is composed of small to medium-sized round cells with scant cytoplasm, hyperchromatic nuclei, inconspicuous nucleoli and show nuclear molding (Fig. 8.11).

In contrast, large cell neuroendocrine carcinoma is composed of tumor cells with nuclear pleomorphism, characterized by large nuclei, some with prominent nucleoli, and variable amounts of cytoplasm (Fig. 8.12). Neuroendocrine carcinomas of the ovary are often associated with an endometrioid, mucinous, Brenner tumor or, rarely, a serous carcinoma component.

Neuroendocrine neoplasms express one or more neuroendocrine markers, including chromogranin, synaptophysin, CD56, and INSM1. They also express cytokeratin and EMA. Areas of intestinal/goblet cell differentiation may express CK20, SATB2, and CDX2, while the thyroid component stains for TTF-1 and thyroglobulin. The cells are generally negative for ER, PR, and WT-1.

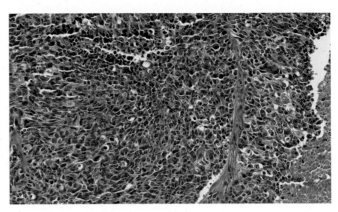

FIG. 8.12 Large cell neuroendocrine carcinoma showing nuclear pleomorphism and abundant cytoplasm.

Neuroendocrine neoplasms of the ovary are thought to be derived from neuroendocrine cells, through transdifferentiation of a surface epithelial tumor, or from mature cystic teratoma. They typically exhibit an aneuploid karyotype.

The possibility of metastatic disease from an extraovarian site should always be considered when evaluating a neuroendocrine neoplasm involving the ovary. Metastatic tumors are usually multinodular and bilateral, while the presence of an associated teratoma favors an ovarian primary. Presence of high-risk HPV subtypes highly favors a cervical origin, though diffuse staining for p16 may occur in neuroendocrine carcinoma arising elsewhere. Staining for TTF-1 or CDX2 does not exclude a gynecological origin.

Granulosa cell tumors can display growth patterns similar to insular and trabecular carcinoids. However, the nuclei of granulosa cells are finely granular, often with nuclear grooves, while neuroendocrine cells are coarsely granular. The tubules of Sertoli cell tumors and Sertoli-Leydig cell tumors (SLCTs) may also resemble carcinoid tumor. The presence of Leydig cells and well-formed tubular growth are useful in distinguishing these entities. Sex cord stromal tumors stain for sex cord markers such as inhibin, calretinin, WT-1, SF-1, and FOXL2, while are negative for neuroendocrine markers (except CD56) and EMA. Small foci of carcinoid tumor may be present in association with other ovarian tumors, such as SLCT. These foci are considered heterologous differentiation rather than a separate primary.[61]

Brenner tumor shows a nested growth pattern that may mimic carcinoid tumor. However, the nuclei often display grooves and the chromatin is finely granular. Brenner tumors are also negative for neuroendocrine markers.

Endometrioid carcinomas may display areas of trabecular or tubular growth pattern, mimicking a carcinoid tumor. Areas of conventional endometrioid morphology are helpful in making the distinction. Endometrioid carcinomas are typically positive for ER and PR, although they can show some staining for neuroendocrine markers.

Similar to epithelial ovarian cancers, NETs are staged according to FIGO staging (Table 8.2). Given the rare nature of these tumors, limited data are available on management of primary ovarian NETs. National Comprehensive Cancer Network (NCCN) guidelines for NETs recommend that the tumor be completely resected with an attempt at attaining negative margins.[62] Most ovarian NETs are confined to the ovary and are usually curable with surgery alone.[54] In rare cases of the diagnosis of NETs being known or suspected prior to the surgery, octreotide should be administered prior to and during the resection of the tumor in order to prevent carcinoid crisis.[54] While fertility-sparing surgery should be considered in women who may be interested in future pregnancy, a more radical approach including hysterectomy and bilateral salpingo-oophorectomy (BSO) may be considered in postmenopausal women or women who have completed childbearing. It is important to remove the tumor en bloc as failure to do so can result in peritoneal seeding and recurrence.[54] There is no current evidence to support adjuvant treatment.[62]

For unresectable or metastatic disease, treatment recommendations are like those for gastroenteropancreatic NETs.[54] Patients with limited metastases should undergo complete resection of the primary tumor and metastases with curative intent.[62] Per NCCN guidelines, unresectable liver metastases should be considered for cryotherapy, radiofrequency ablation or regional embolization.[62] Skeletal metastases can be treated with radiation.[62] Asymptomatic patients with low tumor burden can be observed with imaging and biochemical marker surveillance such as serum serotonin, 5-HIAA (5-hydroxyindoleacetic acid) and chromogranin A.[62] In patients with MEN1, biomarkers should be carefully interpreted as elevation in these biomarkers can represent NETs of other organs and not recurrence of ovarian NETs.[62] Patients with high tumor burden can undergo debulking surgery.[62]

Given the rarity of this disease, limited data are available on prognosis. Studies have found that cyst wall invasion, intraoperative rupture of the ovarian mass, tumor dissemination and adhesions are all unfavorable prognostic factors.[62] If any of these negative prognostic factors are encountered, a more radical surgical approach should be considered. CT imaging and MRI imaging can both be used for diagnosis and surveillance, although MRI has been shown to be superior for initial detection and follow-up of liver metastasis.[63] Somatostatin receptor-based imaging is not well understood and is generally not recommended for surveillance. However, receptor-based imaging can be used as a follow-up to evaluate the activity of any new masses identified on surveillance imaging.

When NET recurrences are diagnosed, somatostatin receptor analogs can be used for systemic treatment of advanced disease in patients with somatostatin receptor positivity on In-111 pentetreotide or ^{68}Ga-DOTATATE PET/CT imaging.[54] Since low-grade NETs frequently express somatostatin receptors on their cell membrane, radio-labeled somatostatin analogs, such as ^{68}Ga-DOTATATE somatostatin analogs, can be used for functional imaging. ^{68}Ga-DOTATATE has high sensitivity and specificity for the diagnosis of NETs, especially in low-grade, moderately differentiated and well-differentiated NETs. Therapies targeting VEGF and mTOR have shown promising results in cases of GI and pancreatic NETs and can be considered for cases of ovarian NETs as well.[54] For patients with ovarian NETs who progress while on treatment, chemotherapy can be used as a salvage option. Active agents include doxo-rubicin, 5-FU, dacarbazine, actinomycin-D, cisplatin, etoposide, and carboplatin which have objective response rates of 20% to 50%.[62] On the other hand, bleomycin, temozolomide, capecitabine, and paclitaxel have not shown compa-rable objective response rates and therefore should not be used. Furthermore, given significant toxicity with unclear benefit, chemotherapy is only used in patients who have progressive disease despite alternative treatment options, such as somatostatin receptor analogs, that have been shown to have more benefit in NETs of other primary sites.

Peptide receptor radionuclide therapy (PRRT) is the newest breakthrough in treatment of NETs. It is a molecular tar-geted therapy used to treat NETs by injection of a radiopeptide that binds to somatostatin receptors and delivers high doses of radiation to the tumor. A phase III trial of treatment options for patients with advanced midgut NETs and progression of disease during first-line somatostatin analogue therapy showed that treatment with ^{177}Lu-Dotatate, a PRRT, resulted in significantly higher response rate and progression-free survival (PFS) compared to high-dose octreotide.[64] While the role of PRRT in ovarian NETs has not yet been studied, it may play a role in the treatment of ovarian disease in the future.

Mesothelioma

Peritoneal malignant mesothelioma is a rare, progressive, and often ultimately fatal disease that can present as either primary peritoneal carcinoma or ovarian cancer.[65] Secondary ovarian involvement in peritoneal malignant mesothelioma is much more common than primary ovarian mesothelioma.[65] Given the extremely rare nature of primary ovarian meso-thelioma, there is little data on the clinical presentation and treatment strategies for it. Instead, most of the information we have is on peritoneal malignant mesothelioma with secondary ovarian involvement.

Mesotheliomas of the abdominal cavity are rare tumors that primarily involve the peritoneum, mesentery, and omentum, with an incidence ranging from 0.2 to 2 cases per one million women.[66] Although the most common site of mesotheliomas is in the pleural cavity, 10% to 30% of cases are found originating in the peritoneum.[67] Although peritoneal malignant mesothelioma with secondary ovarian involvement is more common than primary ovarian mesothelioma, both diseases are extremely rare. Utilizing a United Kingdom data registry over a 24-year period, ovarian mesotheliomas comprised 0.03% of all mesothelioma-related deaths, which is consistent with the very rare nature of this disease.[68] While there is a strong relationship between asbestos exposure and mesothelioma of the lung, given the rarity of primary ovarian mesotheliomas, no such association is known; however, in a patient with asbestos exposure, consideration should be given to an elevated risk of gonadal mesothelioma.[66] Loss of BAP1 protein characterizes peritoneal mesotheliomas and helps to differentiate from high-grade serous carcinomas.[69] Germline mutations in *BAP1* results in a tumor predisposition syndrome that includes mesotheliomas, pleural and peritoneal, as well as uveal melanoma, renal cell carcinomas and other tumors.[70]

Tumors may be unilateral or bilateral and usually involve the ovarian surface. The tumor usually appears as nodules, plaques, or papillary excrescences ranging in size between 5–15 cm with a white, homogeneous, and mostly solid cut surface. The residual ovary, if seen, is often encased by tumor. Malignant mesothelioma often exhibits glandular/tubular and papillary architecture involving the ovarian surface and parenchyma. The epithelioid subtype is most common. Simple papillae are lined by a single layer of polygonal to cuboidal cells, which are often flat or hobnail-like, characteristic of mesothelial differentiation (Fig. 8.13). Areas of solid and cord-like growth may be present. Psammoma bodies can be seen, especially in papillary areas. In the rarer biphasic subtype, spindle cells with fascicular growth are also present. In mesothelioma, the nuclei are typically monotonous and lack significant atypia, and mitotic activity is usually low.

Mesothelial cells express cytokeratins, EMA, WT-1, calretinin (Fig. 8.14 A), and D2–40. A subset of benign mesothelium and malignant mesotheliomas express PAX-8 and ER.[71] The cells are negative for MOC31, Ber-EP4 and CLDN4. Loss of BAP1 expression is seen in approximately half of peritoneal mesothelioma while it is retained in well-differentiated papillary mesothelial tumor, reactive mesothelium, and serous carcinoma (Fig. 8.14 B).[71] Approximately 10% of cases are associated with germline mutations in *BAP1*.[72]

Malignant mesothelioma primarily involving the ovary is very rare and should be distinguished from more common primary ovarian neoplasms. High-grade serous carcinomas display severe cytologic atypia and pleomorphism with abundant mitotic figures while mesotheliomas are typically monotonous without sig-

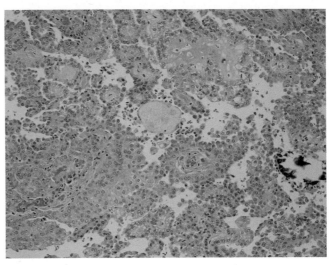

FIG. 8.13 Mesothelioma with papillae lined by monotonous hobnailed epithelioid cells and occasional psammomatous calcification.

nificant cytologic atypia or mitotic activity. Low-grade serous neoplasms are more similar to malignant mesothelioma in terms of cytology. However, hierarchical branching, nuclear pseudostratification, and cell budding are more commonly seen in serous neoplasms. Immunohistochemical stains are also useful to make the distinction between serous and mesothelial neoplasms. While both express WT-1 and can express PAX-8 and ER, serous neoplasms are positive for Ber-EP4 and CLDN4, while mesothelial cells are positive for CK5/6, calretinin and D2–40. The latter are also negative for other markers of adenocarcinoma such as MOC31 and Ber-EP4. A subset of mesotheliomas can show cytoplasmic clearing mimicking clear cell carcinoma (CCC). Immunostains such as MOC31, Ber-EP4, and napsin-A will be positive in CCC, while markers of mesothelial differentiation will be negative in these tumors.

Benign mesothelial proliferations can also involve the ovaries. These include mesothelial hyperplasia, peritoneal inclusion cysts, adenomatoid tumor, and well-differentiated papillary mesothelial tumor. In contrast to malignant mesothelioma, mesothelial hyperplasia and peritoneal inclusion cysts do not infiltrate into the underlying tissue and lack complex architecture. Adenomatoid tumors may have a pseudo-infiltrative appearance; however, they show a smooth lobulated configuration without destructive invasion. Similarly, well-differentiated papillary mesothelial tumors are

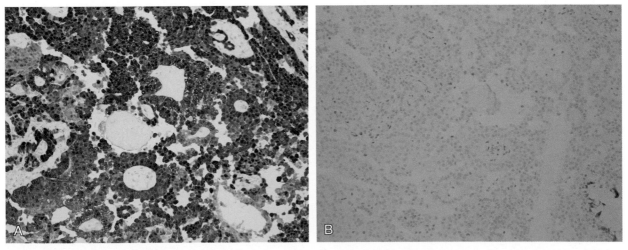

FIG. 8.14 Immunohistochemical staining shows diffuse expression of the mesothelial marker, calretinin (A) and loss of BAP1 expression (B).

noninvasive with delicate papillae lined by a monolayer of mesothelial cells without cytologic atypia or mitotic activity. In difficult cases, BAP1 immunohistochemistry can be of use in distinguishing benign mesothelial proliferations from malignant mesothelioma.

The clinical presentation, diagnostic imaging, and operative findings of peritoneal mesothelioma are often similar to those of ovarian carcinomas. As a primarily peritoneal tumor, the clinical presentation often comprises a variety of nonspecific symptoms as seen in epithelial ovarian cancers. As a primary peritoneal tumor, abdominal symptoms such as ascites, abdominal mass, abdominal pain, or intestinal occlusion are the most frequent presentations.[67] More aggressive mesothelioma subtypes are more likely to present with intestinal obstruction and significant abdominal distension due to a combination of ascites and omental disease.[67] The differential diagnosis includes cystic lymphangioma, cystic forms of endosalpingiosis, endometriosis, and cystic adenomatoid tumors.[66]

Computed tomography (CT) imaging of the chest, abdomen and pelvis is the initial imaging modality of choice. While MRI and PET-CT are other commonly used imaging modalities in cancer work-up, these studies have yet to demonstrate superiority over conventional CT.[67] Diagnostic laparoscopy is increasingly being used to better assess the volume and distribution of the disease and to obtain biopsies for pathologic assessment.[73,74] Formal diagnosis requires histopathological analysis of tissue biopsies, which may be obtained percutaneously or surgically. Percutaneous aspiration and cytology of ascites alone has limited diagnostic potential and is not routinely recommended.[75] Serum CA-125 is not as useful for establishing initial diagnosis but has more of a role in monitoring recurrence.[76]

Like epithelial ovarian cancers, peritoneal or ovarian mesotheliomas are staged according to FIGO staging (Table 8.2). The traditional treatment has been systemic chemotherapy, using the same regimens developed for pleural mesothelioma (commonly a platinum-derivative combined with pemetrexed) combined with palliative debulking procedures to alleviate obstructive symptoms. Studies have found that systemic chemotherapy with or without concomitant palliative surgery has relatively poor response rates and low median survival of approximately 1 year.[77] Given primary peritoneal malignancy is generally confined to the abdominal cavity, treatment by a combination of cytoreductive surgery and HIPEC has been proposed. Yan et al. reported outcomes following cytoreductive surgery and HIPEC in 401 patients with diffuse malignant peritoneal mesothelioma with a median overall survival of 53 months and 1-, 3-, and 5-year survival rates of 81%, 60%, and 47%. Although no prospective, randomized studies have been performed to compare cytoreductive surgery and HIPEC with systemic chemotherapy with or without palliative debulking surgery, the survival outcomes reported by Yan et al. were significantly better than the 12 to 27 months of median survival seen after systemic chemotherapy with or without palliative debulking surgery.[78] More recently, immune-based therapy and CAR-T cells have shown promise in mesothelioma.[79]

The main prognostic factor in this disease is the degree of surgical cytoreduction. The aim of surgery should be complete cytoreduction of macroscopic tumors. Some studies have suggested that complete parietal peritonectomy regardless of macroscopic involvement is associated with better outcomes compared with peritoneal stripping of only macroscopically affected peritoneum, as the risk of microscopic involvement of macroscopically normal peritoneum may be as high as 54%.[80] Given the scarcity of reported cases, the poor prognosis and short overall survival, there are no current recommendations for surveillance and treatment of recurrence. An approach similar to that taken with epithelial ovarian cancer using symptoms to guide surveillance imaging or imaging scheduled every few months initially with longer intervals over time would be reasonable (Fig. 8.4).

Squamous cell carcinoma

Squamous cell carcinoma of the ovary is a very rare tumor that accounts for less than 1% of all primary ovarian malignancies.[81,82] In most cases, ovarian squamous cell carcinomas arise from malignant transformation of mature cystic teratomas, or dermoid cysts.[83] The overall incidence of malignant transformation of dermoid cysts is 1% to 2%.[84] Less commonly, ovarian squamous cell carcinomas are seen in association with endometriosis or Brenner's tumors.[85,86] Most rare among ovarian squamous cell carcinomas are *de novo* cases.

Macroscopic features are nonspecific. Teratomatous elements may be identified grossly in cases of malignant transformation of a mature cystic teratoma. Primary squamous cell carcinoma of the ovary is morphologically identical to squamous cell carcinoma of other sites and is characterized by invasive nests, cords and sheets of malignant squamous

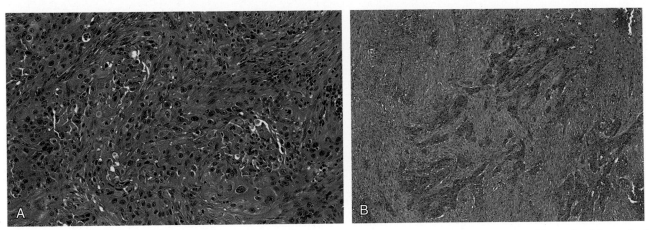

FIG. 8.15 Squamous cell carcinoma demonstrating foci of keratinization (A). Infiltrative nests of squamous cell carcinoma with associated desmoplastic stroma (B).

cells. (Fig. 8.15) Foci of keratinization may be present. Most commonly, invasive squamous cell carcinoma of the ovary arises from malignant transformation of a mature cystic teratoma.

Squamous cell carcinomas of any site stain for cytokeratin 5/6, p40, and p63. Primary squamous cell carcinoma of the ovary is very rare, and metastatic disease from other sites must first be excluded. Features favoring a primary ovarian tumor includes unilateral involvement, large size, and absence of surface involvement. The presence of teratomatous elements also supports a primary ovarian squamous cell carcinoma. Detection of high-risk HPV subtypes by in situ hybridization indicates metastatic HPV-associated squamous cell carcinoma, most commonly from the cervix.

Endometrioid adenocarcinoma with extensive squamous differentiation, either arising in the ovary or metastatic from the endometrium, can rarely mimic squamous cell carcinoma. The presence of conventional endometrioid morphology helps discern the two entities.

There are sparse reports on the demographic and clinical features of ovarian squamous cell carcinomas due to the rarity of the disease. In a review of 22 articles from 1964 to 2018, the average age of diagnosis was 52.9 with a range of 27 to 90.[81] Tumor sizes ranged from 1 to 26 cm and were found to present both unilaterally and bilaterally.[81] While the most frequent presenting symptom was abdominal pain, other commonly reported presenting symptoms included palpable abdominal mass, abdominal distension, vaginal bleeding, cough, rectal bleeding, weight loss, fever, and constipation.[81] The differential diagnosis of ovarian squamous cell carcinomas include those associated with mature cystic teratoma, endometriosis, endometrioid carcinoma with squamous differentiation, ovarian carcinosarcoma (malignant mixed mesodermal tumor) as well as metastasis from another organ or anatomical location.[81]

Like epithelial ovarian cancers, ovarian squamous cell carcinomas are staged according to FIGO staging (Table 8.2). Based on reported cases, the treatment for most patients is surgical including a hysterectomy, BSO, and omentectomy in some cases. A systematic review and meta-analysis showed that there may be a survival benefit associated with performing a pelvic LAD at the time of surgery (mean survival 59.2 months with LAD *versus* 40.4 months without).[83] However, given the small numbers and retrospective nature of existing studies, decision whether to perform pelvic LAD should consider the presence of enlarged lymph nodes on imaging, patient factors that would predispose to complications following LAD, and surgeon preference. In young women desiring future pregnancy, fertility-sparing surgery can be performed in patients with stage I disease with disease grossly limited to the ovary.[84] While there is no clear consensus on management of women with malignant squamous cell carcinoma incidentally identified on postoperative pathology for what was thought to be a benign teratoma, some suggest that restaging is not indicated if disease is microscopically limited to the ovary.[84] Additionally, due to the small number of cases worldwide and the lack of prospective data, there is no well-established role for adjuvant treatment. Current management guidelines are derived from ovarian carcinoma recommendations despite this representing a different histology. For early-stage IA disease, close follow-up is recommended for surveillance.[85,87] Patients with stage IB-IV disease should be treated with adjuvant chemotherapy with or without radiotherapy.[85,87] In 2008, Hackethal et al. found that patients with ovarian squamous cell carcinoma who received adjuvant chemotherapy

TABLE 8.5 5-year survival for ovarian squamous cell carcinoma by FIGO Stage.

Stage	5-Year survival
Stage I	76%
Stage II	34%
Stage III	21%
Stage IV	0%

From: R.M. Glasspool, A. González Martín, D. Millan et al. Gynecologic Cancer InterGroup (GCIG) consensus review for squamous cell carcinoma of the ovary. Int J Gynecol Pathol 12 (1993) 350–4.

with an alkylating agent had an improved overall survival of 57.1 months compared to 25.2 months among those who received a nonalkylating agent.[88] In the same study, no benefit from radiotherapy was shown.[88] On the other hand, in a case series of 17 patients with squamous cell carcinoma of the ovary, the impact of adjuvant chemotherapy with and without radiotherapy was retrospectively studied.[89] The median survival was not reached in the study and therefore no conclusions were made; however, the authors advocated for the use of concurrent platinum-based chemoradiotherapy.[89] While adjuvant chemotherapy has been shown to consistently offer benefit, there is mixed evidence on the utility of radiotherapy.

The two known prognostic factors for survival are stage and optimal debulking. Glasspool et al. found no association between postoperative treatment and survival.[90] Furthermore, the authors report a 5-year survival of 76% for stage I patients, 34% for stage II patients, 21% for stage III patients, and 0% for stage IV patients (Table 8.5).[90] Propensity score matching analysis of SEER data suggests that patients with ovarian squamous cell carcinomas have worse prognosis than those with serous carcinomas.[91] Given the scarcity of reported cases, poor prognosis, and short overall survival, there are no current recommendations for surveillance and treatment of recurrence. Like other ultrarare ovarian tumors, an approach similar to that taken with epithelial ovarian cancer using symptoms to guide surveillance imaging or imaging scheduled every few months initially with longer intervals over time would be reasonable (Fig. 8.4).

Sarcoma

Ovarian sarcomas are rare malignancies that include leiomyosarcoma, rhabdomyosarcomas, fibromyosarcomas, and angiomyosarcomas. Rhabdomyosarcomas, leiomyosarcomas, and angiosarcomas are extremely rare and generally described in case reports or small case series. Rhabdomyosarcomas are extremely aggressive and are most frequently reported as embryonal tumors in children.[92–95] Primary ovarian angiosarcomas are also extremely aggressive and even though long survival for patients with early-stage disease has been described, most patients with advanced stage die in the first year following diagnosis.[96,97] Rhabdomyosarcomas, leiomyosarcomas, and angiosarcomas of the ovary are extremely rare and only a few cases have been reported. While rhabdomyosarcomas of the ovary are more commonly seen in children, leiomyosarcomas and angiosarcomas typically present in postmenopausal women. A misnomer, ovarian carcinosarcomas, or malignant mixed Mullerian tumors (MMMT), are not considered a type of ovarian sarcoma but rather an aggressive subtype of epithelial ovarian cancers and comprise less than 4% of ovarian tumors[98] (see Chapter 3 Ovarian Carcinosarcoma).

Macroscopic features are nonspecific, but tumors tend to be large and unilateral with areas of necrosis. Sarcomas of the ovary resemble their counterparts at other sites and include leiomyosarcoma, adenosarcoma, low-grade endometrioid stromal sarcoma, and undifferentiated sarcoma. Leiomyosarcoma is a high-grade malignant smooth muscle showing fascicular growth with marked nuclear atypia, brisk mitotic activity, and areas of coagulative tumor necrosis. Adenosarcoma is a biphasic neoplasm composed of polypoid projections of cellular stroma lined by Müllerian glandular epithelium. Low-grade endometrioid stromal sarcoma is composed of sheets of uniform cells with scant cytoplasm and round to oval nuclei, with a "tongue-like" pattern of invasion. Undifferentiated sarcoma is a poorly-differentiated malignant neoplasm with no specific line of differentiation. Other rare sarcomas, mostly reported in case reports, include fibrosarcoma, rhabdomyosarcoma, angiosarcoma, myxofibrosarcoma, liposarcoma, and osteosarcoma. Sarcomas arising from a mature teratoma are classified as germ cell tumors with secondary malignant transformation.

Immunohistochemical profiles vary by tumor type. Low-grade endometrioid stromal sarcoma and the stromal component of adenosarcoma are positive for CD10. Smooth muscle markers, including desmin and SMA, are positive in leiomyosarcoma. Though not specific, ER and PR are often positive in gynecologic mesenchymal tumors. Ovarian sarcomas are thought to be derived from metaplastic ovarian stroma or from endometriosis.

Primary ovarian sarcoma should be distinguished from metastasis from the uterus. The possibility of metastatic uterine leiomyosarcoma is supported by a prior clinical history, presence of a uterine mass, and other features of metastatic disease (bilaterality, nodularity, and surface involvement). Endometrial stromal sarcomas have been associated with late recurrences; thus, it is important to consider a metastasis from a uterine primary, even with a remote history of hysterectomy. Ovarian endometrioid stromal sarcoma and adenosarcoma are often associated with endometriosis.

Sex cord-like differentiation may be seen in endometrioid stromal sarcoma and may mimic a sex cord stromal tumor. Both endometrioid stromal sarcoma and sex cord stromal tumors are positive for CD10, and sex cord makers may be positive in areas of sex cord-like differentiation. Correlation with areas of conventional endometrioid stromal sarcoma is helpful, as these areas would be negative for sex cord markers. Clinical correlation can also be useful, as sex cord stromal tumors may be associated with hormonal manifestations.

Ovarian sarcomas typically present with symptoms similar to epithelial ovarian cancer, such as abdominal distension, abdominal pain, and bulk symptoms.[98] Given the data on this disease is limited to rare case reports, there are no clear guidelines on the typical diagnostic workup. Furthermore, most cases are found incidentally after surgery for ovarian masses without a clear preoperative etiology. In any scenario where sarcoma is suspected on imaging of an ovarian mass, full imaging of the chest, abdomen, and pelvis should be pursued to rule out metastasis.

Ovarian rhabdomyosarcomas are typically treated with primary debulking followed by adjuvant chemotherapy, while leiomyosarcomas are treated with primary debulking surgery alone. Bacalbasa et al. describe a case of rhabdomyosarcoma in a 58-year-old patient with stage IIIC ovarian cancer, who underwent primary cytoreductive surgery followed by adjuvant chemotherapy with platinum and taxane. Two months after surgery, she presented with intestinal obstruction due to diffuse peritoneal sarcomatosis. A secondary cytoreduction was performed with macroscopic tumor remaining on the surface of the urinary bladder. She continued adjuvant chemotherapy but died of her disease 4.5 months later. The same authors also described a case of ovarian leiomyosarcoma in a 71-year-old patient who was diagnosed intraoperatively with a stage IIA leiomyosarcoma. After a cytoreductive surgery with no gross residual disease, her postoperative course was uneventful, and she remained disease-free four years later.[99]

Ovarian angiosarcomas are another subtype of ovarian sarcomas, and they are vascular tumors that demonstrate aggressive clinical behavior. Similar to the other ovarian sarcomas, radical surgical excision followed by adjuvant chemotherapy is the typical therapeutic regimen. Guseh et al. described a 40-year-old woman who presented with fatigue, nausea, and increasing abdominal girth and was found to have a pelvic mass, ascites, and omental nodularity on CT imaging along with an elevated CA-125 of 1851 U/mL She underwent an uncomplicated primary cytoreductive surgery followed by adjuvant chemotherapy with doxorubicin and ifosfamide, after which CT imaging showed no evidence of disease and her CA-125 was 18 U/mL. Three months later, her CA-125 remained stable, but 2 months later, she had increasing abdominal girth. CT imaging revealed recurrent disease, for which she was started on weekly paclitaxel with a partial response. Ultimately at 18 months after surgery, she had progressive disease and was receiving palliative chemotherapy.[100] As is shown by this case and other similar cases, patients typically present with advanced disease (FIGO stage III or IV) and have a poor prognosis, with median overall survival being 6 to 7 months (range 1–30 months).

Like epithelial ovarian cancers, ovarian sarcomas are staged according to FIGO staging (Table 8.2). Higher grade, older age, advanced stage, and suboptimal cytoreduction have been shown to be associated with worse prognosis.[98] Given the scarcity of reported cases, there are no current recommendations for surveillance and treatment of recurrence. Surveillance for recurrence and treatment of recurrent disease should be the same as that for epithelial ovarian cancers (Fig. 8.4). In cases of sarcoma, serial surveillance imaging or symptoms-based imaging would be a reasonable approach following surgery.

References

1. Austin RM, Norris HJ. Malignant Brenner tumor and transitional cell carcinoma of the ovary: a comparison. *Int J Gynecol Pathol.* 1987;6:29–39.
2. Nasioudis D, Sisti G, Kanninen TT, Fambrini M, Di Tommaso M. Prognostic significance of transitional cell carcinoma-like morphology of high-grade serous ovarian carcinoma: a comparative study. *Int J Gynecol Cancer.* 2016;26(9):1624–1629. https://doi.org/10.1097/IGC.0000000000000817. 27575630.
3. Austin RM, Norris HJ. Malignant Brenner tumor and transitional cell carcinoma of the ovary: a comparison. *Int J Gynecol Pathol.* 1987;6(1):29–39. https://doi.org/10.1097/00004347-198703000-00004. 3570630.
4. Kommoss F, Kommoss S, Schmidt D, Trunk MJ, Pfisterer J, du Bois A. Arbeitsgemeinschaft Gynaekologische Onkologie Studiengruppe Ovarialkarzinom. Survival benefit for patients with advanced-stage transitional cell carcinomas vs. other subtypes of ovarian carcinoma after chemotherapy with platinum and paclitaxel. *Gynecol Oncol.* 2005;97(1):195–199. https://doi.org/10.1016/j.ygyno.2004.12.047. 15790458.

5. Guseh SH, Rauh-Hain JA, Tambouret RH, et al. Transitional cell carcinoma of the ovary: a case-control study. *Gynecol Oncol.* 2014;132(3):649–653. https://doi.org/10.1016/j.ygyno.2014.01.020. Epub 2014 Jan 21 24462804.

6. Ali RH, Seidman JD, Luk M, Kalloger S, Gilks CB. Transitional cell carcinoma of the ovary is related to high-grade serous carcinoma and is distinct from malignant Brenner tumor. *Int J Gynecol Pathol.* 2013;31(6):499–506.

7. Gershenson DM, Silva EG, Mitchell MF, Atkinson EN, Wharton JT. Transitional cell carcinoma of the ovary: a matched control study of advanced-stage patients treated with cisplatin-based chemotherapy. *Am J Obstet Gynecol.* 1993;168(4):1178–1185.

8. Eichhorn J, Young R. Transitional cell carcinoma of the ovary: pathologic study of 100 cases with emphasis on differential diagnosis. *Am J Surg Pathol.* 2004;28(4):453–463.

9. Soslow RA, Brenton JD, Davidson B, et al. High grade serous carcinoma of the ovary. In: WHO Classification of Tumors Editorial Board, ed. *Female Genital Tumors.* World Health Organization Classification of Tumors. Lyon: IARC Press; 2020:45–47.

10. Folkins AK, Palacios J, Xue WC. Malignant Brenner tumor. In: WHO Classification of Tumors Editorial Board, ed. *Female Genital Tumors.* World Health Organization Classification of Tumors. Lyon: IARC Press; 2020:75–76.

11. Tessier-Cloutier B, Cochrane DR, Karnezis AN, et al. Proteomic analysis of transitional cell carcinoma-like variant of tubo-ovarian high-grade serous carcinoma. *Hum Pathol.* 2020;101:40–52.

12. Lang SM, Mills AM, Cantrell LA. Malignant Brenner tumor of the ovary: review and case report. *Gynecol Oncol Rep.* 2017;22:26–31. https://doi.org/10.1016/j.gore.2017.07.001. PMID: 28971141; PMCID: PMC5608552.

13. Nasioudis D, Sisti G, Holcomb K, et al. Malignant Brenner tumors of the ovary; a population-based analysis. *Gynecol Oncol.* 2016;142(1):44–49. https://doi.org/10.1016/j.ygyno.2016.04.538. Epub 2016 May 11. PMID: 27130406.

14. Quirk JT, Natarajan N. Ovarian cancer incidence in the United States, 1992-1999. *Gynecol Oncol.* 2005;97(2):519–523. https://doi.org/10.1016/j.ygyno.2005.02.007. PMID: 15863154.

15. King L, Gogoi RP, Hummel C, et al. Malignant Brenner tumor: two case reports. *Case Rep Womens Health.* 2018;20, e00082. https://doi.org/10.1016/j.crwh.2018.e00082. PMID: 30364765; PMCID: PMC6197787.

16. Takeuchi T, Ohishi Y, Imamura H, et al. Ovarian transitional cell carcinoma represents a poorly differentiated form of high-grade serous or endometrioid adenocarcinoma. *Am J Surg Pathol.* 2013;37(7):1091–1099.

17. Pfarr N, Darb-Esfahani S, Leichsenring J, et al. Mutational profiles of Brenner tumors show distinctive features uncoupling urothelial carcinomas and ovarian carcinoma with transitional cell histology. *Genes Chromosomes Cancer.* 2017;56(10):758–766.

18. Khani F, Diolombi ML, Khattar P, et al. Benign and malignant Brenner tumors show an absence of TERT promoter mutations that are commonly present in urothelial carcinoma. *Am J Surg Pathol.* 2016;40(9):1291–1295.

19. Zhang Y, Staley SA, Tucker K, et al. Malignant Brenner tumor of the ovary: case series and review of treatment strategies. *Gynecol Oncol Rep.* 2019;28:29–32. https://doi.org/10.1016/j.gore.2019.02.003. PMID: 30815527; PMCID: PMC6378317.

20. Han JH, Kim DY, Lee SW, et al. Intensive systemic chemotherapy is effective against recurrent malignant Brenner tumor of the ovary: an analysis of 10 cases within a single center. *Taiwan J Obstet Gynecol.* 2015;54(2):178–182. https://doi.org/10.1016/j.tjog.2014.03.008. PMID: 25951724.

21. Yamamoto R, Fujita M, Kuwabara M, et al. Malignant Brenner tumors of the ovary and tumor markers: case reports. *Jpn J Clin Oncol.* 1999;29 (6):308–313. https://doi.org/10.1093/jjco/29.6.308. PMID: 10418561.

22. Jung SE, Lee JM, Rha SE, et al. CT and MR imaging of ovarian tumors with emphasis on differential diagnosis. *Radiographics.* 2002;22(6):1305–1325. https://doi.org/10.1148/rg.226025033. PMID: 12432104.

23. Gezginç K, Karatayli R, Yazici F, et al. Malignant Brenner tumor of the ovary: analysis of 13 cases. *Int J Clin Oncol.* 2012;17(4):324–329. https://doi.org/10.1007/s10147-011-0290-7. Epub 2011 Jul 28. PMID: 21796330.

24. Haid M, Victor TA, Weldon-Linne CM, et al. Malignant Brenner tumor of the ovary. Electron microscopic study of a case responsive to radiation and chemotherapy. *Cancer.* 1983;51(3):498–508. https://doi.org/10.1002/1097-142(19830201)51:3<498::aid-cncr2820510323>3.0.co;2-b. PMID: 6821829.

25. Lin DI, Killian JK, Venstrom JM, et al. Recurrent urothelial carcinoma-like FGFR3 genomic alterations in malignant Brenner tumors of the ovary. *Mod Pathol.* 2021;34(5):983–993. https://doi.org/10.1038/s41379-020-00699-1. Epub 2020 Oct 19. PMID: 33077920.

26. Sampson JA. Endometrial carcinoma of the ovary arising in endometrial tissue in that organ. *Arch Surg.* 1925;10:1–72.

27. Parra-Herran C, Lerner-Ellis J, Xu B, et al. Molecular-based classification algorithm for endometrial carcinoma categorizes ovarian endometrioid carcinoma into prognostically significant groups. *Mod Pathol.* 2017;30(12):1748–1759.

28. Aysal A, Karnezis A, Medhi I, et al. Ovarian endometrioid adenocarcinoma: incidence and clinical significance of the morphologic and immunohistochemical markers of mismatch repair protein defects and tumor microsatellite instability. *Am J Surg Pathol.* 2012;36:163–172.

29. Vierkoetter KR, Ayabe AR, VanDrunen M, et al. Lynch syndrome in patients with clear cell and endometrioid cancers of the ovary. *Gynecol Oncol.* 2014;135:81–84.

30. Dominguez-Valentin M, Sampson JR, Seppälä TT, et al. Cancer risks by gene, age, and gender in 6350 carriers of pathogenic mismatch repair variants: findings from the Prospective Lynch Syndrome Database. *Genet Med.* 2020;22(1):15–25. https://doi.org/10.1038/s41436-019-0596-9. Epub 2019 Jul 24. Erratum in: Genet Med. 2020 Sep;22(9):1569 31337882.

31. Hereux SL, Braunstein M, Oza AM, et al. Epithelial ovarian cancer: evolution of management in the era of precision medicine. *CA Cancer J Clin.* 2019;69(4):280–304.

32. Zheng G, Yu H, Kanerva A, et al. Familial risks of ovarian cancer by age at diagnosis, proband type and histology. *PLoS One.* 2018;13(10), e0205000.

33. Bennett JA, Pesci A, Morales-Oyarvide V, et al. Incidence of mismatch repair protein deficiency and associated clinicopathologic features in a cohort of 104 ovarian endometrioid carcinomas. *Am J Surg Pathol.* 2018. https://doi.org/10.1097/PAS.0000000000001165.

34. Storey DJ, Rush R, Stewart M, et al. Endometrioid epithelial ovarian cancer: 20 years of prospectively collected data from a single center. *Cancer.* 2008;112:2211–2220.

35. Chiang YC, Chen CA, Huang CY, Hsieh CY, Cheng WF. Synchronous primary cancers of the endometrium and ovary. *Int J Gynecol Cancer.* 2008; 18(1):159–164.

36. AlHilli MM, Dowdy SC, Weaver AL, et al. Incidence and factors associated with synchronous ovarian and endometrial cancer: a population-based case-control study. *Gynecol Oncol.* 2012;125(1):109–113.

37. Lim D, Murali R, Murray MP, et al. Morphological and immunohistochemical reevaluation of tumors initially diagnosed as ovarian endometrioid carcinoma with emphasis on high-grade tumors. *Am J Surg Pathol.* 2016;40:302–312.

38. Assem H, Rambau PF, Lee S, et al. High-grade endometrioid carcinoma of the ovary: a clinicopathologic study of 30 cases. *Am J Surg Pathol.* 2018;42:534–544.

39. Köbel M, Rahimi K, Rambau PF, et al. An immunohistochemical algorithm for ovarian carcinoma typing. *Int J Gynecol Pathol.* 2016;35(5):430–441.

40. McConechy MK, Ding J, Senz J, et al. Ovarian and endometrial endometrioid carcinomas have distinct CTNNB1 and PTEN mutation profiles. *Mod Pathol.* 2014;27(1):128–134.

41. Wu R, Hendrix-Lucas N, Kuick R, et al. Mouse model of human ovarian endometrioid adenocarcinoma based on somatic defects in the Wnt/beta-catenin and PI3K/Pten signaling pathways. *Cancer Cell.* 2007;11(4):321–333.

42. Reijnen C, Küsters-Vandevelde HVN, Ligtenberg MJL, et al. Molecular profiling identifies synchronous endometrial and ovarian cancers as metastatic endometrial cancer with favorable clinical outcome. *Int J Cancer.* 2020;147(2):478–489.

43. Schultheis AM, Ng CK, De Filippo MR, et al. MAssively Parallel Sequencing-based clonality analysis of synchronous endometrioid endometrial ovarian carcinomas. *J Natl Cancer Inst.* 2016;108(6). djv427. 26832770.

44. Fadare O, Parkash V. Pathology of Endometrioid and clear cell carcinoma of the ovary. *Surg Pathol Clin.* 2019;12(2):529–564. https://doi.org/10.1016/j.path.2019.01.009. 31097114.

45. Peres LC, Cushing-Haugen KL, Köbel M, et al. Invasive epithelial ovarian cancer survival by histotype and disease stage. *J Natl Cancer Inst.* 2018. https://doi.org/10.1093/jnci/djy071.

46. Rambau P, Kelemen LE, Steed H, et al. Association of hormone receptor expression with survival in ovarian endometrioid carcinoma: biological validation and clinical implications. *Int J Mol Sci.* 2017;18(3).

47. Parra-Herran C, Bassiouny D, Vicus D, et al. FIGO versus Silverberg grading systems in ovarian endometrioid carcinoma: a comparative prognostic analysis. *Am J Surg Pathol.* 2018. https://doi.org/10.1097/PAS.0000000000001160.

48. Rambau PF, Vierkant RA, Intermaggio MP, et al. Association of p16 expression with prognosis varies across ovarian carcinoma histotypes: an ovarian tumor tissue analysis consortium study. *J Pathol Clin Res.* 2018. https://doi.org/10.1002/cjp2.109.

49. Heckl M, Schmoeckel E, Hertlein L, et al. The ARID1A, p53 and ß-catenin statuses are strong prognosticators in clear cell and endometrioid carcinoma of the ovary and the endometrium. *PLoS One.* 2018;13(2), e0192881.

50. Liu J, Albarracin CT, Chang KH, et al. Microsatellite instability and expression of hMLH1 and hMSH2 proteins in ovarian endometrioid cancer. *Mod Pathol.* 2004;17(1):75–80. https://doi.org/10.1038/modpathol.3800017. 14631366.

51. Le DT, Uram JN, Wang H, et al. PD-1 blockade in tumors with mismatch-repair deficiency. *N Engl J Med.* 2015;372(26):2509–2520. https://doi.org/10.1056/NEJMoa1500596. Epub 2015 May 30 26028255.

52. Storey DJ, Rush R, Stewart M, et al. Endometrioid epithelial ovarian cancer : 20 years of prospectively collected data from a single center. *Cancer.* 2008;112(10):2211–2220. https://doi.org/10.1002/cncr.23438. 18344211.

53. Duh QY, Hybarger CP, Geist R, et al. Carcinoids associated with multiple endocrine neoplasia syndromes. *Am J Surg.* 1987;142–148. https://doi.org/10.1016/0002-9610(87)90305-9.

54. Jhawar S, Lakhotia R, Suzuki M, et al. Clinical presentation and management of primary ovarian neuroendocrine tumor in multiple endocrine neoplasia type 1. *Endocrinol Diabetes Metab Case Rep.* 2019;2019:19–0040.

55. Spaulding R, Alatassi H, Stewart Metzinger D, Moghadamfalahi M. Ependymoma and carcinoid tumor associated with ovarian mature cystic teratoma in a patient with multiple endocrine neoplasia I. *Case Rep Obstet Gynecol.* 2014;712657. https://doi.org/10.1155/2014/712657.

56. Soga J, Osaka M, Yakuwa Y. Carcinoids of the ovary: an analysis of 329 reported cases. *J Exp Clin Cancer Res.* 2000;271–280.

57. Robboy SJ, Norris HJ, Scully RE. Insular carcinoid primary in the ovary. A clinicopathologic analysis of 48 cases. *Cancer.* 1975;36(2):404–418.

58. Robboy SJ, Scully RE, Norris HJ. Primary trabecular carcinoid of the ovary. *Obstet Gynecol.* 1977;49(2):202–207.

59. Robboy SJ, Scully RE. Strumal carcinoid of the ovary: an analysis of 50 cases of a distinctive tumor composed of thyroid tissue and carcinoid. *Cancer.* 1980;46(9):2019–2034.

60. Baker PM, Oliva E, Young RH, et al. Ovarian mucinous carcinoids including some with a carcinomatous component: a report of 17 cases. *Am J Surg Pathol.* 2001;25(5):557–568. https://doi.org/10.1097/00000478-200105000-00001. PMID: 11342766.

61. Young RH, Prat J, Scully RE. Ovarian Sertoli-Leydig cell tumors with heterologous elements. I. Gastrointestinal epithelium and carcinoid: a clinicopathologic analysis of thirty-six cases. *Cancer.* 1982;50(11):2448–2456.

62. Gardner GJ, Reidy-Lagunes D, Gehrig PA. Neuroendocrine tumors of the gynecologic tract: a Society of Gynecologic Oncology (SGO) clinical document. *Gynecol Oncol.* 2011;190–198. https://doi.org/10.1016/j.ygyno.2011.04.011.

63. Sundin A, Vullierme MP, Kaltsas G, Plockinger U, Mallorca Consensus Conference Participants & European Neuroendocrine Tumor Society. ENETS Consensus Guidelines for the standards of care in neuroendocrine tumors: radiological examinations. *Neuroendocrinology.* 2009;167–183. https://doi.org/10.1159/000184855.

64. Strosberg J, El-Haddad G, Wolin E, et al. Phase 3 Trial of 177Lu-Dotatate for Midgut Neuroendocrine Tumors. *N Engl J Med.* 2017;376(2):125–135. https://doi.org/10.1056/NEJMoa1607427. 28076709. PMC5895095.

65. Taşkın S, Gümüş Y, Kiremitçi S, Kahraman K, Sertçelik A, Ortaç F. Malignant peritoneal mesothelioma presented as peritoneal adenocarcinoma or primary ovarian cancer: case series and review of the clinical and immunohistochemical features. *Int J Clin Exp Pathol.* 2012;5(5):472–478. Epub 2012 May 23 22808303. 3396062.

66. Mani H, Merino MJ. Mesothelial neoplasms presenting as, and mimicking, ovarian cancer. *Int J Gynecol Pathol.* 2010;29(6):523–528. https://doi.org/10.1097/PGP.0b013e3181e6a3ee. 20881862.

67. García-Fadrique A, Mehta A, Mohamed F, Dayal S, Cecil T, Moran BJ. Clinical presentation, diagnosis, classification and management of peritoneal mesothelioma: a review. *J Gastrointest Oncol.* 2017;8(5):915–924. https://doi.org/10.21037/jgo.2017.08.01. 29184697. PMC5674249.

68. Attanoos RL, Gibbs AR. Primary malignant gonadal mesotheliomas and asbestos. *Histopathology.* 2000;37:150–159.

69. Andrici J, Jung J, Sheen A, et al. Loss of BAP1 expression is very rare in peritoneal and gynecologic serous adenocarcinomas and can be useful in the differential diagnosis with abdominal mesothelioma. *Hum Pathol.* 2016;51:9–15. https://doi.org/10.1016/j.humpath.2015.12.012. Epub 2015 Dec 29 27067777.

70. Pilarski R, Carlo M, Cebulla C, Abdel-Rahman M. *BAP1 Tumor Predisposition Syndrome. 2016 Oct 13 [Updated 2020 Sep 17]. In: Adam MP, Ardinger HH, Pagon RA, Wallace SE, Bean LJH, Stephens K, Amemiya a, Editors. GeneReviews® [Internet].* Seattle (WA): University of Washington; 1993–2020. 27748099.

71. Tandon RT, Jimenez-Cortez Y, Taub R, et al. Immunohistochemistry in peritoneal mesothelioma: a single-center experience of 244 cases. *Arch Pathol Lab Med.* 2018;142(2):236–242. https://doi.org/10.5858/arpa.2017-0092-OA. Epub 2017 Oct 19. PMID: 29048219.

72. Panou V, Gadiraju M, Wolin A, et al. Frequency of germline mutations in cancer susceptibility genes in malignant mesothelioma. *J Clin Oncol.* 2018;36(28):2863–2871.

73. Valle M, Federici O, Garofalo A. Patient selection for cytoreductive surgery and hyperthermic intraperitoneal chemotherapy, and role of laparoscopy in diagnosis, staging, and treatment. *Surg Oncol Clin N Am.* 2012;21(4):515–531.

74. Marmor RA, Kelly KJ, Lowy AM, et al. Laparoscopy is safe and accurate to evaluate peritoneal surface metastasis prior to Cytoreductive surgery. *Ann Surg Oncol.* 2016;23:1461–1467. https://doi.org/10.1245/s10434-015-4958-5.

75. Husain AN, Colby T, Ordonez N, et al. Guidelines for pathologic diagnosis of malignant mesothelioma: 2012 update of the consensus statement from the international mesothelioma interest group. *Arch Pathol Lab Med.* 2013;137:647–667. https://doi.org/10.5858/arpa.2012-0214-OA.

76. Baratti D, Kusamura S, Martinetti A, et al. Circulating CA125 in patients with peritoneal mesothelioma treated with cytoreductive surgery and intraperitoneal hyperthermic perfusion. *Ann Surg Oncol.* 2007;14:500–508. https://doi.org/10.1245/s10434-006-9192-8.

77. Vogelzang NJ, Rusthoven JJ, Symanowski J, et al. Phase III study of pemetrexed in combination with cisplatin versus cisplatin alone in patients with malignant pleural mesothelioma. *J Clin Oncol.* 2003;21:2636–2644. https://doi.org/10.1200/JCO.2003.11.136.

78. Yan TD, Deraco M, Baratti D, et al. Cytoreductive surgery and hyperthermic intraperitoneal chemotherapy for malignant peritoneal mesothelioma: multi-institutional experience. *J Clin Oncol.* 2009;27:6237–6242. https://doi.org/10.1200/JCO.2009.23.9640.

79. Zeltsman M, Dozier J, McGee E, Ngai D, Adusumilli PS. CAR T-cell therapy for lung cancer and malignant pleural mesothelioma. *Transl Res.* 2017;187:1–10. https://doi.org/10.1016/j.trsl.2017.04.004. Epub 2017 Apr 26 28502785. PMC5581988.

80. Baratti D, Kusamura S, Cabras AD, et al. Cytoreductive surgery with selective versus complete parietal peritonectomy followed by hyperthermic intraperitoneal chemotherapy in patients with diffuse malignant peritoneal mesothelioma: a controlled study. *Ann Surg Oncol.* 2012;19: 1416–1424. https://doi.org/10.1245/s10434-012-2237-2.

81. Koufopoulos N, Nasi D, Goudeli C, et al. Primary squamous cell carcinoma of the ovary. Review of the literature. *J BUON.* 2019;24(5):1776–1784.

82. McCluggage WG. Morphological subtypes of ovarian carcinoma: a review with emphasis on new develop- ments and pathogenesis. *Pathology.* 2011;43:420–432.

83. Hackethal A, Brueggmann AD, Bohlmann MK, Franke FE, Tinneberg HR, Münstedt K. Squamous cell carcinoma in mature cystic teratoma of the ovary: systematic review and analysis of published data. *Lancet Oncol.* 2008;9:1173–1180.

84. Yoshikawa N, Teshigawara T, Ikeda Y, et al. Fertility-sparing surgery of malignant transformation arising from mature cystic teratoma of the ovary. *Oncotarget.* 2018;9(44):27564–27573. Published 2018 Jun 8 10.18632/oncotarget.25548.

85. Goudeli C, Varytimiadi A, Koufopoulos N, Syrios J, Ter-zakis E. An ovarian mature cystic teratoma evolving in squamous cell carcinoma: a case report and review of the literature. *Gynecol Oncol Rep.* 2016;19:27–30.

86. Acién P, Abad M, Mayol MJ, Garcia S, Garde J. Primary squamous cell carcinoma of the ovary associated with endometriosis. *Int J Gynaecol Obstet.* 2010;108:16–20.

87. Mai KT, Yazdi HM, Bertrand MA, LeSaux N, Cathcart LL. Bilateral primary ovarian squamous cell carcinoma associated with human papilloma virus infection and vulvar and cervical intraepithelial neoplasia. A case report with review of the literature. *Am J Surg Pathol.* 1996;20:767–772.

88. Hackethal, Brueggmann D, Bohlmann MK, Franke FE, Tinneberg HR, Münstedt K. Squamous-cell carcinoma in mature cystic teratoma of the ovary: systematic review and analysis of published data. *Lancet Oncol.* 2008;9:1173–1180.

89. Dos Santos L, Mok E, Iasonos A. Squamous cell carcinoma arising in mature cystic teratoma of the ovary: a case series and review of the literature. *Gynecol Oncol.* 2007;105(2):321–324 [May].

90. Glasspool RM, González Martín A, Millan D, et al. Gy- necologic Cancer InterGroup (GCIG) consensus review for squamous cell carcinoma of the ovary. *Int J Gynecol Pathol.* 1993;12:350–354.

91. Zhang C, Ma T. Poorer prognosis of ovarian squamous cell carcinoma than serous carcinoma: a propensity score matching analysis based on the SEER database. *J Ovarian Res.* 2020;13(1):75. https://doi.org/10.1186/s13048-020-00675-y. 32611433. PMC7329546.

92. Mikami M, Tanaka T, Onouchi M, Komiyama S, Ishikawa M, Hirose T. A case of ovarian adenosarcoma with a heterologous rhabdomyosarcoma component: a brief case report. *Eur J Obstet Gyn R B.* 2004;117:112–114.

93. Nielsen GP, Oliva E, Young RH, Rosenberg AE, Prat J, Scully RE. Primary ovarian rhabdomyosarcoma: a report of 13 cases. *Int J Gynecol Pathol.* 1998;17(2):113–119.

94. Mukherjee S, Sen S, Biswas P, Choudhuri M. Primary pleomorphic sarcoma of the ovary with rhabdomyosarcomatous differentiation. *Indian J Pathol Microbiol.* 2009;52:217–218.

95. Cribbs RK, Shehata BM, Ricketts RR. Primary ovarian rhabdomyosarcoma in children. *Pediatr Surg Int.* 2008;24:593–595.

96. Guseh S, Bradford L, Hariri L, Schorge J. Ovarian angiosarcoma: extended survival following optimal cytoreductive surgery and adjuvant chemotherapy. *Gynecol Oncol Rep.* 2013;4:23–25.

97. Yaqoob N, Nemenqani D, Khoja H, Hafez M, Tulbah A, Al-Dayel F. Ovarian angiosarcoma: a case report and review of the literature. *J Med Case Reports.* 2014;8:47.

98. del Carmen MG, Birrer M, Schorge JO. Carcinosarcoma of the ovary: a review of the literature. *Gynecol Oncol.* 2012;125(1):271–277. https://doi.org/10.1016/j.ygyno.2011.12.418. Epub 2011 Dec 8 22155675.

99. Bacalbasa N, Balescu I, Dima S, Popescu I. Ovarian sarcoma carries a poorer prognosis than ovarian epithelial cancer throughout all FIGO stages: a single-center case-control matched study. *Anticancer Res.* 2014;34(12):7303–7308. 2550316.

100. Guseh SH, Bradford LS, Hariri LP, Schorge JO. Ovarian angiosarcoma: Extended survival following optimal cytoreductive surgery and adjuvant chemotherapy. *Gynecol Oncol Case Rep.* 2012;4:23–25. https://doi.org/10.1016/j.gynor.2012.12.006. 24371666. 3862330.

Section B

Uterine cancers

Chapter 9

Uterine leiomyosarcoma

Emily Hinchcliff, Barrett Lawson, Ravin Ratan, and Pamela Soliman

Clinical case

A 59-year-old nulliparous woman with history of multiple uterine fibroids status post myomectomy for abnormal uterine bleeding 20 years prior and recent total abdominal hysterectomy and salpingo-oophorectomy for recurrent, intermittent postmenopausal bleeding presented for management of pathological diagnosis of leiomyosarcoma. Workup prior to hysterectomy had included endometrial biopsies (EMBs) which were benign and serial pelvic ultrasounds over 18 months demonstrating a stable 5.4 cm uterine fibroid. MRI prior to surgery demonstrated a dominant 5.4 cm myometrial mass concerning for a degenerating leiomyoma vs leiomyosarcoma (Fig. 9.1). Pathology from her surgery was notable for a 5 cm uterine leiomyosarcoma limited to the myometrium with necrosis, marked cytologic atypia and 14 mitoses/10 high-powered fields. Computed tomography (CT) of the chest, abdomen and pelvis demonstrated multiple 1 to 2 mm indeterminate pulmonary nodules. How would you manage this patient?

Epidemiology

While uterine sarcomas are a rare form of uterine malignancy, making up only 3% to 9% of all uterine cancers, they represent a heterogeneous group of uterine tumors.[1] Uterine leiomyosarcoma is the most common, accounting for approximately 70% of uterine sarcomas. The remaining 30% of uterine sarcomas include other histologies such as endometrial stromal sarcoma, adenosarcoma, and perivascular endothelial cell tumor (PEComa) (see Chapter 10).

The median age of diagnosis for uterine leiomyosarcoma is in the mid-50s, and most patients do not have any clear predisposing risk factors. Black women have a two-fold higher risk of uterine leiomyosarcoma than white women, and there have been some reported associations with obesity and diabetes.[2] Hereditary syndromes such as hereditary retinoblastoma have a reported risk of approximately 13% for developing any soft-tissue sarcoma, including uterine leiomyosarcoma, while those with Li–Fraumeni syndrome, a defect in p53, also have a higher risk with one study reporting 7% to 8% of women with Li–Fraumeni syndrome developing leiomyosarcoma.[3,4] Pelvic radiation exposure has also been reported to increase the risk of developing a uterine sarcoma, as has hormone exposure.[5,6] In large registry studies, the percentage of women with uterine corpus cancers postpelvic irradiation was 0.08% to 2.4%; of those malignancies, uterine sarcomas made up 18% to 43%.[7–9] Time interval for postirradiation sarcomas between first and second neoplasm was 132 months (14–396).[5]

Tamoxifen use for greater than 5 years demonstrated significant increase in risk of uterine leiomyosarcoma, while shorter exposure had no association.[10] In one study, the relative risk associated with 5 years of tamoxifen use for all uterine malignancy was 4.1 (1.7–9.5).[11] In National Surgical Adjuvant Breast and Bowel Project (NSABP), secondary malignancies were characterized by organ site and histology specifically; they reported a risk of uterine sarcoma to be 17 per 1000 women years. This compares to a risk of uterine adenocarcinoma reported at 2.2 and 0.71 per 1000 women years for those exposed and unexposed to Tamoxifen respectively.[12] The prognosis of women with uterine sarcoma who had taken tamoxifen was no different than women without exposure to tamoxifen, once stage and histology were controlled for.

Pathology

Leiomyosarcomas (LMS) of the uterus are overall rare but make up the majority of uterine sarcomas.[13] The diagnosis of leiomyosarcoma is based on demonstrating smooth muscle differentiation and criteria for malignancy.

Diagnosis and Treatment of Rare Gynecologic Cancers. https://doi.org/10.1016/B978-0-323-82938-0.00009-4

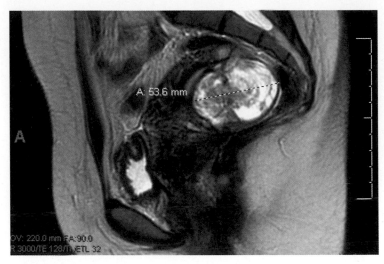

FIG. 9.1   Sagittal view of pelvis showing uterine mass.

Gross description

While leiomyomas are grossly white and whorled on cut surface, LMS are often hemorrhagic with necrosis and soft with a "fish flesh" texture.[14,15] However, this is not always the case, and some may have a firm-to-hard consistency that is predominantly white in color and mimics the appearance of a benign leiomyoma.[15] Tumor size is often greater than 5 cm in greatest dimension, even in early-stage disease.[14,15]

Microscopic description

Overall, the tumor is hypercellular, with a fascicular pattern of growth of elongated, spindled cells, with tumor cells typically easily recognized as with smooth muscle differentiation (Fig. 9.2A and B). The tumors can have spindled, epithelioid, or myxoid features. Other findings such as multinucleated tumor cells, osteoclast-like giant cells, xanthomatous change, and rhabdoid-like cells with inclusion bodies can be seen.[13] While many LMS invade into the surrounding myometrium, some may have a well-circumscribed margin. Lymphovascular invasion can be seen in 10% to 20% of tumors.

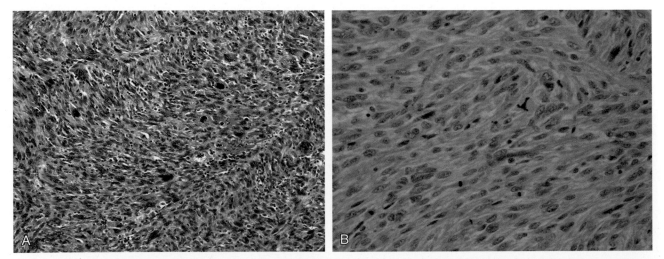

FIG. 9.2   (A) Leiomyosarcoma, tumor cells with smooth muscle differentiation showing severe nuclear atypia and easily identifiable mitotic activity; (B) Another example of leiomyosarcoma, with smooth muscle differentiation with more moderate atypia and numerous mitoses.

TABLE 9.1 Histologic criteria for diagnosis of leiomyosarcoma.

Criteria	Two of 3 criteria needed for conventional leiomyosarcoma
Diffuse Atypia	Moderate to Severe
Mitotic activity	≥10 mitoses/10 HPF
Coagulative tumor cell necrosis	Present

The spectrum of smooth muscle neoplasms can range from benign to uncertain malignant potential to malignant. Due to this wide spectrum, diagnostic criteria are applied to smooth muscle neoplasms to arrive at a correct diagnosis and associated prognosis. The histologic features for criteria include nuclear/cytologic atypia, mitotic index and coagulative tumor cell necrosis (Table 9.1).[16] Once a smooth muscle neoplasm reaches any combination of 2 of the following 3, the diagnosis can be made of a leiomyosarcoma: coagulative tumor cell necrosis, mitotic index ≥10/10 HPF, and diffuse moderate to severe atypia.[13,16] It should be noted that these criteria are only for conventional LMS. Different criteria are applied to variants such as epithelioid leiomyosarcoma and myxoid leiomyosarcoma, which are discussed later. If the neoplasm has atypical features but does not meet 2 of the 3 criteria for leiomyosarcoma, the neoplasm may be categorized as a smooth muscle tumors of unknown malignant potential (STUMP), the criteria of which are covered further in a later chapter.

The correct diagnosis can only be reached if the criteria are appropriately defined and applied. For example, the presence of any necrosis does not suffice for the check box of "necrosis present", but specifically coagulative tumor cell necrosis is needed.[13,16] Coagulative tumor cell necrosis is an abrupt transition between normal and necrotic tissue, with the necrotic cells having the appearance of "ghost" cells of dying but recognizable cells (Fig. 9.3). This contrasts with hyaline or infarct type necrosis, which shows areas of necrosis surrounded by a rim of hyalinization separating necrosis from normal tissue.[13]

Variants

Epithelioid

Epithelioid LMS are smooth-muscle tumors that show a predominant epithelioid-type histology, with the epithelioid cells having an oval or polygonal appearance with abundant eosinophilic to clear cytoplasm.[17] Typical spindled-cells of a conventional leiomyosarcoma may be seen but should be a minor element. Most show coagulative tumor cell necrosis and moderate to severe nuclear atypia. However, in contrast to conventional LMS, the mitotic activity may be as low as 3 mitoses per 10 HPFs.

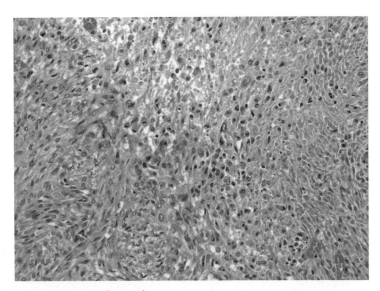

FIG. 9.3 Leiomyosarcoma with coagulative tumor cell necrosis.

Myxoid

Myxoid LMS are usually described grossly as gelatinous, mucoid, or myxoid, being an early indicator of the histologic appearance.[18] These variants typically are diffusely hypercellular or with variable cellularity of hyper/hypocellular areas. Myxoid stroma commonly comprises most of the tumor volume, while the neoplastic cells are arranged in bundles and fascicles. Criteria for diagnosis differ for this variant from conventional leiomyosarcoma as even as low as 2 mitosis per 10 HPF should be considered as worrisome for malignancy.[18,19]

Immunohistochemistry

As LMS are of smooth muscle differentiation, smooth muscle markers such as desmin and h-caldesmon will be positive. In some cases, when the tumor is very high grade, several markers may be needed to establish smooth muscle differentiation, and if all are negative, a diagnosis of high-grade sarcoma, NOS, may be appropriate. LMS of the gynecologic tract are usually positive for estrogen receptor (ER) and progesterone receptor (PR). In challenging cases, p16 and p53 stains may be employed as they can be overexpressed in LMS; however, the stains are not always helpful.

Differential diagnosis

When the tumor shows definitive smooth muscle differentiation, the differential may include the spectrum of smooth muscle neoplasms, including leiomyoma, mitotically active leiomyoma, atypical leiomyoma, and STUMP. In these cases, close histologic evaluation is necessary to determine if criteria of atypia, mitotic activity and necrosis are met to make a definitive diagnosis. If atypical features are seen but a definitive diagnosis cannot be made, consideration should be made for submission of additional sections as features of malignancy may be patchy or only focally seen.

Endometrial stromal sarcomas may mimic leiomyosarcoma but they are characterized by shorter spindle cells, spiral arteriole-like vessels and diffuse CD10 positivity, with the caveat being that this marker is not specific and may be expressed in LMS.

Rhabdomyosarcoma as a pure sarcoma is uncommon in the uterus, and while usually pleomorphic, occasional tumors have a prominent spindled cell component.[13] These tumors can show eosinophilic cytoplasm with cross-striations, the latter being typical of skeletal muscle differentiation. Rhabdomyosarcomas, which can be confirmed by immunohistochemical stains such as myogenin or myo-D1; these markers are negative in LMS.

The sarcomatous component of a carcinosarcoma may resemble a leiomyosarcoma, especially in cases of a predominant sarcomatous component. Sampling the tumor extensively may be necessary to identify a minor carcinomatous component.

Molecular findings

Uterine LMS have been shown to have mutations in *RB1*, *TP53* and *PTEN*, while whole-exome sequencing has also shown frequent alterations in *TP53*, *RB1*, *ATRXZ*, and *MED12*. *MED12* has been shown to be more specific to uterine LMS and those with a favorable prognosis, while *TP53* and *ATRX* mutations have been correlated with poor prognosis.[20]

Diagnosis and workup

Differential diagnosis

The differential diagnosis for uterine mass includes both benign and malignant tumors, with the most common etiology being benign uterine leiomyoma. In terms of malignancy, possibilities including malignancy of endometrial origin or sarcoma, of which leiomyosarcoma is the most common.

Signs and symptoms

It is clinically challenging to distinguish uterine leiomyosarcoma from its benign counterpart, uterine leiomyoma. Both can present with vaginal bleeding, increasing abdominal girth or bloating, pelvic pain and pressure, and/or palpable uterine mass. In a review of these symptoms, approximately half of women with uterine leiomyosarcoma reported abnormal uterine bleeding, a much lower percentage than women with other uterine/endometrial malignancies. Half had increasing girth or a palpable mass.[21,22]

Physical exam findings

In a postmenopausal patients a growing uterine mass or a newly symptomatic uterine fibroid are highly concerning for malignancy. For premenopausal women, neither rapid growth of uterine mass nor overall tumor size is necessarily indicative of increased risk of sarcoma.

Rapid growth of a uterine mass, generally defined as increasing by ≥6-week gestational size within 1 year, has been classically cited as an important delineator between leiomyoma and leiomyosarcoma. However, a literature review of 26 studies reported that only 2.6% of uterine sarcomas had a history of rapid uterine enlargement.[23] One large study of over 1000 women undergoing hysterectomy or myomectomy for presumed uterine leiomyoma also did not support rapid growth of uterine mass as predictive of leiomyosarcoma. In this study, the incidence of sarcoma was low in all patients, with an incidence of 1 in 371 (0.27%) in those with rapid growth and 2 in 961 (0.15%) in those without rapid growth.[23] Additionally, prospective studies of fibroids evaluated with MRI regularly every 3 months for 1 year demonstrated that rapid growth, defined as an increase of >30% over a 3-month period, occurred in 36.6% of tumors.[24]

Data on large uterine size as a predictive factor are more limited, but have also shown no clear association with uterine leiomyosarcoma. A study of women undergoing myomectomy for large uterine size, defined as >16 weeks in size, reported on 91 women and did not describe a single leiomyosarcoma on final pathology.[25] Therefore, the vast majority of premenopausal women with either rapid enlargement or enlarged uterine mass size do not have a leiomyosarcoma.

Tumor markers

There are no routinely used tumor markers to detect or predict uterine leiomyosarcoma. There have been small retrospective studies that indicate that uterine leiomyosarcoma may have a higher level of lactate dehydrogenase (LDH) than uterine leiomyoma; one study of 45 LMS and 180 controls demonstrated an OR for malignancy of 6.5 (95% CI, 2.6–15.8) with an LDH >193.[26,27] Another retrospective study of 2254 women with uterine masses, 43 of which were diagnosed with uterine sarcoma, combined use of LDH isoenzyme subtypes (LDH1, LDH3) predicted sarcoma with 100% sensitivity and 99% specificity, though this has not been replicated in other populations.[28] The use of LDH has subsequently been incorporated into some preoperative prediction modeling with variable success.

Imaging

Workup of a uterine mass often begins with the use of transvaginal ultrasound (Table 9.2). Uterine LMS are described as containing mixed echogenicity, commonly with central necrosis. The use of color Doppler may include irregular vessel distribution with low resistance indices. However, these findings are not unique to leiomyosarcoma and can be found in benign leiomyoma as well. Therefore, concerning features should prompt the use of magnetic resonance imaging (MRI) or CT scan for operative planning. However, these methods have also not been shown to reliably distinguish between uterine leiomyosarcoma and leiomyoma.

For CT or PET/CT, leiomyosarcoma have been shown to generally have higher FDG uptake while leiomyoma tend to have mild FDG uptake; however, this varies by individual tumor. MRI is considered the more useful modality given its improved discrimination for soft tissue. One retrospective study of 19 leiomyosarcoma compared with 22 atypical leiomyoma reported that four qualitative MRI features were most strongly associated leiomyosarcoma: nodular borders, hemorrhage, T2 dark areas (lack of uptake), and central unenhanced areas consistent with central necrosis. The sensitivity and specificity were greatest when a lesion had 3 or greater of these features. Other studies similarly report that a mass with infiltrative margins has been shown to be more likely to be a leiomyosarcoma, and notably, a consistent finding of leiomyosarcoma is a lack of calcifications.

TABLE 9.2 Workup of uterine leiomyosarcoma.
Diagnostic workup
Physical exam Basic laboratory testing including CBC and LDH Imaging—could include pelvic ultrasound, CT, and/or MRI Consider endometrial sampling

When comparing MRI techniques, diagnostic accuracy increases with the use of contrast-enhanced MRI compared with diffusion-weighted imaging (sensitivity 0.94, specificity 0.96). This study also reported that use of diffusion coefficient may provide increased diagnostic precision. A prospective study including 10 patients with leiomyosarcoma and 130 with degenerating fibroids investigated the role of Gd-DTPA contrast enhanced dynamic MRI in combination with serum LDH and reported a 100% specificity and positive predictive value with the use of LDH and dynamic MRI, though this study was limited in sample size and difficult to generalize to a broader patient population.[22] Based on this data, there is no current recommendation for routine MRI prior to surgery for presumed uterine fibroids but concerning clinical or ultrasound findings warrant MRI imaging.

Diagnostic testing

Unfortunately, there are no definitive preoperative diagnostic tests that reliably distinguish uterine leiomyosarcoma from benign leiomyoma. Studies of preoperative endometrial sampling, by dilation and curettage (D&C) or EMB, have reported sensitivity of 30% to 60%.[29,30] While this is a much lower sensitivity than in other endometrial malignancies, sampling may still detect a significant subset of cases and should be considered preoperatively. In practice, women presenting with abnormal uterine bleeding, such as intermenstrual bleeding or menorrhagia, warrant endometrial sampling for pathologic evaluation. The American College of Obstetrics and Gynecology recommends sampling performed in all patients with AUB older than 45 years, or in those younger than 45 years with history of unexposed estrogens, failed medical management, or persistence of their AUB.[31] Thus these criteria should be applied to bleeding in the setting of a uterine mass, though the presence of a uterine mass alone may not warrant sampling.

Staging system

The AJCC staging system for leiomyosarcoma is included in a general staging system for soft-tissue sarcomas in the trunk and extremity (Table 9.3). There is a separate AJCC staging system for sarcomas of the bone. The AJCC staging system is difficult to apply to leiomyosarcoma. Therefore FIGO adopted the TNM system specifically for leiomyosarcoma and endometrial stromal sarcoma (Table 9.4). The latter is more commonly used among gynecologic oncologists.

TABLE 9.3 AJCC staging system for soft-tissue sarcomas in the trunk and extremity of (8th Edition).

AJCC 8th edition	
T1	Tumor ≤5 cm in greatest dimension
T2	Tumor >5 cm and ≤10 cm in greatest dimension
T3	Tumor >10 cm and ≤15 cm in greatest dimension
T4	Tumor >15 cm in greatest dimension
N0	No regional lymph node metastasis or unknown lymph node status
N1	Regional lymph node metastasis
M0	No distant metastasis
M1	Distant metastasis
Stage groups	
Stage IA	T1; N0; M0; G1
Stage IB	T2, T3, T4; N0; M0; G1
Stage II	T1; N0; M0; G2/3
Stage IIIA	T2; N0; M0; G2/3
Stage IIIB	T3, T4; N0; M0; G2/3
Stage IV	Any T; N1; M0; any G Any T; any N; M1; any G

TABLE 9.4 FIGO staging for leiomyosarcoma and endometrial stromal sarcoma.

Stage		Definition
Leiomyosarcomas and endometrial stromal sarcomas		
I		Tumor limited to uterus
	IA	Less than 5 cm
	IB	More than 5 cm
II		Tumor extends beyond the uterus, within the pelvis
	IIA	Adnexal involvement
	IIB	Involvement of other pelvic tissues
III		Tumor invades abdominal tissues (not just protruding into the abdomen).
	IIIA	One site
	IIIB	More than one site
	IIIC	Metastasis to pelvic and/or paraaortic lymph nodes
IV	IVA	Tumor invades bladder and/or rectum
	IVB	Distant metastasis

Prognostic factors

While approximately 60% of women present with uterine confined disease, recurrence rates remain high. As such current staging systems, including FIGO and AJCC, are limited in their ability to predict patient prognosis. This is likely due to the fact that other prognostic features, including age, grade, and menopausal status are not included in staging.[32–35] For example, a SEER national database study reported a four-fold higher incidence in women older than 50 years old (RR 6.4 vs 1.5 per 100,000). In a study from the French Federation of Cancer Centers Sarcoma Group of 1240 patients with sarcoma of various subtypes, histologic grade was associated with prognosis in the 148 included patients with uterine leiomyosarcoma.[36] Additionally, mitotic score and vascular invasion have both been associated with metastasis free interval.[37]

To incorporate these known prognostic features, a nomogram was created and subsequently validated at Memorial Sloan Kettering and can be accessed online.[38] This nomogram was designed based on clinical predictors and included age at diagnosis, tumor size, histologic grade, uterine cervical involvement, extrauterine spread, distant metastases, and mitotic index. The concordance probability of this nomogram was found to be superior to either FIGO or AJCC prognostic prediction.[39,40]

Treatment of primary disease

Surgical resection of uterine leiomyosarcoma is the mainstay of primary treatment. For women with early stage, uterine confined disease a total abdominal hysterectomy with intact removal is recommended. The removal of bilateral fallopian tubes and/or ovaries at time of hysterectomy is often performed but does not seem to impact survival.[33,41] A Surveillance, Epidemiology and End Results (SEER) database study (1988–2003) demonstrated that approximately 60% of surgeries for uterine leiomyosarcoma were performed with oophorectomy. Among women <50 years old with stage I or II disease, 29.6% of women had ovarian preservation; these women had similar survival to those who underwent oophorectomy (5-year disease-specific survival rate of 83.2% vs 83.2%; $P = 0.445$). In a similar study using the National Cancer Database (NCDB), 89% of women underwent oophorectomy at time of hysterectomy and, as expected, women without oophorectomy were younger (median age 46 years vs 55 years). Among women with early leiomyosarcoma, again there was again no difference in survival with oophorectomy compared to ovarian preservation. Therefore, in a premenopausal women, it is reasonable to discuss ovarian preservation.

Routine lymphadenectomy is not recommended as uterine leiomyosarcoma has a greater propensity for hematogenous spread, with rates of lymph node metastases <5%.[35,42] Lymph node beds should be carefully assessed and any clinically enlarged or concerning lymph nodes removed. For those with intra-abdominal metastatic disease, cytoreduction to no gross residual may have improved outcomes.[39,43]

At time of surgery, another consideration is that of frozen section. In a population of 1429 hysterectomies performed in the presence of symptomatic uterine mass with presumed benign disease, histologic diagnosis of uterine leiomyosarcoma was made in 7 women (0.49%). Frozen section only detected suspicion for malignancy in 3 of these 7 (42.8%).[44] Similarly, in a retrospective study of 21 LMS, frozen section revealed the diagnosis in only 1 of the 9 cases in which frozen section was performed.[45] Therefore, frozen section has a significant chance of false negative result and thus only definitive diagnosis of leiomyosarcoma on frozen section should impact surgical approach.

Many uterine leiomyosarcoma diagnoses are discovered on pathologic evaluation following hysterectomy. To allow for minimally invasive approach, the use of power morcellation, or the use of instruments to fragment uterine specimen to allow for laparoscopic removal, increased in popularity in the early 2000s. However, this presents a risk of disruption of occult uterine leiomyosarcoma; due to this risk, the FDA issued a "black box" warning discouraging the use of power morcellation.[46] However, there was criticism of the lack of comprehensive review of the literature and debate regarding the reported risk (1 in 352 for any uterine malignancy and 1 in 498 for uterine leiomyosarcoma).[47,48] Further studies report a much lower incidence of occult leiomyosarcoma at closer to 1 to 7 in 1000,000 women undergoing hysterectomy for presumed benign fibroids.[49,50] Therefore, there has been a spectrum of response to the FDA's black box warning, with some hospitals/departments banning the use of electromechanical morcellation, others recommend a more nuanced approach to counseling and patient selection for whom morcellation may be offered. There have been some studies investigating the potential use of contained tissue extraction, such as in-bag or scalpel-based morcellation, but the optimal method to eliminate morcellation related risk requires further study.[51]

Importantly, specimen fragmentation has been shown to lead to a higher rate of abdominopelvic dissemination. In one study of 56 patients, the rate of dissemination was 44% vs 12.9%, with poorer overall survival on multivariable analysis.[52] The risk of recurrence has been estimated to be up to a four-fold increase for those women whose tumors were fragmented. Notably, literature indicates that approximately 15 to 30% of patients with uterine leiomyosarcoma will be upstaged after reexploration if morcellation was performed.[53–55] Therefore, the management of morcellated leiomyosarcoma remains in debate, though at a minimum patients with history of such a procedure require close radiographic follow up for peritoneal recurrence.

Morcellation is associated not only with high recurrence risk, but with potentially different patterns of recurrence. In one study of 152 patients with stage I leiomyosarcoma, the risk of recurrence was increased (67.2% vs 86.3%) in morcellated specimens.[55] Among patients with intact removal of specimen, the majority (69.4%) recurred at hematogenous sites only with only 18.1% having peritoneal only recurrence. Conversely, patients with morcellated tumors were more likely to recur in the peritoneum with 62.3% recurrences in peritoneum and 28.9% in hematogenous sites.

Adjuvant therapy in early-stage disease

Adjuvant systemic therapy for uterine sarcoma remains a controversial topic as there are no completed prospective, randomized trials evaluating adjuvant therapy in this group of women. Many treatment recommendations are made based on two factors: (1) a high risk of recurrence and (2) therapy that has been shown to be effective in the recurrent or metastatic setting. Incorporating the two of the most effective regimens in the metastatic setting, Sarcoma Alliance for Research through Collaboration (SARC) 005 treated women with early-stage uterine leiomyosarcoma with 4 cycles of adjuvant gemcitabine and docetaxel, followed by 4 cycles of doxorubicin if they remained disease free. The median time to recurrence was 27.4 months, with 57% of patients disease free at 3 years.[56] These data were felt to be promising based on historical controls, and the regimen was subsequently incorporated in a large phase III study that randomized patients to treatment vs observation. Unfortunately, the trial failed to accrue and was ultimately closed.[57,58] Only 38 of the targeted 218 patients enrolled, 20 of whom were assigned to chemotherapy while 18 assigned to observation. There were 8 recurrences in each arm, and the mean recurrence-free survival (RFS) was estimated at 18.1 months in the chemotherapy arm vs 14.6 months in the observation arm. Mean overall survival time was estimated at 34.3 and 46.4 months in the chemotherapy and observation arms respectively, though both of these survival outcomes are not considered statistically meaningful given small sample size. While it remains an accurate statement that no randomized trial has demonstrated a survival benefit with patients with uterine leiomyosarcoma, the difficulty in accruing to a well-designed adjuvant study appears to reflect discomfort among treating providers with randomization of high-risk patients to observation, rather than definitive evidence of lack of efficacy. Meanwhile, a recently presented retrospective study has suggested that treatment with anthracycline-based adjuvant therapy was associated with improvement in DFS (but not OS) over patients treated with gemcitabine and docetaxel in a recent retrospective 111 patient experience.

Turning briefly to the literature for adjuvant therapy of other sarcoma subtypes, adjuvant, or neoadjuvant therapy with an anthracycline and ifosfamide-based regimens has been shown to decrease risk of recurrence in both subtype specific and more heterogeneous patient populations as long as the treated population is at high risk for recurrence. While definition high risk can vary, the Sarculator, a validated nomogram for retroperitoneal and extremity sarcoma has shown some success in identifying a high-risk population that may benefit from adjuvant therapy.[59–62] Consequently, present soft-tissue sarcoma guidelines do recommend consideration of adjuvant systemic therapy for intraabdominal sarcomas at high risk of metastatic disease, and the Sarculator nomogram provides a method for risk stratifying. In uterine LMS, the Memorial Sloan Kettering nomogram provides a method of risk stratification but has not been validated as a tool for selecting patients for adjuvant therapy.[59,60,63] Informed by the experience in sarcomas at other sites, our approach is to have a discussion regarding the pros and cons adjuvant systemic doxorubicin-based therapy to patients with at least stage IB disease, with the important caveat that prevention of recurrence and overall survival has not been definitively demonstrated in this population.[64]

Radiation therapy is commonly used in other uterine cancers. In contrast, sarcomas are generally less radioresponsive, and hematogenous dissemination to distant sites plays a larger role in treatment failure. Retrospective reports of radiation therapy in uterine leiomyosarcoma suggested an improvement in local control. To prospectively examine these findings, EORTC 55874 examined pelvic radiation and surgery vs surgery alone in patients with stage I and II uterine sarcomas (leiomyosarcoma, carcinosarcoma, and endometrial stromal sarcoma). Over 13 years, 224 patients were accrued, with 103 of these having uterine leiomyosarcoma. In the entire study cohort, there was an improvement in local RFS; however, this was not observed in the uterine leiomyosarcoma cohort.[65] A survival benefit was not seen in any of the subgroups. As such, routine application of radiation has not been recommended for early-stage uterine leiomyosarcoma. For more advanced stages, or in specific clinical scenarios that increase risk of local recurrence (intraoperative bisection or morcellation of tumor, invasion of adjacent structures), radiation may be considered on a case by case basis.

Surveillance for recurrence

There is no current standard follow up for patients after the primary treatment of uterine leiomyosarcoma. Due to the high risk of early recurrence and propensity for both intraperitoneal and hematogenous dissemination, we recommend restaging with CT of the chest, abdomen, and pelvis every 3 months for the first two years after surgery, every 4 months for the subsequent two years, every 6 months for the following year, and consideration of annual imaging thereafter.

Survival and patterns of failure

Despite its overall rarity, uterine leiomyosarcoma makes up a large portion of deaths from uterine cancer as a result of its aggressive nature, with high risk of recurrence and overall poor prognosis.[66] Even in the setting of uterine confined disease, recurrence rates are reported to be 50% to 70% following hysterectomy.[67,68] The 5 year survival in early-stage (I–II) disease is 60% to 76%, while late-stage (III–IV) disease is only 29% to 45%.[33] The most common site of first recurrence is the lung (40%–70%), followed by pelvic or peritoneal recurrences (14%–40%), followed by bone (30%) and liver (27%).[69,70] However, the pattern of recurrence may be impacted by the use of morcellation and/or adjuvant therapy as mentioned above.

Treatment of advanced or recurrent disease

In advanced or recurrent disease, surgical management can be considered if disease is felt to be resectable with a goal of no gross residual. A retrospective study of 96 women with advanced leiomyosarcoma demonstrated a complete gross resection (CGR) was achieved in 49% of women, with improved median PFS (14.2 vs 6.8 months) for women in whom CGR was achieved.[71] In multivariate analysis adjusting for disease distribution and use of adjuvant chemotherapy, the presence of no residual disease was independently associated with PFS. Given the often rapid recurrence after surgery, we do not offer surgical therapy to the majority of recurrent patients. Our approach is first to treat with systemic therapy and in a selected, chemoresponsive population with minimal sites of disease and limited morbidity associated with resection, consider surgery after multidisciplinary discussion.

Excluding specific, uncommon situations where local therapies are indicated, palliative chemotherapy is the primary treatment modality for recurrent and metastatic disease (Table 9.5). Since its approval in the early 1970s, doxorubicin-

TABLE 9.5 Key clinical studies in uterine leiomyosarcoma and soft tissue sarcomas.

NCT#	Experimental Arm	Control Arm	Tumor Types	Response Rate	Median PFS	Median OS
NCT0006198	Doxorubicin 75 mg/m^2 Ifosfamide 10 g/m^2	Doxorubicin 75 mg/m^2	High-Grade Soft-Tissue Sarcoma	14% vs 26%	4.6 vs 7.4 mos*	12.8 vs 14.3 mos
NCT00142571	Gemcitabine 900 mg/m^2 Docetaxel 100 mg/m^2	Gemcitabine 1200 mg/m^2	Soft-Tissue Sarcoma	8% vs 16%	3.0 vs 6.2 mos*	11.5 vs 17.9 mos*
NCT00227669	Gemcitabine 900 mg/m^2 Docetaxel 100 mg/m^2	Gemcitabine 1000 mg/m^2	Leiomyosarcoma	Uterine: 19% vs 24%	Uterine: 5.5 vs 4.7 mos	Uterine: 20 vs 23 mos
NCT00752688	Pazopanib 800 mg/m^2	Placebo	Nonadipocytic Soft-Tissue Sarcoma	0% vs 6%	1.6 vs 4.6 mos*	10.7 vs 12.5 mos
NCT101343277	Trabectedin 1.5 mg/m^2	Dacarbazine 1000 mg/m^2	Adipocytic Sarcoma and Leiomyosarcoma	6.9 vs 9.9%	1.5 vs 4.2 mos*	12.9 vs 12.4 mos
NCT01327885	Eribulin 1.4 mg/m^2	Dacarbazine 850–1200 mg/m^2	Adipocytic Sarcoma and Leiomyosarcoma	4% vs 5%	2.6 vs 2.6 mos	11.5 vs 13.5 mos*

Denotes a statistically significant finding.

based therapies have been a cornerstone of treatment for patients with soft-tissue sarcoma.[72,73] From early in its development, a dose response curve was observed in patients with soft-tissue sarcoma, with higher doses of doxorubicin resulting in higher response rates.[74] Consequently, most modern regimens incorporate doxorubicin at a dose of 75 mg/m^2, which is a higher dose than in used in other malignancies.[75,76] For patients with metastatic and relatively asymptomatic disease, single-agent doxorubicin is an acceptable standard of care regimen. Doxorubicin-based combinations have also been studied in an effort to increase response rate and ultimately, overall survival. Historically, these have included combinations to include ifosfamide, dacarbazine, cyclophosphamide, and/or vincristine, with clear increase in response rate over single-agent doxorubicin but no statistically significant improvement in overall survival. For patients with symptomatic disease, combination therapy is more likely to improve disease burden and overall symptoms from the cancer. Doxorubicin-based therapies are generally recommended as first line, supported by data from the GeDDiS trial which demonstrated similar efficacy of gemcitabine and docetaxel vs single-agent doxorubicin in the first-line, with the latter being better tolerated.[77] The median PFS was 23.3 vs 23.7 weeks for those receiving doxorubicin vs gemcitabine/docetaxel, and PFS at 24 weeks did not differ between the groups (46.3% vs 46.4%, respectively). Median overall survival was also similar, at 76.3 weeks in the doxorubicin group and 67.3 weeks in the gemcitabine/docetaxel group.

Gemcitabine, which is often used in other types of uterine cancer, was studied in several phase 2 trials which documented its activity in soft-tissue sarcoma.[78,79] Docetaxel, was also investigated as a single agent, with limited to no activity in soft-tissue sarcoma.[80,81] Given minimal overlapping toxicity, the combination of the two drugs was evaluated in multiple single arm studies, demonstrating a response rate of 14% to 53% in soft-tissue sarcomas and a 53% response rate with patients with ULMS.[82,83] The high response rate in this ULMS study, which included patients pretreated with doxorubicin, was a surprise given the 21% response rate seen with single-agent gemcitabine as second line treatment for ULMS.[84] In two phase II trials of gemcitabine/docetaxel, the median PFS was reported at 4.4 to 6.7 months, and overall survival was found to be 14.7 to 16.1 months.[85,86] While the addition of docetaxel to single-agent gemcitabine was an obvious difference in these two studies, there was also implementation of a prolonged infusion of gemcitabine (over 90 min) in the combination trial. Prolonged infusion of gemcitabine had been shown to increase intracellular concentrations of the drug, and was associated with a higher response rate in other cancers.[87,88]

To determine if the improved response rates were due to the addition of docetaxel vs the modification in gemcitabine infusion, the SARC 002 study randomized patients with soft-tissue sarcoma via a novel Bayesian design to receive either single-agent gemcitabine or the combination of gemcitabine and docetaxel, both with fixed-dose-rate infusion of gemcitabine at 10 mg/m^2/min. Patients receiving combination therapy achieved a 16% response rate in contrast to 8% in patients receiving single-agent gemcitabine, with improved PFS in the combination arm. Notably, combination therapy was significantly more toxic, with more treatment discontinuations due to toxicity.[89] In response to this, the French Sarcoma Group undertook a randomized trial again studying gemcitabine vs gemcitabine and docetaxel, employing a 10 mg/m^2/min fixed dose rate infusion of gemcitabine in both arms and enrolling patients with uterine and nonuterine leiomyosarcoma. In both groups, single-agent gemcitabine and the combination of gemcitabine and docetaxel performed similarly in terms of PFS and OS, with less toxicity in the gemcitabine alone arm.[90] Consequently, while gemcitabine and docetaxel remains the most commonly used gemcitabine-based regimen in the United States, other combinations pairing gemcitabine with vinorelbine, dacarbazine, and other agents have been studied and are considered reasonable alternatives.[91,92]

Trabectedin is a novel DNA binding agent which was originally isolated from a marine tunicate and commonly employed in later lines of therapy for uterine leiomyosarcoma. Multiple phase I and phase II studies lead to approval in Europe as early as 2007. Regulatory authorities in the United States required a phase III study with an overall survival endpoint. This study, randomized patients with liposarcoma and leiomyosarcoma to trabectedin vs single-agent dacarbazine demonstrated an improvement in PFS (4.2 vs 1.5 months) and a response rate of 10% for trabectedin.[93] The drug is approved in the United States for patients with leiomyosarcoma; however, given the overall low RECIST response rates relative to doxorubicin and gemcitabine-based treatments, it is typically used as a second or third line agent.

While not a true targeted agent, the multitargeted anti-VEGF tyrosine kinase inhibitor pazopanib has been studied in, in soft-tissue sarcoma, including uterine leiomyosarcoma. The PALETTE trial randomized patients with pretreated metastatic soft-tissue sarcoma to pazopanib vs placebo. The response rate by RECIST was modest at 6%; however, PFS was improved (4.6 vs 1.6 months) in patients receiving active drug.[94] This study ultimately led to FDA approval of pazopanib for treatment of soft-tissue sarcoma including uterine leiomyosarcoma that has been previously treated with chemotherapy.

Noted to have activity in sarcomas early in its development, dacarbazine remains part of the armamentarium for patients with soft-tissue sarcoma. The drug can be employed in combination with doxorubicin or gemcitabine, and is also used as a single agent. In recent randomized studies where dacarbazine has functioned as a standard of care comparator, an ORR by RECIST of 5% to 7% has been noted with a PFS in the range of 1.5 to 2.6 months, suggesting modest but potentially meaningful activity as a single-agent in patients who have exhausted more efficacious lines of therapy.[93,95]

Uterine leiomyosarcoma, like many malignancies of Mullerian origin, frequently expresses ER and PRs, but the relation of these findings to the biological behavior of the malignancy is not clear. While hormonal blockade has been of some utility in low grade endometrial stromal sarcoma, the evidence for efficacy in uterine leiomyosarcoma is less clear. A phase II study of letrozole in patients with uterine leiomyosarcoma demonstrated stable disease at 12 weeks in 50% of the patients, with >30% being a customary threshold for drugs with possible efficacy in soft-tissue sarcoma patients. No objective responses were seen; however, 3 (11%) out of 27 patients on the study remained on treatment for over 24 weeks, and each of these had >90% ER and PR positivity suggesting that a further selected group of uterine leiomyosarcoma patients may derive some benefit from an aromatase inhibitor.[96]

Potential therapeutic targets

There has been a limited role for targeted therapies outside of anti-VEGF agents like pazopanib in the treatment of leiomyosarcoma. Genomic analysis has demonstrated frequent loss or alteration of *p53, RB1,* and *PTEN* and amplification/upregulation of the PI3K-AKT-MTOR pathway.[97] A study analyzing 83 uterine leiomyosarcoma samples demonstrated top somatic mutated genes were TP53, ATRX, PTEN and MEN1 genes. Interestingly, they demonstrated clinically relevant mutation signatures for homologous recombination deficiency (HRD) in 25% (12/48) of samples, and found that treatment of PDX models harboring HRD signatures with olaparib inhibited tumor growth.[98] A recently reported phase II study combining olaparib with temozolomide in patients with metastatic uterine leiomyosarcoma was encouraging, with an overall response rate (ORR) of 27% and a PFS of 6.9 months in a pretreated patient population.

The 83 patient mutational analysis also demonstrated that 61.4 (51/83) of tumors had PTEN/PIK3CA/AKT/mTOR gene alterations, and treatment with copanlisib (pan-class PI3K inhibitor) also inhibited PDX model tumor growth. Notably, single-agent mTOR inhibition has been evaluated in sarcomas without appreciable clinical benefit, possibly related to AKT activation and also lack of selection for patients with appropriate genetic alterations.[99,100] Combination trials attempting to address paradoxical upregulation of upstream signaling, either with TORC1/TORC2 inhibitors or dual blockade of PI3K and MTOR may be of interest in leiomyosarcoma patients, particularly those with *PTEN* pathway alterations.

Another emerging area is the detection of novel translocations across a subset of sarcomas, including leiomyosarcoma. Novel chromosomal translocations have not been readily identified by next generation sequencing platforms, though improved interrogation of the generated data has led to detection of potentially targetable translocations, including ALK fusions.[101] There has also been a recently described subset of uterine sarcomas with NTRK rearrangements who may benefit from NTRK inhibition with larotrectinib.[102,103]

Immunotherapy targets

Initial efforts at immunotherapy with checkpoint blockade in patients with uterine leiomyosarcoma have been disappointing. While there have been rare case reports suggesting response, no activity was demonstrated with single-agent PD-1 directed therapy in two separate prospective studies.[104,105] Combination therapy has also been studied, with a multicenter phase II study of nivolumab and ipilimumab vs nivolumab alone enrolling 85 patients with broad range of sarcomas, including 29 with uterine or nonuterine leiomyosarcoma. The response rate in the combination arm was 16%, with 1 of the 6 responses in this arm being a patient with uterine leiomyosarcoma.[106] Given the low response rates, checkpoint blockade is not recommended for uterine leiomyosarcoma outside of a clinical trial.

Case resolution

The patient was followed with exam and scans every 3 months however on a subsequent restaging CT scan 6 months after her initial visit, she was found to have multiple (greater than 20) new and enlarging scattered pulmonary nodules, the largest now being 16 mm in size (Fig. 9.4). The patient voiced a desire to be aggressive with her treatment, and was started on doxorubicin 75 mg/m^2 and ifosfamide 10 g/m^2 IV every 3 weeks. Cycle 2 of treatment was complicated by hospital admission for neutropenic fever, and renal insufficiency requiring supplemental IV hydration. Restaging assessments after 2 cycles demonstrated shrinkage of many of her pulmonary nodules. Due to fatigue and renal insufficiency, she was transitioned to therapy with doxorubicin 75 mg/m^2 and dacarbazine 750 mg/m^2. After completing 6 cycles of doxorubicin-based treatment, the patient was noted to have achieved a partial response. She was transitioned to a treatment break and remained progression free for 6 months. She subsequently received two cycles of gemcitabine and docetaxel with progression of disease on restaging studies. She is currently receiving trabectedin 1.5 mg/m^2 with stable disease after 3 cycles (9 weeks) of treatment. She remains on treatment with trabectedin at this time.

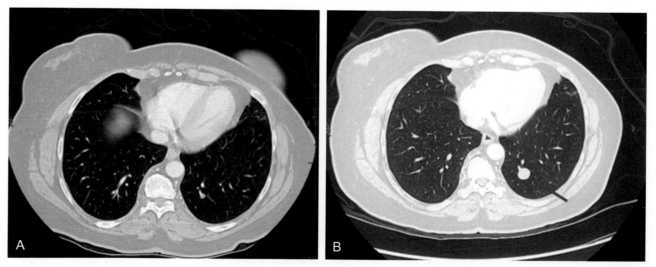

FIG. 9.4　CT scan showing (A) baseline scan with no evidence of disease and (B) 3-month postoperative restaging scan with lung nodule (*red arrow*).

References

1. Amant F, Coosemans A, Debiec-Rychter M, Timmerman D, Vergote I. Clinical management of uterine sarcomas. *Lancet Oncol.* 2009. https://doi.org/10.1016/S1470-2045(09)70226-8.
2. Felix AS, et al. The etiology of uterine sarcomas: a pooled analysis of the epidemiology of endometrial cancer consortium. *Br J Cancer.* 2013. https://doi.org/10.1038/bjc.2013.2.
3. Venkatraman L, Goepel JR, Steele K, Dobbs SP, Lyness RW, McCluggage WG. *Soft tissue, pelvic, and urinary bladder leiomyosarcoma as second neoplasm following hereditary retinoblastoma. J. Clin. Pathol;* 2003. https://doi.org/10.1136/jcp.56.3.233.
4. Ognjanovic S, Olivier M, Bergemann TL, Hainaut P. *Sarcomas in TP53 germline mutation carriers: a review of the iarc tp53 database. Cancer;* 2012. https://doi.org/10.1002/cncr.26390.
5. Robinson E, Neugut AI, Wylie P. Clinical aspects of postirradiation sarcomas. *J Natl Cancer Inst.* 1988. https://doi.org/10.1093/jnci/80.4.233.
6. Abeler VM, Røyne O, Thoresen S, Danielsen HE, Nesland JM, Kristensen GB. Uterine sarcomas in Norway. A histopathological and prognostic survey of a total population from 1970 to 2000 including 419 patients. *Histopathology.* 2009. https://doi.org/10.1111/j.1365-2559.2009.03231.x.
7. Meredith RF, Eisert DR, Kaka Z, Hodgson SE, Johnston GA, Boutselis JG. An excess of uterine sarcomas after pelvic irradiation. *Cancer.* 1986. https://doi.org/10.1002/1097-0142(19861101)58:9<2003::AID-CNCR2820580908>3.0.CO;2-2.
8. Rodriguez J, Hart WR. Endometrial cancers occurring 10 or more years after pelvic irradiation for carcinoma. *Int J Gynecol Pathol.* 1982. https://doi.org/10.1097/00004347-198202000-00002.
9. Czes'nin K, Wronkowski Z. Second malignancies of the irradiated area in patients treated for uterine cervix cancer. *Gynecol Oncol.* 1978. https://doi.org/10.1016/0090-8258(78)90037-9.
10. Lavie O, Barnett-Griness O, Narod SA, Rennert G. The risk of developing uterine sarcoma after tamoxifen use. *Int J Gynecol Cancer.* 2008. https://doi.org/10.1111/j.1525-1438.2007.01025.x.
11. Bernstein L, et al. Tamoxifen therapy for breast cancer and endometrial cancer risk. *J Natl Cancer Inst.* 1999. https://doi.org/10.1093/jnci/91.19.1654.
12. Wickerham DL, Fisher B, Wolmark N, et al. Association of tamoxifen and uterine sarcoma. *J Clin Oncol.* 2002;20:2758–2760.
13. Mills AM, Longacre TA. Smooth muscle tumors of the female genital tract. *Surg Pathol.* 2009;2:625–677.
14. Kempson RL, Hendrickson MR. Smooth muscle, endometrial stromal and mixed Mullerian tumors of the uterus. *Mod Pathol.* 2000;13:328–342.
15. Wang W, Soslow R, Hensley M, et al. Histopathologic prognostic factors in stage I leiomyosarcoma of the uterus: a detailed analysis of 27 cases. *Am J Surg Pathol.* 2011;35:522–529.
16. Bell SW, Kempson RL, Hendrickson MR. Problematic uterine smooth muscle neoplasms: a clinicopathologic study of 213 cases. *Am J Surg Pathol.* 1994;18(6):535–558.
17. Prayson RA, Goldblum J, Hart W. Epithelioid smooth-muscle tumors of the uterus: a clinicopathologic study of 18 patients. *Am J Surg Pathol.* 1997;21(4):383–391.
18. Parra-Herran C, Schoolmeester JK, Yuan L, et al. Myxoid leiomyosarcoma of the uterus: a clinicopathologic analysis of 30 cases and review of the literature with reappraisal of its distinction from other uterine myxoid mesenchymal neoplasms. *Am J Surg Pathol.* 2016;40:283–301.
19. Burch DM, Tavassoli FA. Myxoid leiomyosarcoma of the uterus. *Histopathology.* 2011;59:1144–1155.
20. Tsuyoshi H, Yoshida Y. Molecular biomarkers for uterine leiomyosarcoma and endometrial stromal sarcoma. *Cancer Sci.* 2018;109:1743–1752.
21. D'Angelo E, Prat J. Uterine sarcomas: A review. *Gynecol Oncol.* 2010. https://doi.org/10.1016/j.ygyno.2009.09.023.
22. Ganjoo KN. Uterine sarcomas. *Curr Probl Cancer.* 2019. https://doi.org/10.1016/j.currproblcancer.2019.06.001.
23. Parker WH, Fu YS, Berek JS. Uterine sarcoma in patients operated on for presumed leiomyoma and rapidly growing leiomyoma. *Obstet Gynecol.* 1994.
24. Day Baird D, Garrett TA, Laughlin SK, Davis B, Semelka RC, Peddada SD. Short-term change in growth of uterine leiomyoma: tumor growth spurts. *Fertil Steril.* 2011. https://doi.org/10.1016/j.fertnstert.2010.05.011.
25. West S, Ruiz R, Parker WH. Abdominal myomectomy in women with very large uterine size. *Fertil Steril.* 2006. https://doi.org/10.1016/j.fertnstert.2005.05.073.
26. Zhang G, Yu X, Zhu L, Fan Q, Shi H, Lang J. Preoperative clinical characteristics scoring system for differentiating uterine leiomyosarcoma from fibroid. *BMC Cancer.* 2020. https://doi.org/10.1186/s12885-020-07003-z.
27. Nagai T, et al. Highly improved accuracy of the revised PREoperative sarcoma score (rPRESS) in the decision of performing surgery for patients presenting with a uterine mass. *Springerplus.* 2015. https://doi.org/10.1186/s40064-015-1318-7.
28. Di Cello A, et al. A more accurate method to interpret lactate dehydrogenase (LDH) isoenzymes' results in patients with uterine masses. *Eur J Obstet Gynecol Reprod Biol.* 2019. https://doi.org/10.1016/j.ejogrb.2019.03.017.
29. Bansal N, Herzog TJ, Burke W, Cohen CJ, Wright JD. *The utility of preoperative endometrial sampling for the detection of uterine sarcomas.* Gynecol. Oncol; 2008. https://doi.org/10.1016/j.ygyno.2008.02.026.
30. Hinchcliff EM, et al. The role of endometrial biopsy in the preoperative detection of uterine leiomyosarcoma. *J Minim Invasive Gynecol.* 2016;23(4). https://doi.org/10.1016/j.jmig.2016.01.022.
31. Committee on Practice Bulletins-Gynecology. Practice bulletin no. 128: diagnosis of abnormal uterine bleeding in reproductive-aged women. *Obstet Gynecol.* 2012.
32. Nordal RR, Kristensen GB, Kern J, Stenwig AE, Pettersen EO, Tropé CG. The prognostic significance of stage, tumor size, cellular atypia and DNA ploidy in uterine leiomyosarcoma. *Acta Oncol (Madr).* 1995. https://doi.org/10.3109/02841869509127189.

33. Kapp DS, Shin JY, Chan JK. Prognostic factors and survival in 1396 patients with uterine leiomyosarcomas: Emphasis on impact of lymphadenectomy and oophorectomy. *Cancer.* 2008. https://doi.org/10.1002/cncr.23245.

34. Giuntoli RL, et al. Retrospective review of 208 patients with leiomyosarcoma of the uterus: Prognostic indicators, surgical management, and adjuvant therapy. *Gynecol Oncol.* 2003. https://doi.org/10.1016/S0090-8258(03)00137-9.

35. Pautier P, et al. Analysis of clinicopathologic prognostic factors for 157 uterine sarcomas and evaluation of a grading score validated for soft tissue arcoma. *Cancer.* 2000. https://doi.org/10.1002/(SICI)1097-0142(20000315)88:6<1425::AID-CNCR21>3.0.CO;2-3.

36. Coindre JM, et al. Predictive value of grade for metastasis development in the main histologic types of adult soft tissue sarcomas: A study of 1240 patients from the French Federation of Cancer Centers sarcoma group. *Cancer.* 2001. https://doi.org/10.1002/1097-0142(20010515)91:10<1914::AID-CNCR1214>3.0.CO;2-3.

37. Pelmus M, et al. Prognostic factors in early-stage leiomyosarcoma of the uterus. *Int J Gynecol Cancer.* 2009. https://doi.org/10.1111/IGC.0b013e3181a1bfbc.

38. Fucà G, Fabbroni C, Rosanna M, et al. Anthracycline-based and gemcitabine-based chemotherapy in the adjuvant setting for stage I uterine leiomyosarcoma: a retrospective analysis at two reference centers. *Clin Sarcoma Res.* 2020;10:17.

39. Zivanovic O, et al. A nomogram to predict postresection 5-year overall survival for patients with uterine leiomyosarcoma. *Cancer.* 2012. https://doi.org/10.1002/cncr.26333.

40. Iasonos A, et al. External validation of a prognostic nomogram for overall survival in women with uterine leiomyosarcoma. *Cancer.* 2013. https://doi.org/10.1002/cncr.27971.

41. Seagle BLL, Sobecki-Rausch J, Strohl AE, Shilpi A, Grace A, Shahabi S. Prognosis and treatment of uterine leiomyosarcoma: a National Cancer Database study. *Gynecol Oncol.* 2017. https://doi.org/10.1016/j.ygyno.2017.02.012.

42. Leitao MM, Sonoda Y, Brennan MF, Barakat RR, Chi DS. Incidence of lymph node and ovarian metastases in leiomyosarcoma of the uterus. *Gynecol Oncol.* 2003. https://doi.org/10.1016/S0090-8258(03)00478-5.

43. Dinh TA, Oliva EA, Fuller AF, Lee H, Goodman A. The treatment of uterine leiomyosarcoma. Results from a 10-year xperience (1990–1999) at the Massachusetts General Hospital. *Gynecol Oncol.* 2004. https://doi.org/10.1016/j.ygyno.2003.10.044.

44. Leibsohn S, d'Ablaing G, Mishell DR, Schlaerth JB. Leiomyosarcoma in a series of hysterectomies performed for presumed uterine leiomyomas. *Am J Obstet Gynecol.* 1990. https://doi.org/10.1016/0002-9378(90)91298-Q.

45. Schwartz LB, Diamond MP, Schwartz PE. Leiomyosarcomas: Clinical presentation. *Am J Obstet Gynecol.* 1993. https://doi.org/10.1016/S0002-9378(12)90910-2.

46. FDA and U.S. Food and Drug Administration. *Laparoscopic Uterine Power Morcellation in Hysterectomy and Myomectomy: FDA Safety Communication*; 2014. http://www.fda.gov/MedicalDevices/Safety.

47. Pritts EA, Parker WH, Brown J, Olive DL. Outcome of occult uterine leiomyosarcoma after surgery for presumed uterine fibroids: A systematic review. *J Minim Invasive Gynecol.* 2015. https://doi.org/10.1016/j.jmig.2014.08.781.

48. Kho KA, Lin K, Hechanova M, Richardson DL. Risk of occult uterine sarcoma in women undergoing hysterectomy for benign indications. *Obstet Gynecol.* 2016. https://doi.org/10.1097/AOG.0000000000001242.

49. Wright JD, et al. Uterine pathology in women undergoing minimally invasive hysterectomy using morcellation. *JAMA, J Am Med Assoc.* 2014. https://doi.org/10.1001/jama.2014.9005.

50. Mahnert N, Morgan D, Campbell D, Johnston C, As-Sanie S. Unexpected gynecologic malignancy diagnosed after hysterectomy performed for benign indications. *Obstet Gynecol.* 2015. https://doi.org/10.1097/AOG.0000000000000642.

51. Cohen SL, et al. Contained tissue extraction using power morcellation: Prospective evaluation of leakage parameters. *Am J Obstet Gynecol.* 2016. https://doi.org/10.1016/j.ajog.2015.08.076.

52. Park JY, et al. The impact of tumor morcellation during surgery on the prognosis of patients with apparently early uterine leiomyosarcoma. *Gynecol Oncol.* 2011. https://doi.org/10.1016/j.ygyno.2011.04.021.

53. Oduyebo T, et al. Risk factors for occult uterine sarcoma among women undergoing minimally invasive gynecologic surgery. *J Minim Invasive Gynecol.* 2016;23(1). https://doi.org/10.1016/j.jmig.2015.07.017.

54. Einstein MH, et al. Management of uterine malignancy found incidentally after supracervical hysterectomy or uterine morcellation for presumed benign disease. *Int J Gynecol Cancer.* 2008. https://doi.org/10.1111/j.1525-1438.2007.01126.x.

55. Pedra Nobre S, et al. The impact of tumor fragmentation in patients with stage I uterine leiomyosarcoma on patterns of recurrence and oncologic outcome. *Gynecol Oncol.* 2021. https://doi.org/10.1016/j.ygyno.2020.10.020.

56. Hensley ML, et al. Adjuvant therapy for high-grade, uterus-limited leiomyosarcoma: Results of a phase 2 trial (SARC 005). *Cancer.* 2013. https://doi.org/10.1002/cncr.27942.

57. Pautier P, et al. A randomized clinical trial of adjuvant chemotherapy with doxorubicin, ifosfamide, and cisplatin followed by radiotherapy versus radiotherapy alone in patients with localized uterine sarcomas (SARCGYN study). A study of the French sarcoma group. *Ann Oncol.* 2013. https://doi.org/10.1093/annonc/mds545.

58. Hensley ML, et al. Adjuvant gemcitabine plus docetaxel followed by doxorubicin versus observation for high-grade uterine leiomyosarcoma: A phase III NRG oncology/gynecologic oncology group study. *J Clin Oncol.* 2018. https://doi.org/10.1200/JCO.18.00454.

59. Pasquali S, et al. The impact of chemotherapy on survival of patients with extremity and trunk wall soft tissue sarcoma: revisiting the results of the EORTC-STBSG 62931 randomised trial. *Eur J Cancer.* 2019. https://doi.org/10.1016/j.ejca.2018.12.009.

60. Pasquali S, et al. High-risk soft tissue sarcomas treated with perioperative chemotherapy: improving prognostic classification in a randomised clinical trial. *Eur J Cancer.* 2018. https://doi.org/10.1016/j.ejca.2018.01.071.

61. Pervaiz N, Colterjohn N, Farrokhyar F, Tozer R, Figueredo A, Ghert M. *A systematic meta-analysis of randomized controlled trials of adjuvant chemotherapy for localized resectable soft-tissue sarcoma*; 2008Cancer. https://doi.org/10.1002/cncr.23592.

62. Gronchi A, et al. Histotype-tailored neoadjuvant chemotherapy versus standard chemotherapy in patients with high-risk soft-tissue sarcomas (ISG-STS 1001): an international, open-label, randomised, controlled, phase 3, multicentre trial. *Lancet Oncol.* 2017. https://doi.org/10.1016/S1470-2045(17)30334-0.

63. Gadducci A, et al. Uterine leiomyosarcoma: Analysis of treatment failures and survival. *Gynecol Oncol.* 1996. https://doi.org/10.1006/gyno.1996.0185.

64. Littell RD, et al. Adjuvant gemcitabine-docetaxel chemotherapy for stage I uterine leiomyosarcoma: Trends and survival outcomes. *Gynecol Oncol.* 2017. https://doi.org/10.1016/j.ygyno.2017.07.122.

65. Reed NS, et al. Phase III randomised study to evaluate the role of adjuvant pelvic radiotherapy in the treatment of uterine sarcomas stages I and II: an European Organisation for Research and Treatment of Cancer Gynaecological Cancer group study (protocol 55874). *Eur J Cancer.* 2008. https://doi.org/10.1016/j.ejca.2008.01.019.

66. Ricci S, Stone RL, Fader AN. Uterine leiomyosarcoma: Epidemiology, contemporary treatment strategies and the impact of uterine morcellation. *Gynecol Oncol.* 2017. https://doi.org/10.1016/j.ygyno.2017.02.019.

67. George S, et al. Retrospective cohort study evaluating the impact of intraperitoneal morcellation on outcomes of localized uterine leiomyosarcoma. *Cancer.* 2014. https://doi.org/10.1002/cncr.28844.

68. Raine-Bennett T, et al. Occult uterine sarcoma and leiomyosarcoma: Incidence of and survival associated with morcellation. In: *Obstetrics and Gynecology*; 2016. https://doi.org/10.1097/AOG.0000000000001187.

69. Major FJ, et al. Prognostic factors in early-stage uterine sarcoma: A gynecologic oncology group study. *Cancer.* 1993. https://doi.org/10.1002/cncr.2820710440.

70. Tirumani SH, et al. Metastatic pattern of uterine leiomyosarcoma: Retrospective analysis of the predictors and outcome in 113 patients. *J Gynecol Oncol.* 2014. https://doi.org/10.3802/jgo.2014.25.4.306.

71. Leitao MM, et al. Surgical cytoreduction in patients with metastatic uterine leiomyosarcoma at the time of initial diagnosis. *Gynecol Oncol.* 2012. https://doi.org/10.1016/j.ygyno.2012.02.014.

72. Jacobs EM. Combination chemotherapy of metastatic testicular germinal cell tumors and soft part sarcomas. *Cancer.* 1970. https://doi.org/10.1002/1097-0142(197002)25:2<324::AID-CNCR2820250208>3.0.CO;2-F.

73. Gottlieb JA, et al. Chemotherapy of sarcomas with a combination of adriamycin and dimethyl triazeno imidazole carboxamide. *Cancer.* 1972. https://doi.org/10.1002/1097-0142(197212)30:6<1632::AID-CNCR2820300632>3.0.CO;2-S.

74. O'Bryan RM, et al. Dose response evaluation of adriamycin in human neoplasia. *Cancer.* 1977. https://doi.org/10.1002/1097-0142(197705)39:5<1940::AID-CNCR2820390505>3.0.CO;2-0.

75. Judson I, et al. Doxorubicin alone versus intensified doxorubicin plus ifosfamide for first-line treatment of advanced or metastatic soft-tissue sarcoma: A randomised controlled phase 3 trial. *Lancet Oncol.* 2014. https://doi.org/10.1016/S1470-2045(14)70063-4.

76. Seddon BM, et al. GeDDiS: A prospective randomised controlled phase III trial of gemcitabine and docetaxel compared with doxorubicin as first-line treatment in previously untreated advanced unresectable or metastatic soft tissue sarcomas (EudraCT 2009–014907-29). *J Clin Oncol.* 2015. https://doi.org/10.1200/jco.2015.33.15_suppl.10500.

77. Seddon B, et al. Gemcitabine and docetaxel versus doxorubicin as first-line treatment in previously untreated advanced unresectable or metastatic soft-tissue sarcomas (GeDDiS): a randomised controlled phase 3 trial. *Lancet Oncol.* 2017. https://doi.org/10.1016/S1470-2045(17)30622-8.

78. Merimsky O, et al. Gemcitabine in soft tissue or bone sarcoma resistant to standard chemotherapy: A phase II study. *Cancer Chemother Pharmacol.* 2000. https://doi.org/10.1007/s002800050027.

79. Patel SR, et al. Phase II clinical investigation of gemcitabine in advanced soft tissue sarcomas and window evaluation of dose rate on gemcitabine triphosphate accumulation. *J Clin Oncol.* 2001. https://doi.org/10.1200/JCO.2001.19.15.3483.

80. Verweij J, et al. Phase II studies of docetaxel in the treatment of various solid tumours. EORTC Early Clinical Trials Group and the EORTC Soft Tissue and Bone Sarcoma Group. *Eur J Cancer.* 1995.

81. Verweij J, et al. Randomized phase II study of docetaxel versus doxorubicin in first- and second-line chemotherapy for locally advanced or metastatic soft tissue sarcomas in adults: A study of the European Organization for Research and Treatment of Cancer Soft Tissue and B. *J Clin Oncol.* 2000. https://doi.org/10.1200/JCO.2000.18.10.2081.

82. Hensley ML, et al. Gemcitabine and docetaxel in patients with unresectable leiomyosarcoma: Results of a phase II trial. *J Clin Oncol.* 2002. https://doi.org/10.1200/JCO.2002.11.050.

83. Bay JO, et al. Docetaxel and gemcitabine combination in 133 advanced soft-tissue sarcomas: a retrospective analysis. *Int J Cancer.* 2006. https://doi.org/10.1002/ijc.21867.

84. Look KY, Sandler A, Blessing JA, Lucci JA, Rose PG. Phase II trial of gemcitabine as second-line chemotherapy of uterine leiomyosarcoma: A Gynecologic Oncology Group (GOG) Study. *Gynecol Oncol.* 2004. https://doi.org/10.1016/j.ygyno.2003.11.023.

85. Hensley ML, Blessing JA, Mannel R, Rose PG. Fixed-dose rate gemcitabine plus docetaxel as first-line therapy for metastatic uterine leiomyosarcoma: A Gynecologic Oncology Group phase II trial. *Gynecol Oncol.* 2008. https://doi.org/10.1016/j.ygyno.2008.03.010.

86. Hensley ML, Blessing JA, DeGeest K, Abulafia O, Rose PG, Homesley HD. Fixed-dose rate gemcitabine plus docetaxel as second-line therapy for metastatic uterine leiomyosarcoma: A Gynecologic Oncology Group phase II study. *Gynecol Oncol.* 2008. https://doi.org/10.1016/j.ygyno.2008.02.024.

87. Abbruzzese JL, et al. A phase I clinical, plasma, and cellular pharmacology study of gemcitabine. *J Clin Oncol.* 1991. https://doi.org/10.1200/JCO.1991.9.3.491.

88. Tempero M, et al. Randomized phase II comparison of dose-intense gemcitabine: Thirty-minute infusion and fixed dose rate infusion in patients with pancreatic adenocarcinoma. *J Clin Oncol.* 2003. https://doi.org/10.1200/JCO.2003.09.140.

89. Maki RG, et al. Randomized phase II study of gemcitabine and docetaxel compared with gemcitabine alone in patients with metastatic soft tissue sarcomas: results of sarcoma alliance for research through collaboration study 002. *J Clin Oncol.* 2007. https://doi.org/10.1200/jco.2006.10.4117.

90. Pautier P, et al. Randomized multicenter and stratified phase II study of gemcitabine alone versus gemcitabine and docetaxel in patients with metastatic or relapsed Leiomyosarcomas: A Fédération Nationale Des Centres de Lutte Contre le Cancer (FNCLCC) French Sarcoma Group. *Oncologist.* 2012. https://doi.org/10.1634/theoncologist.2011-0467.

91. Dileo P, et al. Gemcitabine and vinorelbine combination chemotherapy for patients with advanced soft tissue sarcomas: Results of a phase II trial. *Cancer.* 2007. https://doi.org/10.1002/cncr.22609.

92. García-del-Muro X, et al. Randomized phase II study comparing gemcitabine plus dacarbazine versus dacarbazine alone in patients with previously treated soft tissue sarcoma: A Spanish group for research on sarcomas study. *J Clin Oncol.* 2011. https://doi.org/10.1200/JCO.2010.33.6107.

93. Demetri GD, et al. Efficacy and safety of trabectedin or dacarbazine for metastatic liposarcoma or leiomyosarcoma after failure of conventional chemotherapy: Results of a phase III randomized multicenter clinical trial. *J Clin Oncol.* 2016. https://doi.org/10.1200/JCO.2015.62.4734.

94. Van Der Graaf WTA, et al. Pazopanib for metastatic soft-tissue sarcoma (PALETTE): A randomised, double-blind, placebo-controlled phase 3 trial. *Lancet.* 2012. https://doi.org/10.1016/S0140-6736(12)60651-5.

95. Blay JY, et al. Eribulin versus dacarbazine in patients with leiomyosarcoma: subgroup analysis from a phase 3, open-label, randomised study. *Br J Cancer.* 2019. https://doi.org/10.1038/s41416-019-0462-1.

96. George S, et al. Phase 2 trial of aromatase inhibition with letrozole in patients with uterine leiomyosarcomas expressing estrogen and/or progesterone receptors. *Cancer.* 2014. https://doi.org/10.1002/cncr.28476.

97. Abeshouse A, et al. Comprehensive and Integrated Genomic Characterization of Adult Soft Tissue Sarcomas. *Cell.* 2017;171(4):950–965. e28. https://doi.org/10.1016/j.cell.2017.10.014.

98. Choi J, et al. Integrated mutational landscape analysis of uterine leiomyosarcomas. *Proc Natl Acad Sci.* 2021. https://doi.org/10.1073/pnas.2025182118.

99. Okuno S, et al. A phase 2 study of temsirolimus (CCI-779) in patients with soft tissue sarcomas: A study of the mayo phase 2 consortium (P2C). *Cancer.* 2011. https://doi.org/10.1002/cncr.25928.

100. O'Reilly KE, et al. mTOR inhibition induces upstream receptor tyrosine kinase signaling and activates Akt. *Cancer Res.* 2006. https://doi.org/10.1158/0008-5472.CAN-05-2925.

101. Davis LE, et al. Discovery and characterization of recurrent, targetable ALK fusions in leiomyosarcoma. *Mol Cancer Res.* 2019. https://doi.org/10.1158/1541-7786.MCR-18-1075.

102. Chiang S, et al. NTRK fusions define a novel uterine sarcoma subtype with features of fibrosarcoma. *Am J Surg Pathol.* 2018. https://doi.org/10.1097/PAS.0000000000001055.

103. Drilon A, et al. Efficacy of larotrectinib in TRK fusion–positive cancers in adults and children. *N Engl J Med.* 2018. https://doi.org/10.1056/nejmoa1714448.

104. Tawbi HA, et al. Pembrolizumab in advanced soft-tissue sarcoma and bone sarcoma (SARC028): a multicentre, two-cohort, single-arm, open-label, phase 2 trial. *Lancet Oncol.* 2017. https://doi.org/10.1016/S1470-2045(17)30624-1.

105. Ben-Ami E, et al. Immunotherapy with single agent nivolumab for advanced leiomyosarcoma of the uterus: Results of a phase 2 study. *Cancer.* 2017. https://doi.org/10.1002/cncr.30738.

106. D'Angelo SP, et al. Nivolumab with or without ipilimumab treatment for metastatic sarcoma (Alliance A091401): two open-label, non-comparative, randomised, phase 2 trials. *Lancet Oncol.* 2018. https://doi.org/10.1016/S1470-2045(18)30006-8.

Chapter 10

Other rare uterine sarcomas: Adenosarcoma, endometrial stromal sarcoma, STUMP

Emily Hinchcliff, Barrett Lawson, and Nicole D. Fleming

Clinical case

A 51-year-old patient presents with abnormal uterine bleeding and a 6 cm intrauterine, polypoid mass on pelvic ultrasound imaging (Fig. 10.1). Office endometrial biopsy (EMB) was suggestive of uterine adenosarcoma. She was taken to the operating room for a TLH, BSO, and pelvic sentinel lymph node assessment. Final pathology revealed a stage IA uterine adenosarcoma with sarcomatous overgrowth and presence of lymphovascular space invasion. Do you offer this patient any adjuvant therapy and if so what?

Epidemiology

Uterine sarcomas are rare entities, representing only 1% of all gynecologic malignancies, and 3% of all uterine cancers. Uterine sarcomas are comprised of different subtypes, the most common being uterine leiomyosarcoma (25%–60% cases), endometrial stromal sarcoma (10%–20% cases), high-grade undifferentiated sarcoma (HG-US) (3%–5% cases), and uterine adenosarcoma (5%–9% cases).[1–7] The mortality rate associated with uterine sarcomas is much higher than their endometrial cancer counterparts, which has been mostly driven by high-risk uterine leiomyosarcoma. Five-year overall survival rates have been reported between 25% and 80%, depending on sarcoma histologic subtype and stage.[1,6,7] There have been no significant differences in incidences of these rare uterine sarcomas by ethnicity.[4,8,9] Given the limited numbers of patients that incur this diagnosis annually, challenges exist in preoperative diagnosis, workup, and treatment of these rare tumors. Universal adoption of adjuvant treatment strategies following surgical management has also been limited given lack of prospective clinical trials in these tumors. Thus, majority of treatment recommendations have been based on review of available data and consensus agreements.[7,10] In this chapter, we will focus specifically on the rare uterine sarcoma subtypes of adenosarcoma, endometrial stromal sarcoma, and smooth muscle tumors of uncertain malignant potential (STUMP).

Etiology/risk factors

The majority of uterine adenosarcoma diagnoses arise from the uterus, and median age ranges from 41 to 66 years.[7,8,11–14] A large SEER database study reported that 52% of patients were between the age of 40 and 65 years, 39% were older than 65 years, and 10% of patients were younger than 40 years.[8] Müllerian adenosarcomas can also arise from other gynecologic tissues including the ovaries, cervix, vagina, fallopian tubes, and peritoneum.[7] The association between endometriosis and extrauterine adenosarcoma cases has been described; however, a direct causal link has not been established.[15,16] In a large case series of 1000 patients with biopsy-proven endometriosis, the incidence of cancer was 5.5%, with majority of tumors being carcinoma (endometrioid or clear cell) and minority adenosarcoma.[16] Additional risk factors for uterine adenosarcoma identified have included treatment with selective estrogen receptor modulator (SERM) medications such as tamoxifen.[17] However, despite endometrial changes that can occur with SERMs, the relative risk of developing uterine cancer has been shown to be 2.5, of which majority are uterine carcinomas and not adenosarcoma.[18,19] Other potential risk factors for uterine adenosarcoma have included previous pelvic radiation[11] or prolonged exposure to estrogen.[20]

Endometrial stromal sarcomas make up only approximately 0.2% of all uterine malignancies. Notably, ESS are often diagnosed slightly earlier than their higher grade leiomyosarcoma counterparts, usually occurring in women aged 40–55 years old. Additionally, analysis of the National Cancer Database (NCDB) reported that women with ESS often have smaller tumors than those with high-grade sarcomas of the uterus.[5]

Diagnosis and Treatment of Rare Gynecologic Cancers. https://doi.org/10.1016/B978-0-323-82938-0.00010-0

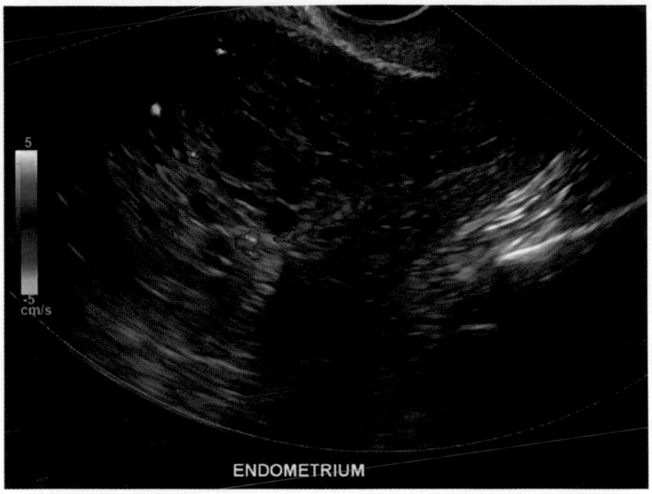

FIG. 10.1 Ultrasound findings of uterine adenosarcoma. Ultrasound features of 6 cm cystic, polypoid endometrial mass with increased vascular flow concerning for malignancy.

STUMP tumors are typically diagnosed in women suspected to have benign uterine leiomyoma on preoperative evaluation. The median age at diagnosis is 41–48 years, with a range of 20–75 years.[9,21,22] There are not clearly defined risk factors for the development of uterine STUMP tumors, and they have not been associated with history of pelvic radiation such as with other uterine sarcomas.[9]

Pathology

Adenosarcoma

Adenosarcomas are, as the name implies, a biphasic tumor, with a benign epithelial component and malignant stromal component.[23] An uncommon tumor, adenosarcoma has been seen in a broad age range with as low as 10 years of age and with incidence highest in perimenopausal and postmenopausal women.

Gross description

The tumor typically is exophytic and polypoid, filling the uterine cavity and may project through the uterine cervix.[23,24] On exam, the lesion may be confused with benign endocervical or endometrial polyps. Tumor size has been reported to range from 1 to 17 cm, with an average size of 5 cm. On cut surface, the tumor can show variable cystic and solid components, with papillary projections into cystic spaces that may be appreciated on gross examination. If there is sarcomatous overgrowth, the tumor may have areas of a more "fleshy" appearance, as is described in other sarcomas.

Microscopic description

On low power examination the tumor may resemble a phyllodes tumor of the breast, with leaf like architecture caused by intraglandular projections (Fig. 10.2).[24] The epithelium is bland, simple Müllerian-type epithelium, usually endometrioid, in the forms of glands or cysts, with no significant architectural complexity or cytologic atypia.[24,25] Metaplastic changes in the epithelium can be seen, including tubal, squamous or mucinous features. The stromal component is malignant and typically is a low-grade spindle cell sarcoma, with no specific differentiation.[23] The stroma will show hypercellular areas around glands, known as periglandular stromal condensation or periglandular cuffing. Mitotic activity was previously required for the diagnosis at a rate of at least 2 per 10 HPF, but as mitotic activity can be very focal or difficult to identify a diagnosis of adenosarcoma can be made when other classical architectural patterns are present.[23a,23b] High-grade stromal component defined as severe nuclear pleomorphism identifiable at low-power magnification can be seen in a subset of cases, without meeting criteria for sarcomatous overgrowth. Regardless, the presence of a high-grade component should be noted, as it may be associated with more aggressive behavior. Heterologous components may also be seen, notably rhabdomyoblastic differentiation (Fig. 10.3), but chondrosarcoma, liposarcoma and sex cord-stromal differentiation have also reported.[23,24]

"Adenosarcoma with sarcomatous overgrowth" is a diagnosis rendered when more than 25% of the tumor shows pure sarcoma without admixed glandular component.[25] The type or grade of sarcoma is not specific to this diagnosis, though typically (approximately 70%) are high grade. This should be reported, as they are associated with extrauterine disease at presentation along with high rates of recurrence and mortality.

Differential diagnosis

Lesions with both epithelial and mesenchymal components dominate the differential, ranging from benign to malignant. Endometrial polyps, adenomyomas, and adenofibromas all have epithelial and mesenchymal components that are histologically benign. As originally described, adenofibroma has similar architectural features to an adenosarcoma, though the stroma is usually hypocellular and fibrotic, and mitoses should be absent. However, the diagnosis of adenofibroma

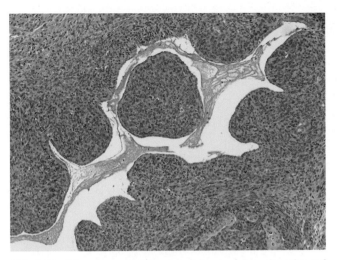

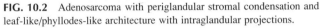

FIG. 10.2 Adenosarcoma with periglandular stromal condensation and leaf-like/phyllodes-like architecture with intraglandular projections.

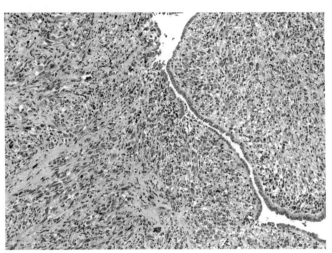

FIG. 10.3 Adenosarcoma, with benign Müllerian type epithelium with underlying high-grade sarcoma component showing rhabdomyoblastic differentiation.

has been removed from the 2020 WHO Classification of Female Genital Tumors as they are either considered to be low-grade adenosarcomas, or polyps with unusual phyllodes architecture or stromal cellularity. When a tumor has an "adenofibroma-like" appearance examination of the entire lesion to identify more typical features of adenosarcoma is warranted.

Carcinosarcoma is another biphasic neoplasm that should be considered. In a subset of cases, carcinosarcoma can have phyllodes like architecture mimicking adenosarcoma. Adequate sampling of the lesion is required to exclude the presence of any malignant epithelium.

Lastly the diagnosis of SMARCA4-deficient undifferentiated sarcoma should be considered in the differential diagnosis. These tumors may have a leaf-like polypoid architecture which can mimic adenosarcoma but is composed essentially of an undifferentiated tumor with prominent rhabdoid morphology.[26] These tumors show loss of SMARCA4 by immunohistochemistry (IHC) and have a very aggressive clinical course.

Molecular findings

Testing of adenosarcomas has shown somatic gene alterations only in the sarcoma component, further supporting these lesions as being primarily a mesenchymal neoplasm.[25] Mutations noted have included *FGFR2, KMT2C,* and *DICER1,* while amplifications in *MDM2/CDK4/HMGA2 and TERT* have been identified along with fusions in *NCOA2/3.* Adenosarcomas with sarcomatous overgrowth have been reported to have *ATRX* mutations, *MYBL1* amplification, higher number of copy number mutations, and more common global chromosomal instability and chromothripsis. And lastly, *TP53* alterations are more common in high-grade adenosarcoma in contrast to low-grade adenosarcomas.

Endometrial stromal sarcoma

Endometrial stromal sarcomas are uncommon tumors, which are broadly classified as either low-grade endometrial stromal sarcoma (LG-ESS) or high-grade endometrial stromal sarcoma (HG-ESS).[27] This entity has evolved over the last several decades from a histologic and molecular standpoint, and now also includes a relatively recent inclusion of HG-ESS with *BCOR* fusion.[28]

Gross description

Typically LG-ESS is superficial and involves the endometrium, grossly seen as a soft, tan to yellow polyp or mass and may show gross necrosis or hemorrhage. As LG-ESS has myometrial invasion by definition, it may show a grossly identifiable infiltrative pattern of growth, with irregular, tan-yellow cords or nodules of tumor extending into the myometrium. Extension into myometrial or parametrial veins may occur and are seen as "worm-like" plugs of tumor. LG-ESS may also grow as well-demarcated, well-circumscribed nodules within the myometrial wall, without definitive gross evidence of invasion. Conversely, it can also have such diffuse invasion of the myometrium that the myometrium is diffusely thickened, without a well-defined tumor seen.

HG-ESS typically forms a polypoid, intracavitary mass and is usually poorly circumscribed.[29] However, there is significant overlap between the gross appearance of LG-ESS and HG-ESS, without definitive features to grossly distinguish the two tumors.

Microscopic description

In LG-ESS, the tumor cells are uniform with scant cytoplasm that resemble the cells of proliferative-phase endometrial stroma, with an arborizing vascular pattern of spiral arterioles and occasionally ropey collagen (Fig. 10.4).[30] Nearly 50% of tumors have mitotic index between 1 and 9 mitoses per 10 HPF, with a range from rare or no mitoses identified to up to over 30. Of note, the mitotic count is neither used for the diagnosis nor grading of these tumors.[30,31] In tumors that appear well-circumscribed, careful sampling of the tumor/myometrial interface is important to identify focal invasion.[27] While endometrial stromal nodules and LG-ESS show similar histology, distinction should be made on the presence of invasion. If the neoplasm shows finger like projections measuring >3 mm in extent from the main mass or >3 in number, then a diagnosis of LG-ESS should be made.[32] Up to 25% of cases exhibit foci of sex cord-like differentiation, resembling uterine tumors with ovarian sex cord-like tumors (UTROSCT) (Fig. 10.5).[27] The two entities are distinguished by the percentage of sex cord-like features being focal in LG-ESS vs greater than 50% in UTROSCT.

HG-ESS usually shows a two cell population, with a mixture of round and spindled cell areas, though tumors with pure components of either can occur.[33] The round cell component is usually highly cellular and arranged in vague nests, with large nuclei (4–6 times the size of background lymphocytes) and scanty to moderate eosinophilic cytoplasm. High mitotic rate (>10 mitoses per 10 HPF, with up to 77 per 10 HPF reported) and tumor necrosis is invariably present. In comparison, the spindle cell component is arranged in loose or intersecting fascicles, with ovoid to oblong nuclei with an overall bland, monomorphic cytologic appearance. In comparison to the round cell component, the spindle cell component shows lower mitotic activity (typically 3 or less mitoses per 10 HPF).

HG-ESS with *BCOR* fusion typically show striking, extensive myxoid stroma, with uniform tumor cells arranged in haphazard fascicles. The cells are predominantly spindled, with spindled or oval to round intermediate sized nuclei.

Immunohistochemistry

Typically LG-ESS is diffusely positive for CD10, though the marker it not entirely specific and can be positive in mimics such as cellular leiomyoma.[34] Smooth muscle markers, such as desmin, may also be positive in LG-ESS, especially those with smooth muscle differentiation; therefore, a panel of CD10 and specific smooth muscle markers such as SMMS-1, calponin, and h-caldesmon should be considered. IHC stains for ER and PR are typically diffuse and strong.

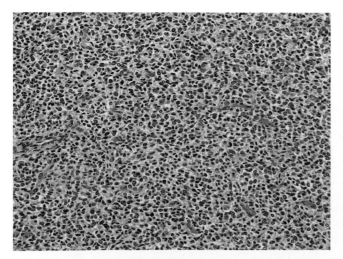

FIG. 10.4   Low-grade endometrial stromal sarcoma with cells resembling that of proliferative phase endometrium and spiral arterioles.

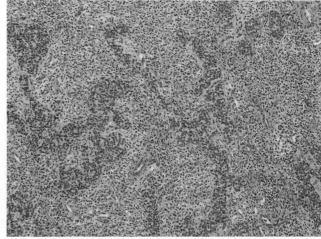

FIG. 10.5   Low-grade endometrial stromal sarcoma with sex-cord like differentiation.

HG-ESS is typically negative or only weakly positive for IHC stains CD10, ER and PR, while cyclin D1 shows strong, diffuse positivity (in >70% of cases), best exhibited in the round cell component.

HG-ESS with *BCOR* fusion shows diffuse staining with CD10 approximately 80% of cases and a similar proportion of cases with exhibiting cyclin-D1 expression. ER and PR staining is variable.

Molecular findings

LG-ESS harbor recurrent chromosomal translocations, the most common of which, occurring in approximately 50% of cases, is the t(7;17)(p15;q21) translocation, producing the *JAZF1-SUZ12* gene fusion.[27] Other reported translocations include *PHF1-JAZF1* t(6;7)(p21;p15), *EPC1-PHF1* t(6;10;10)(p21;q22;p11.2) and *MEAF6-PHF1* t(1;6)(p34;p21).

Usual type HG-ESS will typically harbor the translocation t(10;17)(q22;p13), producing the *YWHAE-NUTM2A*/B (previously known as *FAM22*) gene fusion.[27,28] The newly described *BCOR* HG-ESS is characterized by t(X;22)(p11;q13), resulting in a fusion of *ZC3H7B* and *BCOR*.

Differential diagnosis

The most important differential for classic LG-ESS is an endometrial stromal nodule. Tumors should be well sampled along the tumor-myometrial junction to fully evaluate for the presence of invasion. Areas of smooth muscle metaplasia should not be confused with background myometrium, potentially over calling invasion in an endometrial stromal nodule.[28] The presence of vascular invasion further supports a diagnosis on ESS over a stromal nodule. LG-ESS with significant smooth muscle differentiation may mimic leiomyosarcoma, just as extensive sex cord-like features may mimic UTROSCT. Intravascular leiomyomatosis in which the smooth muscle tumor is cellular can mimic LG-ESS and immunostains for smooth muscle markers may facilitate the correct diagnosis.

The main differential for HG-ESS is an undifferentiated endometrial/uterine sarcoma (UUS), which is characterized by markedly pleomorphic cells with prominent nucleoli in diffuse sheets with no resemblance to proliferative-phase endometrium. The marked cytologic atypia present in UUS is not typically seen in HG-ESS which has more uniform round cell morphology. Furthermore, UUS is typically positive for CD10 and has diffuse cyclin D1 expression, while negative for ER and PR. The differential staining for CD10 further support a diagnosis of UUS over HG-ESS; though expression can be variable and a UUS is essentially a diagnosis of exclusion.

In HG-ESS with *BCOR* the differential focuses on tumors with myxoid change, and includes entities such as myxoid leiomyosarcoma, inflammatory myofibroblastic tumors (IMT), and LG-ESS with fibromyxoid changes. IHC staining with smooth muscle markers and ALK can help distinguish from myxoid leiomyosarcoma and IMT, respectively, while a panel of CD10, ER, PR, and cyclin-D1 may distinguish from LG-ESS.

Smooth muscle tumors of uncertain malignant potential

STUMP represent a subcategory of uterine smooth muscle tumors that cannot be diagnosed unequivocally as benign or malignant.[9,35] Patients range in age from 25 to 75 years of age, with a mean of approximately 44 years of age, distinguishing these patients in age by approximately 10 years before most leiomyosarcomas are diagnosed.[36] While patients diagnosed with uterine STUMPs can be cured by hysterectomy, recurrence or metastasis can occur.

Gross description

The gross appearance of STUMPs is usually similar to a typical leiomyoma. Some tumors may have areas of hemorrhage, necrosis or degenerative type changes.[36] Reported size ranges from 2.5 to 12.2 cm, with a mean of 7.2 cm. The tumors are typically located intramurally but can also be seen submucosal and subserosal.

Microscopic description

The tumor is composed of spindled cells with eosinophilic cytoplasm and blunted elongated nuclei arranged in intersecting fascicles.[36] The diagnosis is based on a combination of atypia, mitotic activity or uncertainty in the type of necrosis, that does not meet the threshold of a leiomyosarcoma. STUMPs can be broadly put into three categories: (1) focal/multifocal or diffuse significant cytologic atypia lacking tumor cell necrosis with a mitotic index of <10 per 10 HPFs, (2) cytologically bland smooth muscle tumors with a mitotic index of less than 10 mitoses per 10 HPFs with the presence of coagulative tumor cell necrosis and (3) cytologically bland smooth muscle tumors with a mitotic index greater than or equal to 15 mitoses per 10 HPFS and lacking tumor cell necrosis.

Differential diagnosis

The differential diagnosis for STUMP primarily includes the spectrum of smooth muscle tumors from benign to malignant. Careful application of the criteria for atypia, mitotic activity and coagulative tumor cell necrosis can help separate tumors into leiomyoma, STUMP and leiomyosarcoma.

Variants of leiomyoma can show focal atypia or necrosis, concerning for a STUMP, but are benign. Apoplectic leiomyoma have foci of necrosis and elevated mitotic activity and can be misdiagnosed as a STUMP; however, awareness of exogenous hormonal therapy as well as recognition that the necrosis is infarct/hyaline necrosis aids in the diagnosis of apoplectic leiomyoma.[36] Fumarate hydratase (FH)-deficient leiomyoma are also on the differential with STUMP, as FH-deficient leiomyomas may have bizarre nuclear features. The presence of staghorn-like vessels, edema, and intracytoplasmic globules/inclusions, along with loss of expression of FH by IHC aids in the diagnosis of an FH-deficient leiomyoma.

IMT can also be on the differential for STUMPs as they can have a combination of cytologic atypia, increased mitotic index and coagulative tumor cell necrosis with positivity for smooth muscle markers. ALK testing by IHC or fluorescent in-situ hybridization can be helpful in this scenario as IMTs are usually positive by one or the other methodology.

Molecular findings

There are no defining molecular findings for STUMP. However, recently genomic profiling has shown the ability to predict potential for aggressive behavior, dividing STUMPs into groups: those that behave more like leiomyoma and those that behave more like leiomyosarcoma, based on a genomic index cut-off of 10.[37]

Diagnosis and workup
Differential diagnosis

Most patients diagnosed with uterine adenosarcoma, endometrial stromal sarcoma, or STUMP tumors present with abnormal uterine bleeding and a pelvic mass diagnosed by imaging. However, patients with uterine adenosarcoma and endometrial stromal sarcoma are more likely to have an endometrial or polypoid like mass, vs STUMP tumors which typically resemble smooth muscle tumors in the myometrium and closely resemble uterine leiomyomas.[6]

Signs and symptoms

The majority of patients with rare uterine sarcoma subtypes will experience abnormal uterine bleeding in 65%–75% of cases. Other associated clinical symptoms include pelvic pain or demonstration of pelvic mass in 10%–30% of cases, and abnormal vaginal discharge in 11% of cases.[12,14]

Physical exam findings

On clinical examination, patients with rare uterine sarcoma subtypes may have an enlarged uterus or palpable pelvic mass, prolapsing uterine mass visible in the vagina, endocervical polyp or cervical mass (Table 10.1).[12,14] Rarely, these tumors are diagnosed and detected on routine Papanicolaou smear examination.[59,60]

Tumor markers

There are no reliable predictive serum biomarkers for the diagnosis of rare subtypes of uterine sarcomas. CA-125 is a membrane glycoprotein associated with coelomic epithelium, including that of the female reproductive tract. It is the most commonly used tumor marker in the diagnosis and follow-up of ovarian cancer. Serum CA-125 has been studied as a biomarker in the workup of uterine and pelvic masses; however, it can be relatively nonspecific and is typically only elevated in cases of advanced stage disease. Serum CA-125 has been a poor differentiator between benign uterine leiomyoma and early-stage sarcomas in some cases, but other studies have shown significantly higher serum CA-125 levels in uterine sarcomas compared to benign myomas.[39–45] Lactate dehydrogenase (LDH) is a pyridine-linked enzyme catalyzing the reduction of free pyruvate to lactate during glycolysis. Malignant cells proliferate rapidly and have an increased rate of glycolysis. Following cell damage, LDH leaks into the bloodstream.[39] Several studies have found higher preoperative serum LDH levels in uterine sarcomas compared to benign myomas.[43–45] Nagamatsu et al. reported significant differences in LDH levels between endometrial carcinomas, uterine sarcomas, and benign leiomyomas. Patients with uterine sarcoma had higher

TABLE 10.1 Diagnosis and work up of uterine adenosarcoma, endometrial stromal sarcoma and STUMP tumors.

Diagnostic tools	Comments
Clinical exam[2]	
Abnormal uterine bleeding	65%–75% Cases
Pelvic or uterine mass	50% Cases
Pelvic pain or discomfort	20% Cases
Abnormal vaginal discharge	11% Cases
Endometrial sampling (EMB or D&C)[37,38]	Sensitivity 52%–85%, Specificity 35%–67%
Tumor markers[39–45]	
Serum CA-125	Limited reliability for primary diagnosis
	Increased sensitivity in recurrent/metastatic (67%–70%)
Serum LDH	Elevated when compared to benign disease
Imaging[46–58]	
Ultrasound	Large, solid lesions, nonhomogeneous, irregularity, increased vascularity
CT scans	Useful for initial staging, assessment for metastatic disease, surveillance
MRI	Higher diagnostic accuracy for evaluation of uterine masses suspicious for sarcoma
PET	Data on utility limited, higher FDG uptake seen in uterine sarcomas, cost considerations

D&C, dilation and curettage; *EMB*, endometrial biopsy.

levels of LDH when compared with endometrial carcinoma ($P = 0.0018$) and benign leiomyoma ($P = 0.0023$).[43] In addition, other studies have demonstrated that the combined use of serum LDH levels with different imaging modalities (PET-CT or MRI) increased the sensitivity and specificity of differentiating between malignant uterine sarcomas and benign myomas.[43,44,61] Nagai et al. proposed a preoperative diagnosis scoring system for uterine sarcomas (PRESS) utilizing age, serum LDH levels, and endometrial cytology results. Patients at risk for sarcoma scored 4 or higher on the scoring tool. The scoring system yielded an accuracy, sensitivity, and specificity of 94%, 80%, and 98%, respectively.[45]

Imaging tests

Most patients for workup of abnormal uterine bleeding or uterine mass will undergo imaging of the abdomen and pelvis with either ultrasound, computed tomography (CT) scan, or magnetic resonance imaging (MRI). Ultrasound has been the gold-standard first line test in workup of abnormal bleeding or uterine mass given its wide availability, low cost, and efficiency as diagnostic tool for gynecologic anatomic abnormalities. Increased vascularity utilizing Doppler has also been useful as a sonographic tool during ultrasound to detect uterine masses concerning for malignancy. Sonographic features of uterine sarcomas on ultrasound can include large, solid lesions with nonhomogeneous echostructure, irregular cystic areas, irregular margins, marked vascularization, and unstructured solid tissue in absence of shadow cones and calcifications (see Fig. 10.1).[6,46–48]

MRI represents the best approach to imaging uterine masses concerning for sarcoma and defining extent of local disease, while CT imaging is preferred for staging assessment of distant metastatic disease and follow-up.[49,50] Features of uterine adenosarcoma on MRI include a well-demarcated mass that is hypointense and heterogeneous on T1, multiseptated cystic appearance on T2, and low signal on diffusion weighted imaging. Masses associated with adenosarcoma can also be polypoid, arising on a stalk, or prolapsing through the endocervical canal which can be seen on MRI imaging (Fig. 10.6).[51–53] On MRI, leiomyosarcomas and STUMP tumors can display high T1-weighted and T2-weighted signals (due to necrosis) and grow more rapidly than their benign counterparts. Areas of increased T2 signal and restriction of diffusion on diffusion-weighted images may indicate hypercellularity or necrosis.[54–56] There is no clear imaging tool to distinguish between leiomyosarcoma and STUMP tumors, as this is a pathologic diagnosis. Contrast-enhanced MRI appears to yield higher diagnostic accuracy and higher specificity compared with diffusion-weighted MRI for

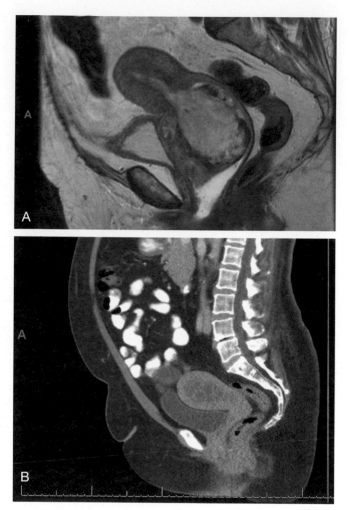

FIG. 10.6 MRI and CT imaging of uterine adenosarcoma. (A) Increased T2-weighted imaging by MRI on prolapsing uterine sarcoma through endo-cervix. (B) CT imaging of uterine adenosarcoma confined to uterine cavity.

discriminating between leiomyosarcoma/STUMP and benign leiomyoma, with comparable high sensitivity. Contrast-enhanced MRI has been shown to be superior to diffusion-weighted MRI based on the area under the ROC (0.92 vs 0.68, $P < 0.01$).[57]

Few data are currently available on utility of F-18-fluorodeoxyglucose (FDG) positron emission tomography (PET) as a diagnostic tool for uterine sarcomas. Ho et al. evaluated utility of PET imaging in a small cohort of patients with rapidly growing uterine masses suspicious for malignancy on ultrasound or MRI. The maximum FDG uptake for leiomyosarcoma and STUMP were higher (SUV max 3.7–11.8, median 11.3) versus benign leiomyomas (SUV max 2.0–9.4; median 3.5, $P = 0.003$), and the metabolic tumor/necrosis ratio was higher in leiomyosarcoma/STUMP compared to benign myomas ($P < 0.001$). All leiomyosarcoma/STUMP tumors had a typical pattern of FDG-uptake with a specific hollow ball sign, reflecting a sharp transition between necrotic and viable, well-preserved cells. This sign was absent in benign leiomyomas.[58]

Diagnostic tests

Most patients with rare uterine sarcomas present with abnormal uterine bleeding (65%–75%), pelvic or uterine mass (50%), pelvic pain or pressure (20%), or abnormal vaginal discharge (11%).[2] While typical epithelial endometrial cancers can be detected with >90 to 95% sensitivity by office EMB or dilation and curettage (D&C), there are no preoperative diagnostic tests that have been consistently utilized to diagnose uterine sarcomas.[37,62–65] In a group of 72 women with a diagnosis of uterine sarcoma, preoperative endometrial sampling suggested an invasive tumor in 86% (62/72) and predicted the correct histologic diagnosis in 64% (46/72). The rate of detection of invasive cancer by preoperative sampling was not significantly different among sarcomas and epithelial tumors (86% vs 84%, $P = 0.76$) and did not differ by sampling method (EMB vs. D&C, $P = 0.84$).[37] A similar, yet smaller study of 68 patients who underwent preoperative endometrial sampling with diagnosis of uterine leiomyosarcoma, showed that 52% of preoperative biopsies showed either uterine leiomyosarcoma or atypical spindle cell proliferation, and 36% confirmed uterine leiomyosarcoma specifically.[38] Thus, it is strongly recommended to perform endometrial sampling when a uterine sarcoma diagnosis is suspected.

Endometrial sampling combined with imaging (MRI preferred) and tumor marker assessment (serum CA-125 and LDH) can increase the detection of suspected early-stage uterine sarcoma preoperatively.[37–58,61–66] However, some uterine sarcomas will be diagnosed at advanced stages by CT, MRI, or PET imaging and thus, endometrial sampling or interventional radiology guided biopsy of a metastatic lesion can also be utilized for diagnostic purposes.

Staging

Staging for uterine sarcomas follows the International Federation of Gynecology and Obstetrics (FIGO) staging 2009 criteria (Table 10.2). Endometrial stromal sarcomas following the same staging guidelines as uterine leiomyosarcoma

TABLE 10.2 2009 FIGO staging of uterine sarcomas.

(1) Leiomyosarcomas and endometrial stromal sarcomas[a]		
I		Tumor limited to uterus
	IA	Less than 5 cm
	IB	More than 5 cm
II		Tumor extends beyond the uterus, within the pelvis
	IIA	Adnexal involvement
	IIB	Involvement of other pelvic tissues
III		Tumor invades abdominal tissues (not just protruding into the abdomen).
	IIIA	One site
	IIIB	More than one site
	IIIC	Metastasis to pelvic and/or paraaortic lymph nodes
IV	IVA	Tumor invades bladder and/or rectum
	IVB	Distant metastasis
(2) Adenosarcomas		
I		Tumor limited to uterus
	IA	Tumor limited to endometrium/endocervix with no myometrial invasion
	IB	Less than or equal to half myometrial invasion
	IC	More than half myometrial invasion
II		Tumor extends beyond the uterus, within the pelvis
	IIA	Adnexal involvement
	IIB	Tumor extends to extrauterine pelvic tissue
III		Tumor invades abdominal tissues (not just protruding into the abdomen).
	IIIA	One site
	IIIB	More than one site
	IIIC	Metastasis to pelvic and/or paraaortic lymph nodes
IV	IVA	Tumor invades bladder and/or rectum
	IVB	Distant metastasis

[a]Simultaneous endometrial stromal sarcomas of the uterine corpus and ovary/pelvis in association with ovarian/pelvic endometriosis should be classified as independent primary tumors.

given that they are pure mesenchymal in origin. Endometrial stromal sarcomas comprise 0.2% of all uterine malignancies and 10%–20% of uterine sarcomas.[2] Endometrial stromal sarcoma is stratified by low-grade (LG-ESS) and high-grade (HG-ESS) based on pathologic criteria. LG-ESS has been characterized by expression of estrogen receptor (ER) in 70% and progesterone receptor (PR) in 90% of cases. CD10 and Ki-67 is expressed in <5% of cells.[67–69] Most LGESS is diagnosed at an early-stage with 65%–85% of cases confined to the uterus. Patients with LG-ESS typically have an indolent course with reported 5-year overall survival rates range from 80% to 100%. However, 40%–50% will recur with possibility of remote recurrences.[2,70,71] HG-ESS is characterized by more destructive growth and necrosis, with only 50% histologically low-grade cells. High-grade cells express cyclin D1, BCOR, ER, PR, and CD10, while low-grade cells are positive for CD10, ER and PR. The majority of patients diagnosed with HG-ESS are diagnosed at advanced stages (70%), with 5-year survival rates between 30% and 35%.[71,72] There is also a subset of rare uterine sarcomas classified as HG-US. These are poorly differentiated sarcomas that do not resemble proliferative-phase endometrial stroma. HG-US is characterized by TP53 mutation, variable CD10 expression, and ER and PR expression is negative.[73] Most patients are diagnosed at advanced stage disease (stage III 10%–13%; stage IV 52%–57%), and only 20%–25% 5-year survival rate.[74–76]

Uterine adenosarcoma comprises 5%–10% of all uterine sarcomas and are characterized as mixed lesions with malignant mesenchymal and benign glandular epithelial components. In most adenosarcomas, the mesenchymal component is low-grade, resembling endometrial stromal sarcoma; however, up to 10%–25% of cases have heterologous sarcoma elements.[2,11,77] Adenosarcoma with greater than 25% of the tumor comprised of pure high-grade sarcoma without a glandular component are designated as adenosarcoma with sarcomatous overgrowth, found in 8%–54% of cases.[2,11,12] The FIGO staging for uterine adenosarcoma is separate from other uterine sarcomas and is also shown in Table 10.2. The majority of patients are diagnosed as stage I in 73%–82% of cases. The 5-year overall survival for stage I patients is 63%–86%, while overall survival is less in stage III (0%–48%) and stage IV (15%) disease.[4,8,12,13,78] The presence of sarcomatous overgrowth is a significant prognostic factor. Recurrence rates in stage I uterine adenosarcoma without sarcomatous overgrowth range from 20% to 30% compared to stage I cases with sarcomatous overgrowth between 45% and 75%.[79–81]

STUMP tumors are defined as neoplasms with pathological features that preclude an equivocal diagnosis of leiomyosarcoma, but do not fulfill criteria for benign leiomyoma or its variants. The histological parameters proposed by the WHO 2014 classification refer to tumor cell necrosis, moderate-to-severe atypia, and mitotic count per 10 HPF for diagnosis of STUMP (Table 10.3).[10,82] Given the borderline malignant nature of STUMP tumors, there is currently no official staging system for these tumors. Even though classified as slow growing tumors, they can occasionally relapse as either a recurrent STUMP or leiomyosarcoma.[10] Recurrence rates range from 0% to 36%, with median time to recurrence of 51 months (15 months to 9 years). Recurrent disease may involve different sites, either local in the abdomen or pelvis, or distant metastases.[9,10,21,22,83] Five-year overall survival in patients with STUMP is 92%–100%.[9,83]

Prognostic factors

Uterine adenosarcoma has typically been seen as a relatively indolent tumor, with low recurrence rate and high survival. However, there is a subset of uterine adenosarcomas that have a higher recurrence rates and worse survival. Recurrence

TABLE 10.3 Uterine smooth muscle tumors of uncertain malignant potential, with spindle morphology.

Tumor cell necrosis	Moderate to severe atypia	[a] Mitoses/mm² (mitoses/10 HPF)	Frequency of recurrence
Absent	Focal/multifocal	<4 (<10)	17% (6 of 35 cases)
Absent	Diffuse	<4 (<10)	12% (10 of 81 cases)
Present	None (or mild atypia)	<4 (<10)	28% (5 of 18 cases)
Absent	None	>6.3 (>15)	0% (0 of 48 cases)

[a]Mitotic counts are given for defined HPF of 0.55 mm in diameter and 0.24 mm² in area; at least 2.4 mm² (10 HPF) should be assessed. Adapted from the 2020 WHO Classification of Female Genital Tumors.[83a]

rates reported in the literature for uterine adenosarcoma vary from 25% to 50%; however, with certain risk factors, including the presence of sarcomatous overgrowth, recurrence rates increase to 45%–75%.[7,11–13,84] The two largest series reported, recurrence rates of 70%–77% for patients with uterine adenosarcoma with sarcomatous overgrowth with significantly worse progression-free and overall survival compared to those with tumors without sarcomatous overgrowth. Thus, presence of sarcomatous overgrowth is a significant prognostic factor in patients with uterine adenosarcoma.

Other prognostic factors in uterine adenosarcoma include increasing age, presence of myometrial invasion, and presence of lymphovascular invasion, all of which have been shown to have significant effects on both disease-free and overall survival (Table 10.4).[7,12,84,85] The rate of lymph node metastasis in uterine adenosarcoma is between 0% and 6.5%. Although a rare occurrence, the presence of lymph node metastases has been shown to be an independent prognostic factor for cause-specific survival (HR 2.34, 95% CI, 1.29–4.25) and overall survival (HR 2.04, 95% CI, 1.20–3.46) in a recent Surveillance, Epidemiology, End Results (SEER) database study. Large tumors, deep myometrial invasion, and sarcomatous overgrowth were associated with increased risk of lymph node metastasis (all, $P < 0.05$).[86] Size of primary tumor may be a prognostic factor and the current 2009 FIGO staging system does delineate tumors $\leq$5 cm as stage IA and >5 cm as stage IB. In recent analysis, patients with tumors >5 cm had a median OS of 5.8 years versus OS was not reached in patients with tumors $\leq$5 cm ($P = 0.0009$). However, on multivariate analysis, size of primary tumor was not a significant prognostic factor.[7,84] Stage of disease is noted to be a prognostic factor in most cancers, which is also true for uterine adenosarcoma. Five-year overall survival differs by stage as follows; stage I (63%–86%), stage II (50%–60%), stage III (0%–48%), and stage IV (15%).[7,8,78] Heterologous elements can also be present in uterine adenosarcoma, including rhabdomyoblasts, sex-cord stromal elements, chondrosarcoma, and liposarcoma elements. Smaller series have suggested worse outcomes with presence of heterologous elements; however, a recent larger series did not show a significant difference in either DFS or OS by presence of heterologous elements.[7]

The prognosis for endometrial stromal sarcomas is dependent on stage of disease, with specific analysis of SEER databases demonstrating significant improved survival in those with tumors <5 cm.[87] Additionally, NCDB analysis demonstrated increasing tumor size, and treatment with adjuvant therapy were significantly associated with survival. However, nodal and metastasis status were not associated with survival in that analysis which is likely reflective of this tumor types' indolent nature and the low number of observed deaths.[5] Other studies have investigated factors including cellular atypia, mitotic count, and margin status but have had mixed results.[88,89] For women with early stage disease, the 5-year overall survival rates are 84% (stage I) and 62% (stage II). However, late recurrence can occur even in early stage disease, with relapse rates described between 36% and 56%. The time to recurrence is much shorter for those with stage III/IV, with median of 9 months for those with advanced stage disease as compared to 65 months for those with stage I disease.[90]

TABLE 10.4 Prognostic factors in uterine adenosarcoma and impact on survival.

Prognostic factor	Impact on survival
Sarcomatous overgrowth[7,12] (presence vs absence)	Recurrence rates 70%–77% vs 20%–23% Median DFS (2.5 years vs 10.9 years, $P < 0.0001$) Median OS (5.2 years vs 14.5 years, $P < 0.0001$)
Increasing age[7,12]	Worse survival (HR 1.02, 95% CI, 1.00–1.04, $P = 0.016$) Median OS (for age < = 53 14.1 years vs 6.4 years for age > 53 years, $P = 0.0017$)
Race	
Myometrial invasion[12] (presence vs absence)	Median DFS (3.7 years vs 12.2 years, $P = 0.0002$) Median OS (5.8 years vs NR, $P = 0.0005$)
Lymphovascular invasion[85] (presence vs absence)	Worse DFS (0.5 years vs 4.8 years, $P = 0.011$) Worse OS (1 year vs 8.9 years, $P = 0.0021$)
Lymph node metastases[86] (presence vs absence)	Cause-specific survival (HR 2.34, 95% CI, 1.29–4.25) OS (HR 2.04, 95% CI, 1.20–3.46)
Stage (5-year OS)[7,8,78]	Stage I 63%–86% Stage II 50%–60% Stage III 0%–48% Stage IV 15%

DFS, disease-free survival; *OS*, overall survival.

The stratification of low-grade vs high-grade endometrial stromal sarcoma is typically based on pathologic factors, including hormone receptor positivity (ER/PR in LG-ESS), presence of JAZF1 fusion rearrangement (low-grade ESS), YWHAE-NUT2A/B gene rearrangement and BCOR gene alterations (HG-ESS). LG-ESS tumors typically follow a more indolent course, while their high-grade and undifferentiated counterparts have a high-risk of recurrent disease and poor prognosis. In high-grade and undifferentiated endometrial stromal sarcoma, prognostic factors reported include age, FIGO stage, optimal surgery, and receipt of chemotherapy and radiation. In LG-ESS, prognostic factors reported include stage and receipt of adjuvant hormonal therapy.[90–98]

STUMP tumors are rare entities that histologically do not meet definition of uterine leiomyosarcoma and are typically indolent tumors; however, they can metastasize and recur as either a STUMP tumor or leiomyosarcoma. Recurrence rates range from 0 and 36% and median time to recurrence is 51 months. However, there has been no prognostic factor reported that discriminates a higher recurrence risk, such as age, ethnicity, or smoking status. Additionally, type of surgery, i.e., hysterectomy or myomectomy, also does not appear to be prognostic. Thus, there are no clearly defined prognostic factors for STUMP tumors.[9,10,22]

Treatment of primary disease

Surgery

The standard treatment for uterine adenosarcoma, endometrial stromal sarcoma and STUMP tumors is surgical resection with total hysterectomy (TAH). Given the increased utilization of minimally invasive surgery for hysterectomy procedures and the tendency for larger uteri when involved with uterine sarcomas, it is recommended that hysterectomy or myomectomy be performed with surgical specimen excised intact without morcellation. Morcellation of uterine sarcomas or STUMP tumors can increase the risk of recurrence or metastases, thus, leading to worse survival outcomes compared to tumors excised intact.[6,62,63,86,99–105]

Bilateral salpingo-oophorectomy (BSO) should be considered for postmenopausal patients diagnosed with uterine sarcomas and STUMP tumors; however, in premenopausal patients, the studies evaluating the benefits of BSO have yielded inconsistent results. In uterine adenosarcoma, the risk of adnexal involvement has been reported in 0%–17% of cases, with one of the largest series reporting an 8% rate of ovarian involvement when gross extrauterine disease was not suspected.[11,12,78] Many uterine adenosarcoma tumors will express estrogen and PRs; however, it is unclear the long-term therapeutic benefit of BSO in these tumors.[4,106] Given the high rate of recurrence with adenosarcoma with sarcomatous overgrowth, BSO procedure should be considered in these cases. In LG-ESS, BSO has benefits of providing staging and prognostic information, and given the consistent expression of both estrogen and PRs in these tumors, eliminates endogenous production of hormones that may stimulate tumor growth. In young premenopausal women with LG-ESS there is uncertain benefit in BSO compared to possible long-term health risks associated with premature surgical menopause.[107] A recent meta-analysis suggested that ovarian preservation was associated with increased tumor recurrence (47% vs 24%, OR 2.70, 95% CI, 1.39–5.28) when compared with BSO, though there was no difference in death rate between groups.[108] However, other studies, including a recent NCDB study in stage I LG-ESS showed no difference in overall survival by BSO (96% vs 97%, $P = 0.50$).[109–113] In HG-ESS and undifferentiated sarcoma, BSO should be considered given the high risk of recurrence and poor survival outcomes.

Fertility sparing treatment options can be considered in select cases of rare uterine sarcomas and STUMP tumors. There have been reported cases of uterine adenosarcoma without sarcomatous overgrowth treated with polypectomy alone or polypectomy with chemotherapy.[11,12,114] However, appropriate counseling and discussion should be performed in these cases that standard of care surgical management is with hysterectomy. Similarly, fertility sparing management of LG-ESS is limited to case series and is not considered standard of care. These case series included hysteroscopic resection, with or without the use of adjuvant hormonal therapy based on hormone receptor status. They report successful pregnancy following this fertility sparing approach; however, several of these cases also recurred following pregnancy.[115] Additional studies and long-term follow-up is needed to determine the safety of fertility sparing treatment in LG-ESS. There are no standard guidelines for the treatment of uterine STUMP tumors. Hysterectomy has been considered gold standard especially in women who have completed childbearing. However, in young women, there have been reported cases of management with myomectomy followed by hysterectomy at the completion of childbearing. This management strategy would require risk–benefit discussion with the patient and close surveillance.[116–118] In the largest review of 76 patients with STUMP tumors who underwent myomectomy, only 5 patients (6.6%) relapsed and only 1 patient (1.3%) died of recurrence.[116]

While lymphadenectomy or sentinel lymph node assessment has been established as standard of care in the surgical staging of endometrial carcinomas, the utility and benefit of lymphadenectomy in uterine sarcomas has not been established.[119] The rate of lymph node metastasis in uterine adenosarcoma has been reported between 0% and 6.5%. Although a rare occurrence, the presence of lymph node metastases has been shown to be an independent prognostic factor for cause-specific survival (HR 2.34, 95% CI, 1.29–4.25) and overall survival (HR 2.04, 95% CI, 1.20–3.46) in a recent Surveillance, Epidemiology, End Results (SEER) database study. Large tumors, deep myometrial invasion, and sarcomatous overgrowth were associated with increased risk of lymph node metastasis (all, $P < 0.05$).[86] In endometrial stromal sarcoma, the rate of lymph node metastases has been reported between 7% and 10%.[86,112,120–123] Although performance of lymphadenectomy itself did not have a prognostic impact on survival in a large SEER database set, those patients with positive lymph nodes had a significantly worse disease-specific survival (35% vs 80%, $P < 0.001$) compared to those patients with negative lymph nodes.[120] The rate of node positivity may be higher in HG-ESS, with reported rates around 20% in two large series.[121,124] Also, it was reported that women with HG-ESS that had a negative lymphadenectomy (removal of at least 1 or more lymph nodes) had superior survival (70.9 vs 46.9 months, $P < 0.001$) compared to those patients that had no surgical node evaluation.[124] Therefore, performance of lymphadenectomy in endometrial stromal sarcoma may provide prognostic information and guide adjuvant therapy choices in certain cases. However, staging lymphadenectomy in tumors grossly confined to the uterus with clinically negative nodes should not be routinely performed. Preoperative imaging may guide those cases to consider lymphadenectomy based on pathologically enlarged lymph nodes. Surgical staging for STUMP tumors is not recommended as there has been no reported prognostic or therapeutic value.[10]

Adjuvant chemotherapy

Given the rare nature of uterine adenosarcoma and endometrial stromal sarcoma, there have been no prospective trials evaluating the role of chemotherapy in these tumors. Additionally, most uterine sarcoma trials (i.e., gemcitabine/docetaxel trial, GOG 277) have excluded tumors such as uterine adenosarcoma. Patients with stage I adenosarcoma without sarcomatous overgrowth and no myometrial invasion, and stage I LG-ESS have good survival outcomes with surgical resection alone, and unlikely to derive any benefit from adjuvant chemotherapy.[7,124,125] Patients with early-stage uterine adenosarcoma with high-risk factors such as sarcomatous overgrowth, deep myometrial invasion, or lymphovascular space invasion, have an increased risk of recurrence and decreased survival, thus adjuvant chemotherapy can be considered on an individual basis.[7] Similarly, patients with early-stage HG-ESS and undifferentiated sarcoma also have an increased risk of recurrence compared to their low-grade counterparts, and adjuvant chemotherapy must be individualized (Fig. 10.7). The current NCCN guidelines, however, support observation in cases of stage I uterine sarcomas regardless of risk factors.[119] Data on benefits of adjuvant chemotherapy in this population is limited due to small numbers of patients; however, it has not shown survival benefit with neoadjuvant or adjuvant chemotherapy in this high-risk population.[6,7,12,13] The previous Gynecologic Oncology Group (GOG) prospective trial comparing adjuvant chemotherapy using single-agent doxorubicin versus no treatment in stage I and II uterine sarcomas did include a small proportion of HG-ESS and undifferentiated sarcomas ($n = 12$). There was no difference in PFS or OS with adjuvant chemotherapy.[126] Another prospective randomized study by SARCGYN, which also included a small cohort of undifferentiated sarcoma patients ($n = 9$), evaluated adjuvant chemotherapy with doxorubicin, ifosfamide, and cisplatin followed by pelvic radiotherapy versus radiotherapy alone. Combined chemotherapy and radiation increased the 3-year disease-free survival (DFS) (55% vs 44%, $P = 0.048$) compared to radiation alone; however, there was no difference in overall survival.[127] Chemotherapeutic agents utilized and reported in the literature include doxorubicin-based regimens and gemcitabine and docetaxel, as these have the highest report efficacy in mesenchymal tumors (Table 10.5).[7] Patients with advanced stage uterine adenosarcoma, and high-grade and undifferentiated endometrial stromal sarcoma should be offered adjuvant chemotherapy with doxorubicin-based regimens or gemcitabine and docetaxel. Patients with advanced stage LG-ESS are preferentially treated with hormonal therapy options first prior to considering chemotherapy based on their hormone receptor positivity and indolent courses.

Adjuvant radiotherapy

Adjuvant radiotherapy may be offered to patients with uterine sarcomas to decrease the risk of local recurrence. Treatment modalities utilized include external beam radiotherapy and brachytherapy. The current NCCN guidelines in uterine cancer recommend adjuvant radiation be considered in patients with stage II to IVA HG-ESS, undifferentiated sarcoma, and leiomyosarcoma.[119] However, radiation has only been cautiously used in select cases of uterine sarcoma following the results

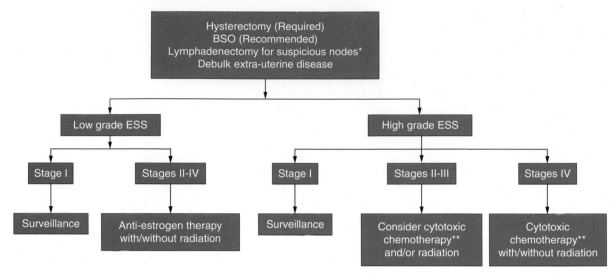

FIG. 10.7   Treatment of newly diagnosed endometrial stromal sarcoma.

TABLE 10.5 Adjuvant chemotherapy in high-risk uterine sarcomas.

Chemotherapy regimens	Dosing
Adriamycin alone	60–75 mg/m^2/21-day cycle
Adriamycin + Ifosfamide	60–75 mg/m^2/21-day cycle 7.5–10 g/m^2/21-day cycle
Adriamycin + Dacarbazine	60–75 mg/m^2/21-day cycle 750 to 1000 mg/m^2/21-day cycle
Gemcitabine + Docetaxel	675–900 mg/m^2 (day 1, 8) 75–100 mg/m^2/21-day cycle

of a phase III trial of adjuvant pelvic radiotherapy in stage I and II uterine sarcoma (leiomyosarcoma, carcinosarcoma, and endometrial stromal sarcoma) failed to demonstrate any benefit in progression-free or overall survival. This study did not include uterine adenosarcoma patients. There was a significant reduction in loco-regional recurrence ($P = 0.004$), but this finding may be due to a large number of carcinosarcoma patients in the study. Also, there is a high risk for distant metastatic disease with high-risk uterine sarcomas, thus radiation has no impact on these outcomes.[128] In some of the largest series reported in uterine adenosarcoma, utilization of pelvic radiation or brachytherapy has been reported in 17%–24% of cases. However, these studies did not show any survival benefit with adjuvant radiation in uterine adenosarcoma.[8,12] A recent study published by the French Sarcoma Group, evaluated the utility of adjuvant chemotherapy and radiation in 39 patients with stage I to III HG-ESS and undifferentiated sarcoma. The authors found a significant survival benefit on multivariate analysis in both disease-free (HR 0.22, 95% CI, 0.05–0.91, $P = 0.036$) and overall survival (HR 0.13, 95% CI, 0.13–0.63, $P = 0.012$) with adjuvant radiotherapy and significant benefit in overall survival (HR 0.13, 95% CI, 0.13–0.86, $P = 0.034$) with adjuvant chemotherapy.[127] Thus, adjuvant radiotherapy can be considered in select cases of high-risk uterine sarcomas at increased risk of local recurrence (i.e., positive margins following local surgical resection), however, should not be routinely used as adjuvant therapy in early-stage tumors with pathologic complete resection.

Adjuvant hormonal therapy

ER and PR expression is most notable in LG-ESS tumors,[90] however, have been seen in some cases of uterine adeno-sarcoma.[12,92] Although hormonal therapy is not considered standard adjuvant therapy for patients with stage I LG-ESS, patients with advanced or metastatic disease may benefit from hormonal therapies including progestin-based therapies and aromatase inhibitors.[93–95,112,113] Leath et al. presented a retrospective, multiinstitutional series of 30 patients with LG-ESS treated with postoperative hormonal therapy (megestrol acetate or medroxyprogesterone acetate). The median overall survival with hormonal therapy was 94 months versus observation 72 months ($P = 0.07$). Hormonal therapy was associated with improved survival with risk of death higher in observation arm (HR 3.5, 95% CI, 0.91–8.3).[113] Deshmukh et al. published a series of 39 patients with LG-ESS, of which majority had stage I disease ($n = 30$) and evaluated outcomes and responses to progestin vs aromatase inhibitor therapies in the adjuvant setting. They found that disease recurred in 70% of patients not receiving hormonal therapy compared to 14.3% receiving aromatase inhibitors, and 7.7% receiving progestins ($P = 0.003$). In stage I patients, mean recurrence-free survival (RFS) was 153 months for aromatase inhibitors, 306 months with progestins, and 91 months for no hormonal therapy. In stage II to IV patients, mean RFS was 148 months for aromatase inhibitors compared to 121 months for progestin therapy. In this series, 69% of stage I patients stopped or reduced progestin therapy due to side effects, compared to none of the patients taking aromatase inhibitor therapy.[96] Other studies have also confirmed overall well tolerability of aromatase inhibitor therapy, with letrozole being the most commonly used medication.[97] The current NCCN guidelines suggest adjuvant hormonal therapy (aromatase inhibitor therapy preferred) for patients with stage II-IV LG-ESS.[119] There have been a small number of cases of responses to hormonal therapy in uterine adenosarcoma that have correlated with ER/PR expression with responses noted between 10 months to 7 years.[12,92] Hormonal therapies to consider in these cases are listed in Table 10.6.

Surveillance for recurrence

While serial imaging is typically not recommended in the routine surveillance of endometrial cancers, the risk of recurrence with uterine sarcomas is much greater and occur in distant metastatic sites as the lungs and liver more frequently than their epithelial counterparts.[129] Thus, based on this, the current NCCN guidelines support follow up with clinical examination and chest, abdominal, and pelvic CT scans every 3–6 months for the first 3 years, then every 6–12 months for the next 2 years. Depending on histology, grade, and initial stage, there can be consideration of annual to bi-annual imaging thereafter up to an additional 5 years.[119] These surveillance guidelines can be adjusted based on risk of recurrence, especially in early-stage indolent tumors such as LG-ESS and uterine adenosarcoma without sarcomatous overgrowth. Uterine STUMP tumors also follow a typical indolent course and most relapses occur after 5 years of diagnosis. Given the rarity of this diagnosis and lack of data on risk factors for recurrence, it is unclear appropriate surveillance guidelines. Given the risk of recurrence as either a STUMP tumor or leiomyosarcoma, a suggested follow-up has been every 6 months for the first 5 years, followed by annual for another 5 years.[130]

TABLE 10.6 Adjuvant hormonal therapy for low-grade endometrial stromal sarcoma and sarcomas expressing ER/PR.

Hormonal regimens	Dosing
Progestins	
Megestrol acetate[a]	160 mg total PO daily (80 mg BID or 40 mg QID)
Medroxyprogesterone acetate	250 mg PO daily
Aromatase inhibitors	
Letrozole[a]	2.5 mg PO daily
Anastrozole	1 mg PO daily
Exemestane	25 mg PO daily
GnRH analogs	
Leuprolide acetate	3.75 mg IM monthly or 11.25 mg IM q 3 months

[a]Recommended based on available data and response rates.

Survival and patterns of failure

The majority of patients with uterine adenosarcoma are diagnosed with early-stage disease (73%–82%); however, recurrence rates are not only associated with stage at diagnosis, but also high-risk factors such as sarcomatous overgrowth.[7] Five-year survival rates by stage are as follows; stage I: 65%–85%, stage II: 50%–70%, stage III: 25%–50%, and stage IV: 15%.[8,78] Presence of sarcomatous overgrowth represents one of the greatest prognostic factors for recurrence in uterine adenosarcoma with recurrence rates reported in 45$–75% cases.[7,11–13,84] The most common location for recurrence in uterine adenosarcoma is either locally within the pelvis or another site in the abdominal cavity. Distant metastases are less common than local; however, they can be seen mostly involving the liver and lung, but can affect other distant sites.[7]

Most endometrial stromal sarcomas will also present with early-stage disease (65%–86%), and risk of recurrence is driven by stage at diagnosis and tumor grade (low-grade vs. high-grade).[90] Patients with stage I to II disease have a 5-year disease-specific survival of 89.3% compared to patients with stage III to IV disease of 50.3% ($P < 0.001$). Tumor grade was associated with survival with grade 1 and 2 tumors having 5-year survival of 91.4% and 95.4% compared to grade 3 tumors of 42.1% ($P < 0.001$).[120] Risk of recurrence with LG-ESS can be up to 40%–50%, with a risk of remote relapses even after 20 years, which is typically in the pelvis, abdomen, or lungs.[2,70,71] High-grade endometrial stromal and undifferentiated sarcomas have a higher rate of presenting with metastatic disease at diagnosis (57%–70%), and are associated with poor prognosis with 5-year survival rates of 20%–35%.[71,72,75,76]

Uterine STUMP recurrence rates are around 10%, and relapses are usually histologically consistent with either a STUMP tumor or leiomyosarcoma. Time to recurrence has been reported from 2 to 194 months, with mean value of 54 months in accordance with their typical indolent behavior. The lungs are a frequent metastatic site, thus careful attention should be made on follow-up imaging with at least annual chest X-ray imaging.[117,131,132]

Treatment of recurrent disease

Surgery

Secondary surgical cytoreduction can be considered in select cases of local recurrence or isolated distant metastases in patients with uterine adenosarcoma, endometrial stromal sarcoma and STUMP tumors. The benefit of secondary cytoreduction in uterine adenosarcoma was suggested in two series. Carroll et al. reported out of 34 uterine adenosarcoma recurrences, 62% underwent secondary surgery with an overall survival benefit of 58.4 vs 30.1 months (HR 0.68, 95% CI, 0.28–1.67, $P = 0.4$).[12] A second series showed an increase time to second recurrence for those patients who underwent secondary surgery (29.7 vs 12.7 months, $P = 0.37$).[78] Thus, when a patient presents with an isolated recurrence, secondary surgery can be considered.[7] Similarly, in LG-ESS, given the indolent and low-grade nature of these tumors and efficacy of hormonal therapies, surgical cytoreduction in either an upfront metastatic diagnosis or at the time of recurrence should be considered.[133] Given the aggressive nature and tendency for widespread metastatic disease with high-grade and undifferentiated sarcomas, secondary surgery may be of less benefit. Relapse of STUMP tumors can also be considered for secondary surgery for diagnostic (differentiate between STUMP versus leiomyosarcoma) and therapeutic purposes.[117]

Radiation

Stereotactic radiation can be proposed for oligometastatic recurrent uterine sarcoma lesions that cannot be surgically resected or depending on patient performance status. Also, radiotherapy can be utilized for palliative purposes to isolated lesions (i.e., bone) that are symptomatic, typically utilizing hypofractionated schedules with 1–10 fractions according to metastatic extension, whether local disease is controlled, the patient health, and overall life expectancy.[6]

Chemotherapy

Most clinical trials evaluating chemotherapeutic options in the second-line setting focus on soft-tissue sarcomas (nongynecologic) or uterine leiomyosarcoma, and rarely include patients with uterine adenosarcoma, high-grade endometrial stromal or undifferentiated sarcomas. Treatment of recurrent high-grade sarcomas have utilized chemotherapy regimens including doxorubicin/ifosfamide, doxorubicin/dacarbazine, gemcitabine/docetaxel, liposomal doxorubicin, trabectedin, and pazopanib (Table 10.7).[134–150]

TABLE 10.7 Second-line chemotherapy regimens in recurrent setting.

Chemotherapy regimens[a]	Dosing
Adriamycin alone	60–75 mg/m^2/21-day cycle
Adriamycin + Ifosfamide	60–75 mg/m^2/21-day cycle 7.5–10 g/m^2/21-day cycle
Adriamycin + Dacarbazine	60–75 mg/m^2/21-day cycle 750–1000 mg/m^2/21-day cycle
Gemcitabine + Docetaxel	675–900 mg/m^2 (day 1, 8) 75–100 mg/m^2/21-day cycle
Liposomal doxorubicin	40–50 mg/m^2/28-day cycle
Trabectedin	1.5 mg/m^2 IV over 24 h/21-day cycle
Pazopanib	800 mg PO once daily[b]

[a]All chemotherapeutic regimens in the recurrent setting can be given as single agents based on patient performance status and toxicity profile.
[b]See prescribing information for laboratory monitoring frequency.

Hormonal therapy

Patients with recurrent LG-ESS or ER/PR expressing uterine adenosarcomas can be considered for hormonal therapy. High-grade endometrial stromal and undifferentiated sarcomas rarely express ER/PR receptors, thus hormonal therapy is typically not efficacious in this population. Most commonly used hormonal regimens include progestin-based therapies and aromatase inhibitors (Table 10.6).

Immunotherapy

Given the rarity of these tumors, the role for immune targeting therapeutic approaches remains unknown. Thus far, only case reports have described potential for benefit and the remaining literature is limited to larger studies which include multiple sarcoma subtypes. Thus far, even in the more common uterine leiomyosarcoma subtype, immune checkpoint blockage has demonstrated low response rates thus is not recommended at this time outside of a clinical trial. Endometrial stromal sarcoma may be a slightly more attractive target for immune therapy, due to its genetic makeup with translocation and gene fusion. The mechanism for oncogenesis due to translocation remains poorly understood, but the subsequent chromatin remodeling and translocation fusion proteins may provide potential tumor-specific targets.

Only a limited number of studies have evaluated the efficacy and utility of immunotherapy in uterine sarcomas. Uterine leiomyosarcoma exhibits moderate expression of PD-1 (47%) and PD-L1 (36%).[151] A phase 2 trial of single-agent nivolumab in advanced leiomyosarcoma showed no objective responses. PD-1 expression was seen in 20%, PD-L1 expression in 20%, and PD-L2 expression in 90% of samples from this study.[152] A phase II trial of single agent Pembrolizumab (SARC028) in advanced soft-tissue sarcomas showed no responses in a small cohort of leiomyosarcoma patients ($n = 10$).[153] However, combination of nivolumab 3 mg/kg plus ipilimumab 1 mg/kg every 3 weeks did demonstrate responses in one uterine leiomyosarcoma and one nonuterine leiomyosarcoma case.[154] Combination anti–PD-L1 and anti–CTLA-4 therapies have also been studied in advanced sarcomas. A phase II trial of durvalumab (1500 mg) and tremelimumab (75 mg) every 4 weeks in advanced soft tissue sarcomas was reported in abstract form, which included a small cohort of leiomyosarcoma patients which had minimal response to therapy.[155] Combination of checkpoint inhibition and chemotherapy with pembrolizumab and metronomic dosing of cyclophosphamide in patients with advanced sarcoma (included 15 leiomyosarcoma and 3 endometrial stromal sarcoma patients) showed limited utility with only one objective response in the entire study.[156] There is a strong correlation between tumor mutational burden and response to PD-1 blocking antibodies. Sarcomas in general are associated with low tumor mutational burden, thus immunotherapy may not have utility in sarcomas and additional research on targeted therapies and biomarkers in sarcomas is needed.[157]

Clinical case resolution

In this case of stage IA uterine adenosarcoma with presence of sarcomatous overgrowth and lymphovascular invasion; both are significant prognostic factors for worse progression-free and overall survival. However, there is limited data on the benefit of adjuvant systemic chemotherapy and/or radiation in stage I tumors, and should be individualized. The current NCCN guidelines, supports observation in cases of stage I uterine sarcomas regardless of risk factors.

References

1. El-Khalfaoui K, du Bois A, Heitz F, Kurzeder C, Sehouli J, Harter P. Current and future options in the management and treatment of uterine sarcoma. *Ther Adv Med Oncol.* 2014;6:21–28.

2. D'Angelo E, Prat J. Uterine sarcomas: a review. *Gynecol Oncol.* 2010;116:131–139.

3. Major FJ, Blessing JA, Silverberg SG, et al. Prognostic factors in early-stage uterine sarcoma. A Gynecologic Oncology Group study. *Cancer.* 1993;71(4 suppl):1702–1709.

4. Brooks SE, Zhan M, Cote T, Baquet CR. Surveillance, epidemiology, and end results analysis of 2677 cases of uterine sarcoma 1989-1999. *Gynecol Oncol.* 2004;93:204–208.

5. Seagle BL, Sobecki-Rausch J, Strohl AE, Shilpi A, Grace A, Shahabi S. Prognosis and treatment of uterine leiomyosarcoma: a National Cancer Database study. *Gynecol Oncol.* 2017;145:61–70.

6. Ferrandina G, Aristei C, Bionetti PR, et al. Italian consensus conference on management of uterine sarcomas on behalf of S.I.G.O. (Societa' italiana di Ginecologia E Ostetricia). *Eur J Cancer.* 2020;139:149–168.

7. Nathenson MJ, Ravi V, Fleming N, Wang W, Conley A. Uterine adenosarcoma: a review. *Curr Oncol Rep.* 2016;18:68.

8. Arend R, Bagaria M, Lewin SN, et al. Long-term outcome and natural history of uterine adenosarcomas. *Gynecol Oncol.* 2010;119:305–308.

9. Guntupalli SR, Ramirez PT, Anderson ML, Milam MR, Bodurka DC, Malpica A. Uterine smooth muscle tumor of uncertain malignant potential: a retrospective analysis. *Gynecol Oncol.* 2009;113:324–326.

10. Gadducci A, Zannoni GF. Uterine smooth muscle tumors of unknown malignant potential: a challenging question. *Gynecol Oncol.* 2019;154:631–637.

11. Clement PB, Scully RE. Müllerian adenosarcoma of the uterus: a clinicopathologic analysis of 100 cases with review of the literature. *Hum Pathol.* 1990;21:363–381.

12. Carroll A, Ramirez PT, Westin SN, et al. Uterine adenosarcoma: an analysis on management, outcomes, and risk factors for recurrence. *Gynecol Oncol.* 2014;135:455–461.

13. Bernard B, Clarke BA, Malowany JI, et al. Uterine adenosarcoma: a dual-institution update on staging, prognosis, and survival. *Gynecol Oncol.* 2013;131:634–639.

14. Verschraegen CF, Vasuratna A, Edwards C, et al. Clinicopathologic analysis of Müllerian adenosarcoma: the M.D. Anderson cancer center experience. *Oncol Rep.* 1998;5:939–944.

15. Kondi-Pafiti A, Spanidou-Carvouni H, Papadias K, et al. Malignant neoplasms arising in endometriosis: clinicopathologic study of 14 cases. *Clin Exp Obstet Gynecol.* 2004;31:302–304.

16. Stern RC, Dash R, Bentley RC, Snyder MJ, Haney AF, Robboy SJ. Malignancy in endometriosis: frequency and comparison of ovarian and extra-ovarian types. *Int J Gynecol Pathol.* 2001;20:133–139.

17. Arenas M, Rovirosa A, Hernandez V, et al. Uterine sarcomas in breast cancer patients treated with tamoxifen. *Int J Gynecol Cancer.* 2006;16:861–865.

18. Kennedy MM, Baigrie CF, Manek S. Tamoxifen and the endometrium: review of 102 cases and comparison with HRT-related and non-HRT-related endometrial pathology. *Int J Gynecol Pathol.* 1999;18:130–137.

19. Fisher B, Constantino JP, Wickerham DL, et al. Tamoxifen for prevention of breast cancer: report of the National Surgical Adjuvant Breast and Bowel Project P-1 Study. *J Natl Cancer Inst.* 1998;90:1371–1388.

20. Press MF, Scully RE. Endometrial "sarcomas" complicating ovarian thecoma, polycystic ovarian disease and estrogen therapy. *Gynecol Oncol.* 1985;21:135–154.

21. Basaran D, Usubutun A, Salman MC, et al. The clinicopathological study of 21 cases with uterine smooth muscle tumors of uncertain malignant potential: centralized review can purify the diagnosis. *Int J Gynecol Cancer.* 2018;28:233–240.

22. Gupta M, Laury AL, Nucci MR, Quade BJ. Predictors of adverse outcome in uterine smooth muscle tumours of uncertain malignant potential (STUMP): a clinicopathologic analysis of 22 cases with a proposal for the inclusion of additional histological parameters. *Histopathology.* 2018;73:284–298.

23. Pinto A, Howitt B. Uterine adenosarcoma. *Arch Pathol Lab Med.* 2016;140:286–290.

23a. McCluggage WG. Mullerian Adenosarcoma of the Female Genital Tract. *Adv Anat Pathol.* 2010;17:122–129.

23b. Howitt BE, Carlson JW, Quade BJ. Adenosarcoma of uterine corpus. Edited by the WHO Classification of Tumors Editorial Board. Female Genital Tumors. World Health Organization Classification of Tumors, Lyon: IARC Press, 2020; 305–306.

24. Friedlander ML, Covens A, Glasspool RM, et al. Gynecologic Cancer InterGroup (CGIG) consensus review for Müllerian adenosarcoma of the female genital tract. *Int J Gynecol Cancer.* 2014;24:S78–S82.

25. Parra-Herran C, Howitt BE. Uterine mesenchymal tumors: update on classification, staging, and molecular features. *Surg Pathol Clin.* 2019;12:363–396.

26. Kolin DL, Dong F, Baltay M, et al. SMARCA4-deficient undifferentiated uterine sarcoma (malignant rhabdoid tumor of the uterus): a clinicopathologic entity distinct from undifferentiated carcinoma. *Mod Pathol.* 2018;31(9):1442–1456.

27. Conklin CMJ, Longacre TA. Endometrial stromal tumors: the new WHO classification. *Adv Anat Pathol.* 2014;21:383–393.

28. Hoang L, Chiang S, Lee CH. Endometrial stromal sarcomas and related neoplasms: new developments and diagnostic considerations. *Pathology.* 2018;50(2):162–177.

29. Nucci MR. Practical issues related to uterine pathology: endometrial stromal tumors. *Mod Pathol.* 2016;29:S92–S103.

30. Chang KL, Crabtree GS, Lim-Tan SK, et al. Primary uterine endometrial stromal neoplasms. A clinicopathologic study of 117 cases. *Am J Surg Pathol.* 1990;14(5):415–438.

31. Evans HL. Endometrial stromal sarcoma and poorly differentiated endometrial sarcoma. *Cancer*. 1982;50:2170–2182.

32. Nucci MR, O'Connell JT, Huettner PC, et al. h-Caldesmon expression effectively distinguishes endometrial stromal tumors from uterine smooth muscle tumors. *Am J Surg Pathol*. 2001;25(4):455–463.

33. Lee CH, Marino-Enriquez A, Ou W, et al. The clinicopathologic features of YWHAE-FAM22 endometrial stromal sarcomas: a histologically high-grade and clinically aggressive tumor. *Am J Surg Pathol*. 2012;36:641–653.

34. Chu PG, Arber DA, Weiss LM, et al. Utility of CD10 in distinguishing between endometrial stromal sarcoma and uterine smooth muscle tumors: an immunohistochemical comparison of 34 cases. *Mod Pathol*. 2001;14(5):465–471.

35. Ip PPC, Cheung ANY, Clement PB. Uterine smooth muscle tumors of uncertain malignant potential (STUMP): a clinicopathologic analysis of 16 cases. *Am J Surg Pathol*. 2009;33:992–1005.

36. Devereaux KA, Schoolmeester JK. Smooth muscle tumors of the female genital tract. *Surg Pathol*. 2019;12:397–455.

37. Croce S, Ducoulombier A, Ribeiro A, et al. Genome profiling is an efficient tool to avoid the STUMP classification of uterine smooth muscle lesions: a comprehensive array-genomic hybridization analysis of 77 tumors. *Mod Pathol*. 2018;31:816–828.

38. Bansal N, Herzog TJ, Burke W, Cohen CJ, Wright JD. The utility of preoperative endometrial sampling for the detection of uterine sarcomas. *Gynecol Oncol*. 2008;110:43–48.

39. Hinchcliff EM, Esselen KM, Watkins JC, et al. The role of endometrial biopsy in the preoperative detection of uterine leiomyosarcoma. *J Minim Invasive Gynecol*. 2016;23:567–572.

40. Glorie N, Baert T, Van Den Bosch T, Coosemans A. Circulating protein biomarkers to differentiate uterine sarcomas from leiomyomas. *Anticancer Res*. 2019;39:3981–3989.

41. Duk JM, Bouma J, Burger GTN, Nap M, De Brujin HW. CA 125 in serum and tumor from patients with uterine sarcoma. *Int J Gynecol Cancer*. 1994;4:156–160.

42. Juang CM, Yen SM, Horng CH, Twu NF, Yu HC, Hsu WL. Potential role of preoperative serum CA125 for the differential diagnosis between uterine leiomyoma and uterine leiomyosarcoma. *Eur J Gynaecol Oncol*. 2006;27:370–374.

43. Yilmaz N, Sahin I, Kilic S, Ozgu E, Gungor T, Bilge U. Assessment of the predictivity of preoperative serum CA 125 in the differential diagnosis of uterine leiomyoma and uterine sarcoma in the Turkish female population. *Eur J Gynaecol Oncol*. 2009;30:412–414.

44. Nagamatsu A, Umesaki N, Li L, Tanaka T. Use of F-18-fluorodeoxyglucose positron emission tomography for diagnosis of uterine sarcomas. *Oncol Rep*. 2010;23:1069–1076.

45. Kusunoki S, Terao Y, Ujhira T, et al. Efficacy of PET/CT to exclude leiomyoma in patients with lesions suspicious for uterine sarcoma on MRI. *Taiwan J Obstet Gynecol*. 2017;56:508–513.

46. Nagai T, Takai Y, Akahori T, et al. Highly improved accuracy of the revised PREoperative sarcoma socre (rPRESS) in the decision of performing surgery for patients presenting with a uterine mass. *SpringerPlus*. 2015;4:520.

47. Kim JH, Kim HJ, Kim SH, et al. Sonographic and clinical characteristics of uterine sarcoma initially misdiagnosed as uterine fibroid in women in late reproductive age. *J Menopausal Med*. 2019;25:164–171.

48. Oh J, Park SB, Park HJ, Lee ES. Ultrasound features of uterine sarcomas. *Ultrasound Q*. 2019;35:376–384.

49. Ludovisi M, Moro F, Pasciuto T, et al. Imaging in gynecological disease (15): clinical and ultrasound characteristics of uterine sarcoma. *Ultrasound Obstet Gynecol*. 2019;54:676–687.

50. Suzuki A, Aoki M, Miyagawa C, et al. Differential diagnosis of uterine leiomyoma and uterine sarcoma using magnetic resonance images: a literature review. *Healthcare (Basel)*. 2019;7(4).

51. Brocker KA, Alt CD, Eichbaum M, Sohn C, Kauczor HU, Hallscheidt P. Imaging of female pelvic malignancies regarding MRI, CT, and PET/CT: part 1. *Strahlenther Onkol*. 2011;187:611–618.

52. Santos P, Cunha TM. Uterine sarcomas: clinical presentation and MRI features. *Diagn Interv Radiol*. 2015;21:4–9.

53. Takeuchi M, Matsuzaki K, Yoshida S, et al. Adenosarcoma of the uterus: magnetic resonance imaging characteristics. *Clin Imaging*. 2009;33:244–247.

54. Tirumani SH, Ojili V, Shanbhogue AK, Fasih N, Ryan JG, Reinhold C. Current concepts in imaging of uterine sarcoma. *Abdom Imaging*. 2013;38:397–411.

55. Tamai K, Koyama T, Saga T, et al. The utility of diffusion-weighted MR imaging for differentiating uterine sarcomas from benign leiomyomas. *Eur Radiol*. 2008;18:723–730.

56. DeMulder D, Ascher SM. Uterine leiomyosarcoma: can MRI differentiate leiomyosarcoma from benign leiomyoma before treatment? *Am J Roentgenol*. 2018;211:1405–1415.

57. Gaetke-Udager K, McLean K, Sciallis AP, et al. Diagnostic accuracy of ultrasound, contrast-enhanced CT, and conventional MRI for differentiating leiomyoma from leiomyosarcoma. *Acad Radiol*. 2016;23:1290–1297.

58. Lin G, Yang LY, Huang YT, et al. Comparison of the diagnostic accuracy of contrast-enhanced MRI and diffusion-weighted MRI in the differentiation between uterine leiomyosarcoma/smooth muscle tumor with uncertain malignant potential and benign leiomyoma. *J Magn Reson Imaging*. 2016;43:333–342.

59. Ho KC, Dean Fang YH, Lin G, et al. Presurgical identification of uterine smooth muscle malignancies through the characteristic FDG uptake pattern on PET scans. *Contrast Media Mol Imaging*. 2018;7890241.

60. Lai CR, Hsu CY, Li AF. Uterine adenosarcoma detected by conventional Papanicolaou smear: a case report with emphasis on integrating the immu-nocytochemical staining. *Diagn Cytopathol*. 2012;40:920–924.

61. Pasternak S, MacIntosh R. Uterine adenosarcoma detected by Papanicolaou smear: a case report. *Diagn Cytopathol*. 2006;34:495–498.

62. Goto A, Takeuchi S, Sugimura K, Maruo T. Usefulness of Gd-DTPA contrast-enhanced dynamic MRI and serum determination of LDH and its isoenzymes in the differential diagnosis of leiomyosarcoma from degenerated leiomyoma of the uterus. *Int J Gynecol Cancer*. 2002;12:354–361.

63. ACOG Committee Opinion No. 770. Uterine morcellation for presumed leiomyomas. *Obstet Gynecol.* 2019;133:604–605.

64. Ricci S, Stone RL, Fader AN. Uterine leiomyosarcoma: epidemiology, contemporary treatment strategies and the impact of uterine morcellation. *Gynecol Oncol.* 2017;145:208–216.

65. Diagnosis of abnormal uterine bleeding in reproductive-aged women. Practice Bulletin No. 128. American College of Obstetricians and Gynecologists. *Obstet Gynecol.* 2012;120:197–206.

66. Kho KA, Lin K, Hechanova M, Richardson DL. Risk of occult uterine sarcoma in women undergoing hysterectomy for benign indications. *Obstet Gynecol.* 2016;127:468–473.

67. Umesaki N, Tanaka T, Miyama M, et al. Positron emission tomography with 18(F)-fluorodeoxyglucose of uterine sarcoma: a comparison with magnetic resonance imaging and power Doppler imaging. *Gynecol Oncol.* 2001;80:372–377.

68. Reich O, Regauer S. Aromatase expression in low-grade endometrial stromal sarcomas: an immunohistochemical study. *Mod Pathol.* 2004;17:104–108.

69. Abeler VM, Nenodovic K. Diagnostic immunohistochemistry in uterine sarcomas: a study of 397 cases. *Int J Gynecol Pathol.* 2011;30:236–243.

70. Thiel FC, Halmen S. Low-grade endometrial stromal sarcoma-a review. *Oncol Res Treat.* 2018;41:687–692.

71. Gadducci A. Prognostic factors in uterine sarcoma. *Best Pract Res Clin Obstet Gynaecol.* 2011;25:783–795.

72. Seagle BL, Shilpi A, Buchanan S, Goodman C, Shahabi S. Low-grade and high-grade endometrial stromal sarcoma: a National Cancer Database study. *Gynecol Oncol.* 2017;146:254–262.

73. Ferreira J, Felix A, Lennerz JK, Oliva E. Recent advances in histological and molecular classification of endometrial stromal neoplasms. *Virchows Arch.* 2018;473:665–678.

74. Philip CA, Pautier P, Duffaud F, Ray-Coquard I. High-grade undifferentiated sarcomas of the uterus: diagnosis, outcomes, and new treatment approaches. *Curr Oncol Rep.* 2014;16:405.

75. Malouf GG, Lhomme C, Duvillard P, Morice P, Haie-Meder C, Pautier P. Prognostic factors and outcome of undifferentiated endometrial sarcoma treated by multimodal therapy. *Int J Gynaecol Obstet.* 2013;122:57–61.

76. Tanner EJ, Garg K, Leitao Jr MM, Soslow RA, Hensley ML. High grade undifferentiated uterine sarcoma: surgery, treatment, and survival outcomes. *Gynecol Oncol.* 2012;127:27–31.

77. McCluggage WG. Müllerian adenosarcoma of the female genital tract. *Adv Anat Pathol.* 2010;17:122–129.

78. Tanner EJ, Toussaint T, Leitao Jr MM, et al. Management of uterine adenosarcomas with and without sarcomatous overgrowth. *Gynecol Oncol.* 2013;129:140–144.

79. Ulrich UA, Denschlag D. Uterine adenosarcoma. *Oncol Res Treat.* 2018;41:693–696.

80. Seagle BL, Kanis M, Strohl AE, Shahabi S. Survival of women with Müllerian adenosarcoma: a national cancer database study. *Gynecol Oncol.* 2016;143:636–641.

81. Nathenson MJ, Conley AP, Lin H, Fleming N, Ravi V. Treatment of recurrent or metastatic uterine adenosarcoma. *Sarcoma.* 2017;2017:4680273.

82. Oliva E, Carcangiu ML, Carinelli SG, et al. Mesenchymal tumours. Smooth muscle tumour of uncertain malignant potential. In: Kurman RJ, Carcangui ML, Herrington CS, Young RH, eds. *WHO classification of tumours of female reproductive organs.* Lyon: IARC; 2014:135–147.

83. Peters 3rd WA, Howard DR, Andersen WA, Figge DC. Uterine smooth muscle of uncertain malignant potential. *Obstet Gynecol.* 1994;83:1015–1020.

83a. Ip PPC, Croce S, Gupta M. Uterine smooth muscle tumors of uncertain malignant potential of the uterine corpus. In: WHO Classification of Tumors Editorial Board, ed. *Female Genital Tumors.* World Health Organization Classification of Tumors. Lyon: IARC Press; 2020: 279–280.

84. Nathenson MJ, Conley AP. Prognostic factors for uterine adenosarcoma: a review. *Expert Rev Anticancer Ther.* 2018;18:1093–1100.

85. Nathenson MJ, Conley AP, Lin H, et al. The importance of lymphovascular invasion in uterine adenosarcoma. *Int J Gynecol Cancer.* 2018;28:1297–1310.

86. Machida H, Nathenson MJ, Takiuchi T, Adams CL, Garcia-Sayre J, Matsuo J. Significance of lymph node metastasis on survival of women with uterine adenosarcoma. *Gynecol Oncol.* 2017;144:524–530.

87. Garg G, Shah JP, Toy EP, Bryant CS, Kumar S, Morris RT. Stage IA vs. IB endometrial stromal sarcoma: does the new staging system predict survival. *Gynecol Oncol.* 2010;118:8–13.

88. Nordal RR, Kristensen GB, Kaern J, et al. The prognostic significance of surgery, tumor size, malignancy grade, menopausal status, and DNA ploidy in endometrial stromal sarcoma. *Gynecol Oncol.* 1996;62:254–259.

89. Bodner K, Bodner-Adler B, Obermair A, et al. Prognostic parameters in endometrial stromal sarcoma: a clinicopathologic study in 31 patients. *Gynecol Oncol.* 2001;81:160–165.

90. Amant F, Coosemans A, Debiec-Rychter M, Timmerman D, Vergote I. Clinical management of uterine sarcomas. *Lancet Oncol.* 2009;10:1188–1198.

91. Meurer M, Floquet A, Ray-Coquard I, et al. Localized high grade endometrial stromal sarcoma and localized undifferentiated uterine sarcoma: a retrospective series of the French Sarcoma Group. *Int J Gynecol Cancer.* 2019;29:691–698.

92. Amant F, Schurmans K, Steenkiste E, et al. Immunohistochemical determination of estrogen and progesterone receptor positivity in uterine adenosarcoma. *Gynecol Oncol.* 2004;93:680–685.

93. Cheng X, Yang G, Schmeler KM, et al. Recurrence patterns and prognosis of endometrial stromal sarcoma and the potential of tyrosine kinase-inhibiting therapy. *Gynecol Oncol.* 2011;121:323–327.

94. Reich O, Nogales FF, Regauer S. Gonadotropin-releasing hormone receptor expression in endometrial stromal sarcomas: an immunohistochemical study. *Mod Pathol.* 2005;18:573–576.

95. Chu MC, Mor G, Lim C, Zheng W, Parkash V, Schwartz PE. Low-grade endometrial stromal sarcoma: hormonal aspects. *Gynecol Oncol.* 2003;90:170–176.

96. Deshmukh U, Black J, Perez-Irizarry J, et al. Adjuvant hormonal therapy for low-grade endometrial stromal sarcoma. *Reprod Sci.* 2019;26:600–608.

97. Ryu H, Choi Y, Song I, et al. Long-term treatment of residual or recurrent low-grade endometrial stromal sarcoma with aromatase inhibitors: a report of two cases and a review of literature. *Oncol Lett.* 2015;10:3310–3314.

98. Cabrera S, Bebia V, Acosta U, et al. Survival outcomes and prognostic factors of endometrial stromal sarcoma and undifferentiated sarcoma. *Clin Transl Oncol.* 2020. Online ahead of print.

99. Nobre SP, Hensley ML, So M, et al. The impact of tumor fragmentation in patients with stage I uterine leiomyosarcoma on patterns of recurrence and oncologic outcome. *Gynecol Oncol.* 2021;160:99–105.

100. Park JY, Kim DY, Kim JH, Kim YT, Nam JH. The impact of tumor morcellation during surgery on the outcomes of patients with apparently early low-grade endometrial stromal sarcoma of the uterus. *Ann Surg Oncol.* 2011;18:3453–3461.

101. Park JY, Park SK, Kim DY, et al. The impact of tumor morcellation during surgery on the prognosis of patients with apparently early uterine leiomyosarcoma. *Gynecol Oncol.* 2011;122:255–259.

102. George S, Barysauskas C, Serrano C, et al. Retrospective cohort study evaluating the impact of intraperitoneal morcellation on outcomes of localized uterine leiomyosarcoma. *Cancer.* 2014;120:3154–3158.

103. Raspagliesi F, Maltese G, Bogani G, et al. Morcellation worsens survival outcomes in patients with undiagnosed uterine leiomyosarcoma: a retrospective MITO group study. *Gynecol Oncol.* 2017;144:90–95.

104. Xu X, Lin H, Wright JD, et al. Association between power morcellation and mortality in women with unexpected uterine cancer undergoing hysterectomy or myomectomy. *J Clin Oncol.* 2019;37:3412–3424.

105. Benito V, Lubrano A, Leon L, Molano F, Pinar B. Does iatrogenic tumor rupture during surgery have prognostic implications for the outcome of uterine sarcomas? *Int J Gynecol Cancer.* 2020;30:1726–1732.

106. Amant F, Schurmans K, Steenkiste E, et al. Immunohistochemical determination of estrogen and progesterone receptor positivity in uterine adenosarcoma. *Gynecol Oncol.* 2004;93:680–685.

107. Kodaman PH. Early menopause: primary ovarian insufficiency and surgical menopause. *Semin Reprod Med.* 2010;28:360–369.

108. Nasioudis D, Ko EM, Kolovos G, Vagios S, Kalliouris D, Giuntoli RL. Ovarian preservation for low-grade endometrial stromal sarcoma: a systematic review of the literature and meta-analysis. *Int J Gynecol Cancer.* 2019;29:126–132.

109. Nasioudis D, Mastroyannis SA, Latif NA, et al. Effect of bilateral salpingo-oophorectomy on the overall survival of premenopausal patients with stage I low-grade endometrial stromal sarcoma; a National Cancer Database analysis. *Gynecol Oncol.* 2020;157:634–638.

110. Bai H, Yang J, Cao D, et al. Ovary and uterus-sparing procedures for low-grade endometrial stromal sarcoma: a retrospective study of 153 cases. *Gynecol Oncol.* 2014;132:654–660.

111. Nasioudis D, Chapman-Davis E, Frey M, Holcomb K. Safety of ovarian preservation in premenopausal women with stage I uterine sarcoma. *J Gynecol Oncol.* 2017;28, e46.

112. Amant F, De Knijf A, Van Calster B, et al. Clinical study investigating the role of lymphadenectomy, surgical castration and adjuvant hormonal treatment in endometrial stromal sarcoma. *Br J Cancer.* 2007;97:1194–1199.

113. Leath 3rd CA, Huh WK, Hyde Jr J, et al. A multi-institutional review of outcomes of endometrial stromal sarcoma. *Gynecol Oncol.* 2007;105:630–634.

114. Zaloudek CJ, Norris HJ. Adenofibroma and adenosarcoma of the uterus: a clinicopathologic study of 35 cases. *Cancer.* 1981;48:354–366.

115. Zheng Y, Yin Q, Yang X, Dong R. Fertility-sparing management of low-grade endometrial stromal sarcoma: analysis of an institutional series, a population-based analysis and review of the literature. *Ann Transl Med.* 2020;8:1358.

116. Vilos GA, Marks J, Ettler HC, Vilos AG, Prefontaine M, Abu-Rafea B. Uterine smooth muscle tumors of uncertain malignant potential: diagnostic challenges and therapeutic dilemmas. Report of 2 cases and review of the literature. *J Minim Invasive Gynecol.* 2012;19:288–295.

117. Rizzo A, Ricci AD, Saponara M, et al. Recurrent uterine smooth-muscle tumors of uncertain malignant potential (STUMP): state of the art. *Anticancer Res.* 2020;40:1229–1238.

118. Sahin H, Karatas F, Coban G, et al. Uterine smooth muscle tumor of uncertain malignant potential: fertility and clinical outcomes. *J Gynecol Oncol.* 2019;30, e54.

119. Abu-Rustum NR, Yashar CM, Bradley K, et al. *NCCN clinical practice guidelines in oncology uterine neoplasms version 1.2021.* National Comprehensive Cancer Network; 2021. Available from: https://www.nccn.org/professionals/physician_gls/pdf/uterine.pdf.

120. Chan JK, Kawar NM, Shin JY, et al. Endometrial stromal sarcoma: a population-based analysis. *Br J Cancer.* 2008;99:1210–1215.

121. Shah JP, Bryant CS, Kumar S, et al. Lymphadenectomy and ovarian preservation in low-grade endometrial stromal sarcoma. *Obstet Gynecol.* 2008;112:1102–1108.

122. Riopel J, Plante M, Renaud MC, Roy M, Tetu B. Lymph node metastases in low-grade endometrial stromal sarcoma. *Gynecol Oncol.* 2005;96:402–406.

123. Si M, Jia L, Song K, Zhang Q, Kong B. Role of lymphadenectomy for uterine sarcoma: a meta-analysis. *Int J Gynecol Cancer.* 2017;27:109–116.

124. Seagle BL, Shilpi A, Buchanan S, Goodman C, Shahabi S. Low-grade and high-grade endometrial stromal sarcoma: a National Cancer Database study. *Gynecol Oncol.* 2017;146:254–262.

125. Thiel FC, Halmen S. Low-grade endometrial stromal sarcoma-a review. *Oncol Res Treat.* 2018;41:687–692.

126. Omura GA, Blessing JA, Major F, et al. A randomized clinical trial of adjuvant Adriamycin in uterine sarcomas: a Gynecologic Oncology Group Study. *J Clin Oncol.* 1985;3:1240–1245.

127. Pautier P, Rey A, Haie-Meder C, et al. Adjuvant chemotherapy with cisplatin, ifosfamide, and doxorubicin followed by radiotherapy in localized uterine sarcomas: results of a case-control study with radiotherapy alone. *Int J Gynecol Cancer.* 2004;14:1112–1117.

128. Reed NS, Mangioni C, Malmstrom H, et al. Phase III randomized study to evaluate the role of adjuvant pelvic radiotherapy in the treatment of uterine sarcomas stages I and II: an European Organisation for Research and Treatment of Cancer Gynaecological Cancer Group Study (protocol 55874). *Eur J Cancer.* 2008;44:808–818.

129. Salani R, Khanna N, Frimer M, Bristow RE, Chen LM. An update on post-treatment surveillance and diagnosis of recurrence in women with gynecologic malignancies: Society of Gynecologic Oncology (SGO) recommendations. *Gynecol Oncol.* 2017;146:3–10.

130. Ip PPC, Tse KY, Tam KF. Uterine smooth muscle tumors other than the ordinary leiomyomas and leiomyosarcomas: a review of selected variants with emphasis on recent advances and unusual morphology that may cause concern for malignancy. *Adv Anat Pathol.* 2010;17:91–112.

131. Bell SW, Kempson RL, Hendrickson MR. Problematic uterine smooth muscle neoplasms. a clinicopathologic study of 213 cases. *Am J Surg Pathol.* 1994;18:535–558.

132. Dall'Asta A, Gizzo S, Musaro A, et al. Uterine smooth muscle tumors of uncertain malignant potential (STUMP): pathology, follow-up and recurrence. *Int J Clin Exp Pathol.* 2014;7:8136–8142.

133. Thomas MB, Keeney GL, Podratz KC, Dowdy SC. Endometrial stromal sarcoma: treatment and patterns of recurrence. *Int J Gynecol Cancer.* 2009;19:253–256.

134. Desar IME, Ottevanger PB, Benson C, van der Graaf. Systemic treatment in adult uterine sarcomas. *Crit Rev Oncol Hematol.* 2018;122:10–20.

135. Judson I, Verweij J, Gelderblom H, et al. Doxorubicin alone versus intensified doxorubicin plus ifosfamide for first-line treatment of advanced or metastatic soft-tissue sarcoma: a randomized controlled phase 3 trial. *Lancet Oncol.* 2014;15:415–423.

136. Seddon B, Strauss SJ, Whelan J, et al. Gemcitabine and docetaxel versus doxorubicin as first-line treatment in previously untreated advanced unresectable or metastatic soft-tissue sarcomas (GeDDiS): a randomized controlled phase 3 trial. *Lancet Oncol.* 2017;18:1397–1410.

137. Ray-Coquard I, Rizzo E, Blay JY, et al. Impact of chemotherapy in uterine sarcoma (UtS): review of 13 clinical trials from the EORTC Soft Tissue and Bone Sarcoma Group (STBSG) involving advanced/metastatic UtS compared to other soft tissue sarcoma (STS) patients treated with first line chemotherapy. *Gynecol Oncol.* 2016;142:95–101.

138. Pautier P, Floquet A, Penel N, et al. Randomized multicenter and stratified phase II study of gemcitabine alone versus gemcitabine and docetaxel in patients with metastatic or relapsed leiomyosarcomas: a Federation Nationale des Centres de Lutte Contre le Cancer (FNCLCC) French Sarcoma Group Study (TAXOGEM study). *Oncologist.* 2012;17:1213–1220.

139. Okuno S, Edmonson J, Mahoney M, Buckner JC, Frytak S, Galanis E. Phase II trial of gemcitabine in advanced sarcomas. *Cancer.* 2002;94:3225–3229.

140. Look KY, Sandler A, Blessing JA, Lucci III JA, Rose PG. Gynecologic Oncology Group (GOG) Study. Phase II trial of gemcitabine as second-line chemotherapy of uterine leiomyosarcoma: a Gynecologic Oncology Group (GOG) study. *Gynecol Oncol.* 2004;92:644–647.

141. Demetri GD, Von Mehren M, Jones RL, et al. Efficacy and safety of trabectedin or dacarbazine for metastatic liposarcoma or leiomyosarcoma after failure of conventional chemotherapy: results of a phase III randomized multicenter clinical trial. *J Clin Oncol.* 2016;34:786–793.

142. Garcia-del-Muro X, Lopez-Pousa A, Maurel J, et al. Randomized phase II study comparing gemcitabine plus dacarbazine versus dacarbazine alone in patients with previously treated soft tissue sarcoma: a Spanish group for research on sarcomas study. *J Clin Oncol.* 2011;29:2528–2533.

143. Hensley M, Patel SR, von Mehren M, et al. Efficacy and safety of trabectedin or dacarbazine in patients with advanced uterine leiomyosarcoma after failure of anthracycline-based chemotherapy: subgroup analysis of a phase 3, randomized clinical trial. *Gynecol Oncol.* 2017;146:531–537.

144. Benson C, Ray-Coquard I, Sleijfer S, et al. Outcome of uterine sarcoma patients treated with pazopanib: a retrospective analysis based on two European Organisation for Research and Treatment of Cancer (EORTC) Soft Tissue and Bone Sarcoma Group (STBSG) clinical trials 62043 and 62072. *Gynecol Oncol.* 2016;142:89–94.

145. van der Graaf WT, Blay JY, Chawla SP, et al. EORTC Soft Tissue and Bone Sarcoma Group; PALETTE study group. Pazopanib for metastatic soft-tissue sarcoma (PALETTE): a randomized, double-blind, placebo-controlled phase 3 trial. *Lancet.* 2012;379:1879–1886.

146. Cesne AL, Bauer S, Demetri GD, et al. Safety and efficacy of pazopanib in advanced soft tissue sarcoma: PALETTE (EORTC 62072) subgroup analyses. *BMC Cancer.* 2019;19:794.

147. Pautier P, Penel N, Ray-Coquard I, et al. A phase II trial of gemcitabine combined with pazopanib followed by pazopanib maintenance, as second-line treatment in patients with advanced leiomyosarcomas: a unicancer French Sarcoma Group study (LMS03 study). *Eur J Cancer.* 2020;125:31–37.

148. Grunwald V, Karch A, Schuler M, et al. Randomized comparison of pazopanib and doxorubicin as first-line treatment in patients with metastatic soft tissue sarcoma age 60 years or older: results of a German intergroup study. *J Clin Oncol.* 2020;38:3555–3564.

149. Schmoll HJ, Lindner LH, Reichardt P, et al. Efficacy of Pazopanib with or without gemcitabine in patients with anthracycline- and/or ifosfamide-refractory soft tissue sarcoma: final results of the PAPAGEMO phase 2 randomized clinical trial. *JAMA Oncol.* 2020;23, e206564.

150. Somaiah N, Van Tine BA, Wahlquist AE, et al. A randomized, open-label, phase 2, multicenter trial of gemcitabine with pazopanib or gemcitabine with docetaxel in patients with advanced soft-tissue sarcoma. *Cancer.* 2020. Online ahead of print.

151. Herzog T, Arguello D, Reddy S, Gatalica Z. PD-1 and PD-L1 expression in 1599 gynecological cancers: implications for immunotherapy. *Gynecol Oncol.* 2015;137(suppl. 1):204–205.

152. Ben-Ami E, Barysauskas CM, Solomon S, et al. Immunotherapy with single agent nivolumab for advanced leiomyosarcoma of the uterus: results of a phase 2 study. *Cancer.* 2017;123:3285–3290.

153. Tawbi HA, Burgess M, Bolejack V, et al. Pembrolizumab in advanced soft-tissue sarcoma and bone sarcoma (SARC028): a multicenter, two-cohort, single-arm, open-label, phase 2 trial. *Lancet Oncol.* 2017;18:1493–1501.

154. D'Angelo SP, Mahoney MR, Van Tine BA, et al. Nivolumab with or without ipilumumab treatment for metastatic sarcoma (Alliance A091401): two open-label, non-comparative, randomized, phase 2 trials. *Lancet Oncol.* 2018;19:416–426.

155. Somaiah N, Conley AP, Lin HY, et al. A phase II multi-arm study of durvalumab and tremelimumab for advanced or metastatic sarcomas. *J Clin Oncol.* 2020;38(15_suppl):11509.

156. Toulmonde M, Penel N, Adam J, et al. Use of PD-1 targeting, macrophage infiltration, and IDO pathway activation in sarcomas. A phase 2 clinical trial. JAMA. *Oncologia.* 2018;4:93–97.

157. Klemen ND, Kelly CM, Bartlett EK. The emerging role of immunotherapy for the treatment of sarcoma. *J Surg Oncol.* 2020. Online ahead of print.

Chapter 11

Uterine carcinosarcoma

Leigh A. Cantrell, Barrett Lawson, and Katherine Peng

Clinical case

A 75-year-old African American woman presents to your clinic with complaints of new onset vaginal bleeding. She has a past medical history significant for obesity and history of breast cancer managed with tamoxifen maintenance. On pelvic exam, she is noted to have a 7 cm tumor prolapsing through the cervix into the vaginal canal (Fig. 11.1). Pelvic ultrasound confirms a hyperechoic mass in the uterus with associated expansion of the endometrial canal suspicious for malignancy. Endometrial biopsy (EMB) is performed that is consistent with a diagnosis of uterine carcinosarcoma (UCS). A computed tomography (CT) of the chest, abdomen, and pelvis is ordered that demonstrates a large heterogeneous mass within the uterus and no obvious lymphadenopathy or other metastatic disease. The patient underwent a robotic assisted total hysterectomy (TAH), bilateral salpingo-oophorectomy (BSO), and pelvic lymphadenectomy. Her final pathology was consistent with a stage II UCS. What adjuvant therapy do you recommend?

Epidemiology

Incidence and mortality

While endometrioid carcinomas are the most common gynecologic malignancy in developed countries, a diagnosis of UCS, a subtype of endometrial cancer, is rare. UCS historically known as malignant mixed Mullerian tumor or malignant mixed mesodermal tumor (MMMT), is now considered one of the high-grade histologies of uterine cancer. In the past, carcinosarcomas were treated and studied as sarcomas. Table 11.1 outlines uterine cancer subtypes and their frequencies. The worldwide annual incidence of UCS ranges between 0.5 and 3.3 cases per 100,000 women with the age-adjusted incidence rate rising from 1.0 per 100,000 in 2000 to 1.4 per 100,000 in 2016.[1] UCS accounts for only 5% of all uterine tumors, yet it is responsible for 15% of all deaths from uterine corpus malignancies.[2] For all stages, the median overall survival is less than 2 years, and the 5-year overall survival rate is 33.4%.[3,4] When comparing survival by stage of disease, even women with stage I disease have poor survival outcomes. The 5-year survival rates for stages I/II, III, and IV disease are 59%, 22%, and 9%, respectively.[5] In comparison, the 5-year survival rate for stage I high-grade uterine endometrioid cancer is over 80%.[6] Women with stage IV UCS have a median overall survival of only several months.

Etiology and risk factors

The pathogenesis of UCS is controversial but the currently accepted theory is that UCS originates from the metaplastic transformation of a single cell.[7,8] While UCS was previously included and studied in the sarcoma category, it is now categorized as a high-grade dedifferentiated carcinoma. UCS is comprised of both carcinomatous (epithelial) and mesenchymal (stromal) components.[2] The epithelial components are graded as either low grade or high grade and are most likely to metastasize and be the source of recurrence as opposed to the sarcomatous component.[9–11] The stromal component can be graded as homologous or heterologous. Examples of homologous sarcomas include leiomyosarcoma, fibrosarcoma, and endometrial stromal sarcoma; examples of heterologous sarcomas include rhabdomyosarcoma, chondrosarcoma, and osteosarcoma.[12] The distinction between homologous and heterologous is based on whether the stromal component is comprised of cell types native to the uterus.

Age is a significant risk factor in the development of UCS. Carcinosarcomas are more commonly found in older women, with usual age of onset in the seventh decade of life.[3] Black women are also noted to be at increased risk of developing UCS. A 2003 SEER analysis showed that black women had significantly higher incidence rates than white non-Hispanic

Diagnosis and Treatment of Rare Gynecologic Cancers. https://doi.org/10.1016/B978-0-323-82938-0.00011-2

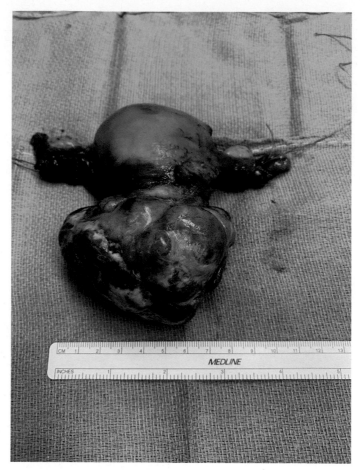

FIG. 11.1 Uterine carcinosarcoma prolapsing through cervix.

TABLE 11.1 Uterine cancer subtypes and incidence.

Histology	Percentage of total cases	Cases/year in US[a]
Endometrioid–Grade 1/2/3	75%–80%	49,900–53,000
Serous	10%	6657
Clear cell	<5%	3300
Carcinosarcoma	<5%	3300

Undifferentiated, mesonephric and squamous cell carcinomas of the endometrium are extremely rare.
[a]*http://cancerstatisticscenter.cancer.org.*

women (RR 2.33 [1.99–2.72]).[13] This was concordant with a 2004 SEER study that found the age-adjusted incidence rate of carcinosarcoma to be twofold greater in black women as compared to white women.[14]

Additional risk factors for UCS parallel risk factors for endometrial adenocarcinoma, including nulliparity, obesity, and use of exogenous estrogen.[15] Multiple small series demonstrated the relationship between tamoxifen exposure and development of UCS with median time from initiation of tamoxifen to diagnosis of UCS averaging around 9 years. In the National Surgical Adjuvant Breast and Bowel Project (NSABP) P-1 trial, the risk of endometrial cancer in those women 50 or older on tamoxifen was higher than those taking placebo after 7 years of follow up (RR 5.33 [2.47–13.17]). The incidence of endometrial cancer in the 13,388 women studied was 15.64 vs 4.68/1000 woman-years in those on tamoxifen vs placebo. Most commonly, these cancers are low grade endometrioid cancers and stage 1. Tamoxifen-related

TABLE 11.2 Prognostic factors in uterine carcinosarcoma.

Factor	Improved survival	Worsened survival
Stage	I/II (59% at 5 years)	III/IV (22 and 9% at 5 years)
Lymphovascular space Invasion	Negative	Positive
Age	<40 years	>40 years
Race	Asian/Caucasian	African-American
Carcinoma component		Serous, clear cell
Sarcoma component		Rhabdomyosarcomatous
CA125 elevation		Postoperative elevation

carcinosarcomas are estimated to comprise approximately 8% of all carcinosarcomas.[16–19] Prior pelvic radiation is also associated with the development of UCS. In one retrospective study examining the diagnosis of endometrial cancer following pelvic radiotherapy for cervical cancer, 35% of women were diagnosed with UCS which was a significant increase from the baseline sporadic rate of 6%.[20] Prognostic factors in UCS include those similar to all malignancies such as age, stage, and presence of lymphovascular space invasion. In carcinosarcoma, the carcinoma component of serous or clear cell and the sarcoma component of rhabdomyosarcoma portend a worse prognosis. Predictors of improved survival in UCS include age <40, Asian race followed by white, followed by African American, the utilization of postoperative radiotherapy, undergoing lymphadenectomy, and early stage of disease.[21] Table 11.2 demonstrates prognostic factors in uterine carcinosarcoma.

Pathology
Gross description

Tumors are typically polypoid, pedunculated and soft, though color and consistency are variable secondary to various quantity of necrosis and hemorrhage.[22] Tumors that are significantly polypoid may protrude through the cervix and may appear as a primary cervical neoplasm.[23] The median size is 5.6 cm with a range from 2.5 to 20 cm.

Microscopic description

UCS, also known as MMMT, are malignant neoplasms composed of both a malignant carcinomatous component and a malignant sarcomatous component. These neoplasms are in contrast with adenosarcoma that while having epithelial and mesenchymal elements, only the latter component is malignant.

The carcinoma and sarcoma areas are intermixed, with components that may appear well differentiated to highly anaplastic. Just over half of all UCS are predominantly composed of the sarcomatous component.[24]

The carcinoma component may include one or more of the following histotypes: endometrioid, serous, undifferentiated or dedifferentiated carcinoma, or clear cell carcinoma (Fig. 11.2).[25] Of these the most common epithelial component is serous carcinoma. Rarely, the epithelial component can be a mesonephric-like carcinoma. The sarcomatous component may be composed of homologous and/or heterologous components. Homologous components are those in which the mesenchymal differentiation is that of native uterine corpus mesenchymal elements such as a leiomyosarcoma, fibrosarcoma, endometrial stromal sarcoma or high-grade undifferentiated sarcoma. Heterologous components are those in which the differentiation of the sarcoma is not native to the uterine corpus, including rhabdomyosarcoma, chondrosarcoma, liposarcoma, or osteosarcoma (Figs. 11.3A, B, and 11.4). While carcinosarcomas are overall considered high grade, the presence of the heterologous sarcomatous components needs to be noted, as these have an even worse prognosis, particularly if rhabdomyosarcoma.[24] Rarely somatically derived germ cell tumors such as yolk sac tumor may be present. UCS are usually deeply myoinvasive; however, some tumors may be confined to a polyp. The metastases are usually composed of only the carcinomatous component (90%), sometimes of only the sarcomatous component, or can be mixed.

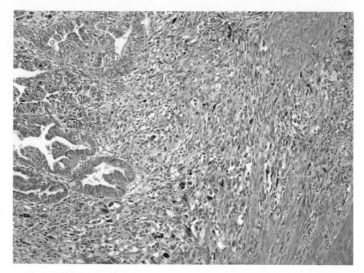

FIG. 11.2 Uterine carcinosarcoma with endometrioid type glands (*left*) with underlying malignant spindled cells.

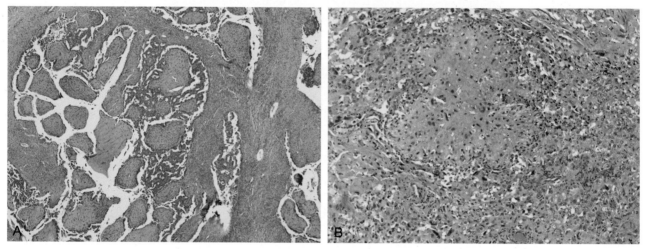

FIG. 11.3 (A) A case of uterine carcinosarcoma, with only the carcinoma component present in this field. (B) Same case of carcinosarcoma with cartilaginous differentiation in a separate field.

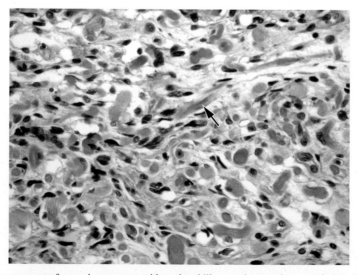

FIG. 11.4 Rhabdomyosarcoma component of a carcinosarcoma, with eosinophilic cytoplasm and cross striations (*arrow*).

Immunohistochemistry

The epithelial component is positive for keratin markers while the sarcomatous component is usually negative. The epithelial component is usually positive for PAX-8, and variably positive for hormone receptors, depending on the subtype. Both epithelial (if serous carcinoma) and sarcoma components can show aberrant expression of p53.

Differential diagnosis

The differential diagnosis includes tumors in which the carcinoma or sarcoma element can mimic the other, including carcinomas with spindle cell features, uterine adenosarcoma and pure malignant mesenchymal tumors with an epithelioid appearance.[25] Epithelial tumors with spindle features such as sarcomatoid carcinoma or endometrioid carcinomas with spindle morphology are usually diffusely positive for cytokeratins, which are typically negative in the sarcoma component. Histologically, carcinomas with spindle morphology merge with one another whereas in carcinosarcoma, there is an abrupt transition between the two components. Furthermore, markers such as CD10, WT1 or desmin may stain the sarcomatous component.

Uterine adenosarcomas are also biphasic with epithelial and mesenchymal elements; however, only the latter is malignant. The epithelial component can be glandular, dilated or slit-like and typically have a leaf-like or phyllodes architecture.[26] The epithelium may show focal atypia, few mitoses or metaplastic/hyperplastic changes; however, no malignant epithelium should be present to make this diagnosis. The stromal component is composed of spindled or rounded cells, with stromal cells aggregating against the epithelial component, called "periglandular cuffing." While higher or lower grade sarcomatous elements can be seen in either, the sarcoma in adenosarcoma is usually low grade, as opposed to the sarcoma component seen in carcinosarcoma, which is frequently high grade.[25,26]

Because either the carcinomatous or sarcomatous element can be minor, consideration must be given to adequate tumor sampling at the time of gross examination. Consequently another important differential diagnosis includes uterine sarcomas such as leiomyosarcoma or undifferentiated sarcoma, when the epithelial component is minor. Also of note, if a tumor is predominantly one component, an EMB may only sample the primary component, and the second component may only be recognized on the hysterectomy specimen.

Molecular findings

Molecular alterations in carcinosarcomas include *TP53, FBXW7, PIK3CA, PPP2R1A, PTEN, CHD4, ARID1A,* and *KRAS.* While *TP53* has been found to be the most common (up to 91%), no one mutation molecular defines carcinosarcoma.[23] While in other endometrial tumors *PTEN* and *TP53* are typically mutually exclusive, the majority of carcinosarcomas appear to have both mutations. Also, in contrast to other endometrial tumors, no evidence currently exists for traditional molecular subgroups, though a minor group of carcinosarcomas show molecular features of an endometrioid subtype, including mutations in *PTEN* and *KRAS.*

Diagnosis and workup

Differential diagnosis

UCS presents similarly to other uterine adenocarcinomas and is indistinguishable based on signs and symptoms alone; however, an accurate diagnosis is essential as the treatment and prognosis in endometrial adenocarcinoma vs carcinosarcoma is significantly different. The diagnosis of UCS is ultimately a histologic diagnosis (see Section "Pathology" above). Clinicians should have a high level of suspicion for UCS in women who present with postmenopausal bleeding and a rapidly enlarging uterine mass or concern for extrauterine disease spread. The differential diagnosis for postmenopausal bleeding is vast and ranges from benign etiologies such as endometrial hyperplasia, polyps, and atrophy to malignant etiologies, including carcinosarcoma. Table 11.3 summarizes the recommendations for the diagnostic workup of a woman suspected to have carcinosarcoma.

Signs and symptoms

Women with UCS typically have disease detected after presentation with postmenopausal bleeding, abdominal pain, or uterine enlargement. Approximately 15% of women diagnosed with UCS have cervical involvement which can be identified through biopsy or endocervical curettage.[15] UCS is an aggressive, fast-growing cancer, and as such, many patients

TABLE 11.3 Initial work-up of newly diagnosed uterine carcinosarcoma.

Physical exam	Complete physical exam with pelvic and rectovaginal examinations
Imaging	Pelvic ultrasound Consider CT or MRI for extrauterine disease spread
Laboratories	CBC to evaluate for anemia Consider CA-125

with UCS have extrauterine disease at presentation. Women with metastatic spread may develop pain or weight loss in addition to the abovementioned symptoms.

Less commonly, patients with endometrial cancer, including women with UCS, may be asymptomatic and have their disease detected on routine pap test screening. Pap test cytology findings may include endometrial cells (in patients ≥40 years of age), atypical glandular cells, or adenocarcinoma. The sensitivity of a Pap test for detection of endometrial cancer ranges between 40% and 65% based on conventional versus liquid-based preparation but does not convey information on the presence or absence of sarcomatous features.[27]

Physical exam findings

Physical exam findings for UCS mimic findings in women with endometrial adenocarcinomas. A pelvic exam may reveal a bulky, enlarged uterus or a mass prolapsing through the cervical canal; however, it is also possible that a physical exam may not reveal any abnormalities. A complete pelvic exam should include a rectovaginal exam to evaluate for extent of disease spread.

Tumor markers

There are no validated serum tumor markers for women with UCS. One single institution study of 54 patients with UCS found an association between elevated preoperative CA125 levels and more advanced disease. In this study, elevated preoperative CA125 levels were associated with extrauterine disease ($P < 0.001$) and deep myometrial invasion ($P < 0.001$). More than 75% of those with elevated CA125 had serous histology. Additionally, elevated postoperative CA125 levels were associated with poor survival (HR = 5.725, $P = 0.009$).[28,29] These findings have not been confirmed on follow-up studies. Surveillance with CA125 has not been studied specifically in UCS; however, studies in serous uterine cancer could be extrapolated and CA125 surveillance could be considered in women with preoperative elevation of CA125.

Imaging

The first-line imaging study for any patient with concern for a uterine malignancy is pelvic ultrasonography. Carcinosarcomas appear hyperechoic on ultrasound and can appear as large polypoid masses extending from the endometrial canal to the cervical OS. Over 10% of patients with UCS and apparently early-stage disease will present with lymph node metastases.[30] Given the high rate of extrauterine disease, comprehensive imaging is often used to guide patient counseling and treatment planning.

On gadolinium-enhancing magnetic resonance imaging (MRI), carcinosarcoma often appears as a heterogeneous bulky polypoid mass with prolonged enhancement. On CT, UCS presents as an ill-defined, hypodense mass with associated dilatation of the endometrial canal. Positron emission tomography (PET)/CT may also be used in place of a CT scan; however, there are insufficient data to suggest a PET/CT is superior to CT. Both MRI and CT can help detect myometrial invasion, nodal involvement, or presence of metastatic disease. Ultimately, the use of preoperative imaging is clinician dependent as there is insufficient evidence that preoperative imaging is useful or cost effective.

Diagnostic tests

The diagnosis of UCS is made after surgical resection and complete pathological analysis. Prior to definitive treatment, endometrial sampling with either EMB or dilation and curettage (D&C) is recommended, and yet, endometrial sampling does not always identify malignancy or the correct histology. Carcinosarcomas, versus true uterine sarcomas, arise from the endometrial lining and are therefore amenable to diagnosis by sampling; however, even when endometrial sampling does identify malignant features, it does not always confirm UCS. It is not infrequent for only the epithelial component to be sampled and present on endometrial biopsy; therefore, a negative EMB does not rule out carcinosarcoma. The final pathology is dependent on examination of the entire surgical specimen for the presence of both carcinomatous and sarcomatous elements (see Section "Pathology" above).

Staging system

UCS is surgically staged utilizing the 2017 International Federation of Gynecology and Obstetrics (FIGO)/ Tumor, Node, Metastasis (TNM) system used for endometrial carcinoma (Table 11.4). This is the same staging system used for epithelial adenocarcinoma of the uterus and no the staging system used for uterine sarcomas (see Chapters 9 and 10). Differences in treatment algorithm depend on stage of disease with early-stage disease typically referring to stage IA disease (see Section "Treatment" below).

Prognostic factors

The diagnosis of UCS is associated with an overall poor prognosis. Known prognostic factors for women with UCS include stage at diagnosis and race. The higher the stage of disease, the more likely a woman is to succumb to the disease. The 5-year survival rate for stage III and stage IV disease is 22% and 9%, respectively, and a diagnosis of stage IV UCS is associated with a median OS of months. Black race is also associated with poor survival. Analysis of the results of Gynecologic Oncology Group (GOG) 150 (a Phase 3 randomized study of whole abdominal radiotherapy (WAR) versus chemotherapy with ifosfamide/mesna and cisplatin in optimally debulked stages I–IV UCS) found no difference in survival between black and white women with advanced stage disease; however, both progression-free and overall survival were significantly worse in black women when only early-stage disease was considered.[31]

Other prognostic factors, including optimal cytoreductive surgery, myometrial invasion, serum CA125 levels and lymphovascular space invasion, are still under investigation. A retrospective multiinstitutional study performed through the Japanese GOG assessed a number of these factors. They found that higher disease stage, abnormal serum CA125 levels and LVSI were associated with worse disease-free survival (DFS); however, the authors could not find a significant impact of lymphovascular space invasion on overall survival. Additionally, as mentioned above, there is no validated serum tumor marker for women with carcinosarcoma. The authors also found that higher disease stage, poorer performance status, increased myometrial depth of invasion, and suboptimal tumor debulking with residual tumor >1 cm were associated with worse overall survival[32] (Table 11.2).

Treatment of primary disease

The diagnosis of UCS is not always known at the time of initial treatment planning. Thus, patients may undergo surgery for endometrial cancer without preoperative imaging. However, if the UCS diagnosis is made preoperatively, consideration of comprehensive imaging is warranted as 60% of patients will have extrauterine disease which may preclude primary surgery.[33] As with all endometrial cancers, if the patient's health and imaging allow, full surgical staging should be performed, including hysterectomy, BSO, lymph node dissection (sentinel lymph node dissection is permissible) and removal of all gross metastatic disease (Fig. 11.5).[34–39] Laparoscopic or robotic surgery should be considered.[40] The goal of surgery for patients with UCS is optimal cytoreduction. Interestingly, the endometrial cancer studies that support aggressive surgical cytoreduction did not include patients with carcinosarcoma. However, a retrospective review of cytoreductive surgery in 44 patients with stages III–IV disease showed a survival benefit to complete resection (52.3 months vs 8.6 months; $P < 0.0001$).[41–44] The histology of UCS is often known only after surgery, when the full tumor can be examined. The poor prognosis should be discussed with the patient as treatment should be aggressive.

Most Gynecologic Oncology experts agree that the preferred treatment for all patients with UCS, regardless of stage, is systemic chemotherapy and consideration of radiation (vaginal cuff brachytherapy (VCBT) or external beam radiotherapy (EBRT)). Historically, UCS was thought to be a uterine sarcoma and was treated with ifosfamide/cisplatin. However, research supporting UCS as an endometrial cancer, has led to inclusion in treatment studies of endometrial cancer. GOG 261 was a randomized control trial of paclitaxel and carboplatin versus paclitaxel and ifosfamide that revealed that

TABLE 11.4 TNM and FIGO staging for Corpus uteri: Carcinoma and carcinosarcoma.

Corpus uteri: Carcinoma and carcinosarcoma TNM staging AJCC UICC 8th edition

	Primary tumor (T)	
T category	**FIGO stage**	**T criteria**
TX		Primary tumor cannot be assessed
T0		No evidence of primary tumor
T1	I	Tumor confined to the corpus uteri, including endocervical glandular involvement
T1a	IA	Tumor limited to the endometrium or invading less half the myometrium
T1b	IB	Tumor invading one half or more of the myometrium
T2	II	Tumor invading the stromal connective tissue of the cervix but not extending beyond the uterus. Does NOT include endocervical glandular involvement.
T3	III	Tumor involving serosa, adnexa, vagina, or parametrium
T3a	IIIA	Tumor involving the serosa and/or adnexa (direct extension or metastasis)
T3b	IIIB	Vaginal involvement (direct extension or metastasis) or parametrial involvement
T4	IVA	Tumor invading the bladder mucosa and/or bowel mucosa (bullous edema is not sufficient to classify a tumor as T4)

The definitions of the T categories correspond to the stages accepted by the International Federation of Gynecology and Obstetrics (FIGO). Both systems are included for comparison.

T suffix (m) if synchronous primary tumors are found in a single organ.

	Regional lymph nodes (N)	
N category	**FIGO stage**	**N criteria**
NX		Regional lymph nodes cannot be assessed
N0		No regional lymph node metastasis
N0(i+)		Isolated tumor cells in regional lymph node(s) no greater than 0.2 mm
N1	IIIC1	Regional lymph node metastasis to pelvic lymph nodes
Nmi	IIIC1	Regional lymph node metastasis (greater than 0.2 mm but not greater than 2.0 mm in diameter) to pelvic lymph nodes
N1a	IIIC1	Regional lymph node metastasis (greater than 0.2 mm but not regular than 2.0 mm in diameter) to pelvic lymph nodes
N2	IIIC2	Regional lymph node metastasis para-aortic lymph nodes, with or without positive pelvic lymph nodes
N2mi	IIIC2	Regional lymph node metastasis (greater than 0.2 mm but not regular than 2.0 mm in diameter) to para-aortic lymph nodes, with or without positive pelvic lymph nodes
N2a	IIIC2	Regional lymph node metastasis (greater 2.0 mm in diameter) to para-aortic lymph nodes, with or without positive pelvic lymph nodes

Suffix (sn) added to the N category when lymph node metastasis is identified by sentinel lymph node biopsy only.
Suffix (f) is added to the N category when metastasis is identified by fine needle aspiration (FNA) or core needle biopsy only.

	Distant metastasis (M)	
M category	**FIGO stage**	**M criteria**
cM0		No distant metastasis
cM1	IVB	Distant metastasis (includes inguinal lymph nodes, intraperitoneal disease, lung, liver, or bone). (it excludes metastasis to pelvic or para-aortic lymph nodes, vagina, uterine serosa, or adnexa.)

Continued

TABLE 11.4 TNM and FIGO staging for Corpus uteri: Carcinoma and carcinosarcoma—cont'd

Prognostic stage groups			
When T is...	And N is...	And M is...	Then FIGO stage is...
T1	N0	M0	I
T1a	N0	M0	IA
T1b	N0	M0	IB
T2	N0	M0	II
T3	N0	M0	III
T3a	N0	M0	IIIA
T3b	N0	M0	IIIB
T1-T3	N1/N1mi/N1a	M0	IIIC1
T1-T3	N2/N2mi/N2a	M0	IIIC2
T4	Any N	M0	IVA
Any T	Any N	M1	IVB

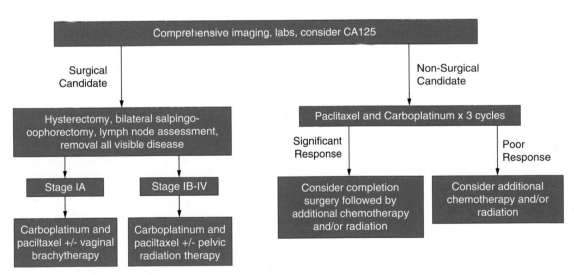

FIG. 11.5 Primary treatment of uterine carcinosarcoma.

patients with stages I–IV persistent or recurrent UCS had at least equivalent outcomes with the less toxic carboplatin and paclitaxel. Thus, contemporary recommendation is that paclitaxel and carboplatin should be used as first-line chemotherapy, even in early-stage disease.[44,45] Recent data utilizing tumor molecular detailing have shown that serous carcinomas may have a HER2 mutation. In patients with UCS in which the epithelial component is serous, HER2 testing is advisable, and if positive, it would allow for the addition of trastuzumab to upfront or recurrent therapy.[46]

Radiation therapy can be used to target sites of known or suspected disease. Some experts only use chemotherapy as adjuvant therapy, and there are no data to support radiation therapy alone as sufficient to treat UCS. For stage IA UCS, VCBT may be considered to target the upper vagina. In patients with stages IB–IV disease, EBRT is directed to the pelvis and may include the para-aortic region based on imaging or surgical findings. EBRT doses for microscopic disease are generally 45–50 Gy and IMRT (intensity-modulated radiation therapy) for sparing of normal tissue is often utilized. If gross residual disease, including gross nodal disease, is present after surgery, a RT boost of up to 60–70 Gy may be given.

In patients who cannot undergo upfront surgery, neoadjuvant chemotherapy with paclitaxel and carboplatin or neoadjuvant radiation can be given. Neoadjuvant radiation is generally 45–50 Gy with consideration of 1–2 high-dose rate (HDR) insertions to a total dose of 75–80 Gy.[21,47,48]

Surveillance

Patients with carcinosarcoma, after primary surgery and treatment, should be followed closely for 5 years. Patients are most likely to recur in the first 2 years after diagnosis and initial treatment and should be examined more frequently during that timeframe. In general, patients should be seen every 3–6 months for the first 2 years and every 6 months until 5 years. In women with elevated preoperative CA125, this level may be followed during surveillance. Women should be counseled to communicate any symptoms of recurrence, including vaginal bleeding, pelvic pain or changes in bowel or bladder function. Regardless of stage, patients have a high risk of recurrence. Surveillance should include pelvic exams, with speculum, bimanual and rectal exams, for local recurrence. The use of a pap smear is not necessary.[49] Patients should be counseled that distant recurrences are not uncommon; therefore, symptoms such as abdominal pain, difficulty with bowel movements or persistent cough should prompt imaging to evaluate for distant recurrence.

It is common for patients to experience physical and psychosocial effects following treatment for UCS. Surgery may cause adhesions, pelvic floor dysfunction, and lymphedema. Chemotherapy may cause neurotoxicity, cardiac toxicity, and cognitive dysfunction. Immunotherapy long-term effects are still unknown. Radiation may cause vulvovaginal atrophy and fibrosis. Given these possibilities, all patients should receive general medical care focused on treatment of chronic diseases and healthy lifestyles. The long-term effects of a specific patient's treatment course should be addressed at surveillance visits and appropriate specialty referrals placed.[50,51]

Recurrent disease

Survival and patterns of failure

As stated previously, for all stages of UCS, the median overall survival is less than 2 years, and the median 5-year overall survival rate is 33.4%.[3] Even women with stage I disease have poor survival outcomes. The 5-year survival rates for stages I/II, III, and IV disease are 59%, 22%, and 9%, respectively.[5]

UCS can recur both locally and distantly. Local pelvic recurrences often present with vaginal bleeding, pelvic pain or change in bowel or bladder function (change in caliber of stool, hematuria, etc.). Pelvic recurrence is generally diagnosed on pelvic exam. If a visible lesion is noted, a biopsy should be obtained. Distant recurrences are frequent and may be asymptomatic. Any concerning symptoms, such as cough, early satiety, pain, should be promptly evaluated with imaging. It is not infrequent for patients to present with multifocal recurrent disease. Clinical trials have shown that patterns of recurrence may vary by prior treatment. GOG 150 (206 women with UCS, 70% with extrauterine disease) revealed that: compared with WAR therapy, chemotherapy alone was associated with a higher incidence of vaginal recurrence (10 vs 4 patients) and serious (grade 3/4) neuropathy (9 vs 0 patients). WAR therapy was associated with a higher incidence of abdominal relapse (29 vs 19 patients), metastases to other distant sites (13 vs 10 patients), and grade 2 or worse gastrointestinal (GI) events (10 vs 0).

Treatment of recurrent disease

Recurrent disease is rarely cured. However, there are treatment options when UCS recurs. Prognosis should be discussed with the patient as best supportive care with no additional treatment is a reasonable option. For patients who opt to proceed with treatment of recurrent disease, there are several standard chemotherapy regimens, as well as newly identified immunotherapy targets. Clinical trials should always be considered and discussed with the patient. In some cases (local recurrence), surgery or targeted radiation therapy may be reasonable options. There are no studies on secondary cytoreduction in this population. Refer to Table 11.5 for dosing of the regimens discussed.

For a patient with recurrent, metastatic UCS who has not been treated with paclitaxel and carboplatin, this regimen should be utilized. If the time since treatment is longer than 6 months (platinum sensitive), then this regimen can again be considered. Often, patients recur quickly after adjuvant therapy with paclitaxel and carboplatin, and options for chemotherapy include those used for all endometrial cancer.[44] Ifosfamide, with or without paclitaxel or cisplatin, has effectiveness in carcinosarcoma, but it does have possible significant side effects (10%–30% have central nervous system toxicity).[52,53] Other options for recurrent treatment include carboplatin/docetaxel, cisplatin/doxorubicin, carboplatin/paclitaxel/bevucizumab, doxorubicin, liposomal doxorubicin or topotecan.[52,54–59] Any agent used in a combination therapy may be used as a single agent. Some recommend only using single-agent therapy in the recurrent setting to minimize toxicity in the treatment of an incurable disease. These agents and dosing are outlined in Table 11.5.

Molecular testing should be considered for patients with UCS in the recurrent setting if not performed upfront. Biomarker-directed therapies include Lenvatinib/pembroluzimab, pembrolizumab (in patients with mismatch repair deficient (MMR-D) tumors and TMB-H (>10 mutations/megabase), nivolumab, lartrectinib, and entrectinib [53–56]. Nivolumab has recently been shown to be effective (ORR 36% with an additional 21% having stable disease) in a small study of dMMR tumors, 4 of which were UCS [53]. Recent data have shown a small percentage of UCS are MMR-D (4%) and that most have low to moderate tumor mutational load [57] (Tables 11.5 and 11.6).

Case resolution

Postoperatively, she completed a combination of 6 cycles of carboplatin and paclitaxel and consolidation whole pelvic radiation therapy. Risk factors for development of UCS included her age, African American race, obesity, and possibly her prior history of tamoxifen use. Her prognosis is worse than that of a woman with another histology of uterine cancer and poorer due to her race. With a stage II UCS, data would suggest that her 5-year survival rate is 59%.

TABLE 11.5 Recurrent disease treatment options.

Recurrence characteristics	Commonly used	Less commonly used
No Prior therapy, multifocal	Paclitaxel + Carboplatin[a] (175 mg/m^2) + (AUC 5–6) every 3 weeks With consideration of RT[a]	Ifosfamide + Paclitaxel every 3 weeks $(1.6 \text{ g/m}^2/\text{d} \times 3\text{d})$ + $(135 \text{ mg/m}^2 \text{ d } 1)$ Ifosfamide + Cisplatin $(1.5 \text{ g/m}^2/\text{d} \times 5 \text{ d})$ + $(20 \text{ mg/m}^2/\text{d} \times 5\text{d})$ every 3 weeks
Prior therapy, multifocal	Paclitaxel + Carboplatin[a] (175 mg/m^2) + (AUC 5–6) every 3 weeks With consideration of RT[a] Paclitaxel + Carboplatin + Bevucizumab (175 mg/m^2) + (AUC 5–6) + (15 mg/m^2) every 3 weeks Ifosfamide[b] 1–2 $\text{g/m}^2/\text{d} \times 3$–5 d every 3 weeks Paclitaxel 175 mg/m^2 every 3 weeks 80 mg/m^2 weekly Carboplatin AUC 5–6 every 3–4 weeks Bevucizumab 15 mg/m^2 every 3 weeks or 10 mg/m^2 every 2 weeks Liposomal doxorubicin 35–40 mg/m^2 every 4 weeks	Doxorubicin 60 mg/m^2 every 21 days [MAX dose 420 mg/m^2] Albumin bound paclitaxel (off label) 260 mg/m2 every 3 weeks Topotecan (from ovarian cancer regimens) $1.5 \text{ mg/m}^2/\text{d} \times 5$ days every 21 days Temsirolimus (off label) 25 mg IV weekly
Prior therapy, multifocal with known biomarker	Pembroluzimab (if dMMR, MSI-H or HMB) 200 mg every 3 weeks or 400 mg every 6 weeks Lenvatinib + Pembro (if dMMR, MSI-H) 20 mg oral daily + Pembro dosing above	Nivolumab (if dMMR, MSI-H) 3 mg/kg IV every 2 weeks

[a]*If more than 6 months since primary treatment. Consider external beam radiotherapy if not used previously or if only vaginal cuff brachytherapy in past.*
[b]*All ifosfamide regimens should be given with Mesna uroprotection at 120 mg/m²/IV bolus, then 1.5 g/m²/24hr.*

TABLE 11.6 Biomarker-driven therapies

Biomarker	Agent	Dose
dMMR, MSI-H, HMB	Pembroluzimab (Pembro)	200 mg q 3 weeks 400 mg q 6 weeks
dMMR, MSI-H	Pembro + Lenvatinib	Above + 20 mg po daily
dMMR, MSI-H	Nivolumab	3 mg/kg q 2 weeks
HER2 amplification	Trastuzumab	
KRAS mutation	Selumetinib	
EGFR amplification	Lapatinib Cabozantinib	
PTEN, PIK3CA mutation F8XW7 mutation CCNE1 amplification ARIDIA mutation	Everolimus Temsirolimus Buparlisib MK2206 Adavosertib Ribociclib Palbociclib BAY 1895344 Tazemetostat	

References

1. Matsuzaki S, et al. Uterine carcinosarcoma: contemporary clinical summary, molecular updates, and future research opportunity. *Gynecol Oncol.* 2021 Feb;160(2):586–601.
2. Cantrell LA, Blank SV, Duska LR. Uterine carcinosarcoma: a review of the literature. *Gynecol Oncol.* 2015;137(3):581–588.
3. Matsuo K, et al. Trends of uterine carcinosarcoma in the United States. *J Gynecol Oncol.* 2018;29(2), e22.
4. Toboni MD, et al. State of the science: uterine carcinosarcomas: from pathology to practice. *Gynecol Oncol.* 2021 Jul;162(1):235–241.
5. Odei B, et al. Chemoradiation versus chemotherapy in uterine Carcinosarcoma: patterns of care and impact on overall survival. *Am J Clin Oncol.* 2018;41(8):784–791.
6. Soslow RA, et al. Clinicopathologic analysis of 187 high-grade endometrial carcinomas of different histologic subtypes: similar outcomes belie distinctive biologic differences. *Am J Surg Pathol.* 2007;31(7):979–987.
7. Gotoh O, et al. Clinically relevant molecular subtypes and genomic alteration-independent differentiation in gynecologic carcinosarcoma. *Nat Commun.* 2019;10(1):4965.
8. Zhao S, et al. Mutational landscape of uterine and ovarian carcinosarcomas implicates histone genes in epithelial-mesenchymal transition. *Proc Natl Acad Sci U S A.* 2016;113(43):12238–12243.
9. Artioli G, et al. Rare uterine cancer: carcinosarcomas. Review from histology to treatment. *Crit Rev Oncol Hematol.* 2015;94(1):98–104.
10. Sreenan JJ, Hart WR. Carcinosarcomas of the female genital tract. A pathologic study of 29 metastatic tumors: further evidence for the dominant role of the epithelial component and the conversion theory of histogenesis. *Am J Surg Pathol.* 1995;19(6):666–674.
11. Hecht JL, Mutter GL. Molecular and pathologic aspects of endometrial carcinogenesis. *J Clin Oncol.* 2006;24(29):4783–4791.
12. de Jong RA, et al. Molecular markers and clinical behavior of uterine carcinosarcomas: focus on the epithelial tumor component. *Mod Pathol.* 2011; 24(10):1368–1379.
13. Sherman ME, Devesa SS. Analysis of racial differences in incidence, survival, and mortality for malignant tumors of the uterine corpus. *Cancer.* 2003;98(1):176–186.
14. Brooks SE, et al. Surveillance, epidemiology, and end results analysis of 2677 cases of uterine sarcoma 1989-1999. *Gynecol Oncol.* 2004;93(1): 204–208.
15. Denschlag D, Ulrich UA. Uterine Carcinosarcomas - diagnosis and management. *Oncol Res Treat.* 2018;41(11):675–679.
16. Kloos I, et al. Tamoxifen-related uterine carcinosarcomas occur under/after prolonged treatment: report of five cases and review of the literature. *Int J Gynecol Cancer.* 2002;12(5):496–500.
17. Fisher B, et al. Tamoxifen for the prevention of breast cancer: current status of the National Surgical Adjuvant Breast and bowel project P-1 study. *J Natl Cancer Inst.* 2005;97(22):1652–1662.

18. Matsuo K, et al. Tumor characteristics and survival outcomes of women with tamoxifen-related uterine carcinosarcoma. *Gynecol Oncol.* 2017;144 (2):329–335.

19. Uehara T, et al. Prognostic impact of the history of breast cancer and of hormone therapy in uterine carcinosarcoma. *Int J Gynecol Cancer.* 2012;22 (2):280–285.

20. Pothuri B, et al. Radiation-associated endometrial cancers are prognostically unfavorable tumors: a clinicopathologic comparison with 527 sporadic endometrial cancers. *Gynecol Oncol.* 2006;103(3):948–951.

21. Wright JD, et al. The role of radiation in improving survival for early-stage carcinosarcoma and leiomyosarcoma. *Am J Obstet Gynecol.* 2008;199(5). 536 e1–8.

22. Norris HJ, Taylor HB. Mesenchymal tumors of the uterus III. A clinical and pathologic study of 31 carcinosarcomas. *Cancer.* 1966;19:1459–1465.

23. Cherniack AD, Shen H, Walter V, et al. Integrated molecular characterization of uterine carcinosarcoma. *Cancer Cell.* 2017;31:411–423.

24. Ferguson SE, Tornos C, Hummer A, et al. Prognostic features of surgical stage I uterine carcinosarcoma. *Am J Surg Pathol.* 2007;31:1653–1661.

25. Lopez-Garcia M, Palacios J. Pathologic and molecular features of uterine carcinosarcomas. *Semin Diagn Pathol.* 2010;27:274–286.

26. McCluggage WG. Mullerian adenosarcoma of the female genital tract. *Adv Anat Pathol.* 2010;17:122–129.

27. Guidos BJ, Selvaggi SM. Detection of endometrial adenocarcinoma with the ThinPrep pap test. *Diagn Cytopathol.* 2000;23(4):260–265.

28. Huang GS, et al. Serum CA125 predicts extrauterine disease and survival in uterine carcinosarcoma. *Gynecol Oncol.* 2007;107(3):513–517.

29. Rose PG, et al. Serial serum CA 125 measurements for evaluation of recurrence in patients with endometrial carcinoma. *Obstet Gynecol.* 1994; 84(1):12–16.

30. Hosh M, et al. Uterine sarcoma: analysis of 13,089 cases based on surveillance, epidemiology, and end results database. *Int J Gynecol Cancer.* 2016; 26(6):1098–1104.

31. Erickson BK, et al. Black race independently predicts worse survival in uterine carcinosarcoma. *Gynecol Oncol.* 2014;133(2):238–241.

32. Harano K, et al. Prognostic factors in patients with uterine carcinosarcoma: a multi-institutional retrospective study from the Japanese gynecologic oncology group. *Int J Clin Oncol.* 2016;21(1):168–176.

33. Boruta 2nd DM, et al. Management of women with uterine papillary serous cancer: a Society of Gynecologic Oncology (SGO) review. *Gynecol Oncol.* 2009;115(1):142–153.

34. Hernandez E. ACOG practice bulletin number 65: management of endometrial cancer. *Obstet Gynecol.* 2006;107(4):952 [author reply 952-3].

35. Holloway RW, et al. Sentinel lymph node mapping and staging in endometrial cancer: a Society of Gynecologic Oncology literature review with consensus recommendations. *Gynecol Oncol.* 2017;146(2):405–415.

36. Leitao Jr MM, et al. Impact of incorporating an algorithm that utilizes sentinel lymph node mapping during minimally invasive procedures on the detection of stage IIIC endometrial cancer. *Gynecol Oncol.* 2013;129(1):38–41.

37. Rossi EC, et al. A comparison of sentinel lymph node biopsy to lymphadenectomy for endometrial cancer staging (FIRES trial): a multicentre, prospective, cohort study. *Lancet Oncol.* 2017;18(3):384–392.

38. Schiavone MB, et al. Survival of patients with uterine Carcinosarcoma undergoing sentinel lymph node mapping. *Ann Surg Oncol.* 2016;23(1): 196–202.

39. Soliman PT, et al. A prospective validation study of sentinel lymph node mapping for high-risk endometrial cancer. *Gynecol Oncol.* 2017;146 (2):234–239.

40. Walker JL, et al. Laparoscopy compared with laparotomy for comprehensive surgical staging of uterine cancer: gynecologic oncology group study LAP2. *J Clin Oncol.* 2009;27(32):5331–5336.

41. Chi DS, et al. The role of surgical cytoreduction in stage IV endometrial carcinoma. *Gynecol Oncol.* 1997;67(1):56–60.

42. Landrum LM, et al. Stage IVB endometrial cancer: does applying an ovarian cancer treatment paradigm result in similar outcomes? A case-control analysis. *Gynecol Oncol.* 2009;112(2):337–341.

43. Tanner EJ, et al. The role of cytoreductive surgery for newly diagnosed advanced-stage uterine carcinosarcoma. *Gynecol Oncol.* 2011;123(3): 548–552.

44. Powell MA, et al. A randomized phase 3 trial of paclitaxel (P) plus carboplatin (C) versus paclitaxel plus ifosfamide (I) in chemotherapy-naive patients with stage I-IV, persistent or recurrent carcinosarcoma of the uterus or ovary: An NRG Oncology trial. *Am J Clin Oncol.* 2019;**37**(15_suppl):5500.

45. Cantrell LA, et al. A multi-institutional cohort study of adjuvant therapy in stage I-II uterine carcinosarcoma. *Gynecol Oncol.* 2012;127(1):22–26.

46. Fader AN, et al. Randomized phase II trial of carboplatin-paclitaxel versus carboplatin-paclitaxel-Trastuzumab in uterine serous carcinomas that over-express human epidermal growth factor receptor 2/neu. *J Clin Oncol.* 2018;36(20):2044–2051.

47. Einstein MH, et al. Phase II trial of adjuvant pelvic radiation "sandwiched" between combination paclitaxel and carboplatin in women with uterine papillary serous carcinoma. *Gynecol Oncol.* 2012;124(1):21–25.

48. Galaal K, et al. Adjuvant radiotherapy and/or chemotherapy after surgery for uterine carcinosarcoma. *Cochrane Database Syst Rev.* 2013;2, CD006812.

49. Salani R, et al. An update on post-treatment surveillance and diagnosis of recurrence in women with gynecologic malignancies: Society of Gynecologic Oncology (SGO) recommendations. *Gynecol Oncol.* 2017;146(1):3–10.

50. Colombo N, et al. ESMO-ESGO-ESTRO consensus conference on endometrial Cancer: diagnosis, treatment and follow-up. *Ann Oncol.* 2016;27 (1):16–41.

51. Elit L, Reade CJ. Recommendations for follow-up Care for Gynecologic Cancer Survivors. *Obstet Gynecol.* 2015;126(6):1207–1214.

52. Homesley HD, et al. A randomized phase III trial in advanced endometrial carcinoma of surgery and volume directed radiation followed by cisplatin and doxorubicin with or without paclitaxel: a gynecologic oncology group study. *Gynecol Oncol.* 2009;112(3):543–552.

53. Sutton G, et al. A phase III trial of ifosfamide with or without cisplatin in carcinosarcoma of the uterus: a gynecologic oncology group study. *Gynecol Oncol.* 2000;79(2):147–153.

54. Aghajanian C, et al. Phase II trial of bevacizumab in recurrent or persistent endometrial cancer: a gynecologic oncology group study. *J Clin Oncol.* 2011;29(16):2259–2265.

55. Homesley HD, et al. Phase III trial of ifosfamide with or without paclitaxel in advanced uterine carcinosarcoma: a gynecologic oncology group study. *J Clin Oncol.* 2007;25(5):526–531.

56. Oza AM, et al. Phase II study of temsirolimus in women with recurrent or metastatic endometrial cancer: a trial of the NCIC clinical trials group. *J Clin Oncol.* 2011;29(24):3278–3285.

57. Rose PG, et al. Paclitaxel, carboplatin, and bevacizumab in advanced and recurrent endometrial carcinoma. *Int J Gynecol Cancer.* 2017;27(3):452–458.

Chapter 12

Uterine serous carcinoma

Diana Miao, Lora Hedrick Ellenson, and Amanda N. Fader

Clinical case

A 64-year-old female presents to the Gynecologic Oncology clinic for a second opinion regarding a new diagnosis of uterine serous carcinoma. She originally presented to her gynecologist within the last 3 months complaining of postmenopausal vaginal spotting. Pelvic ultrasound demonstrated a 3 mm endometrial stripe and endometrial sampling was deferred. However, the spotting persisted, and hysteroscopy, dilation and curettage (D&C) was performed. Final pathology demonstrated uterine serous carcinoma in an endometrial polyp. Computed tomography (CT) of the chest/abdomen/pelvis demonstrated no obvious evidence of metastatic disease. Surgical staging was performed with minimally invasive total hysterectomy (TAH), bilateral salpingo-oophorectomy (BSO), and pelvic and aortic lymph node lymphadenectomies. Final pathology demonstrated serous endometrial cancer without lymphovascular space invasion. However, one of the right pelvic lymph nodes was positive for disease. The patient presents to clinic inquiring about additional recommended workup and suggestions for adjuvant treatment.

Epidemiology

Incidence/mortality

Uterine corpus cancer is the third most common cancer in women in the United States, with approximately 65,620 new cases in the United States in 2020 and 12,590 estimated deaths.[1] Endometrial cancers can broadly be classified into two groups. Cancers of endometrioid histology are common (about 80% of cases), are associated with obesity and estrogen exposure, and generally have good prognosis. Nonendometrioid cancers are more rare (~20%), are less hormone dependent, and have poorer prognosis.[2]

Endometrial cancer incidence has been steadily rising in the United States and many other areas internationally, with an average annual percent change in the United States of 1.4%–3.1%.[3] Analysis of the SEER database in the United States has suggested that this increase is largely driven by nonendometrioid cancers.[4]

Uterine serous carcinoma is the most common form of nonendometrioid uterine corpus cancer. Data from the Surveillance, Epidemiology, and End Results (SEER) database from 1988 to 2001 suggest uterine serous carcinoma accounted for about 10% of uterine cancers but 39% of deaths.[5] Uterine serous carcinoma is more likely to be stage III or IV at presentation (52% of cases), even compared with other high-risk endometrial cancer histologies (36% for clear cell and 29% for grade 3 endometrioid carcinoma). Median age at diagnosis is in the 60s[6] (Table 12.1).

Etiology/risk factors

When first described, uterine serous carcinoma was noted for its histological similarity to ovarian papillary serous carcinoma. Prominent features included marked nuclear pleomorphism, complex papillary architecture, fibrous stalks, prominent tumor necrosis, and frequent psammoma bodies. Additionally, disease was often noted within the myometrium, ovarian lymphatics, or vascular channels without evidence of gross disease.

Later studies also observed that within uterine serous carcinoma, different histological subtypes are apparent, including disease admixed with other histologies such as endometrioid or clear cell and disease confined to endometrial polyps.[7] Overall, the authors found that these tumors were clinically similar in their aggressive behavior and shared hobnail-shaped cells with high-grade nuclei with foci of papillary or glandular architecture. These findings led them to propose renaming the disease to uterine serous carcinoma. Subsequent studies have found that mixed adenocarcinomas with serous

Diagnosis and Treatment of Rare Gynecologic Cancers. https://doi.org/10.1016/B978-0-323-82938-0.00012-4

TABLE 12.1 Comparative features of endometrioid and non-endometrioid carcinomas of the cervix.

	Endometrioid endometrial carcinomas	Non-endometrioid, including uterine serous, carcinomas
Risk factors	Obesity Exposure to unopposed estrogen Insulin resistance	Older age History of breast cancer
Pattern of recurrence	Locoregional: Vaginal/pelvic	Distant: Extrapelvic
Precursor lesion	Complex atypical hyperplasia / endometrial intraepithelial neoplasia	
Histologic grade	Largely grade 1/2	Always high grade
Stage I/II at diagnosis	70%–80%	50%–60%
5-year OS for stage I/II disease	70%–95%	50%–85%
Molecular features	PTEN inactivation Microsatellite instability	*TP53* mutation *HER2* amplification Mutations in *PIK3CA, PPP2R1, FBXW7, CHD4*

Table adapted from A. N. Fader, A. D. Santin, P. A. Gehrig, Early stage uterine serous carcinoma: management updates and genomic advances. Gynecol Oncol 129 (2013) 244–250.

components, even if they contained some endometrioid or clear cell components, should be treated similarly to uterine serous carcinoma as the presence of a serous component was associated with worse prognosis.[8]

The relationship between myometrial invasion and disease severity also differs in uterine serous carcinoma compared to endometrioid endometrial cancer. While extrauterine spread is rare in low-grade endometrioid endometrial cancer with limited myometrial invasion and small tumor size,[9] early studies found that patients with non-invasive uterine serous carcinoma had a high risk of stages III–IV disease and high rates of death from disease.[7] Subsequent studies have affirmed these findings. Noninvasive or early invasive forms of uterine serous carcinoma have been variably termed "intraepithelial serous carcinoma" and "endometrial intraepithelial carcinoma" or "superficial serous carcinoma," respectively, and have previously been felt to represent earlier forms of disease. However, in one study, 3 of 9 (33%) patients with noninvasive disease and 15 of 31 (48%) patients with early invasive disease had extrauterine spread.[10] Considering these groups together as "minimal uterine serous carcinoma" to highlight the invasive potential of these uterine lesions, 5-year survival was 94% for patients without extrauterine spread vs 56% with extrauterine spread. Thus, even for apparently polyp-confined disease, complete surgical staging with detailed pathological scrutiny to rule out extrauterine spread is advised. Though noninvasive disease does not rule out extrauterine spread, larger studies have found that depth of myometrial invasion does predict worse outcome, with 38% of patients with noninvasive disease having stages III–IV disease vs 80% of patients with depth of invasion ≥50%.[6]

Efforts at identifying a true precursor lesion to uterine serous carcinoma led to description of a distinct entity termed endometrial glandular dysplasia in 2004.[11,12] This is morphologically distinct from both benign endometrium and uterine serous carcinoma, has molecular features shared with subsequently diagnosed uterine serous carcinoma, and can be diagnosed by EMB or D&C.[13] The clinical implications of this pathological entity are still unclear, but point to key steps in the development of uterine serous carcinoma.

New capabilities in molecular characterization have further helped elucidate the biological underpinnings of uterine serous carcinoma. Mutations in *TP53* are the most common genetic alteration in uterine serous carcinoma, present in over 90% of cases.[14] While *TP53* mutations are never observed in resting endometrium, they occur in 43% of endometrial glandular dysplasia and 72% of serous endometrial intraepithelial carcinoma, suggesting an early role of TP53 in uterine serous carcinoma carcinogenesis. An even earlier lesion termed "p53 signature glands" may represent an even earlier form of disease identifiable only by immunoassay rather than histological change.[15] As *TP53* is the most commonly mutated gene in human cancer,[16] improved understanding of the biology of uterine serous carcinoma may yield insights into other cancer types, and vice versa. Other recurrently mutated genes in uterine serous carcinoma include *PIK3CA*, *FBXW7*, and *PPP2R1A*.[17,18]

Risk factors for uterine serous carcinoma include African-American race, older age, and multiparity. Overall, uterine serous carcinoma is approximately twice as common in non-Hispanic black women than in other populations (non-Hispanic white, Hispanic, Asian) in a US study population from 2000 to 2011.[19] In addition, while rates of low-grade endometrioid endometrial cancer decreased slightly in non-Hispanic whites (annual percent change or APC = -0.8) and increased slightly in non-Hispanic blacks (APC = 1.0), rates of uterine serous carcinoma are increasing in all racial groups. However, the increase in rate is more pronounced in minority populations, with rates of increase ranging from APC = 2.8 in non-Hispanic Whites to 3.8 in non-Hispanic blacks to 4.5 in Hispanics and 9.0 in Asians. Non-Hispanic blacks face worse outcomes in endometrial cancer even controlling for histology and stage of disease, and this trend sadly is also true in uterine serous carcinoma. Non-Hispanic white, Asian, and Hispanic populations experience 5-year survival rates of about 80%, 40%, and 20% for localized, regional, and distant disease. Analogous figures for non-Hispanic black populations are approximately 70%, 30%, and 10%. The reasons behind the rising rates and racial disparities seen in uterine serous carcinoma are poorly understood and likely multifactorial.

An area of much controversy is the association between *BRCA1/2* alterations and risk of development of uterine serous carcinoma. Past studies have linked a history of breast cancer with increased risk of subsequent development of uterine serous carcinoma.[20] *BRCA1* alterations are disproportionately common in patients with uterine serous carcinoma[21,22] and may predispose to both breast and uterine cancers. Specifically, loss-of-heterozygosity events have been seen in uterine serous carcinoma in a *BRCA1* germline carrier, suggesting a causal role for this mutation.[23] That said, the risk of developing uterine serous carcinoma in women who are germline positive for BRCA remains undefined. The recommendation for a hysterectomy at the time of risk reducing bilateral salpingo-oophorectomy (RR-BSO) in women with germline *BRCA1* mutation remains controversial but should be discussed with patients.

The oncogenic potential of the human epidermal growth factor receptor 2 (HER2) is well known. HER2, encoded by the gene *ERBB2*, is receptor tyrosine kinase. Among all four HER family proteins, HER2 has the strongest catalytic kinase activity and functions as the most active signaling complex of the HER family after dimerization with other HER family members [1, 2]. Overexpression of HER2 leads to increased homodimerization (HER2:HER2) and heterodimerization (e.g., HER2:HER3), which initiates a strong pro-tumorigenic signaling cascade [3]. Overexpression of this oncogene plays an important role in the development and progression of certain aggressive types of breast, gastric and uterine cancers [4–7]. While the protein has become an important biomarker and target of therapy for approximately 30% of breast cancer patients, has also been identified that 25%–30% of women with uterine scrous carcinoma also overexpress HER2.

Pathology

Gross appearance

Serous carcinoma of the endometrium most commonly occurs in atrophic uteri and can present with grossly identifiable tumor or as microscopic disease, often involving endometrial polyps. Myometrial invasion as well as adnexal involvement may be grossly evident or only identified microscopically.

Microscopic features

Uterine serous carcinoma can demonstrate glandular (Fig. 12.1A), papillary (Fig. 12.1B) or solid architecture.[24] Although there can be substantial variability in the cytologic features, marked cytologic atypia is a hallmark of serous carcinoma (Fig. 12.1A). The tumor cells may have eosinophilic cytoplasm or cytoplasmic clearing, sometimes with hobnail features. Many, if not all, of the tumor cells show nuclear pleomorphism, hyperchromasia, and prominent eosinophilic nucleoli. Mitotic figures, including abnormal mitotic figures, are easily identified, as are smudged nuclei. When serous carcinoma arises in an endometrial polyp, the tumor cells line the surface of the polyp and may show extension into underlying glands with no associated stromal invasion. This phenomenon can also be seen in the native endometrium. This lesion was previously called serous endometrial intraepithelial carcinoma. However, given that the purely intraepithelial carcinoma can be associated with metastatic disease, it is now recommended to simply refer to it as serous carcinoma. Uterine serous carcinomas are all considered high grade, thus the use of "high grade" to further describe these tumors is considered redundant and not recommended. Lymphovascular invasion can be focal or extensive. Careful attention to exclude other mixed components including endometrioid carcinoma, clear cell carcinoma and sarcoma is necessary.

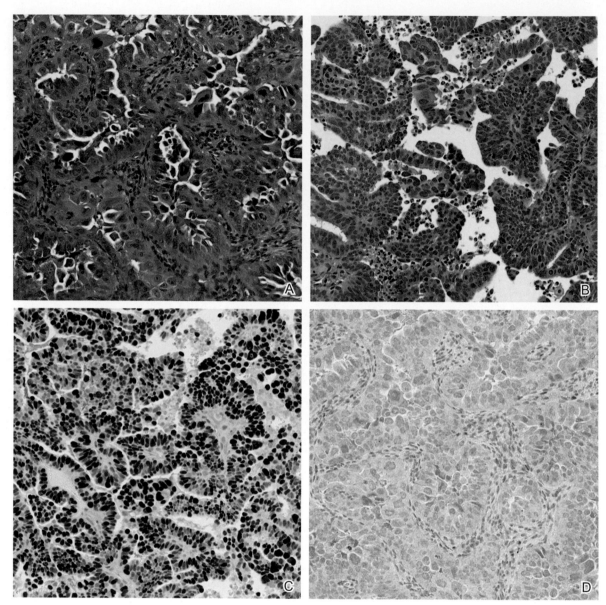

FIG. 12.1 (A) Glandular pattern of uterine serous carcinoma (USC) with marked cytologic atypia. (B) Papillary pattern of USC with marked nuclear heterochromasia. (C) Immunohistochemistry for p53 showing an aberrant (strong, diffuse) staining pattern. (D) Immunohistochemistry for p53 showing an aberrant (null) staining pattern.

Immuohistochemistry

Serous carcinomas express epithelial markers such as keratins and EMA, PAX-8, and hormone receptors though the latter show decreased expression compared to endometrioid carcinomas. The most common pattern of aberrant expression of p53 is diffuse strong nuclear staining in >75% of the tumor cells (Fig. 12.1C).[14] However, in a subset of cases, there is complete loss of staining consistent with a null-phenotype (Fig. 12.1D). In the latter, positive staining in internal controls is necessary to ensure authenticity of the absent staining. More recently diffuse cytoplasmic staining has also been recognized as a pattern of aberrant p53 expression.

Differential diagnosis

The most critical differential is distinguishing serous carcinoma from any low-grade form of endometrioid carcinoma which can also demonstrate papillary and glandular growth patterns. However, the presence of marked cytologic atypia and frequent mitoses favor serous carcinoma. Ancillary p53 and p16 immunohistochemical (IHC) studies can help in this distinction. The vast majority of endometrial serous carcinomas show aberrant staining for p53 along with intense, block-like staining for p16, whereas the vast majority of low-grade endometrioid tumors will show wild-type p53 staining and heterogeneous staining for p16.[25] It is important to record the IHC stains in a manner that can be definitively interpreted from the report. It is recommended that p53 IHC be reported as aberrant with either diffuse, strong nuclear staining or as a complete lack (null-pattern) of staining. Both staining patterns are reliable predictors of *TP53* mutations in serous carcinoma. Results of p16 IHC should be reported as diffuse, block-like staining or as patchy staining. In addition, some serous carcinomas show overlapping features with clear cell carcinoma, as serous carcinoma can show cytoplasmic clearing and clear cell carcinoma can consist largely of cells with eosinophilic cytoplasm similar to serous carcinoma. However, serous carcinomas lack a tubulocystic growth pattern and eosinophilic, hyalinized stroma usually seen in clear cell carcinoma. In addition, immunohistochemistry can aid in this distinction as clear cell carcinomas are usually negative for ER/PR expression while many serous carcinomas are at least focally positive. In addition, HNF-1B and napsin-A are often expressed in clear cell carcinoma. Of note, p53 staining can show aberrant expression in a subset of clear cell carcinomas.

Molecular findings

Serous carcinomas are defined by alterations in the *TP53* gene. The high incidence of this alteration results in the usefulness of p53 immunohistochemistry as an ancillary test in the diagnosis of serous carcinoma. In over 75% of cases p53 immunohistochemistry will show an aberrant staining pattern usually with strong, diffuse nuclear staining with fewer cases showing a complete absence (null pattern) of staining.[14] In addition, the genomes of serous carcinomas exhibit numerous copy number alterations, hence the designation as copy number high tumors in The Cancer Genome Atlas (TCGA) classification of endometrial carcinoma. A number of other genes (*PIK3CA*, *PPP2R1A*, *FBXW7*, *PIK3R1*) are commonly mutated in serous carcinoma and *CCNE1* is amplified in approximately 20% of cases. Importantly, approximately 18% of serous carcinomas show amplification of *ERBB2* and are, thus, potentially amenable to targeted therapy. Consequently, HER2 immunostaining with HER2 FISH studies, if indicated, are recommended for all metastatic or recurrent cases of serous carcinoma.

Diagnosis and workup

Differential diagnosis

Uterine serous carcinoma presents similarly to other uterine adenocarcinomas and is indistinguishable based on signs and symptoms alone; however, an accurate diagnosis is essential as the treatment and prognosis in endometrial adenocarcinoma vs uterine serous carcinoma is significantly different. The diagnosis of uterine serous carcinoma is ultimately a histologic diagnosis (see Section "Pathology" above). The differential diagnosis for postmenopausal bleeding is vast and ranges from benign etiologies such as endometrial hyperplasia, polyps, and atrophy to malignant etiologies, including uterine serous carcinoma.

Signs and symptoms

Women with uterine serous carcinoma typically have disease detected after presentation with postmenopausal bleeding, abdominal pain, or uterine enlargement. Uterine serous carcinoma is an aggressive, fast-growing cancer, and as such, many patients with uterine serous carcinoma have extrauterine disease at presentation. Women with metastatic spread may develop pain or weight loss in addition to the above-mentioned symptoms.

Physical exam findings

As with other forms of endometrial cancer, postmenopausal bleeding is the most common presenting symptom for uterine serous carcinoma. Because many women with uterine serous carcinoma have extrauterine disease at diagnosis, presenting symptoms may also include abdominal pain or bloating as in ovarian serous carcinomas.[26] Differential diagnosis includes other uterine/endometrial cancers, including carcinosarcoma, which often include a serous epithelial component.

Tumor markers

Given the histological similarities between epithelial ovarian cancer and uterine serous carcinoma, the serum marker cancer antigen 125 (CA-125) has been proposed as a marker of uterine serous carcinoma disease activity, though this is controversial. Three retrospective studies of CA-125 in the preoperative, posttreatment, and recurrent setting have found that as in epithelial ovarian cancer, pretreatment CA-125 levels are positively correlated with risk of extrauterine and recurrent disease, CA-125 falls substantially following initial treatment, and CA-125 rise after treatment is correlated with disease recurrence.[27-29] However, there are no prospective studies evaluating CA-125 monitoring in uterine serous carcinoma, and whether CA-125 monitoring improves overall or progression-free survival (PFS) in this disease is unclear. However, our practice is to monitor CA-125 as part of surveillance after initial treatment.

Imaging

Given the high risk of extrauterine spread even in apparently polyp-confined disease, imaging with CT of the chest, abdomen, and pelvis or whole-body positron emission tomography (PET) can be considered to evaluate for the presence of metastatic disease.[30,31] Magnetic resonance imaging (MRI) of the pelvis may also be considered. Unlike in endometrioid cancer, where the primary role goal of preoperative MRI is to assess risk of lymphatic spread by measuring depth of myometrial invasion, endometrial cavity thickness and tumor thickness, and presence of lymphadenopathy, the goal of MRI in uterine serous carcinoma is to assess for signs of invasion into the cervical stroma, parametrial structures, or bladder and rectum that may impact initial surgical planning.[32] In the initial work-up of a newly diagnosed patient, we typically perform CT scan of the chest, abdomen, and pelvis. We may add a MRI if there is concern for cervical or parametrial involvement on physical exam or CT scan (Table 12.2).

Diagnostic tests

Office-based Pipelle biopsy has approximately 99% sensitivity for detection of uterine serous carcinoma, though specificity is lower due to potential under-sampling disease that features mixed histology with clear cell or endometrioid components as described above.[33] Additionally, ultrasound may not be able to exclude uterine serous carcinoma as a cause of postmenopausal bleeding even when endometrial stripe thickness is <5 mm, as has been described for endometrioid endometrial cancers.[34]

Staging system

Uterine serous carcinoma is surgically staged utilizing the 2017 International Federation of Gynecology and Obstetrics (FIGO)/Tumor, Node, Metastasis (TNM) system used for endometrial carcinoma[35] (Table 12.3). All uterine serous carcinoma is considered grade 3 or high-grade disease. Differences in treatment algorithm depend on stage of disease with early-stage disease typically referring to stage IA disease.

Prognostic factors

The overall 5-year survival rate for uterine serous carcinoma is approximately 18%–27%.[36] This is largely attributable to the high rate of extrauterine disease at initial presentation of 60%–70%, and complete surgical staging, as discussed below, is a crucial component of prognostication and treatment planning.[6] In an FIGO Annual Report, stages II–IV disease was noted at diagnosis in 46% of women with uterine serous carcinoma compared with 21% of women with the more common endometrioid adenocarcinoma.[37] However, even controlling for disease-stage, uterine serous has a less favorable 5-year disease-specific survival rate compared to grade 3 endometrioid endometrial carcinoma (stage I/II, 74% vs 85%, $P < 0.0001$; stage III/IV, 33 vs 54%, $P < 0.0001$) (Table 12.4).[5] The surgical pathology protocol GOG 210 provides a

---

TABLE 12.2 Work-up of newly diagnosed uterine serous carcinoma.

Endometrial sampling (office-based biopsy or dilation and curettage)
Once diagnosis is histologically confirmed, consider measuring baseline CA-125 and obtaining preoperative imaging (CT scan, possible MRI)

TABLE 12.3 TNM and FIGO staging for Corpus uteri: Carcinoma and carcinosarcoma.

Corpus uteri: Carcinoma and carcinosarcoma TNM staging AJCC UICC 8th edition

Primary tumor (T)

T category	FIGO stage	T criteria
TX		Primary tumor cannot be assessed
T0		No evidence of primary tumor
T1	I	Tumor confined to the corpus uteri, including endocervical glandular involvement
T1a	IA	Tumor limited to the endometrium or invading less half the myometrium
T1b	IB	Tumor invading one half or more of the myometrium
T2	II	Tumor invading the stromal connective tissue of the cervix but not extending beyond the uterus. Does NOT include endocervical glandular involvement.
T3	III	Tumor involving serosa, adnexa, vagina, or parametrium
T3a	IIIA	Tumor involving the serosa and/or adnexa (direct extension or metastasis)
T3b	IIIB	Vaginal involvement (direct extension or metastasis) or parametrial involvement
T4	IVA	Tumor invading the bladder mucosa and/or bowel mucosa (bullous edema is not sufficient to classify a tumor as T4)

The definitions of the T categories correspond to the stages accepted by the International Federation of Gynecology and Obstetrics (FIGO). Both systems are included for comparison.

T suffix (m) if synchronous primary tumors are found in a single organ.

Regional lymph nodes (N)

N category	FIGO stage	N criteria
NX		Regional lymph nodes cannot be assessed
N0		No regional lymph node metastasis
N0(i+)		Isolated tumor cells in regional lymph node(s) no greater than 0.2 mm
N1	IIIC1	Regional lymph node metastasis to pelvic lymph nodes
Nmi	IIIC1	Regional lymph node metastasis (greater than 0.2 mm but not greater than 2.0 mm in diameter) to pelvic lymph nodes
N1a	IIIC1	Regional lymph node metastasis (greater than 0.2 mm but not regular than 2.0 mm in diameter) to pelvic lymph nodes
N2	IIIC2	Regional lymph node metastasis para-aortic lymph nodes, with or without positive pelvic lymph nodes
N2mi	IIIC2	Regional lymph node metastasis (greater than 0.2 mm but not regular than 2.0 mm in diameter) to para-aortic lymph nodes, with or without positive pelvic lymph nodes
N2a	IIIC2	Regional lymph node metastasis (greater 2.0 mm in diameter) to para-aortic lymph nodes, with or without positive pelvic lymph nodes

Suffix (sn) added to the N category when lymph node metastasis is identified by sentinel lymph node biopsy only.
Suffix (f) is added to the N category when metastasis is identified by fine needle aspiration (FNA) or core needle biopsy only.

Distant metastasis (M)

M category	FIGO stage	M criteria
cM0		No distant metastasis
cM1	IVB	Distant metastasis (includes inguinal lymph nodes, intraperitoneal disease, lung, liver, or bone). (it excludes metastasis to pelvic or para-aortic lymph nodes, vagina, uterine serosa, or adnexa.)

Continued

TABLE 12.3 TNM and FIGO staging for Corpus uteri: Carcinoma and carcinosarcoma—cont'd

Prognostic stage groups			
When T is...	And N is...	And M is...	Then FIGO stage is...
T1	N0	M0	I
T1a	N0	M0	IA
T1b	N0	M0	IB
T2	N0	M0	II
T3	N0	M0	III
T3a	N0	M0	IIIA
T3b	N0	M0	IIIB
T1-T3	N1/N1mi/N1a	M0	IIIC1
T1-T3	N2/N2mi/N2a	M0	IIIC2
T4	Any N	M0	IVA
Any T	Any N	M1	IVB

TABLE 12.4 Prognosis of newly diagnosis uterine serous carcinoma.

Stage	5-year overall survival	5-year progression-free survival
IA – no myometrial invasion ($N = 19$)	81.5%	80.9%
IA – myometrial invasion <50% ($N = 26$)	58.6%	59.3%
IB ($N = 7$)	34.3%	No data
II ($N = 5$)	100%	100%
IIIA ($N = 14$)	35.1%	30%
IIIB ($N = 1$)	100%	100%
IIIC ($N = 26$)	35.8%	36.9%
IV ($N = 31$)	19.9%	0%

Data from Slomovitz et al. 2003, Gynecologic Oncology.

large dataset of uterine serous carcinoma tumors from women who were surgically staged.[38] Notably, the risk of pelvic nodal metastasis in GOG 210 was nearly 8% for noninvasive uterine serous carcinoma tumors, 18% for minimally invasive, and 44% for deeply invasive tumors. Rates of aortic nodal metastases were also high at 4.2%, 11.3%, and 32.4%, respectively, underscoring the importance of a comprehensive lymph node assessment in this setting.

Focusing on stage I/II disease, in analysis of 206 comprehensively surgically staged patients, recurrence risk was related to stage at diagnosis, ranging from 11% in stage IA disease without myometrial invasion to 40% in stage IIB When disease recurrence occurs, around 80% are extrapelvic. In multivariate analysis, chemotherapy significantly decreased recurrence rate and increased overall and PFS ($P = 0.006$), while increasing age and greater stage were associate with decreased overall survival.[39] Percentage of cells with serous histology, presence of lymphovascular space invasion, and primary tumor size, and ethnicity were not associated with recurrence or survival. The authors suggest that adjuvant chemotherapy should be considered even in early-stage disease based on the above findings, but that clear risk factors for recurrence remained unclear. More recent studies have identified the presence of HER2 overexpression as a significant risk factor for recurrence of stage I uterine serous carcinoma (50% vs 17%, $P < 0.001$).[40] Some studies have suggested that African-American women with uterine serous carcinoma are more likely to harbor HER2 overexpression,[41] potentially

TABLE 12.5 Risk factors for disease recurrence in stage I/II uterine serous carcinoma.

Stage	Recurrence Rate
IA - no myometrial invasion ($N = 54$)	11.1%
IA - myometrial invasion <50% ($N = 70$)	14.3%
IB ($N = 27$)	29.6%
IIA ($N = 20$)	30%
IIB ($N = 35$)	40%
Treatment	**Recurrence Rate**
Observation ($N = 45$)	31.1%
Radiation alone ($N = 47$)	38.3%
Chemotherapy +/− radiation ($N = 114$)	10.5%

Data from Fader et al. 2009, Gynecologic Oncology.

partially explaining poorer disease-specific outcomes in endometrial among African-American compared to Caucasian women in general, though this has not been affirmed in all study populations[40] (Table 12.5).

Five-year survival for stage III/IV uterine sarcoma is associated with an even higher risk of recurrence (~70%) and 5-year survival of approximately 26% in a population of 260 women from a single institution. This was despite an initial complete response rate of 69% with primary therapy. Features protective against recurrence including initial surgical cytoreduction to no gross residual or ≤ 0.5 cm (compared to >0.5 cm), earlier stage, and platinum sensitivity. Additionally, the authors found that treatment with a combination of surgery, radiation, and chemotherapy was associated with longer recurrence-free survival (RFS) and overall survival compared to surgery and chemotherapy alone.[42] A similar study from two institutions comprising 79 patients with stage IIIC/IV disease also found that greater age and more advanced stage were associated with shorter disease-free survival (DFS) and overall survival, while optimal cytoreduction and administration of adjuvant chemotherapy or radiation were associated with longer disease-free and overall survival.[43] An additional study of 119 patients in an international population in Taiwan affirmed the importance of optimal cytoreduction as a positive prognostic factor at all stages, with optimal cytoreduction and postoperative treatment with chemotherapy and/or combination chemoradiation associated with improved overall and PFS in stage III/IV disease.[44]

Treatment of primary disease

Given the substantially poorer prognosis associated with higher-stage disease and potential for precision-based treatment in this setting, multiple studies have emphasized the importance of careful and complete surgical staging for uterine serous carcinoma, which includes TAH, BSO, a pelvic and para aortic lymph node evaluation, pelvic washings and an omental biopsy (Fig. 12.2). A minimally invasive surgical approach is considered standard for the treatment of early-stage disease based upon the results of the GOG randomized trial, LAP2, and an ad hoc analysis of LAP2, demonstrating that those with higher-grade endometrial cancers, including uterine serous carcinoma, had similar survival outcomes but improved quality of life with minimally invasive vs open hysterectomy.[45] The extent of omentectomy and pelvic and/or para-aortic lymphadenectomy required to fully evaluate extrauterine spread of disease is more controversial.

Metastatic lymphatic disease is among the most important prognostic factors in endometrial cancer. Both the National Comprehensive Cancer Network (NCCN) and the Society for Gynecologic Oncology (SGO) support the use of sentinel lymph node biopsy in the staging of apparent uterine-confined endometrial cancer. However, these recommendations are informed primarily by retrospective and prospective studies performed in women with low-grade endometrial cancer.[46] The use of sentinel lymph node biopsy in women with high-grade endometrial cancer, including uterine serous carcinoma, remains a matter of debate. Soliman et al. were the first to perform a validation study of sentinel node in 123 women with high-risk endometrial cancer, including patients with serous carcinoma.[47] The authors found an overall sensitivity of 95% the sentinel node procedure when compared with standard of care complete lymphadenectomy to the renal vessels. The study was not designed to follow for recurrence or survival. The SENTOR study, which included 156 patients, 80% of who had high grade endometrial cancer, is the first prospective trial adequately powered to evaluate the accuracy of sentinel

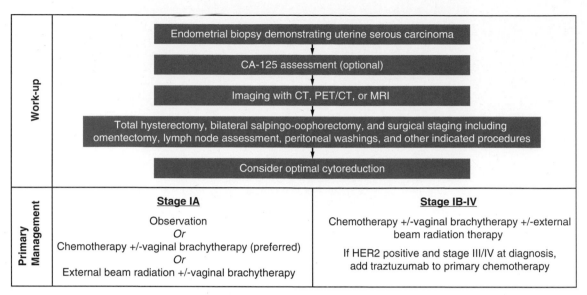

FIG. 12.2 Treatment algorithm for women with newly diagnosed uterine serous carcinoma.

lymph node biopsy in women with high-grade endometrial carcinoma (though not specifically for women with uterine serous carcinoma), with a sensitivity of 97.4% and negative predictive value of 99%.[48] However, the SENTOR study was not adequately powered to evaluate recurrence and survival outcomes. A more recent study retrospectively reviewed 245 cases of uterine serous carcinoma with 79 women undergoing sentinel lymph node only and 166 undergoing complete pelvic and para-aortic lymphadenectomy.[49] There was no difference in detection of metastatic disease to lymph nodes (stage III disease) nor was there any difference in 2-year overall survival between the sentinel node and complete lymphadenectomy groups. Although complete lymphadenectomy certainly remains within the standard of care, surgeons may consider sentinel lymph node biopsy only as an alternative.

The surgical treatment of advanced-stage disease includes hysterectomy, BSO and surgical cytoreduction to minimal disease residual, when possible. Pelvic and aortic lymph node basins should be evaluated and bulky nodal disease should be removed. Several retrospective studies suggest that cytoreductive surgery may also confer a survival benefit in women with metastatic uterine serous carcinoma (see above Section "Prognostic factors").

In part because of its rarity, the optimal management of uterine serous carcinoma is both controversial and understudied. The high recurrence rates and the propensity for extra-pelvic, multisite disease suggest a strong rationale for systemic chemotherapy. Historically women with uterine serous carcinoma have been included in large uterine carcinoma trials, including GOG-0209, GOG-0249, and GOG-0258, and overall, represent approximately 15%–20% of the study populations of these cooperative group trials. Prior to 2018, GOG-0209 established that the standard postsurgical chemotherapy regimen for advanced stage endometrial cancer, including uterine serous carcinoma, should be carboplatin and paclitaxel, given its noninferiority to doxorubicin/cisplatin/paclitaxel.[50] The dosing used in GOG-0209 was paclitaxel 175 mg/m^2 and carboplatin AUC 6 (day 1) every 21 days for 7 cycles with a dose reduction to paclitaxel 135 mg/m^2 and carboplatin AUC 5 for patients with a history of pelvic or spine irradiation.

In early-stage disease, while GOG-0249 did not demonstrated the superiority of vaginal brachytherapy and chemotherapy compared with pelvic external beam radiotherapy, only 14.6% of the study population consisted of women with stages I–II uterine serous carcinoma; therefore, the study was not powered to draw conclusions in women with early-stage disease.[51] However, several large, retrospective studies enriched with patients diagnosed with uterine serous carcinoma support the survival benefit of chemotherapy for treatment of uterine serous carcinoma, even in early-stage disease.[39,52] Nevertheless, recurrence rates remain high, even in those with early-stage disease.

The role for external beam radiation therapy in the treatment of advanced staged disease is less clear. The Phase III PORTEC 3 trial included women with stages IA–III uterine serous carcinoma, which made up 16% of the total study population. Patients were randomly assigned to chemoradiotherapy with cisplatin during pelvic external beam radiotherapy followed by systemic paclitaxel and carboplatin for 4 additional cycles vs pelvic external beam radiotherapy alone.[53] In an exploratory ad hoc analysis, patients with uterine serous carcinoma experienced significantly improved survival from chemoradiotherapy with a 5-year overall survival of 71.4% compared with 52.8% for external beam radiotherapy alone (HR 0.48, 95% CI 0.24–0.96); however, the primary driver of better response here was the addition of chemotherapy. Adding to this, GOG-0258 which evaluated patients with high risk endometrial cancers by randomizing patients to receive carboplatin and paclitaxel vs chemoradiotherapy as described for PORTEC 3 above, enrolled patients with stages IA–II uterine serous carcinoma with positive washings (<3% of the total population) as well as patients with stages III–IVA disease.[54] Overall, patients with uterine serous carcinoma made up 18% of the total study population. The primary endpoint was relapse-free survival, and no significant difference was observed between the two treatment arms. A subgroup analysis of the patients with uterine serous carcinoma failed to identify any factors that would favor chemoradiotherapy over chemotherapy alone. Thus, the current standard for treatment of advanced-stage disease remains cytotoxic chemotherapy.

HER2 positive disease

Molecular characterization of endometrial cancer has emerged as an important prognostic tool to help guide treatment recommendations. In patients with HER2 positive disease, which represent 25%–30% of all uterine serous carcinoma cases, the addition of anti-HER2 therapy appears to improve survival outcomes. A randomized phase II study of 58 patients demonstrated that the addition of trastuzumab—a monoclonal anti-HER2 antibody—to carboplatin/paclitaxel chemotherapy and as maintenance therapy thereafter, significantly improved progression-free and overall survival in patients with HER2 positive, primary uterine serous carcinoma[55,56] (Table 12.6). This is now considered the care standard for women with HER2 positive, stages III–IV disease based on the NCCN guidelines. A retrospective report also demonstrated that up to 26% of patients with stage I uterine serous carcinoma also have overexpressed or amplified HER2 in their tumors and experience a worse progression-free and overall survival as a result compared to patients of similar stage with HER2 negative tumors.[40]

Surveillance for recurrence

The majority of disease recurrence or progression in uterine serous carcinoma occurs within 2 years of conclusion of primary therapy.[57] As in other forms of endometrial cancer, clinical surveillance includes a pelvic exam every 3 months for 2 years followed by every 6 months for 5 years, than annually. Imaging with CT of the chest, abdomen, pelvis, MRI of the pelvis, or whole-body positron emitted tomography (PET) can be considered if patients endorse concerning symptoms (e.g., bloating, abdominal pain, nausea) or physical exam findings (pelvic or vaginal mass, lymphadenopathy). As discussed in Section "Tumor Markers", some retrospective studies have demonstrated correlation between CA-125 level and disease recurrence, though its use as a prospective tool has not been evaluated.

TABLE 12.6 Advances in treatment of uterine serous carcinoma.

Drug[56,60]	Mechanism	Study Design	Study population	Sample Size	Findings
Single arm with adavosertib monotherapy	WEE1 inhibitor	Phase II	Recurrent uterine serous carcinoma	34	ORR 29.4% Median PFS 6.1 months
Single arm with lenvatinib + pembrolizumab KEYNOTE-146[59]	Multikinase inhibitor + monoclonal antibody to PD-L1	Phase II	Advanced or recurrent endometrial carcinoma	108	ORR at week 24 38% overall, reaching 63.6% in MSI-H tumors vs 36.2% in MSS tumors
Randomization to carboplatin and paclitaxel with or without trastuzumab	Monoclonal antibody to HER2 receptor (ERBB2)	Phase II	Advanced or recurrent uterine serous carcinoma	58	Median survival 12.9 months in trastuzumab arm vs 8.0 months in control arm (HR 0.46, $P = 0.005$)

ORR: objective response rate; *PFS*: progression-free survival; *MSI-H*: microsatellite-instability high; *MSS*: microsatellite stable.

Survival and patterns of failure

Even controlling for stage, 5-year survival rates in uterine serous carcinoma are poor, with rates of 74% in stages I–II disease and 33% in stages III–IV disease. Comparatively, clear cell endometrial cancers and grade 3 endometrioid cancers have survival rates of around 80% for stages I–II disease and 40%–50% for stages III–IV disease.[37]

While a preponderance of recurrent disease in endometrioid endometrial cancers present at the vaginal cuff, recurrent disease in uterine serous carcinoma commonly occurs at extrapelvic sites. In the absence of myometrial invasion, observation after primary surgical management yields recurrence rates of 0%–30%. If any degree of myometrial invasion is present, this rate increases to 29%–30%. Given the high likelihood of distant disease, localized adjuvant therapy is rarely indicated.[26] In a sample of 119 patients with pure uterine serous carcinoma, 37% of recurrences occurred in the vagina or pelvis, 18% in the abdomen, and 8% in the lymph nodes, 12% in the lungs or brain, and 21% at multiple sites.[44]

Treatment of recurrent disease

Therapeutic regimens to consider in women with recurrence for biomarker unselected uterine serous carcinoma include cytotoxic chemotherapy (i.e., consideration of a re-challenge with platinum/taxane-based therapy in the setting of a prolonged disease-free interval, pegylated liposomal doxorubicin (PLD) with or without bevacizumab, weekly paclitaxel, among others recommended by the NCCN Uterine Cancer Guidelines)[58] (Table 12.7). As for primary therapy for uterine serous carcinoma, many of the treatment recommendations for recurrent disease are based on treatment paradigms derived from advanced or recurrent uterine cancers of other histologies.

Given the rarity of and lack of direct evidence in management in recurrent serous carcinoma, numerous clinical trials are ongoing to further investigate therapeutic options.

The same randomized phase II study of trastuzumab discussed above included patients with recurrent, HER2 positive uterine serous carcinoma; the addition of trastuzumab resulted in significantly improved progression-free, but not overall, survival[55,56] (Fig. 12.3). The family of anti-HER2 agents has expanded recently, with the addition of small molecule inhibitors (i.e., lapatinib), antibodies (i.e., pertuzumab with or without trastuzumab), and an antibody-drug conjugate (ADC) (i.e., ado-trastuzumab emtansine, T-DM1). Though no anti-HER2 therapy has been FDA-approved for use in women with

TABLE 12.7 Treatment options in recurrent uterine serous carcinoma.

Study	Disease setting	Serous histology	Experimental arm	Control arm	Outcome
GOG 177: Fleming 2004[63] (N = 263)	Advanced/recurrent	17%	TAP	AP	ORR: 57% vs 34%* PFS: 8.3 vs 5.3 mo* OS: 15.3 vs 12.3 mo*
GOG 209: Miller 2020[64] (N = 1381)	Advanced/recurrent	Unknown	CT	TAP	ORR: 51% vs NR PFS: 14 vs 14 mo (HR, 1.03) OS: 32 vs 38 mo (HR, 1.01) CT noninferior to TAP
GOG 3007: Slomovitz 2018[65] (N = 74)	Advanced/recurrent	Unknown	EL or MT	NA	ORR (chemo-naive): EL: 53%; MT: 43%
Fader 2020[56] (N = 61)	Advanced/recurrent, HER2-positive, serous	100%	CT +trastuzumab	CT	Median-PFS, recurrent disease: 7.0 vs 9.2 mos*
GOG 86P: Aghajanian 2018[66] (N = 116)	Advanced/recurrent	14%	CT + bevacizumab	Historical control (GOG 209)	ORR: 60% vs 51% PFS: NS OS: HR, 0.71 (95% CI, 0.55–0.91)*

Table adapted from R. A. Brooks et al., Current recommendations and recent progress in endometrial cancer. CA Cancer J Clin 69 (2019) 258–279.
TAP: Doxorubin, paclitaxel, cisplatin; *AP:* Doxorubicin, cisplatin; *CT:* Carboplatin, paclitaxel; *EL:* Everolimus/letrozole; *MT:* megestrol acetate/tamoxifen (MT); *mo:* months; *NS:* Not significant.

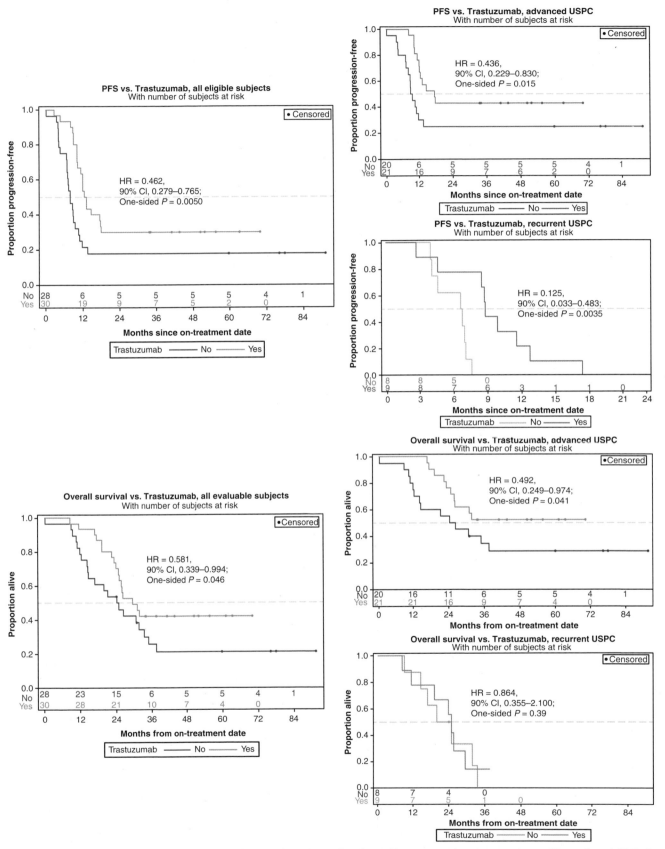

FIG. 12.3 PFS and OS benefit with addition of trastuzumab to chemotherapy for advanced/recurrent uterine serous carcinoma. *Figures from A. N. Fader et al., Randomized phase II trial of carboplatin–paclitaxel compared with carboplatin–paclitaxel–trastuzumab in advanced (stage III–IV) or recurrent uterine serous carcinomas that overexpress her2/neu (NCT01367002): updated overall survival analysis. Clin Cancer Res 26 (2020) 3928–3935.*

HER2 positive uterine serous carcinoma, these treatments are all considerations in this setting if a patient has already received trastuzumab.

In addition, lenvatinib in combination with pembrolizumab[59] and the single agent Wee inhibitor, adavosertib have emerged as exciting treatment options for women with uterine serous disease[60]. In the former study, although immunotherapy is an exciting treatment option for select women with uterine cancer, uterine serous carcinoma appears to be less immunogenic compared to other uterine cancer subtypes. Biomarkers that often predict response to immunotherapy—microsatellite instability (MSI) and PD-L1 expression—are not frequently seen in this cancer subtype. Specifically, PD-L1 positivity was only seen in about 30% of uterine serous carcinomas compared to 62% of low-grade, MSI high endometrioid cancers, 70% of high-grade endometrioid cancers, and 70% of uterine carcinosarcomas.[61] Comprehensive molecular classification of endometrial cancers has instead placed serous cancers in a category characterized by low mutational burden, frequent copy number alterations, low ER/PR levels, and frequent *TP53* mutations.[62]

However, in the KEYNOTE-146 trial, women with recurrent uterine serous disease showed a profound and durable response to the combination of pembrolizumab and lenvatinib, a multikinase inhibitor. Of the 33 women with uterine serous carcinoma, almost 50% had either a partial or complete response to therapy, which was a remarkable response rate. Grade 3 hypertension appears to be one of the most common high-grade adverse events, however. In the latter study of adavosertib, 34 evaluable patients, 10 total responses (one confirmed complete response, eight confirmed partial responses, and one unconfirmed partial response) were observed with adavosertib monotherapy, for an ORR of 29.4% (95% CI, 15.1–47.5) and 16 patients were progression-free at 6 months, for a PFS6 rate of 47.1% (95% CI, 29.8–64.9). Frequent treatment-related adverse events included diarrhea (76.5%), fatigue (64.7%), nausea (61.8%), and hematologic issues.

Case resolution

Based on the patient's diagnosis of stage IIIC uterine serous carcinoma, additional tumor pathology studies with IHC (immunohistochemistry) and FISH (fluorescence in situ hybridization) for HER2 and assessment of mismatch repair status are ordered. The patient's tumor is HER2 positive, microsatellite stable. You recommend six cycles of IV carboplatin (AUC5–6), paclitaxel (175 mg/m^2) with trastuzumab (8 mg/kg loading dose followed by 6 mg/mg IV with subsequent cycles) and subsequent trastuzumab maintenance for primary adjuvant therapy. You continue to follow her every 3 months without evidence of disease progression, and she remains on trastuzumab with minimal side effects at 2-year follow-up.

References

1. Siegel RL, Miller KD, Jemal A. Cancer statistics, 2020. *CA Cancer J Clin.* 2020;70:7–30.
2. Broaddus RR. Endometrial cancer. *N Engl J Med.* 2020;383:2053–2064.
3. Lortet-Tieulent J, Ferlay J, Bray F, Jemal A. International patterns and trends in endometrial Cancer incidence, 1978–2013. *J Natl Cancer Inst.* 2018;110:354–361.
4. Clarke MA, Devesa SS, Harvey SV, Wentzensen N. Hysterectomy-corrected uterine Corpus Cancer incidence trends and differences in relative survival reveal racial disparities and rising rates of Nonendometrioid cancers. *J Clin Oncol.* 2019;37:1895–1908.
5. Hamilton CA, et al. Uterine papillary serous and clear cell carcinomas predict for poorer survival compared to grade 3 endometrioid corpus cancers. *Br J Cancer.* 2006;94:642–646.
6. Slomovitz BM, et al. Uterine papillary serous carcinoma (UPSC): a single institution review of 129 cases. *Gynecol Oncol.* 2003;91:463–469.
7. Sherman ME, Bitterman P, Rosenshein NB, Delgado G, Kurman RJ. Uterine serous carcinoma a morphologically diverse neoplasm with unifying Clinicopathologic features. *Am J Surg Pathol.* 1992;16:600–610.
8. Goff BA, et al. Uterine papillary serous carcinoma: patterns of metastatic spread. *Gynecol Oncol.* 1994;54:264–268.
9. Milam MR, et al. Nodal metastasis risk in endometrioid endometrial cancer. *Obstet Gynecol.* 2012;119:286–292.
10. Hui P, Kelly M, O'Malley DM, Tavassoli F, Schwartz PE. Minimal uterine serous carcinoma: a clinicopathological study of 40 cases. *Mod Pathol.* 2005;18:75–82.
11. Liang SX, et al. Endometrial glandular dysplasia: a putative precursor lesion of uterine papillary serous carcinoma. Part II: molecular features. *Int J Surg Pathol.* 2004;12:319–331.
12. Zheng W, et al. Endometrial glandular dysplasia: a newly defined precursor lesion of uterine papillary serous carcinoma. Part I: morphologic features. *Int J Surg Pathol.* 2004;12:207–223.
13. Zheng W, Xiang L, Fadare O, Kong B. A proposed model for endometrial serous carcinogenesis. *Am J Surg Pathol.* 2011;35.
14. Tashiro H, et al. p53 gene mutations are common in uterine serous carcinoma and occur early in their pathogenesis. *Am J Pathol.* 1997;150:177–185.
15. Zhang X, et al. Molecular identification of "latent precancers" for endometrial serous carcinoma in benign-appearing endometrium. *Am J Pathol.* 2009;174:2000–2006.
16. Hainaut P, Pfeifer GP. Somatic TP53 mutations in the era of genome sequencing. *Cold Spring Harb Perspect Med.* 2016;6:a026179.

17. Kuhn E, et al. Identification of molecular pathway aberrations in uterine serous carcinoma by genome-wide analyses. *J Natl Cancer Inst.* 2012;104:1503–1513.

18. Zhao S, et al. Landscape of somatic single-nucleotide and copy-number mutations in uterine serous carcinoma. *Proc Natl Acad Sci.* 2013;110:2916.

19. Cote ML, Ruterbusch JJ, Olson SH, Lu K, Ali-Fehmi R. The growing burden of endometrial cancer: a major racial disparity affecting black women. *Cancer Epidemiol Biomark Prev.* 2015;24:1407.

20. Gehrig PA, et al. Association between uterine serous carcinoma and breast cancer. *Gynecol Oncol.* 2004;94:208–211.

21. De Jonge M, et al. Linking uterine serous carcinoma to BRCA1/2-associated cancer syndrome: a meta-analysis and case report. *Eur J Cancer.* 2017;72:215–225.

22. Pennington KP, et al. BRCA1, TP53, and CHEK2 germline mutations in uterine serous carcinoma. *Cancer.* 2013;119:332–338.

23. Hornreich G, et al. Is uterine serous papillary carcinoma a BRCA1-related disease? Case report and review of the literature. *Gynecol Oncol.* 1999;75:300–304.

24. Ellenson, LH, Prakash V, Stewart CJR. Serous carcinoma of the uterine corpus. In: WHO Classification of Tumors Editorial Board, ed. Female Genital Tumors. World Health Organization Classification of Tumors. Lyon: IARC Press; 2020:256–257.

25. Sherman ME, Bur ME, Kurman RJ. p53 in endometrial cancer and its putative precursors: evidence for diverse pathways of tumorigenesis. *Hum Pathol.* 1995;26(11):1268–1274. https://doi.org/10.1016/0046-8177(95)90204-x. PMID: 7590703.

26. Fader AN, Santin AD, Gehrig PA. Early stage uterine serous carcinoma: management updates and genomic advances. *Gynecol Oncol.* 2013;129: 244–250.

27. Abramovich D, Markman M, Kennedy A, Webster K, Belinson J. Serum CA-125 as a marker of disease activity in uterine papillary serous carcinoma. *J Cancer Res Clin Oncol.* 1999;125:697–698.

28. Ross MS, et al. Cancer antigen 125 is associated with disease status in uterine carcinosarcoma. *Rare Tumors.* 2019;11. 2036361319884159.

29. Frimer M, Hou JY, McAndrew TC, Goldberg GL, Shahabi S. The clinical relevance of rising CA-125 levels within the normal range in patients with uterine papillary serous cancer. *Reprod Sci.* 2013;20:449–455.

30. Bansal N, et al. The utility and cost effectiveness of preoperative computed tomography for patients with uterine malignancies. *Gynecol Oncol.* 2008;111:208–212.

31. Lin MY, Dobrotwir A, McNally O, Abu-Rustum NR, Narayan K. Role of imaging in the routine management of endometrial cancer. *Int J Gynecol Obstet.* 2018;143:109–117.

32. Nougaret S, et al. Endometrial Cancer MRI staging: updated guidelines of the European Society of Urogenital Radiology. *Eur Radiol.* 2019;29: 792–805.

33. Huang GS, et al. Accuracy of preoperative endometrial sampling for the detection of high-grade endometrial tumors. *Am J Obstet Gynecol.* 2007;196:243. e241–243. e245.

34. Wang J, et al. Thin endometrial echo complex on ultrasound does not reliably exclude type 2 endometrial cancers. *Gynecol Oncol.* 2006;101:120–125.

35. S. G. O. C. P. E. C. W. Group, et al. Endometrial cancer: a review and current management strategies: part I. *Gynecol Oncol.* 2014;134(385–392).

36. Sagae S, et al. Gynecologic Cancer InterGroup (GCIG) consensus review for uterine serous carcinoma. *Int J Gynecol Cancer.* 2014;24:S83–S89.

37. Creasman WT, Kohler MF, Odicino F, Maisonneuve P, Boyle P. Prognosis of papillary serous, clear cell, and grade 3 stage I carcinoma of the endometrium. *Gynecol Oncol.* 2004;95:593–596.

38. Creasman WT, et al. Surgical-pathological findings in type 1 and 2 endometrial cancer: an NRG oncology/gynecologic oncology group study on GOG-210 protocol. *Gynecol Oncol.* 2017;145:519–525.

39. Fader AN, et al. An updated clinicopathologic study of early-stage uterine papillary serous carcinoma (UPSC). *Gynecol Oncol.* 2009;115:244–248.

40. Erickson BK, et al. Human epidermal growth factor 2 (HER2) in early stage uterine serous carcinoma: a multi-institutional cohort study. *Gynecol Oncol.* 2020;159:17–22.

41. Santin AD, et al. Racial differences in the overexpression of epidermal growth factor type II receptor (HER2/neu): a major prognostic indicator in uterine serous papillary cancer. *Am J Obstet Gynecol.* 2005;192:813–818.

42. Holman LL, et al. Factors prognostic of survival in advanced-stage uterine serous carcinoma. *Gynecol Oncol.* 2017;146:27–33.

43. Rauh-Hain JA, et al. Prognostic determinants in patients with stage IIIC and IV uterine papillary serous carcinoma. *Gynecol Oncol.* 2010;119: 299–304.

44. Huang C-Y, et al. Impact of management on the prognosis of pure uterine papillary serous cancer—a Taiwanese gynecologic oncology group (TGOG) study. *Gynecol Oncol.* 2014;133:221–228.

45. Walker JL, et al. Laparoscopy compared with laparotomy for comprehensive surgical staging of uterine cancer: gynecologic oncology group study LAP2. *J Clin Oncol.* 2009;27:5331.

46. Rossi EC, et al. A comparison of sentinel lymph node biopsy to lymphadenectomy for endometrial cancer staging (FIRES trial): a multicentre, prospective, cohort study. *Lancet Oncol.* 2017;18:384–392.

47. Soliman PT, Westin SN, Dioun S, et al. A prospective validation study of sentinel lymph node mapping for high-risk endometrial cancer. *Gynecol Oncol.* 2017;146(2):234–239. https://doi.org/10.1016/j.ygyno.2017.05.016. Epub 2017 May 18. PMID: 28528918; PMCID: PMC5860676.

48. Cusimano MC, et al. Assessment of sentinel lymph node biopsy vs lymphadenectomy for intermediate- and high-grade endometrial Cancer staging. *JAMA Surg.* 2021;156:157–164.

49. Basaran D, Bruce S, Aviki EM, et al. Sentinel lymph node mapping alone compared to more extensive lymphadenectomy in patients with uterine serous carcinoma. *Gynecol Oncol.* 2020;156(1):70–76. 10.1016/j.ygyno.2019.10.005. Epub 2019 Nov 16. PMID: 31739992; PMCID: PMC6980657.

50. Miller D, et al. *Gynecologic Oncology.* 125. San Diego, CA: Academic Press Inc. Elsevier Science; 2012:771.

51. Randall ME, et al. Phase III trial: adjuvant pelvic radiation therapy versus vaginal brachytherapy plus paclitaxel/carboplatin in high-intermediate and high-risk early-stage endometrial cancer. *J Clin Oncol.* 2019;37:1810.

52. Boothe D, et al. The addition of adjuvant chemotherapy to radiation in early-stage high-risk endometrial Cancer: survival outcomes and patterns of care. *Int J Gynecol Cancer.* 2017;27:912.

53. de Boer SM, et al. Adjuvant chemoradiotherapy versus radiotherapy alone for women with high-risk endometrial cancer (PORTEC-3): final results of an international, open-label, multicentre, randomised, phase 3 trial. *Lancet Oncol.* 2018;19:295–309.

54. Matei D, et al. Adjuvant chemotherapy plus radiation for locally advanced endometrial Cancer. *N Engl J Med.* 2019;380:2317–2326.

55. Fader AN, et al. Randomized phase II trial of carboplatin-paclitaxel versus carboplatin-paclitaxel-trastuzumab in uterine serous carcinomas that over-express human epidermal growth factor receptor 2/neu. *J Clin Oncol.* 2018;36(20):2044–2051.

56. Fader AN, et al. Randomized phase II trial of carboplatin–paclitaxel compared with carboplatin–paclitaxel–trastuzumab in advanced (stage III–IV) or recurrent uterine serous carcinomas that overexpress her2/neu (NCT01367002): updated overall survival analysis. *Clin Cancer Res.* 2020;26:3928–3935.

57. Bogani G, et al. Uterine serous carcinoma. *Gynecol Oncol.* 2021.

58. Koh W-J, et al. Uterine neoplasms, version 1.2018, NCCN clinical practice guidelines in oncology. *J Natl Compr Cancer Netw.* 2018;**16**:170–199.

59. Makker V, et al. Lenvatinib plus Pembrolizumab in patients with advanced endometrial Cancer. *J Clin Oncol.* 2020;38:2981–2992.

60. Liu JF, et al. Phase II study of the WEE1 inhibitor Adavosertib in recurrent uterine serous carcinoma. *J Clin Oncol.* 2021;39:1531–1539.

61. Bregar A, et al. Characterization of immune regulatory molecules B7-H4 and PD-L1 in low and high grade endometrial tumors. *Gynecol Oncol.* 2017;145:446–452.

62. Levine DA. Integrated genomic characterization of endometrial carcinoma. *Nature.* 2013;497:67–73.

63. Fleming GF, et al. Phase III trial of doxorubicin plus cisplatin with or without paclitaxel plus filgrastim in advanced endometrial carcinoma: a gynecologic oncology group study. *J Clin Oncol.* 2004;22:2159–2166.

64. Miller DS, et al. Carboplatin and paclitaxel for advanced endometrial Cancer: final overall survival and adverse event analysis of a phase III trial (NRG oncology/GOG0209). *J Clin Oncol.* 2020;38:3841–3850.

65. Slomovitz BM, et al. GOG 3007, a randomized phase II (RP2) trial of everolimus and letrozole (EL) or hormonal therapy (medroxyprogesterone acetate/tamoxifen, PT) in women with advanced, persistent or recurrent endometrial carcinoma (EC): a GOG foundation study. *Gynecol Oncol.* 2018;149:2.

66. Aghajanian C, et al. A phase II study of frontline paclitaxel/carboplatin/bevacizumab, paclitaxel/carboplatin/temsirolimus, or ixabepilone/carboplatin/bevacizumab in advanced/recurrent endometrial cancer. *Gynecol Oncol.* 2018;150:274–281.

Chapter 13

Other rare uterine cancers: neuroendocrine tumors, yolk sac tumors, choriocarcinoma

Anne Knisely, Barrett Lawson, and Jason D. Wright

Neuroendocrine tumors

Epidemiology

Incidence and mortality

Neuroendocrine carcinomas (NEC) of the endometrium, which includes both small-cell and large-cell variants, are rare, highly aggressive tumors that account for approximately 0.8% of endometrial carcinomas. They generally present with advanced stage disease. The literature consists of only case reports and small case series. In one case series, 32% of patients presented with early (stages I–II) disease, whereas 68% presented with advanced stage disease, with a predominance of incidence in the sixth and seventh decades of life.[1] Another case series reports 26%, 5%, 36%, and 33% of patients present with stages I, II, III, and IV, respectively.[2]

Median survival has been reported as 17 months with a 5-year survival of 38.3%.[3] Stage for stage, 5-year survival for uterine neuroendocrine tumors (NETs) is significantly worse than survival for women with endometrioid adenocarcinoma of the uterus (Table 13.1). Mean survival ranges from 12 months for advanced stage disease to 22 months for early stage disease.[1,4] In a cohort of 25 patients, seven attained 5-year survival, of which three patients had stage I disease and four had stage III disease.[1]

Etiology and risk factors

NEC of the endometrium are a histologically distinct subtype of endometrial carcinoma with a propensity of metastatic infiltration and an unfavorable prognosis. They tend to form bulky, intraluminal masses with deep myometrial involvement. They are subdivided into small- and large-cell tumors according to nuclear size. Endometrial NEC are often combined with other epithelial neoplasms, with 50%–80% of cases admixed with FIGO grade 1 or 2 endometrioid carcinoma.[5]

Based on the largest population-based study ($N = 364$) from the National Cancer Database (NCDB), compared to women with poorly differentiated endometrial cancer, women with NEC were more often black (13.7% neuroendocrine vs. 10.7% poorly differentiated endometrial cancer) and Hispanic (8.0% neuroendocrine vs. 5.3% poorly differentiated endometrial cancer).[3] Additionally, as with other endometrial carcinomas, postmenopausal status is a known risk factor.[6]

Pathology

Gross description

Grossly the tumors are large, endometrial based and typically with deep myometrial invasion. Tumor size ranges from 0.8 to 12 cm with a median tumor size of 6.0 cm.[1] No gross pathognomonic features have been described.[7]

Microscopic description

Small-cell neuroendocrine carcinoma (SCNECa) resembles that of pulmonary small-cell carcinoma, with "salt and pepper chromatin" and scant cytoplasm with nuclear molding.[7] Large-cell neuroendocrine carcinoma (LCNECa) typically have neuroendocrine growth pattern, such as organoid/nesting (Fig. 13.1A), trabecular or corded. LCNECa characteristically have polygonal cells with abundant cytoplasm and prominent nucleoli (Fig. 13.1B). The tumors frequently have

Diagnosis and Treatment of Rare Gynecologic Cancers. https://doi.org/10.1016/B978-0-323-82938-0.00013-6

TABLE 13.1 Five-year survival rate by FIGO stage for uterine neuroendocrine carcinoma vs. endometrioid adenocarcinoma.

Stage	Neuroendocrine carcinoma	Endometrioid carcinoma
IA	76.4%	85.4%
IB	65.0%	72.7%
II	37.5%	67.1%
IIIA	16.1%	58.2%
IIIB	45.0%	46.4%
IIIC	34.2%	53.1%
IVA	0.0%	28.8%
IVB	15.4%	27.7%

Adopted from Schlechtweg et al., GYN Onc, 2019.

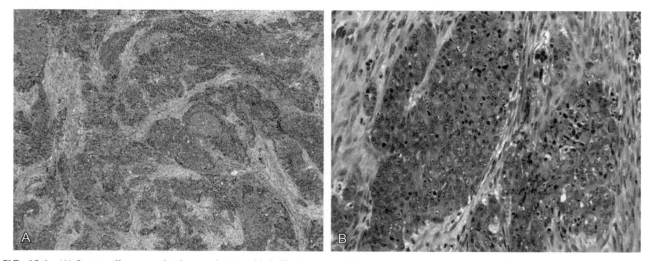

FIG. 13.1 (A) Large-cell neuroendocrine carcinoma with infiltrating nested pattern and foci of central necrosis. (B) Large-cell neuroendocrine carcinoma with large polygonal cells, abundant cytoplasm and prominent nucleoli.

central geographic necrosis, numerous mitotic figures and apoptotic bodies. Tumors may show pure SCNECa or LCNECa or may show mixed small and large-cell morphology. NEC can also be mixed with other histotypes, including endometrioid adenocarcinomas, serous carcinomas and carcinosarcomas.[8]

Immunohistochemistry

Epithelial markers such as a pankeratin cocktail should be positive, while rare tumors that are negative for pancytokeratin cocktail may have expression of cytokeratin 18. In some cases, several markers may be necessary to establish epithelial origin. NEC are positive for at least one neuroendocrine marker in at least 10% of the tumor cells, including synaptophysin, chromogranin, and CD56.[1,7] It should be noted though that non-NECs, such as an endometrioid FIGO grade 3 or undifferentiated carcinoma may show staining for any one of the neuroendocrine markers, and that interpretation of IHC should be in the context of the overall morphology. In some cases where the morphology and or IHC are not characteristic, a diagnosis of neuroendocrine differentiation or features may be used by the pathologist. p16 can be positive in a patchy or diffuse pattern, with no evidence of infection with high-risk HPV.[1]

Differential diagnosis

The differential diagnosis includes NEC from other primary sites, such as extension from the cervix or rarely metastases from other sites. In large tumors that involve the cervix and endometrium, establishing the primary site requires immunohistochemical staining, as the tumors are histologically similar. p16, which is usually a surrogate marker of HPV infection, can be diffusely expressed by non-HPV associated pathways and is not helpful in this distinction. Therefore, testing for HR-HPV is usually required and a negative result would favor endometrial primary in the correct clinical setting. High-grade carcinomas with a solid or nested growth pattern, such as FIGO grade 3 endometrioid carcinoma or serous carcinoma, may warrant consideration of a NEC. While neuroendocrine markers may be exhibited in these tumors, IHC is focal and less than 10% of tumor cells. Undifferentiated/de-differentiated carcinoma is also a consideration, usually lacking a nested architecture and with a diffuse, sheet-like pattern of growth. Like other NEC, focal staining for neuroendocrine markers may be seen but should be less than 10% of tumor cells.

Molecular findings

Approximately 40% of a series of endometrial NEC showed loss of expression of mismatch repair proteins, with the most common pattern being loss of MLH1/PMS2.[1,3] Molecular analysis on a separate series shows that endometrial NEC also classify into The Cancer Genome Atlas (TCGA) groups, with *POLE*-mutated/ultramutated (7%), MSI/hypermuted (43%) and *TP53* mutated/copy number high (14%).[9] Some SCNECa may show similar molecular profiles to those expected in typical pulmonary SCNECa (*RB1* deletion and *TP53* mutations).

Diagnosis and workup

The differential diagnosis for NEC is broad and includes undifferentiated/dedifferentiated endometrial carcinoma, carcinosarcoma, poorly differentiated endometrioid carcinoma, serous carcinoma with a solid growth pattern and massive necrosis, primitive neuroectodermal tumors (PNETs), and carcinoid tumor.[1,5] Additionally, NEC is often associated with tumors of other histologic types, including complex atypical hyperplasia, endometrioid carcinoma, carcinosarcoma, or serous carcinoma.[2]

In a 25 patient series, the most common presenting symptom was vaginal bleeding (15 of 25 patients) with other less common presenting symptoms including abdominal pain, symptoms related to metastasis, and abnormal Pap test.[1] Additional common presenting symptoms include postmenopausal bleeding and pelvic pain.[10] Of note, in very rare cases, NEC can also present with signs of paraneoplastic disease and/or Cushing's syndrome.[11,12]

Workup begins with a complete physical exam including pelvic and rectovaginal examinations (Table 13.2). The most common physical exam findings include abnormal vaginal bleeding,[6,13,14] abdominal pain,[14] and an enlarged uterus and/or a palpable pelvic mass.[10,15] There is not a typical tumor marker that is elevated in NEC. CA-125 may be elevated in the setting of a mixed tumor, but this marker is not specific to NETs.[10,15]

Data on the optimal pretreatment imaging are limited. Consideration can be given to obtaining a transvaginal pelvic ultrasound and a chest radiograph. If there is an abnormality on chest radiograph, a chest computed tomography (CT) can be obtained to further evaluate. If there is concern for high-grade carcinoma (e.g., if already diagnosed as high-grade tumor by an endometrial biopsy (EMB)), it is reasonable to obtain a CT of the chest, abdomen, and pelvis to evaluate for metastatic disease. Other initial imaging may be obtained based on symptoms and/or clinical concern for specific metastatic sites.[16]

In some cases, an MRI abdomen and pelvis may be obtained. MRI findings are similar to other poorly differentiated carcinomas, with an ill-defined endometrial-myometrial border and heterogeneity of the mass indicating necrosis and hemorrhage.[10] Consideration can also be given to positron emission tomography (PET).

TABLE 13.2 Basic workup and testing for neuroendocrine carcinoma of the endometrium.

Component of workup	Specific tests/considerations
Physical exam	Pelvic and abdominal exams
Tumor markers	Consider CA-125
Imaging	– TVUS, CXR – CT C/A/P if high-grade carcinoma – Consider MRI A/P or PET
Diagnostic tests	Endometrial biopsy or dilation and curettage

CXR: chest radiograph; *CT C/A/P*: computed tomography of chest/abdomen/pelvis; *MRI A/P*: magnetic resonance imaging of abdomen/pelvis; *PET*: positron emission tomography; *TVUS*: transvaginal ultrasound.

Similar to other endometrial cancers, the gold standard for initial diagnosis is by pathologic diagnosis obtained from either an EMB or endometrial curettings obtained from a dilation and curettage (D&C).[10]

Staging system

Uterine NEC is surgically staged utilizing the 2017 International Federation of Gynecology and Obstetrics (FIGO)/ Tumor, Node, Metastasis (TNM) system used for endometrial carcinoma (Table 13.3).

Prognostic factors

Factors associated with death in a NCDB series include: diagnosis at 80 years of age or older, stage (diagnosis at stage II or higher compared to stage I), and not receiving adjuvant chemotherapy.[3] Women over the age of 80 have a hazard ratio for death of 2.4 compared to women less than 50 years old and patients who receive chemotherapy have a hazard ratio for death of 0.36 compared to those who do not get chemotherapy. In a smaller study of 42 patients, performance status, FIGO stage, surgery, and histologic subtype (pure type with worse prognosis than mixed type) were significant prognostic factors; in a multivariate analysis, only surgery and histologic subtypes remained significant. There was also a better prognosis in complete surgery cases (versus no surgery or incomplete surgery).[2]

Prognostic factors for small-cell NETs in general (not specific to endometrial origin) include early detection and prompt surgical and adjuvant therapy.[17]

Treatment of primary disease

Standard treatment guidelines do not exist given the rarity of NEC and lack of prospective data to guide therapy. Treatment regimens are largely based on traditional treatments of endometrial cancer and small-cell lung cancer. The majority of reported treatment regimens in the literature include surgical resection and adjuvant therapy with platinum-based chemotherapy with or without radiation therapy.[3,4] Treatment usually begins with surgery for women without metastatic disease (Fig. 13.2). Surgery generally includes hysterectomy, bilateral salpingo-oophorectomy (BSO), and lymph node assessment. For younger women, fertility preserving surgery can be considered on an individual basis but most patients should undergo BSO.

Adjuvant treatment is reasonable to consider given aggressive nature of this cancer type with high risk of recurrence and metastasis. In the largest reported series of cases, all patients underwent surgery, 60% received chemotherapy, and 28% received radiation. Compared to women with poorly differentiated endometrial carcinoma, those with NEC were more likely to receive adjuvant chemotherapy, likely owing to the tendency to present with later stage disease.[3] In another series, all patients underwent surgery and 80% received adjuvant therapy.[1] All patients undergoing surgery with the majority also receiving adjuvant chemotherapy is consistent with smaller series and case studies.[14]

TABLE 13.3 Staging for neuroendocrine carcinoma of the endometrium.

Stage	Description
I	Tumor confined to uterus IA: <50% myometrial invasion IB: >50% myometrial invasion
II	Involvement of cervical stroma
III	Involvement of serosa, adnexa, vagina, parametrium, or locoregional lymph nodes IIIA: serosa and/or adnexa IIIB: vagina or parametrium IIIC: locoregional lymph nodes IIIC1: pelvic lymph nodes IIIC2: para-aortic lymph nodes
IV	Involvement of bladder/bowel mucosa, or distant metastases IVA: bladder/bowel mucosa IVB: distant metastases

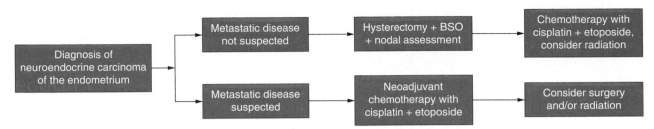

FIG. 13.2 Treatment of newly diagnosed uterine neuroendocrine carcinoma. *BSO*: bilateral salpingo-oophorectomy.

The most common reported chemotherapy regimens include cisplatin and etoposide.[14,17] The following dosage regimen has been reported in the literature and is reasonable to consider for adjuvant treatment: cisplatin (80 mg/m^2 on day 1) and etoposide (80–120 mg/m^2 on days 1–3) over a 3-week interval.[15,18] Of note, adjuvant treatment regimens used for NEC are largely based on data from small-cell lung cancer and neuroendocrine cervical cancer.[19,20] A case series of SCNECa of the cervix demonstrated 83% recurrence-free survival (RFS) at 3 years with use of adjuvant etoposide and cisplatin.[19] Indications for neoadjuvant chemotherapy are similar to those in other endometrial cancer types, and may be considered in the setting of advanced stage disease, though its use is rare in the reported literature.[10]

In conclusion, there are no evidence-based therapeutic regimens for NEC due to its rarity, but surgery followed by adjuvant chemotherapy (most commonly cisplatin and etoposide) has been used with several patients obtaining long-term survival in case reports.[21,22]

Surveillance for recurrence

Based on recommendations for surveillance of endometrial carcinoma, it is reasonable to consider physical exam every 3–6 months for 2–3 years and then every 6 months or annually with thorough review of systems and tumor markers (if initially elevated) at each visit, as well as imaging if clinically indicated.[16] Evidence-based recommendations for surveillance are lacking.

Survival and patterns of failure

A large case series reports 5-year progression-free survival (PFS) and overall survival (OS). Five-year PFS is 81.8%, 50%, 32.5%, and 14.3% for FIGO stages I, II, III, and IV, respectively. OS is 88.9%, 100%, 46.7%, and 21.4% for FIGO stages I, II, III, and IV, respectively. Recurrence occurred in 50% of cases with a higher rate of hematogenous recurrence compared to lymphogenous or local recurrence.[2]

Treatment of recurrent disease

There are no standard regimens due to rarity of the disease (Table 13.4). One report in the literature describes the use of salvage chemotherapy with cisplatin (75 mg/m^2) and ifosfamide (5 g/m^2).[15] Second-line therapies can be considered based on cervical and lung cancer data: cyclophosphamide/doxorubicin/vincristine (CAV), irinotecan/platinum (IP), or topotecan.[23–26]

TABLE 13.4 Treatment of recurrence for neuroendocrine carcinoma of the endometrium.

Treatment options for recurrent disease	Specific regimens/agents
Salvage chemotherapy	Cisplatin and ifosfamide
Second-line therapies (used in cervical and lung cancer)	Cyclophosphamide/doxorubicin/vincristine (CAV), irinotecan/platinum (IP), or topotecan
Targeted therapies	PI3K and MEK inhibitors
Immunotherapy	Nivolumab (PD-1 receptor inhibitor)

Based on preliminary data from NEC of the cervix, PI3K and MEK inhibitors are targeted therapies that may have therapeutic potential for treatment of endometrial NEC.[27] One study looked at a newly established neuroendocrine cervical carcinoma cell line and found that when etoposide and cisplatin were combined with a PI3K inhibitor (which functions in the mTOR pathway), the growth of tumor cells was significantly reduced.[28] Another study examined a MEK inhibitor, trametinib, which functions in the RAS pathway and is FDA-approved for treatment of unresectable or metastatic melanoma in patients with *BRAF* mutations, in the treatment of a patient with recurrent cervical neuroendocrine carcinoma with a *KRAS* mutation; she has been on trametinib for 8 cycles and is without evidence of disease.[29] Based on data from pulmonary small-cell tumors, a number of other targeted therapies have been studied including angiogenesis inhibitors, mTOR inhibitors, and PARP inhibitors.[30–33]

There is a case report evaluating the use of a programmed cell death 1 (PD-1) receptor inhibitor, nivolumab, in the treatment of a patient with recurrent, metastatic SCNECa of the cervix. The patient experienced a complete response and remained free of disease 4 months after stopping treatment.[34] Further research is needed to see if immunotherapy is a reasonable approach to recurrent NEC of the cervix and/or endometrium.

Yolk sac tumors

Epidemiology

Incidence and mortality

Yolk sac tumors (YSTs), also known as endodermal sinus tumors, are malignant germ cell tumors that secrete alpha-fetoprotein (AFP). The most common origin is gonadal, but 20% of cases arise from various extra-gonadal sites (mediastinum, retroperitoneum, sacrococcygeal region, pelvis, liver, stomach, vulva, vagina, and cervix).[35] The most common extra-gonadal site in the female genital tract is the vagina.[36]

Primary YSTs of the endometrium are very rare with fewer than 20 case reports in the literature. The median survival for endometrial YSTs is 28 months (range, 8–72 months).[37] In review of the existing case reports, only 3 (out of 19) reported mortality[36–38]; however, periods of follow up were variable. Five-year survival rates for ovarian YSTs, which are much more common than those of endometrial origin, for stages I, II, III, and IV are 95%, 75%, 30%, and 25%, respectively.[39]

Etiology and risk factors

Four possible mechanisms for germ cell tumors in the endometrium have been proposed: aberrant lateral migration of primordial germ cells during embryogenesis, metastases from an occult focus in the ovary, tumor origination from residual fetal tissue after incomplete abortion, or aberrant differentiation of somatic cells.[40] Given the rarity of this tumor, specific risk factors have not been determined.

Pathology

Extragonadal YSTs are exceedingly rare. YST, in comparison to other germ cell tumors, displays diverse histologic patterns. Due to this variability, YSTs can commonly mimic somatic tumors, posing a significant diagnostic challenge, even more so in extragonadal sites.

Gross description

Due to the rarity of these tumors, there is a paucity of information regarding the gross appearance of uterine YSTs. YSTs have been described as tan-yellow, soft, friable and hemorrhagic. Most patients present with abnormal vaginal bleeding and some with a uterine mass. Approximately 70% of uterine YSTs present with FIGO stage II or higher.

Microscopic description

YSTs have various histologic patterns, including microcystic/reticular, glandular, solid, papillary and hepatoid (Fig. 13.3).[41] Approximately one-third of cases have only a single identifiable histologic pattern, while the rest show an admixture of patterns with a predominant pattern that is typically microcystic/reticular, glandular or solid. Schiller–Duval bodies, while useful as a histologic clue for YSTs, are typically rare, both in the percentage of cases they are present in, as well as within the tumors themselves.[41,42] Approximately 70% of uterine YSTs present with an associated somatic component that may represent <10% to 90% of the total sampled tumor, including the following histotypes: complex atypical hyperplasia, serous carcinoma, carcinosarcoma, and mixed high-grade carcinomas.[41]

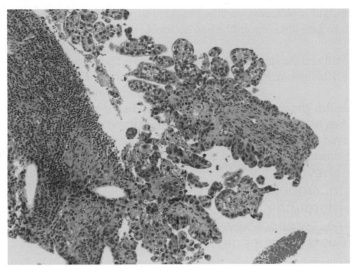

FIG. 13.3   Yolk sac tumor showing prominent papillary morphology.

Immunohistochemistry

YSTs are typically positive for SALL4, AFP, and Glypican-3, while they show focal or no staining for cytokeratin 7 and PAX-8 (Fig. 13.4).[41,42] YSTs, especially those with glandular pattern, may express markers typically associated with a somatic tumor, including villin, CDX2 and cytokeratin 20, and pose a diagnostic pitfall.

Molecular findings

There are very few studies evaluating the molecular characteristics of uterine YSTs. A case report of a pure uterine YST showed allelic copy gains at STR loci on chromosomes 2, 3, 4, 5, 8, 13, and 15, with copy loss at chromosome 1, with no point mutations or indels identified in a 155 gene panel.[43] Overall, these findings are suggestive of a germ cell origin for this one case, rather than a somatic stem cell. On the other hand, a more recent study that performed next generation sequencing in a case of endometrial mixed clear cell carcinoma and YSTs showed *ARID1A* and *TP53* mutations in both components, supporting a somatic derivation for the YST component.[44] It is likely that some uterine YSTs are of germ cell origin and others are somatically derived.

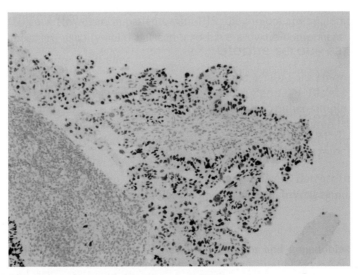

FIG. 13.4   Yolk sac tumor with diffuse immunohistochemical positivity for SALL-4.

Differential diagnosis

The differential diagnosis includes somatic carcinomas in the uterus that may show glandular or clear cell changes, including endometrioid adenocarcinoma, clear cell carcinoma, serous carcinoma or carcinosarcomas. Careful attention to the histology and awareness of the varied histology of YSTs can at the least trigger an IHC panel to rule in or rule out the presence of a YST component. Another important pitfall includes colorectal adenocarcinoma as YSTs can express CK20, CDX2, villin, which are markers of intestinal differentiation.

Diagnosis and workup

Histologically, YSTs are often confused with endometrial clear cell carcinoma.[35,36] However, patients with clear cell carcinomas are typically older. Other conditions that can cause an elevated AFP include hepatitis, extensive hepatic metastasis from an alternative primary tumor, and various malignancies of the gastrointestinal (GI) tract.[38]

The most common symptom associated with endometrial YSTs is abnormal uterine bleeding or postmenopausal bleeding.[35,37,38,40,45–53] Additional presenting symptoms that have been reported in the literature include abdominal and pelvic pain[36,37,54,55] and watery vaginal discharge.[56]

Workup begins with a complete physical exam including pelvic and rectovaginal examinations (Table 13.5). Physical exam findings include bulky/enlarged uterus,[35,38,45,47,49,51,56] prolapsing uterine tumor,[40] and pelvic/abdominal fullness.[37,54,55] A minority of cases in the literature also report unremarkable pelvic exams.[48,50]

YSTs commonly present with elevated AFP. In case reports in the literature, AFP at time of diagnosis ranges from 291.9 to 38,366 ng/mL (normal reference range 1.01–7.10 ng/mL).[57] There are two case reports with normal AFP.[47] If there is a mixed germ cell tumor, other tumor markers including beta-human chorionic gonadotropin (hCG), CA-125, and CEA may be elevated.

The most commonly used imaging modalities include pelvic ultrasound followed by CT and magnetic resonance imaging (MRI). A minority of studies assessed for metastatic disease with chest imaging in the absence of pulmonary symptoms.[37,48] Pelvic imaging commonly shows a thickened endometrial stripe and/or an intrauterine mass.

Similar to other endometrial cancers, the gold standard for initial diagnosis is by pathologic diagnosis obtained from either an EMB or endometrial curettings obtained from a D&C.

Staging system

Similar to uterine NEC described above, uterine YSTs are surgically staged utilizing the 2017 FIGO/TNM system used for endometrial carcinoma (Table 13.3).

Prognostic factors

There are too few case reports of endometrial YSTs to determine prognostic factors with any degree of certainty. However, one can extrapolate from ovarian YSTs for prognostic factors, with the knowledge that the tumors may behave in slightly different ways.

A series of ovarian YSTs found that patients with early stage disease, ascites volume less than 100 cc, and residual tumor less than 1 cm after surgery had a more favorable prognosis.[58] Another retrospective review found the following factors to be associated with a more favorable prognosis: early stage, size of residual tumor less than 2 cm, absence of ascites or less than 100 cc in

TABLE 13.5 Basic workup and testing for yolk sac tumors of the endometrium.

Component of workup	Specific tests/considerations
Physical exam	Pelvic and abdominal exams
Tumor markers	Alpha-fetoprotein (AFP); consider β-hCG, CA-125, CEA
Imaging	– TVUS – Consider CXR, CT C/A/P if concern for metastatic disease
Diagnostic tests	Endometrial biopsy or dilation and curettage

CXR: chest radiograph; *CT C/A/P*: computed tomography of chest/abdomen/pelvis; *TVUS*: transvaginal ultrasound.

volume, and use of chemotherapy with cisplatin (versus without). This study did not find pre-operative AFP level or lymph node status to be prognostic indicators.[39] However, both studies are limited by small sample size.

Treatment of primary disease

Treatment has not been standardized due to the rarity of YSTs of the endometrium. The general consensus regarding the treatment approach for YSTs of the endometrium is a combination of surgery and chemotherapy[35]; this has largely been extrapolated from germ cell tumors in other locations (Fig. 13.5).

In terms of surgical procedures, all case reports document hysterectomy, and the majority also include BSO, though ovarian preservation is noted in two case reports.[46,51] Given the rarity of these tumors there is little data on fertility preserving surgical options. Some case reports include lymph node dissection but this is not a universal practice. Studies from ovarian YSTs have shown that lymph node dissection is not associated with improved prognosis.[39]

The preferred adjuvant chemotherapy regimen, largely extrapolated from treatment of ovarian YSTs, is bleomycin, etoposide, and cisplatin (BEP) every 21 days for 3–4 cycles.[39] Standard regimen is bleomycin 30 units IV per week, etoposide 100 mg/m^2 IV daily on days 1–5, and cisplatin 20 mg/m^2 IV daily on days 1–5.[59] The role of adjuvant radiotherapy is uncertain. There is one case report of a patient who refused adjuvant chemotherapy and instead received postoperative radiation therapy in the setting of stage I disease with no evidence of recurrence.[48]

Surveillance for recurrence

Based on recommendations for surveillance of endometrial carcinoma, it is reasonable to consider physical exam every 3–6 months for 2–3 years and then every 6 months or annually with thorough review of systems and tumor markers (if initially elevated) at each visit, as well as imaging if clinically indicated.[16]

Survival and patterns of failure

In review of published case reports of endometrial YSTs ($N = 19$), there are five reports of persistent or recurrent disease. Documented sites of recurrence include para-aortic lymph nodes[56] and the liver.[38,55] The other two cases were persistent disease in the setting of incomplete primary cytoreductive surgery that subsequently progressed. There are three reported deaths.[36–38]

Treatment of recurrent disease

Given how rare endometrial YSTs are, there are no standardized regimens for treatment of recurrent disease (Table 13.6). In the literature, various approaches have been documented including additional chemotherapy with or without external beam radiation therapy[36,53] and secondary cytoreductive surgery followed by second-line chemotherapy.[55,56] One case report documents salvage chemotherapy with floxuridine, dactinomycin, etoposide, and vincristine.[53] Considerations for treatment of recurrent disease in ovarian YSTs include secondary surgery if definitive residual disease or chemotherapy with paclitaxel, ifosfamide, cisplatin (TIP), or high-dose chemotherapy (HDC).[60,61]

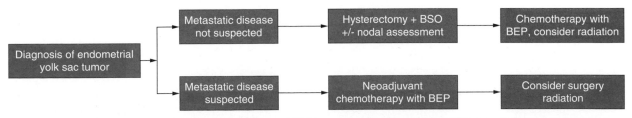

FIG. 13.5   Treatment of newly diagnosed uterine yolk sac tumor. *BEP*: bleomycin, etoposide, cisplatin; *BSO*: ilateral salpingo-oophorectomy.

TABLE 13.6 Treatment of recurrence for yolk sac tumors of the endometrium.

Treatment options for recurrent disease	Specific regimens/agents
Second-line therapies	Consider radiation, secondary cytoreductive surgery, additional chemotherapy
Salvage chemotherapy	Floxuridine, dactinomycin, etoposide, and vincristine
Targeted therapies	N/A
Immunotherapy	N/A

Choriocarcinoma

Epidemiology

Incidence and mortality

Gestational trophoblastic neoplasia (GTN) includes invasive mole, choriocarcinoma, placental site trophoblastic tumor (PSTT), and epithelioid trophoblastic tumor (ETT). Invasive moles are the most common, representing 75% of GTN, with choriocarcinoma and the other more rare types of GTN comprising the remaining 25%.[62,63] Postmolar GTN (invasive mole and choriocarcinoma) develops in 15%–20% of complete molar pregnancies but only 1%–5% of partial molar pregnancies.[64]

The incidence of choriocarcinoma is 1 in 40,000 pregnancies and 1 in 40 hydatiform moles in Europe and North America. In Southeast Asia and Japan, the incidence is 9.2 and 3.3 per 40,000 pregnancies, respectively.[64]

Cure rates for choriocarcinoma approach 100%. For high-risk GTN in general, cure rates are 90% for all stages and 70% for stage IV disease.[62,63]

Etiology and risk factors

Choriocarcinoma is a malignant epithelial tumor that develops from the villous trophoblast and is therefore generally seen in reproductive age women. It can occur with different types of pregnancy events, with 50% of cases arising from hydatiform moles, 25% from term or preterm gestations, and 25% from tubal pregnancies or abortions.[64] In general, 2%–3% of hydatiform moles progress to choriocarcinoma.[65] Choriocarcinoma is characterized by abnormal trophoblastic hyperplasia and anaplasia, hCG production, absence of chorionic villi, hemorrhage, and necrosis, with direct invasion into the myometrium and vascular invasion resulting in spread to distant sites, most commonly to the lungs, brain, liver, pelvis and vagina, kidneys, intestines, and spleen.[64–66]

Risk factors for choriocarcinoma include Asian, American Indian, and African American race, prior HM (100 fold increased risk), advanced age, long-term oral contraceptive pill use, and blood type A.[64] Risk factors for development of choriocarcinoma among those with low-risk GTN include higher parity, pretreatment β-hCG levels >100,000 mIU/mL, longer duration of disease, and higher FIGO scores.[67]

Pathology

Gross description

Gestational choriocarcinoma typically presents as a bulky, destructive mass with easily identifiable hemorrhage and necrosis. Deep myometrial invasion is common and uterine perforation may occur. Gestational choriocarcinomas associated with pregnancy may arise intra-placental or extra-placental.[68] Nongestational choriocarcinoma is also grossly described as bulky with "crumbly tumor tissue" and can present as tissue protruding through the cervical os.[71]

Microscopic description

Choriocarcinoma histologically shows proliferating, malignant appearing trophoblasts, consisting of intermediate trophoblasts and cytotrophoblasts, rimmed by multinucleated syncytiotrophoblastic cells.[68,69] Cytologic atypia is typically marked, with nuclear enlargement and brisk mitoses. Hemorrhage and necrosis are common and typically centrally located, with viable tumor cells more towards the periphery. Lymphovascular invasion is also commonly noted.

Immunohistochemistry

Choriocarcinoma is typically positive for hCG and HSD3B1 diffusely in the neoplastic syncytiotrophoblastic cells, while the intermediate trophoblasts express Mel-CAM, HLA-G, and MUC-4.[69,70]

Differential diagnosis

The differential diagnosis of choriocarcinoma, in a way, includes itself; as choriocarcinoma must be determined to be gestational or nongestational. Careful attention to history can help guide determination, as nongestational choriocarcinomas commonly occur in children or young adults, and a choriocarcinoma in nulligravidae is nongestational by default. Sampling of the tumor specimen may also help, as nongestational choriocarcinomas in postmenopausal patients are typically a component of a mixed carcinoma. Syncytiotrphblast-like giant cells can be seen in high-grade tumors such as serous carcinoma and carcinosarcoma; however, a diagnosis of choriocarcinoma can only be made when there is an accompanying intermediate/cytotrophoblastic component. Establishing a diagnosis in an EMB can be particularly challenging. Distinguishing choriocarcinoma from intermediate trophoblastic tumors (PSTT and ETT) can typically be done by histology characteristics and history (serum beta-hCG levels). Additionally immunohistochemistry for beta-hCG should show diffuse staining in choriocarcinomas, while in intermediate trophoblastic tumors hCG expression should be positive only in scattered syncytiotrophoblasts.[69,70]

Molecular findings

Genotyping of gestational choriocarcinomas shows a predominance for purely androgenetic tumors, with approximately 25% biparental.[68] DNA polymorphism analysis on nongestational choriocarcinomas will show identical polymorphic pattern between the tumor and the patient's alleles at all short tandem repeat loci.[71]

Diagnosis and workup

The differential diagnosis for choriocarcinoma includes PSTT, seminoma, mixed germ cell tumor, solid variant of YST and embryonal carcinoma.[64,72]

The majority of patients present with abnormal uterine bleeding. For patients with choriocarcinoma arising after a molar pregnancy, the most common presentation is irregular bleeding after initial treatment. Other possible presenting symptoms include abdominal pain/distension and hyperthyroidism (given elevated β-hCG). In the setting of metastatic disease, patients may present with pulmonary symptoms (e.g., chest pain, shortness of breath, hemoptysis), neurologic symptoms (e.g., headache, seizures, focal neurologic findings on exam), or GI symptoms.[64]

Workup begins with a complete physical exam including pelvic and rectovaginal examinations (Table 13.7). Common physical exam findings in choriocarcinoma include vaginal bleeding, an enlarged or irregular uterus, and bilateral ovarian enlargement. Rarely, a vaginal mass may be appreciated in the setting of vaginal metastasis.[64,66,73]

β-hCG is elevated in the setting of choriocarcinoma. Postmolar GTN is typically diagnosed by β-hCG surveillance, per FIGO guidelines according to any of the following criteria: β-hCG levels plateau for 4 consecutive values over ≥3 weeks, β-hCG levels rise ≥10% for 3 values over ≥2 weeks, or β-hCG persistence 6 months or more after molar evacuation.[74]

The first-line imaging is pelvic ultrasound, which can confirm the absence of pregnancy, measure uterine size, and delineate volume and vasculature of the tumor. In the setting of choriocarcinoma confirmed by pathology, one should obtain a metastatic work-up including chest radiograph, chest/abdominal/pelvic CT with contrast. If pulmonary metastases are present, then brain imaging with brain MRI (preferred) or CT with contrast is indicated. If negative and no other signs/symptoms concerning for metastatic disease, no further imaging is required prior to treatment.[75,76]

Diagnostic tests

The diagnosis of postmolar GTN is made based on β-hCG levels (see Section "Tumor Markers" above).[74] The diagnosis of choriocarcinoma is ultimately a pathologic diagnosis, with tissue obtained from endometrial sampling (usually D&C) or, in more rare cases, hysterectomy. Once choriocarcinoma is diagnosed, the NCCN also recommends obtaining a complete blood count in addition to liver, renal, and thyroid function testing.[76]

TABLE 13.7 Basic workup and testing for choriocarcinoma.

Component of workup	Specific tests/considerations
Physical exam	Pelvic and abdominal exams
Tumor markers	β-hCG
Imaging	TVUS, CXR, CT C/A/P; add MRI brain if pulmonary metastases present
Diagnostic tests	Dilation and curettage or hysterectomy

CXR: chest radiograph; *CT C/A/P*: computed tomography of chest/abdomen/pelvis; *TVUS*: transvaginal ultrasound.

Staging system

Anatomic staging for choriocarcinoma follows the FIGO staging system for gestational trophoblastic disease (Table 13.8). Stage I disease is confined to the uterus. Stage II disease reflects metastases to the vagina or other gynecologic organs. Stage III disease refers specifically to lung metastases, while stage IV disease refers to other visceral spread.

Prognostic factors

A prognostic scoring index has been developed for GTN based on individual risk factors that have been shown to be predictive of resistance to single-agent chemotherapy[34,74,77,78] (Table 13.9). Factors that portend a more favorable prognosis include age < 40, antecedent pregnancy of HM (versus abortion or term pregnancy), <4 months from pregnancy, pretreatment β-hCG <1000 IU/L, largest tumor size <3 cm (including uterus), and no metastases; however, if present, those with metastases to lung (versus spleen/kidney, GI tract, brain/liver) have more favorable prognoses.

A total score < 7 indicates low-risk GTN, whereas a total score of ≥7 indicates high-risk GTN. A clinicopathologic diagnosis of choriocarcinoma should be considered a poor prognostic factor in low-risk GTN, as choriocarcinoma is associated with initial treatment failure in this cohort.[67]

Treatment of primary disease

Choriocarcinoma is uniquely sensitive to chemotherapy, which is the major treatment modality. In the treatment of high-risk disease, other modalities such as surgery and radiation therapy may be indicated.

In the setting of low-risk disease (based on prognostic scoring outlined above), treatment can start with single-agent chemotherapy with methotrexate or dactinomycin (Fig. 13.6). There is no consensus in the literature regarding which chemotherapeutic agent is superior. Some prefer methotrexate as initial treatment due to similar efficacy, decreased toxicity, and increased cost effectiveness.[79–83] However, some studies, including a Cochrane meta-analysis that included six randomized controlled trials, have demonstrated higher cure rates for dactinomycin compared to methotrexate.[83,84] The standard dosing regimen for dactinomycin is a 5-day regimen (10–12 µg/kg or flat 0.5 mg dose IV, q2wk). Common methotrexate dosing includes both 5- and 8-day regimens. The 5-day regimen is 0.4 mg/kg IV or IM daily × 5 days, repeated every 2 weeks. The 8-day regimen is methotrexate 1.0–1.5 mg/kg IM on days 1, 3, 5, and 7, alternating with folinic acid (leucovorin) 15 mg PO on days 2, 4, 6, and 8, repeated every 14 days.[85] Treatment should continue until complete remission

TABLE 13.8 FIGO anatomic staging of GTD.

FIGO anatomic staging
Stage I: Disease is only in the uterus
Stage II: GTD extends outside the uterus but is limited to the genital structures.
Stage III: GTD extends to the lungs and may or may not involve the genital tract.
Stage IV: GTD has extended to other distant sites.

TABLE 13.9 Prognostic scoring index for GTN[34,75].

	Risk score			
Prognostic factor	**0**	**1**	**2**	**4**
Age (years)	<40	≥40	–	–
Antecedent pregnancy	Hydatidiform mole	Abortion	Term pregnancy	–
Interval from index pregnancy (months)	<4	4–6	7–12	>12
Pretreatment β-hCG (IU/L)	$<10^3$	10^3 to $<10^4$	10^4 to 10^5	$\geq10^5$
Largest tumor size, including uterus (cm)	<3	3–5	>5	–
Site of metastases	Lung	Spleen, kidney	Gastrointestinal tract	Brain, liver
Number of metastases	0	1–4	5–8	>8
Previous failed chemotherapy	–	–	Single drug	Two or more drugs
Total score	–	–	–	–

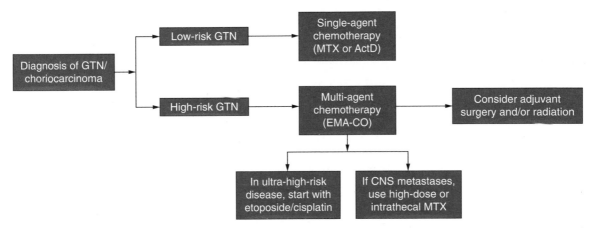

FIG. 13.6 Treatment of newly diagnosed uterine choriocarcinoma. *GTN*: gestational trophoblastic neoplasm; *MTX*: methotrexate; *ActD*: dactinomycin; *CNS*: central nervous system; *EMA-CO*: etoposide, methotrexate, actinomycin D, cyclophosphamide, vincristine.

is obtained (hCG level remains undetectable for 3 consecutive weeks); after remission, consolidation therapy (three additional courses) should be administrated to prevent relapse.[86]

Based on data that initial treatment failure is higher in low-risk choriocarcinoma (compared to invasive mole), one may consider going straight to a multiagent chemotherapy regimen in the setting of choriocarcinoma regardless of prognostic score.[67]

The initial approach to high-risk GTN, defined as stages II–III disease with a prognostic score ≥ 7 or stage IV disease, is multiagent chemotherapy with or without adjuvant surgery or radiation. The preferred regimen is etoposide, methotrexate (MTX), plus dactinomycin (ActD) alternating with cyclophosphamide and vincristine (EMA-CO). This regimen has demonstrated complete response rates of 62%–78% and long-term survival of 85%–94%.[87–94] Compared to other less frequently used regimens including MA (MTX, ActD), CHAMOCA (MTX, ActD, cyclophosphamide, doxorubicin, melphalan, hydroxyurea, vincristine), and MAC (MTX, ActD, chlorambucil), EMA-CO has demonstrated higher remission rates and lower mortality, supporting its use as primary treatment for high-risk GTN.[95] EMA-CO should be administrated every 2–3 weeks until the hCG level becomes undetectable and remains undetectable for 3 consecutive weeks, followed by three cycles of consolidation therapy as with single-agent regimens.[86] The following standard dosing regimen can be used for EMA-CO[88]:

Etoposide – 100 mg/m^2 IV over 30 min on days 1 and 2.
MTX – 100 mg/m^2 IV bolus followed by 200 mg/m^2 IV over 12 h on day 1.
ActD – 0.5 mg IV bolus on days 1 and 2.
Leucovorin calcium – 15 mg orally every 12 h for four doses, starting 24 h after start of MTX.
Cyclophosphamide – 600 mg/m^2 IV on day 8.
Vincristine – 1.0 mg/m^2 IV on day 8.

In ultra-high-risk disease, defined as widespread metastatic disease with prognostic score $\geq$ 12, initiation of standard combination chemotherapy can lead to tumor collapse with hemorrhage, acidosis, septicemia, multiple organ failure, and rapid mortality. Therefore, induction chemotherapy with etoposide and cisplatin is recommended prior to initiating EMA/CO. The dosing is etoposide 100 mg /m^2 IV and cisplatin 20 mg/m^2 IV on days 1 and 2, every 7 days for 1–3 courses.[87,96]

In cases of central nervous system metastases (20% of patients with choriocarcinoma), first line treatment should include combination chemotherapy plus consideration of whole brain irradiation, stereotactic radiosurgery, and/or craniotomy with surgical excision.[97–101] Additionally, EMA/CO should be modified to include high-dose MTX (1 g/m^2) or addition of intrathecal MTX.[85,100]

Hysterectomy can be considered as a primary treatment modality in patients with stage I choriocarcinoma if fertility preservation is not desired to avoid toxicity associated with chemotherapy, with cure rates not quite as high as with chemotherapy but still over 80%.[102–104] This should be combined with one course of single-agent chemotherapy at the time of hysterectomy to increase remission rates.[105]

Surveillance for recurrence

During treatment, β-hCG level should be assessed every 1–2 weeks. Upon normalization of β-hCG and completion of therapy, β-hCG level should be checked monthly for a year, combined with reliable contraception, with oral contraception preferred.[63,66,85,106] This should be combined with routine history and physical exam to evaluate for any new symptoms or exam findings concerning for recurrent disease.

Survival and patterns of failure

Low risk choriocarcinoma is associated with a survival of almost 100% in women treated with chemotherapy, while high-risk choriocarcinoma patients have 91%–93% survival after multi-agent chemotherapy with or without radiation and surgery.[62]

There are two different types of treatment failure: (1) good initial response followed by plateau or rapid rise in β-hCG level (>10% change), and (2) poor response to initial therapy. Chemotherapy resistance is indicated by a plateau in β-hCG over 3 consecutive cycles or a rise in β-hCG over two consecutive cycles.[63,75,106] For disease that is resistant to single-agent chemotherapy, assessment of metastatic disease should be repeated and patients should be transitioned to second-line chemotherapy.[62,66] About 30%–40% of high-risk GTN patients will have an incomplete response to first-line therapy or experience relapse from remission.[107,108]

Treatment of recurrent disease

For low-risk GTN, there are no randomized controlled trial data on second-line therapy. In cases of a good response to initial therapy followed by β-hCG plateau or re-elevation, one can consider switching to the single agent chemotherapeutic not used initially (MTX or dactinomycin) and consider hysterectomy with salpingectomy; if the patient continues to have plateau or rise in β-hCG, initiation of a multi-agent chemotherapy regimen should be considered as the next step (Table 13.10). In cases of a good response to initial therapy followed by a rapid rise in β-hCG level or in cases of a poor response to initial therapy, the recommendation is to move straight to multi-agent chemotherapy (EMA/CO).[75,87,109,110]

For high-risk GTN, treatment considerations in the setting of recurrent disease include adjuvant surgery, interventional procedures for symptom control, and salvage chemotherapy. Adjuvant surgery is especially useful for patients with isolated disease in the uterus or lungs with hysterectomy or thoracotomy, respectively.[104,111,112] Interventional procedures, including selective arterial embolization, may be utilized in this patient population to prevent or control hemorrhage if clinically indicated.[113–115] Salvage chemotherapy drug combination regimens that have been utilized with success often employ etoposide and a platinum agent with methotrexate and actinomycin D (EMA-EP), bleomycin (BEP), ifosfamide (VIP, ICE) or paclitaxel (TP/TE).[116,117] Salvage therapy with one of these regimens, often in conjunction with surgery and brain radiation, was successful in achieving cure in 80%–90% of high-risk GTN patients.[116,118]

TABLE 13.10 Treatment of recurrence for choriocarcinoma.

Risk category	Treatment options for recurrent disease	Specific regimens/agents
Low-risk GTN	Alternative single agent chemotherapeutic	MTX or ActD
	Multi-agent chemotherapy regimen	EMA-CO
High-risk GTN	Adjuvant surgery	Hysterectomy or thoracotomy if isolated recurrence
	Salvage chemotherapy	EMA-EP, BEP, VIP, ICE, or TP/TE
All GTN	Immunotherapy	Pembrolizumab

ActD: dactinomycin; *BEP*: bleomycin, etoposide, and cisplatin; *EMA-CO*: etoposide, methotrexate, dactinomycin, alternating with cyclophosphamide and vincristine; *EMA-EP*: etoposide, methotrexate, dactinomycin, alternating with etoposide and cisplatin; *GTN*: gestational trophoblastic neoplasia; *MTX*: methotrexate; *ICE*: ifosfamide, carboplatin, etoposide; *VIP*: etoposide, ifosfamide, cisplatin; *TP/TE*: paclitaxel/cisplatin alternating with paclitaxel/etoposide.

A chemotherapy regimen including paclitaxel, ifosfamide, and cisplatin (TIP) has been used for salvage chemotherapy in germ cell tumors, including those with choriocarcinoma components, with acceptable cure rate and safety profile demonstrated in multiple studies.[60,119–121] This regimen may therefore be considered in the setting of recurrent gestational choriocarcinoma.

A case series has been published investigating the use of pembrolizumab, a PD-L1 inhibitor, for drug-resistant GTN. The two patients with choriocarcinoma in the series remained in remission 5–24 months after treatment completion.[122] Further research is needed to elucidate the potential role of immunotherapy in the treatment of chemotherapy-resistant choriocarcinoma.

References

1. Pocrnich CE, Ramalingam P, Euscher ED, Malpica A. Neuroendocrine carcinoma of the endometrium: a Clinicopathologic study of 25 cases. *Am J Surg Pathol.* 2016;40:577–586.
2. Matsumoto H, Shimokawa M, Nasu K, et al. Clinicopathologic features, treatment, prognosis and prognostic factors of neuroendocrine carcinoma of the endometrium: a retrospective analysis of 42 cases from the Kansai clinical oncology group/Intergroup study in Japan. *J Gynecol Oncol.* 2019;30, e103.
3. Schlechtweg K, Chen L, St Clair CM, et al. Neuroendocrine carcinoma of the endometrium: disease course, treatment, and outcomes. *Gynecol Oncol.* 2019;155:254–261.
4. Atienza-Amores M, Guerini-Rocco E, Soslow RA, Park KJ, Weigelt B. Small cell carcinoma of the gynecologic tract: a multifaceted spectrum of lesions. *Gynecol Oncol.* 2014;134:410–418.
5. Chun YK. Neuroendocrine tumors of the female reproductive tract: a literature review. *J Pathol Transl Med.* 2015;49:450–461.
6. Hu R, Jiang J, Song G, et al. Mixed large and small cell neuroendocrine carcinoma of the endometrium with serous carcinoma: a case report and literature review. *Medicine.* 2019;98, e16433.
7. Howitt BE, Kelly P, McCluggage WG. Pathology of neuroendocrine tumors of the female genital tract. *Curr Oncol Rep.* 2017;19:59.
8. Mulvany NJ, Allen DG. Combined large cell neuroendocrine and endometrioid carcinoma of the endometrium. *Int J Gynecol Pathol.* 2008;27:49–57.
9. Howitt BE, Dong F, Vivero M, et al. Molecular characterization of neuroendocrine carcinomas of the endometrium representation of all 4 TCGA groups. *Am J Surg Pathol.* 2020;44:1541–1548.
10. Jenny C, Kimball K, Kilgore L, Boone J. Large cell neuroendocrine carcinoma of the endometrium: a report and review of the literature. *Gynecol Oncol Rep.* 2019;28:96–100.
11. Sato H, Kanai G, Kajiwara H, Itoh J, Osamura RY. Small-cell carcinoma of the endometrium presenting as Cushing's syndrome. *Endocr J.* 2010;57:31–38.
12. Meydanli MM, Erguvan R, Altinok MT, Ataoglu O, Kafkasli A. Rare case of neuroendocrine small cell carcinoma of the endometrium with paraneoplastic membranous glomerulonephritis. *Tumori.* 2003;89:213–217.
13. Abaid LN, Cupp JS, Brown 3rd JV, Goldstein BH. Primary small cell neuroendocrine carcinoma of the endometrium. *Case Rep Oncol.* 2012;5:439–443.
14. Akgor U, Kuru O, Sakinci M, et al. Neuroendocrine carcinoma of the endometrium: a very rare gynecologic malignancy. *J Gynecol Obstet Hum Reprod.* 2020;101897.
15. Tu YA, Chen YL, Lin MC, Chen CA, Cheng WF. Large cell neuroendocrine carcinoma of the endometrium: a case report and literature review. *Taiwan J Obstet Gynecol.* 2018;57:144–149.
16. Se Hyun Nam WYK. Comparison of surgical outcomes between laparoscopy and laparotomy for early-stage ovarian cancer. *Eur J Gynaecol Oncol.* 2019;40:262–267.

17. Brudie LA, Khan F, Radi MJ, Ahmad S. Serous carcinoma of endometrium in combination with neuroendocrine small-cell: a case report and literature review. *Gynecol Oncol Rep.* 2016;17:79–82.

18. Satoh T, Takei Y, Treilleux I, et al. Gynecologic Cancer InterGroup (GCIG) consensus review for small cell carcinoma of the cervix. *Int J Gynecol Cancer.* 2014;24:S102–S108.

19. Zivanovic O, Leitao Jr MM, Park KJ, et al. Small cell neuroendocrine carcinoma of the cervix: analysis of outcome, recurrence pattern and the impact of platinum-based combination chemotherapy. *Gynecol Oncol.* 2009;112:590–593.

20. Eba J, Kenmotsu H, Tsuboi M, et al. A phase III trial comparing irinotecan and cisplatin with etoposide and cisplatin in adjuvant chemotherapy for completely resected pulmonary high-grade neuroendocrine carcinoma (JCOG1205/1206). *Jpn J Clin Oncol.* 2014;44:379–382.

21. Matsumoto H, Takai N, Nasu K, Narahara H. Small cell carcinoma of the endometrium: a report of two cases. *J Obstet Gynaecol Res.* 2011;37:1739–1743.

22. Sawada M, Matsuzaki S, Yoshino K, et al. Long-term survival in small-cell carcinoma of the endometrium with liver and brain metastases. *Anticancer Drugs.* 2016;27:138–143.

23. Makihara N, Maeda T, Nishimura M, et al. Large cell neuroendocrine carcinoma originating from the uterine endometrium: a report on magnetic resonance features of 2 cases with very rare and aggressive tumor. *Rare Tumors.* 2012;4, e37.

24. Matsumoto H, Nasu K, Kai K, Nishida M, Narahara H, Nishida H. Combined large-cell neuroendocrine carcinoma and endometrioid adenocarcinoma of the endometrium: a case report and survey of related literature. *J Obstet Gynaecol Res.* 2016;42:206–210.

25. Shepherd FA, Evans WK, MacCormick R, Feld R, Yau JC. Cyclophosphamide, doxorubicin, and vincristine in etoposide- and cisplatin-resistant small cell lung cancer. *Cancer Treat Rep.* 1987;71:941–944.

26. O'Brien ME, Ciuleanu TE, Tsekov H, et al. Phase III trial comparing supportive care alone with supportive care with oral topotecan in patients with relapsed small-cell lung cancer. *J Clin Oncol.* 2006;24:5441–5447.

27. Frumovitz M, Burzawa JK, Byers LA, et al. Sequencing of mutational hotspots in cancer-related genes in small cell neuroendocrine cervical cancer. *Gynecol Oncol.* 2016;141:588–591.

28. Lai ZY, Yeo HY, Chen YT, et al. PI3K inhibitor enhances the cytotoxic response to etoposide and cisplatin in a newly established neuroendocrine cervical carcinoma cell line. *Oncotarget.* 2017;8:45323–45334.

29. Lyons YA, Frumovitz M, Soliman PT. Response to MEK inhibitor in small cell neuroendocrine carcinoma of the cervix with a KRAS mutation. *Gynecol Oncol Rep.* 2014;10:28–29.

30. Allen JW, Moon J, Redman M, et al. Southwest oncology group S0802: a randomized, phase II trial of weekly topotecan with and without ziv-aflibercept in patients with platinum-treated small-cell lung cancer. *J Clin Oncol.* 2014;32:2463–2470.

31. Byers LA, Wang J, Nilsson MB, et al. Proteomic profiling identifies dysregulated pathways in small cell lung cancer and novel therapeutic targets including PARP1. *Cancer Discov.* 2012;2:798–811.

32. Spigel DR, Townley PM, Waterhouse DM, et al. Randomized phase II study of bevacizumab in combination with chemotherapy in previously untreated extensive-stage small-cell lung cancer: results from the SALUTE trial. *J Clin Oncol.* 2011;29:2215–2222.

33. Morabito A, Carillio G, Daniele G, et al. Treatment of small cell lung cancer. *Crit Rev Oncol Hematol.* 2014;91:257–270.

34. Paraghamian SE, Longoria TC, Eskander RN. Metastatic small cell neuroendocrine carcinoma of the cervix treated with the PD-1 inhibitor, nivolumab: a case report. *Gynecol Oncol Res Pract.* 2017;4:3.

35. Abhilasha N, Bafna UD, Pallavi VR, Rathod PS, Krishnappa S. Primary yolk sac tumor of the endometrium: a rare entity. *Indian J Cancer.* 2014;51:446.

36. Clement PB, Young RH, Scully RE. Extraovarian pelvic yolk sac tumors. *Cancer.* 1988;62:620–626.

37. Qzler A, Dogan S, Mamedbeyli G, et al. Primary yolk sac tumor of endometrium: report of two cases and review of literature. *J Exp Ther Oncol.* 2015;11:5–9.

38. Pileri S, Martinelli G, Serra L, Bazzocchi F. Endodermal sinus tumor arising in the endometrium. *Obstet Gynecol.* 1980;56:391–396.

39. Nawa A, Obata N, Kikkawa F, et al. Prognostic factors of patients with yolk sac tumors of the ovary. *Am J Obstet Gynecol.* 2001;184:1182–1188.

40. Joseph MG, Fellows FG, Hearn SA. Primary endodermal sinus tumor of the endometrium. A clinicopathologic, immunocytochemical, and ultrastructural study. *Cancer.* 1990;65:297–302.

41. Ravishankar S, Malpica A, Ramalingam P, et al. Yolk sac tumor in extragonadal pelvic sites: still a diagnostic challenge. *Am J Surg Pathol.* 2017;41:1–11.

42. Fadare O, Shaker N, Alghamdi A, et al. Endometrial tumors with yolk sac tumor-like morphologic patterns or immunophenotypes: an expanded appraisal. *Mod Pathol.* 2019;32:1847–1860.

43. Simpson S, Simoni M, Hui P, et al. Extragonadal yolk sac tumor limited to the myometrium: report of a case with potential fertility preservation and molecular analysis suggesting germ cell origin. *Int J Gynecol Pathol.* 2020;39:247–253.

44. Acosta AM, Sholl LM, Cin PD, et al. Malignant tumours of the uterus and ovaries with Mullerian and germ cell or trophoblastic components have a somatic origin and are characterised by genomic instability. *Histopathology.* 2020;77(5):788–797.

45. Ohta M, Sakakibara K, Mizuno K, et al. Successful treatment of primary endodermal sinus tumor of the endometrium. *Gynecol Oncol.* 1988;31:357–364.

46. Rossi R, Stacchiotti D, Bernardini MG, Calvieri G, Lo VR. Primary yolk sac tumor of the endometrium: a case report and review of the literature. *Am J Obstet Gynecol.* 2011;204:e3–e4.

47. Song L, Wei X, Wang D, et al. Primary yolk sac tumor originating from the endometrium: a case report and literature review. *Medicine.* 2019;98, e15144.

48. Spatz A, Bouron D, Pautier P, Castaigne D, Duvillard P. Primary yolk sac tumor of the endometrium: a case report and review of the literature. *Gynecol Oncol.* 1998;70:285–288.

49. Wang C, Li G, Xi L, Gu M, Ma D. Primary yolk sac tumor of the endometrium. *Int J Gynaecol Obstet.* 2011;114:291–293.

50. Li JK, Yang KX, Zheng Y. Endometrial yolk sac tumor with omental metastasis. *Chin Med J (Engl).* 2017;130:2007–2008.

51. Lu T, Qi L, Ma Y, Lu G, Zhang X, Liu P. Primary yolk sac tumor of the endometrium: a case report and review of the literatures. *Arch Gynecol Obstet.* 2019;300:1177–1187.

52. Lin SW, Hsieh SW, Huang SH, Liang HS, Huang CY. Yolk sac tumor of endometrium: a case report and literature review. *Taiwan J Obstet Gynecol.* 2019;58:846–848.

53. Ji M, Lu Y, Guo L, Feng F, Wan X, Xiang Y. Endometrial carcinoma with yolk sac tumor-like differentiation and elevated serum β-hCG: a case report and literature review. *Onco Targets Ther.* 2013;6:1515–1522.

54. Pasternack T, Shaco-Levy R, Wiznitzer A, Piura B. Extraovarian pelvic yolk sac tumor: case report and review of published work. *J Obstet Gynaecol Res.* 2008;34:739–744.

55. Patsner B. Primary endodermal sinus tumor of the endometrium presenting as "recurrent" endometrial adenocarcinoma. *Gynecol Oncol.* 2001;80:93–95.

56. Oguri H, Sumitomo R, Maeda N, Fukaya T, Moriki T. Primary yolk sac tumor concomitant with carcinosarcoma originating from the endometrium: case report. *Gynecol Oncol.* 2006;103:368–371.

57. Zhang GM, Guo XX, Ma XB, Zhang GM. Reference intervals of alpha-fetoprotein and carcinoembryonic antigen in the apparently healthy population. *Med Sci Monit.* 2016;22:4875–4880.

58. Umezu T, Kajiyama H, Terauchi M, et al. Long-term outcome and prognostic factors for yolk sac tumor of the ovary. *Nagoya J Med Sci.* 2008;70:29–34.

59. NCCN. *Clinical Practice Guidelines in Oncology: Ovarian Cancer (Version 2.2019);* 2019.

60. Kondagunta GV, Bacik J, Donadio A, et al. Combination of paclitaxel, ifosfamide, and cisplatin is an effective second-line therapy for patients with relapsed testicular germ cell tumors. *J Clin Oncol.* 2005;23:6549–6555.

61. Einhorn LH, Williams SD, Chamness A, Brames MJ, Perkins SM, Abonour R. High-dose chemotherapy and stem-cell rescue for metastatic germ-cell tumors. *N Engl J Med.* 2007;357:340–348.

62. Lurain JR. Gestational trophoblastic disease II: classification and management of gestational trophoblastic neoplasia. *Am J Obstet Gynecol.* 2011;204:11–18.

63. Brown J, Naumann RW, Seckl MJ, Schink J. 15 years of progress in gestational trophoblastic disease: scoring, standardization, and salvage. *Gynecol Oncol.* 2017;144:200–207.

64. Lurain JR. Gestational trophoblastic disease I: epidemiology, pathology, clinical presentation and diagnosis of gestational trophoblastic disease, and management of hydatidiform mole. *Am J Obstet Gynecol.* 2010;203:531–539.

65. Lurain JR. Gestational trophoblastic tumors. *Semin Surg Oncol.* 1990;6:347–353.

66. Seckl MJ, Sebire NJ, Berkowitz RS. Gestational trophoblastic disease. *Lancet (London, England).* 2010;376:717–729.

67. Strohl AE, Lurain JR. Postmolar choriocarcinoma: an independent risk factor for chemotherapy resistance in low-risk gestational trophoblastic neoplasia. *Gynecol Oncol.* 2016;141:276–280.

68. Savage J, Adams E, Veras E, et al. Choriocarcinoma in women analysis of a case series with genotyping. *Am J Surg Pathol.* 2017;41:1593–1606.

69. Hui P. Gestational trophoblastic tumors. *Arch Pathol Lab Med.* 2019;143:65–74.

70. Kalhor N, Ramirez PT, Deavers MT, et al. Immunohistochemical studies of trophoblastic tumors. *Am J Surg Pathol.* 2009;33:633–638.

71. Hirata Y, Yanaihara N, Yanagida S, et al. Molecular genetic analysis of nongestational choriocarcinoma in a postmenopausal woman: a case report and literature review. *Int J Gynecol Pathol.* 2012;31:364–368.

72. Ali TZ, Parwani AV. Benign and malignant neoplasms of the testis and Paratesticular tissue. *Surgical Pathol Clin.* 2009;2:61–159.

73. May T, Goldstein DP, Berkowitz RS. Current chemotherapeutic management of patients with gestational trophoblastic neoplasia. *Chemother Res Pract.* 2011;2011:806256.

74. FIGO Oncology Committee. FIGO staging for gestational trophoblastic neoplasia 2000. *Int J Gynaecol Obstet.* 2002;77:285–287.

75. NCCN. *Clinical Practice Guidelines in Oncology: Gestational Trophoblastic Neoplasia (Version 2.2020);* 2020.

76. Rotmensch S, Cole LA. False diagnosis and needless therapy of presumed malignant disease in women with false-positive human chorionic gonadotropin concentrations. *Lancet (London, England).* 2000;355:712–715.

77. Ngan HY, Bender H, Benedet JL, Jones H, Montruccoli GC, Pecorelli S. Gestational trophoblastic neoplasia, FIGO 2000 staging and classification. *Int J Gynaecol Obstet.* 2003;83(Suppl 1):175–177.

78. Goldstein DP, Berkowitz RS, Horowitz NS. Optimal management of low-risk gestational trophoblastic neoplasia. *Expert Rev Anticancer Ther.* 2015;15:1293–1304.

79. Yarandi F, Mousavi A, Abbaslu F, et al. Five-day intravascular methotrexate versus biweekly Actinomycin-D in the treatment of low-risk gestational trophoblastic neoplasia: a clinical randomized trial. *Int J Gynecol Cancer.* 2016;26:971–976.

80. Schink JC, Filiaci V, Huang HQ, et al. An international randomized phase III trial of pulse actinomycin-D versus multi-day methotrexate for the treatment of low risk gestational trophoblastic neoplasia; NRG/GOG 275. *Gynecol Oncol.* 2020;158:354–360.

81. Garrett AP, Garner EO, Goldstein DP, Berkowitz RS. Methotrexate infusion and folinic acid as primary therapy for nonmetastatic and low-risk metastatic gestational trophoblastic tumors. 15 years of experience. *J Reprod Med.* 2002;47:355–362.

82. Shah NT, Barroilhet L, Berkowitz RS, Goldstein DP, Horowitz N. A cost analysis of first-line chemotherapy for low-risk gestational trophoblastic neoplasia. *J Reprod Med.* 2012;57:211–218.

83. Lawrie TA, Alazzam M, Tidy J, Hancock BW, Osborne R. First-line chemotherapy in low-risk gestational trophoblastic neoplasia. *Cochrane Database Syst Rev.* 2016;2016, Cd007102.

84. Osborne RJ, Filiaci V, Schink JC, et al. Phase III trial of weekly methotrexate or pulsed dactinomycin for low-risk gestational trophoblastic neoplasia: a gynecologic oncology group study. *J Clin Oncol.* 2011;29:825–831.

85. Ngan HYS, Seckl MJ, Berkowitz RS, et al. Update on the diagnosis and management of gestational trophoblastic disease. *Int J Gynaecol Obstet.* 2018;143(Suppl 2):79–85.

86. Lybol C, Sweep FC, Harvey R, et al. Relapse rates after two versus three consolidation courses of methotrexate in the treatment of low-risk gestational trophoblastic neoplasia. *Gynecol Oncol.* 2012;125:576–579.

87. Alifrangis C, Agarwal R, Short D, et al. EMA/CO for high-risk gestational trophoblastic neoplasia: good outcomes with induction low-dose etoposide-cisplatin and genetic analysis. *J Clin Oncol.* 2013;31:280–286.

88. Lurain JR, Singh DK, Schink JC. Primary treatment of metastatic high-risk gestational trophoblastic neoplasia with EMA-CO chemotherapy. *J Reprod Med.* 2006;51:767–772.

89. Newlands ES, Bagshawe KD, Begent RH, Rustin GJ, Holden L. Results with the EMA/CO (etoposide, methotrexate, actinomycin D, cyclophosphamide, vincristine) regimen in high risk gestational trophoblastic tumours, 1979 to 1989. *Br J Obstet Gynaecol.* 1991;98:550–557.

90. Matsui H, Suzuka K, Iitsuka Y, Seki K, Sekiya S. Combination chemotherapy with methotrexate, etoposide, and actinomycin D for high-risk gestational trophoblastic tumors. *Gynecol Oncol.* 2000;78:28–31.

91. Escobar PF, Lurain JR, Singh DK, Bozorgi K, Fishman DA. Treatment of high-risk gestational trophoblastic neoplasia with etoposide, methotrexate, actinomycin D, cyclophosphamide, and vincristine chemotherapy. *Gynecol Oncol.* 2003;91:552–557.

92. Turan T, Karacay O, Tulunay G, et al. Results with EMA/CO (etoposide, methotrexate, actinomycin D, cyclophosphamide, vincristine) chemotherapy in gestational trophoblastic neoplasia. *Int J Gynecol Cancer.* 2006;16:1432–1438.

93. Lu WG, Ye F, Shen YM, et al. EMA-CO chemotherapy for high-risk gestational trophoblastic neoplasia: a clinical analysis of 54 patients. *Int J Gynecol Cancer.* 2008;18:357–362.

94. Cagayan MS. High-risk metastatic gestational trophoblastic neoplasia. Primary management with EMA-CO (etoposide, methotrexate, actinomycin D, cyclophosphamide and vincristine) chemotherapy. *J Reprod Med.* 2012;57:231–236.

95. Kim SJ, Bae SN, Kim JH, et al. Effects of multiagent chemotherapy and independent risk factors in the treatment of high-risk GTT–25 years experiences of KRI-TRD. *Int J Gynaecol Obstet.* 1998;60(Suppl 1):S85–S96.

96. Bolze PA, Riedl C, Massardier J, et al. Mortality rate of gestational trophoblastic neoplasia with a FIGO score of ≥13. *Am J Obstet Gynecol.* 2016;214. 390.e1–8.

97. Newlands ES, Holden L, Seckl MJ, McNeish I, Strickland S, Rustin GJ. Management of brain metastases in patients with high-risk gestational trophoblastic tumors. *J Reprod Med.* 2002;47:465–471.

98. Savage P, Kelpanides I, Tuthill M, Short D, Seckl MJ. Brain metastases in gestational trophoblast neoplasia: an update on incidence, management and outcome. *Gynecol Oncol.* 2015;137:73–76.

99. Gavanier D, Leport H, Massardier J, et al. Gestational trophoblastic neoplasia with brain metastasis at initial presentation: a retrospective study. *Int J Clin Oncol.* 2019;24:153–160.

100. Neubauer NL, Latif N, Kalakota K, et al. Brain metastasis in gestational trophoblastic neoplasia: an update. *J Reprod Med.* 2012;57:288–292.

101. Piura E, Piura B. Brain metastases from gestational trophoblastic neoplasia: review of pertinent literature. *Eur J Gynaecol Oncol.* 2014;35:359–367.

102. Clark RM, Nevadunsky NS, Ghosh S, Goldstein DP, Berkowitz RS. The evolving role of hysterectomy in gestational trophoblastic neoplasia at the New England trophoblastic disease center. *J Reprod Med.* 2010;55:194–198.

103. Bolze PA, Mathe M, Hajri T, et al. First-line hysterectomy for women with low-risk non-metastatic gestational trophoblastic neoplasia no longer wishing to conceive. *Gynecol Oncol.* 2018;150:282–287.

104. Alazzam M, Hancock BW, Tidy J. Role of hysterectomy in managing persistent gestational trophoblastic disease. *J Reprod Med.* 2008;53:519–524.

105. Goldstein DP, Berkowitz RS. Current management of gestational trophoblastic neoplasia. *Hematol Oncol Clin North Am.* 2012;26:111–131.

106. Mangili G, Lorusso D, Brown J, et al. Trophoblastic disease review for diagnosis and management: a joint report from the International Society for the Study of trophoblastic disease, European organisation for the treatment of trophoblastic disease, and the gynecologic Cancer InterGroup. *Int J Gynecol Cancer.* 2014;24:S109–S116.

107. Powles T, Savage PM, Stebbing J, et al. A comparison of patients with relapsed and chemo-refractory gestational trophoblastic neoplasia. *Br J Cancer.* 2007;96:732–737.

108. Hoekstra AV, Lurain JR, Rademaker AW, Schink JC. Gestational trophoblastic neoplasia: treatment outcomes. *Obstet Gynecol.* 2008;112:251–258.

109. Sita-Lumsden A, Short D, Lindsay I, et al. Treatment outcomes for 618 women with gestational trophoblastic tumours following a molar pregnancy at the Charing cross hospital, 2000-2009. *Br J Cancer.* 2012;107:1810–1814.

110. Alazzam M, Tidy J, Osborne R, Coleman R, Hancock BW, Lawrie TA. Chemotherapy for resistant or recurrent gestational trophoblastic neoplasia. *Cochrane Database Syst Rev.* 2016;2016, Cd008891.

111. Fleming EL, Garrett L, Growdon WB, et al. The changing role of thoracotomy in gestational trophoblastic neoplasia at the New England trophoblastic disease center. *J Reprod Med.* 2008;53:493–498.

112. Kanis MJ, Lurain JR. Pulmonary resection in the Management of High-Risk Gestational Trophoblastic Neoplasia. *Int J Gynecol Cancer.* 2016;26:796–800.

113. Lim AK, Agarwal R, Seckl MJ, Newlands ES, Barrett NK, Mitchell AW. Embolization of bleeding residual uterine vascular malformations in patients with treated gestational trophoblastic tumors. *Radiology.* 2002;222:640–644.

114. Tse KY, Chan KK, Tam KF, Ngan HY. 20-year experience of managing profuse bleeding in gestational trophoblastic disease. *J Reprod Med.* 2007;52:397–401.

115. McGrath S, Harding V, Lim AK, Burfitt N, Seckl MJ, Savage P. Embolization of uterine arteriovenous malformations in patients with gestational trophoblastic tumors: a review of patients at Charing cross hospital, 2000-2009. *J Reprod Med.* 2012;57:319–324.

116. Lurain JR, Schink JC. Importance of salvage therapy in the management of high-risk gestational trophoblastic neoplasia. *J Reprod Med.* 2012;57:219–224.

117. Mao Y, Wan X, Lv W, Xie X. Relapsed or refractory gestational trophoblastic neoplasia treated with the etoposide and cisplatin/etoposide, methotrexate, and actinomycin D (EP-EMA) regimen. *Int J Gynaecol Obstet.* 2007;98:44–47.

118. Anantharaju AA, Pallavi VR, Bafna UD, et al. Role of salvage therapy in chemo resistant or recurrent high-risk gestational trophoblastic neoplasm. *Int J Gynecol Cancer.* 2019;29:547–553.

119. Feldman DR, Hu J, Dorff TB, et al. Paclitaxel, Ifosfamide, and cisplatin efficacy for first-line treatment of patients with intermediate- or poor-risk germ cell tumors. *J Clin Oncol.* 2016;34:2478–2483.

120. Mardiak J, Rejlekova K, Mego M, et al. Determination of efficacy of TIP combination (paclitaxel, ifosfamide, cisplatin) as first salvage therapy for patients with relapsed germ cell tumors in a poor prognosis group. *J Clin Oncol.* 2009;27, e16049.

121. Motzer RJ, Sheinfeld J, Mazumdar M, et al. Paclitaxel, ifosfamide, and cisplatin second-line therapy for patients with relapsed testicular germ cell cancer. *J Clin Oncol.* 2000;18:2413–2418.

122. Ghorani E, Kaur B, Fisher RA, et al. Pembrolizumab is effective for drug-resistant gestational trophoblastic neoplasia. *Lancet (London, England).* 2017;390:2343–2345.

Section C

Cervical cancers

Chapter 14

High grade neuroendocrine carcinoma of the cervix

Gloria Salvo, Preetha Ramalingam, and Michael Frumovitz

Clinical case

A 32-year-old G0 female presents with a newly diagnosed small cell neuroendocrine carcinoma (NEC) of the cervix. On physical exam, she is noted to have a 1.5 cm lesion on the anterior lip of the cervix with no evidence of vaginal or parametrial involvement. MRI of the pelvis reveals an isolated 1 cm lesion on the anterior lip of the cervix and confirms no vaginal or parametrial involvement. A PET scan shows no evidence of metastatic disease (Fig. 14.1). The patient desires fertility sparing treatment for her disease. How do you treat this patient?

Epidemiology

Incidence and mortality

The broad category of NEC accounts for a variety of tumor subtypes. Carcinoid and atypical carcinoid tumors are considered low grade and most frequently found in the gastrointestinal (GI) tracks. Although there are case reports of these low grade tumors arising in the cervix, they are almost always metastatic sites from a GI primary and a full workup in search of a GI site should be undertaken.[1] In the cervix, almost all primary neuroendocrine tumors (NETs) are high grade lesions (see Section "Pathology").

High grade NEC of the cervix account for 1%–2% of cervical cancer diagnoses. The World Health Organization (WHO) further classifies high grade NEC of the cervix into two categories—small cell and large cell carcinomas. As there will be 14,480 cases of cervical cancer in the United States in 2021, a rough calculation will find approximately 150–200 cases/year for the entire country.[2] The median age at diagnosis for patients with high grade NEC of the cervix is 48 years old which is younger than the age for those women diagnosed with squamous or adenocarcinomas of the cervix.[3] Women with high grade NETs are also more likely to present with advanced stage disease than women with squamous or adenocarcinomas of the cervix. Although almost a third of patients will present with clinical stage I disease, an almost equivalent number will have stage IV disease at diagnosis (Table 14.1).[4]

Stage for stage, women with NEC have significantly worse outcomes than those with squamous or adenocarcinomas of the cervix (Table 14.1). Even in those women where disease is clinically limited to the cervix, the 5-year overall survival is only 55% compared to 80%–85% for squamous and adenocarcinomas of the cervix. This speaks to the aggressiveness of the disease as 40% of patients with tumors <4 cm and clinically limited to the cervix will have metastatic disease to pelvic nodes compared to only 10%–15% of similarly sized tumors that are squamous cell or adenocarcinoma histologies.[5] Women with early disease (stages IA–IIA) high grade NEC of the cervix have a hazard ratio for death of 2.96 when compared to patients with squamous cell carcinoma at the same stage. When comparing women with high grade neuroendocrine and squamous cell carcinomas of the cervix who have locally advanced disease (stages IIB–IVA), the hazard ratio for death is 1.70 if the patient has high grade NEC.[4]

Diagnosis and Treatment of Rare Gynecologic Cancers. https://doi.org/10.1016/B978-0-323-82938-0.00014-8

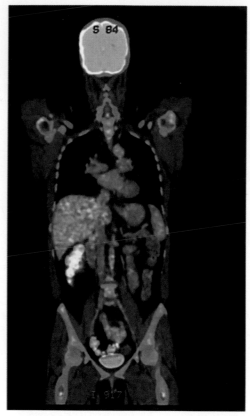
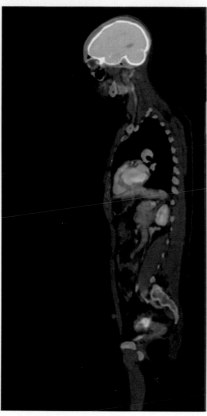

FIG. 14.1   PET/CT imaging (coronal and sagittal views) of patient with stage IB1 high grade neuroendocrine carcinoma of the cervix.

TABLE 14.1 Stage at diagnosis and overall survival of 1739 patients with high grade neuroendocrine carcinoma of the cervix.

Stage[a]	Percent of cases	5 Year overall survival
IA	2.8%	82%
IB	29.8%	55%
IIA	0.8%	—[b]
IIB	10.8%	22%
IIIA	1.4%	—[b]
IIIB	21.8%	24%
IVA	3.2%	4%
IVB	25.7%	7%
IV NOS	3.7%	

[a]Stage utilizing 2008 FIGO staging.
[b]Not enough patients to calculate.
Adapted from Margolis B, Tergas AI, Chen L, et al. Natural history and outcome of neuroendocrine carcinoma of the cervix. *Gynecol Oncol.* 2016;141(2):247–254. https:/doi.org/10.1016/j.ygyno.2016.02.008.

Etiology and risk factors

Risk factors and the etiology of high grade NEC of the cervix continue to be investigated. Whole exome sequencing has compared high grade NEC of the cervix to that same histology in the lung and bladder as well as to cervical squamous cell carcinoma and adenocarcinoma. Investigators found that tumor specimens from women with high grade NEC of the cervix were genetically more similar to the common HPV-associated cervical cancers (squamous and adenocarcinomas) than they were to the high grade NEC of the lung and bladder.[6] The role of HPV in the development of high grade neuroendocrine cervical cancer has been investigated. A meta-analysis found that 85% of patients with small cell neuroendocrine carcinoma (SCNEC) of the cervix were HPV positive with HPV18 being the most common subtype detected.[7] In women with large cell neuroendocrine carcinoma (LCNEC) of the cervix, 88% were found to have HPV with seemingly equal distributions of HPV16 and HPV18 detected. Although HPV may be detected in tumor samples from patients with high grade neuroendocrine cervical cancer, a causative relationship has not been clearly established as it has for squamous cell carcinoma and adenocarcinoma. As many high grade NEC are mixed with squamous and adenocarcinoma and as HPV is commonly found in sexually active women it is unknown whether the virus detected is simply a bystander infection or a causative agent in the disease process.

Pathology

Gross

The gross appearance of the tumor is variable and can be either small or large involving the entire cervix. The tumors can be polypoid or indurated with tan-white cut surface and necrosis.

Microscopic findings

The 2020 WHO Classification of Female Genital Tumors proposes a standardized nomenclature for all NETs, regardless of the site of involvement. While the etiology may differ at various anatomic sites (i.e., cervix, endometrium, and vulva) the histologic appearance is similar and these tumors should be classified uniformly. Neuroendocrine neoplasms are broadly classified as NET which encompasses low grade (grade 1) and intermediate grade tumors (grade 2), i.e., typical and atypical carcinoid; and high grade NEC that include SCNEC, LCNEC, and mixed carcinomas.

The discussion in this chapter is limited to high grade NEC. SCNEC is characterized by sheets of markedly atypical cells with high nuclear-cytoplasmic ratio, and hyperchromatic nuclei without prominent nucleoli (Fig. 14.2). Nuclei show "salt and pepper" chromatin, nuclear molding with marked crush artifact, numerous apoptotic bodies, geographic necrosis, and

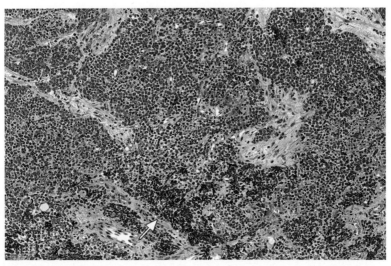

FIG. 14.2 Small cell neuroendocrine carcinoma showing tumor cells with high nuclear-cytoplasmic ratio and crush artifact (arrow).

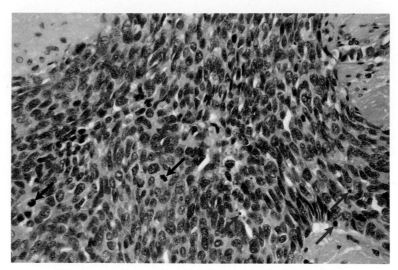

FIG. 14.3   Small cell neuroendocrine carcinoma showing tumor cells with high N/C ratio, salt and pepper chromatin, frequent mitoses (*black arrows*), and apoptotic bodies (*red arrows*).

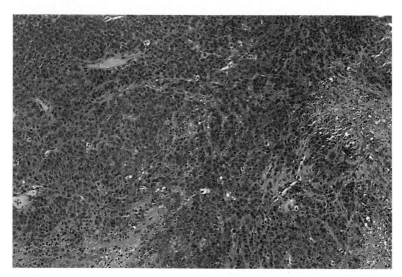

FIG. 14.4   Large cell neuroendocrine carcinoma showing nested and trabecular pattern composed of cells with moderate amounts of cytoplasm and prominent nucleoli.

frequent mitoses are typical (Fig. 14.3).[8] LCNEC on the other hand is composed of tumor cells that are arranged in a nested pattern, with moderate amounts of cytoplasm and prominent nucleoli (Fig. 14.4). Trabecular, pseudoglandular, and insular patterns are frequent.[9] NEC, either small or large cell type, may be admixed with other components such as adenocarcinoma or squamous carcinoma.

Ancillary testing

The diagnosis of NEC is made based on a combination of morphology and immunohistochemical stains. Markers of NEC include synaptophysin (Fig. 14.5A), chromogranin (Fig. 14.5B), CD56, neuron-specific enolase (NSE), and insulinoma-associated protein 1 (INSM1). CD56 and NSE are not very specific, and if they are the only positive markers a diagnosis of NEC should not be made in the absence of characteristic morphology. NEC are variably positive for cytokeratins and sometimes use of more than one keratin marker is necessary to confirm epithelial differentiation. NEC usually display block-like staining for p16, and the majority are positive for high-risk HPV. The latter supports a diagnosis of NEC, when epithelial markers are negative.

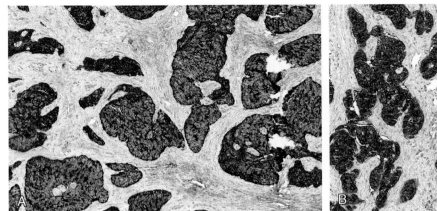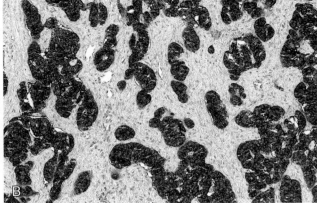

FIG. 14.5   Small cell neuroendocrine carcinoma showing diffuse staining for synaptophysin (A) and chromogranin (B).

Differential diagnosis

NEC can mimic poorly differentiated squamous carcinoma with small cell morphology, and the pseudoglandular pattern may be mistaken for adenocarcinoma. In curettage specimens they can also mimic high grade squamous intraepithelial lesion (HSIL). Making the distinction between squamous carcinomas with basaloid/small cell features and NEC can be challenging, and a low threshold to perform neuroendocrine stains is prudent when frequent mitoses and apoptotic bodies are seen, to ensure the correct diagnosis. Squamous carcinomas are diffusely positive for p40 and p63 and negative for neuroendocrine markers. Adenocarcinomas are more diffusely positive for keratin markers and negative for neuroendocrine marker expression. Another important differential diagnosis is primitive neuroectodermal tumor (PNET) as they have histologic overlap with NEC and express neuroendocrine markers. In such cases positivity for epithelial markers and high-risk HPV would support a diagnosis of NEC over PNET.

Molecular alterations

A subset of SCNEC can have recurrent genetic alterations in TP53/BRCA, PI3K/AKT/mTOR, and MAPK pathways. Loss of heterozygosity in the short arm of chromosome 3 (3p) has been reported.[10,11]

Diagnosis and workup

Signs and symptoms

Women with high grade NEC of the cervix may have their disease detected by routine Pap screening or gynecologic exam. In these patients, disease is typically asymptomatic. As this disease tends to effect younger women, some may have diagnosis made during pregnancy (see Section "Special considerations"). In those women who present with grossly evident disease, symptoms are similar to those found in patients with other large cervical tumors. These include postcoital bleeding, irregular bleeding, or discharge. Women with metastatic disease may experience pain or weight loss. Common sites for metastatic disease outside the pelvis include the liver, lung, and brain. Disease metastatic to these sites are typically asymptomatic but obviously large volume disease in the brain can cause significant neurologic symptoms.

Physical exam findings

For the minority of women with lesions found on screening cytology, physical exam may not reveal obvious abnormalities. However, most women will have grossly evident tumor on pelvic examination. In fact, over 80% of women will have a tumor >2 cm at time of presentation.[12] A thorough pelvic exam including a rectovaginal examination is important to determine extent of disease within the pelvis (Table 14.2). Physical exam findings are similar to those found in women with more common squamous cell or adenocarcinomas and largely related to extent of disease spread. For example, women with large, bulky tumors may have unilateral leg swelling/lymphedema if tumor has spread to pelvic lymph nodes or compresses the pelvic sidewall. As mentioned, common sites for metastatic disease outside the pelvis include the liver, lung, and brain. Disease in these sites may cause symptoms but are unlikely to present with findings on physical exam.

TABLE 14.2 Initial workup of newly diagnosed high grade neuroendocrine carcinoma of the cervix.

Physical exam	Complete physical exam with pelvic and rectovaginal examinations
Imaging	CT, PET, or PET/CT MRI pelvis MRI brain[a]
Laboratories	Serum neuron-specific enolase

[a]MRI of the brain only if patient has metastatic disease to liver and/or lung or neurologic symptoms.

Differential diagnosis

Accurate diagnosis of high grade NEC of the cervix is exceedingly important as therapeutic approaches are different than those for more common squamous cell and adenocarcinomas (see Section "Treatment of primary disease"). Most times the diagnosis will be made on pathologic review of cervical specimens (see Section "Pathology"). High grade NETs are frequently mixed with squamous cell or adenocarcinoma.[5] When both subtypes of cervix cancer are present, treatment recommendations should follow algorithms for the neuroendocrine component as opposed to the squamous cell or adenocarcinoma components of the mixed tumor. Clinicians should have a high level of suspicion for high grade NEC of the cervix in patients who present with widely metastatic disease particularly with multiple tumors in the liver and/or lung.

Primary NEC from other sites metastatic to the cervix should also be ruled out. As mentioned, primary carcinoid or atypical carcinoid tumors of the cervix are very rare, and a complete GI workup should be performed to rule out a GI source before assigning the cervix as primary site. For high grade NEC, isolated metastases from other primary sites to the cervix are equally rare. Therefore, high grade NEC found on just the cervix and in the lungs is likely a primary cervical lesion as opposed to a primary lung cancer. Small cell lung cancer will almost always spread to the liver, adrenal glands, bone, and brain before the cervix; however, small cell cervical cancer may metastasize to the lung before other sites of disease are evident.

Tumor markers

There are no validated serum tumor markers for women with high grade NEC of the cervix. However, as high grade NEC of the cervix are histologically similar to small cell lung cancer, some have suggested utilizing serum NSE as a tumor marker for these patients.[13] NSE is a neuro- and neuroendocrine-specific isoenzyme of enolase which localizes to neurons and neuroendocrine cells. This serum marker can be found elevated in people with several types of tumors of neuronal or neuroendocrine origin including small cell lung cancer. In patients with small cell lung cancer, serum NSE is frequently elevated at diagnosis, normalizes with response to primary therapy, and may rise again with recurrence. Small cell lung cancer patients with elevated serum NSE at diagnosis have worse progression free and overall survival compared to those with normal levels.[14]

Imaging studies

As a large percentage of women with high grade NEC of the cervix will have metastatic disease outside the pelvis at time of diagnosis, it is important to perform comprehensive imaging to determine disease stage and appropriate treatment recommendations (see Section "Treatment of primary disease"). As part of initial workup, all women with newly diagnosed disease should undergo either computed tomography (CT scan) of the chest, abdomen, and pelvis, positron emission tomography (PET scan) from skull to thigh, or a combined PET/CT scan. Although combination PET/CT scan is preferred by most, there are no studies showing that it is superior to CT scan in patients with high grade NEC of the cervix.

For patients with disease limited to the cervix, magnetic resonance imaging (MRI) of the pelvis should be performed to evaluate tumor size and to rule out parametrial involvement. In women with cervical cancer, this modality has been shown to be the more accurate in assessing tumor size and parametrial involvement than CT or PET scans.[15] Transrectal ultrasonography is another option for determining these factors; however, this approach requires technical experience and expertise not common at most centers.[16] Confirming that tumors are <4 cm in size without parametrial invasion, and no suspicious lymph nodes is important in determining who might be a surgical candidate (see Section "Treatment of primary disease").

Routine MRI of the brain at time of diagnosis is not necessary. Metastatic disease at initial diagnosis is a rare event with one retrospective study showing no occurrences in 31 patients.[17] However, it should be performed if the patient is having neurologic symptoms or if PET and/or CT scans detect metastatic disease in the liver and/or lung. Oligometastatic disease to the brain in the absence of disease spread to the liver, lung, or other sites is a rare event occurring in only 3% of patients.[18]

DOTATATE scans are frequently used to detect disease in patients with well and moderately differentiated NEC of the GI track. These scans utilize DOTA-peptides (DOTATAC, DOTANOC, and DOTATATE) that specifically bind to somatostatin receptors on the surface of GI NETs. In patients with somatostatin expressing tumors, DOTATATE scans have with a sensitivity of 97% in detection of metastatic disease and are more sensitive than CT scans.[19] Although there are no studies in the ability of DOTATATE to detect disease in women with high grade NEC of the cervix, it is unlikely that this type of scan would be of use in these patients as these tumors are almost always negative for the somatostatin receptor.[20]

Diagnostic testing

Similar to squamous cell and adenocarcinoma of the cervix, diagnosis of high grade NEC of the cervix is made pathologically with a biopsy. This is commonly a biopsy of grossly evident tumor on the cervix but may also require colposcope directed biopsies if an abnormality was detected on screening cytology. Occasionally a LEEP or cone specimen for what was thought to be squamous cell or adenocarcinoma will return with a high grade neuroendocrine component as almost 50% of women with high grade NEC will have a mixed tumor.[21] When this occurs, patients should be treated with the therapeutic approaches for high grade NEC as opposed to those for squamous cell or adenocarcinoma as the neuroendocrine component is significantly more aggressive and drives prognosis (see Section "Treatment of primary disease").

Staging system

Staging for high grade NEC of the cervix most commonly utilizes the FIGO staging system for cervical cancer (Table 14.3). Unlike prior versions of the FIGO staging system for cervical cancer, the 2018 version allows for incorporation of imaging and pathologic findings into the stage. This is an important improvement in regards to women with high grade NEC due to the high rate of metastatic disease to lymph nodes at diagnosis, it more accurately reflects true extent of disease as compared to the old staging system that was based solely on clinical findings. When considering treatment algorithms, early stage disease typically encompasses stages IA1–IB2 while locally advanced disease usually refers to stages IB3–IVA and metastatic disease is defined as stage IVB. The Tumor, Node, Metastasis (TNM) staging system (Table 14.4) may also be used to describe extent of disease but this is employed less often among gynecologic oncologists.

Prognostic factors

Clinical stage has been consistently shown to be the most important prognostic factor.[12,22–24] Early studies utilized the old FIGO staging system which only took into account clinical stage. When comparing patients by clinical stage, locally advanced disease (stages IIB–IVA) has a hazard ratio for death of 2.52 compared to early stage disease (stages IA–IIA).[12] When applying the more recent 2018 FIGO staging system to patients with these tumors, relative to patients with stage I disease, those with stage II have a hazard ratio for death of 1.4 those with stage III a hazard ratio of 2.8 and those with stage IV of 8.5.[24] Each of the individual components that make up the 2018 FIGO staging also predict prognosis. For example, T2 tumors have a hazard ratio for death of 1.9 compared to T1 tumors and T3/T4 tumors have a hazard ratio for death of 4.5 compared to T1 tumors. Compared to tumors <2 cm in size, tumors 2–4 cm in size have a hazard ratio for death of 2.2 and those with tumors >4 cm have a hazard ratio for death of 4.2. If pelvic lymph nodes are positive, the hazard ratio for death is 2.4 and if paraaortic nodes are positive, it rises to 4.5. Distant metastases increase the hazard ratio for death to 4.5 when compared to those with local disease only.[24]

For patients with local disease (stages I–II), studies comparing surgical resection to primary chemoradiation have shown conflicting results. In one study, patients who underwent primary radiation had a hazard ratio for death of 4.7 when compared to those who had primary surgery.[25] However, as this was a retrospective study that did not randomize patients to treatment, these data may be confounded by the fact that patients with early stage disease who were dispositioned to radiation instead of surgery may have had worrisome clinical findings such as poor performance status or larger tumors that did not allow for surgery. Additional studies have shown that the ability to treat with radical surgery predicts a better prognosis than those who did not have surgery.[12] Other studies, however, have not shown surgery to be superior to chemoradiation for early stage disease. In one study, 5-year failure free survival trended toward improvement with radiation over surgery (60.5% vs 41.2%, $P = 0.09$) while another study showed a significant improvement in those who underwent

TABLE 14.3 FIGO staging for cervical cancer.

Stage	Description
I	The carcinoma is strictly confined to the cervix (extension to the uterine corpus should be disregarded)
IA	Invasive carcinoma that can be diagnosed only by microscopy, with maximum depth of invasion <5mm[a]
IA1	Measured stromal invasion ≤3 mm in depth
IA2	Measured stromal invasion >3 mm and ≤5 mm in depth
IB	Invasive carcinoma with measured deepest invasion >5 mm (greater than Stage IA), lesion limited to the cervix uteri
IB1	Invasive carcinoma >5 mm depth of stromal invasion, and ≤2 cm in greatest dimension
IB2	Invasive carcinoma >2 cm and ≤4 cm in greatest dimension
IB3	Invasive carcinoma >4 cm in greatest dimension
II	The carcinoma invades beyond the uterus, but has not extended onto the lower third of the vagina or to the pelvic wall
IIA	Involvement limited to the upper two-thirds of the vagina without parametrial involvement
IIA1	Invasive carcinoma ≤4 cm in greatest dimension
IIA2	Invasive carcinoma >4 cm in greatest dimension
IIB	With parametrial involvement but not up to the pelvic wall
III	The carcinoma involves the lower third of the vagina and/or involves pelvic and/or para-aortic lymph nodes[b]
IIIA	The carcinoma involves the lower third of the vagina, with no extension to the pelvic wall
IIIB	Extension to the pelvic wall and/or hydronephrosis or nonfunctioning kidney (unless known to be due to another cause)
IIIC	Involvement of pelvic and/or para-aortic lymph nodes (including micrometastases), irrespective of tumor size and extent (with r and p notations)[b]
IIIC1	Pelvic lymph node metastasis only
IIIC2	Para-aortic lymph node metastasis
IV	The carcinoma has extended beyond the true pelvis or has involved (biopsy proven) the mucosa of the bladder or rectum. (A bullous edema, as such, does not permit a case to be allotted to Stage IV.)
IVA	Spread to adjacent pelvic organs
IVB	Spread to distant organs

International Federation of Gynecology and Obstetrics (FIGO) staging of cancer of the cervix uteri (2018).

When in doubt, the lower staging should be assigned.

[a]*Imaging and pathology can be used, where available, to supplement clinical findings with respect to tumor size and extent, in all stages.*
[b]*Adding notation of r (imaging) and p (pathology) to indicate the findings that are used to allocate the case to Stage IIIC. Example: If imaging indicates pelvic lymph node metastasis, the stage allocation would be Stage IIIC1r, and if confirmed by pathologic findings, it would be Stage IIIC1p. The type of imaging modality or pathology technique used should always be documents.*
The involvement of vascular/lymphatic spaces does not change the staging. The lateral extent of the lesion is no longer considered.
From: N. Bhatla, D. Aoki, D.N. Sharma, Sankaranarayanan R. *Cancer* of the cervix uteri. Int J Gynaecol Obstet 143 (2018) S2:22. Available at: https:/obgyn. onlinelibrary.wiley.com/doi/full/10.1002/igo.12611. Reproduced under the terms of the Creative Commons License 4.0. Updated with information from: Corrigendum to "Revised FIGO Staging for Carcinoma of the Cervix Uteri." Int J Gynaecol Obstet 147 (2019) 279.

chemoradiation instead of surgery (median event free survival not reached for radiation compared to 18 months for surgery, $P = 0.04$).[26] In both these studies, however, there was no difference in overall survival.

No matter what the primary treatment for early stage disease, the addition of concurrent or adjuvant chemotherapy is integral for reducing recurrence and death due to the high propensity for distant metastases at time of recurrence (see Section "Survival and patterns of failure"). For patients with early stage disease who undergo surgery, those who receive adjuvant chemotherapy have a hazard ratio for recurrence of 0.37 when compared to those who do not. In addition, patients seem to have better outcomes when chemotherapy regimens include cisplatin and etoposide and when patients receive ≥5 cycles.[27] After surgery for early stage disease, women who received ≥5 cycles of cisplatin and etoposide had a 5-year RFS of 68% compared to only 21% for those who received other treatments. Patients who received ≥5 cycles of other

TABLE 14.4 Cervix uteri TNM staging AJCC UICC 8th edition.

Primary tumor (T)	
T category	**T criteria**
TX	Primary tumor cannot be assessed
T0	No evidence of primary tumor
T1	Cervical carcinoma confined to the uterus (extension to corpus should be disregarded)
T1a	Invasive carcinoma diagnosed only by microscopy. Stromal invasion with a maximum depth of 5.0 mm measured from the base of the epithelium and a horizontal spread of 7.0 mm or less. Vascular space involvement, venous or lymphatic, does not affect classification
T1a1	Measured stromal invasion of 3.0 mm or less in depth and 7.0 mm or less in horizontal spread
T1a2	Measured stromal invasion of more than 3.0 mm and not more than 5.0 mm, with a horizontal spread of 7.0 mm or less
T1b	Clinically visible lesion confined to the cervix or microscopic lesion greater than T1a/IA2. Includes all macroscopically visible lesions, even those with superficial invasion
T1b1	Clinically visible lesion 4.0 cm or less in greatest dimension
T1b2	Clinically visible lesion more than 4.0 cm in greatest dimension
T2	Cervical carcinoma invading beyond the uterus but not the pelvic wall or to lower third of the vagina
T2a	Tumor without parametrial invasion
T2a1	Clinically visible lesion 4.0 cm or less in greatest dimension
T2a2	Clinically visible lesion more than 4.0 cm in greatest dimension
T2b	Tumor with parametrial invasion
T3	Tumor extending to the pelvic sidewall[a] and/or involving the lower third of the vagina and/or causing hydronephrosis or nonfunctioning kidney
T3a	Tumor involving the lower third of the vagina but not extending to the pelvic wall
T3b	Tumor extending to the pelvic wall and/or causing hydronephrosis or nonfunctioning kidney
T4	Tumor invading the mucosa of the bladder or rectum and/or extending beyond the true pelvis (bullous edema is not sufficient to classify a tumor as T4)
Regional lymph nodes (N)	
N category	**N criteria**
NX	Regional lymph nodes cannot be assessed
N0	No regional lymph node metastasis
N0(i+)	Isolated tumor cells in regional lymph node(s) no greater than 0.2 mm
N1	Regional lymph node metastasis
Distant metastasis (M)	
M category	**M criteria**
M0	No distant metastasis
M1	Distant metastasis (including peritoneal spread or involvement of the supraclavicular, mediastinal, or distant lymph nodes; lung; liver; or bone)

Continued

TABLE 14.4 Cervix uteri TNM staging AJCC UICC 8th edition—cont'd

Prognostic stage groups		
When T is...	And M is...	Then the stage group is...
T1	M0	I
T1a	M0	IA
T1a1	M0	IA1
T1a2	M0	IA2
T1b	M0	IB
T1b1	M0	IB1/2
T1b2	M0	IB3
T2	M0	II
T2a	M0	IIA
T2a1	M0	IIA1
T2a2	M0	IIA2
T2b	M0	IIB
T3	M0	III
T3a	M0	IIIA
T3b	M0	IIIB
T4	M0	IVA
Any T	M1	IVB

[a]*The pelvic sidewall is defined as the muscle, fascia, neurovascular structures, and skeletal portions of the bony pelvis. On rectal examination, there is no cancer-free space between the tumor and pelvic sidewall.*

From Bhatla N, Aoki D, Sharma DN, Sankaranarayanan R. Cancer of the cervix uteri. *Int J Gynaecol Obstet.* 2018;143(S2):22. Available at https:/obgyn.onlinelibrary.wiley.com/doi/full/10.1002/igo.12611. Reproduced under the terms of the Creative Commons License 4.0.Updated with information from Corrigendum to "Revised FIGO staging for carcinoma of the cervix uteri." *Int J Gynaecol Obstet.* 2019;147:279.
Used with permission of the American College of Surgeons, Chicago, IL. The original source for this information is the *AJCC Cancer Staging Manual.* 8th ed. Springer International Publishing; 2017.

chemotherapy regimens had a hazard ratio for recurrence of 3.4 compared to those who received ≥ 5 cycles of cisplatin and etoposide and those who received no chemotherapy after surgery had a hazard ratio for recurrence of 5.4 compared to those who received ≥ 5 cycles of cisplatin and etoposide.[27] Even for those patients with locally advanced disease undergoing chemoradiation, there appears to be an advantage of giving ≥ 5 cycles of cisplatin and etoposide. In one study, patients with stages IIB–IVB disease who received ≥ 5 cycles of cisplatin and etoposide concurrently with radiation had significantly better 5-year failure free survival (63% vs 13%) and 5-year cancer specific survival (75% vs 17%) when compared to women with similar stage disease who did not get ≥ 5 cycles of cisplatin and etoposide with their radiation.[26]

Treatment of primary disease

Primary therapy for women with high grade neuroendocrine is based on extent of disease at diagnosis. Patients can be categorized into three groups: early stage disease (stages IA1–IB2), locally advanced disease (stages IB3–IVA), and metastatic disease (stage IVB). General treatment algorithms for each of these groups can be seen in Fig. 14.6. Many of the treatment approaches and therapeutics utilized for primary therapy have been adopted from those used to treat small cell lung cancer as high grade NEC of the cervix appears to be similar histologically and in clinical behavior. In patients with small cell lung cancer, prophylactic brain irradiation is frequently recommended to address occult disease. However, for patients with high grade NEC of the cervix, this is not recommended as occult disease to the brain is rare in the absence of metastatic disease to the liver and/or lung.[18]

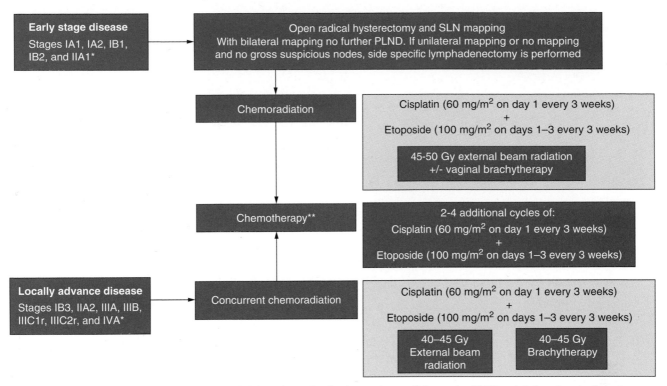

FIG. 14.6 Treatment algorithm for newly diagnosed high grade neuroendocrine carcinoma of the cervix. *PLND*: pelvic lymph node dissection.

Early stage disease

For patients with disease limited to the cervix and measuring <4 cm, open radical hysterectomy, bilateral salpingectomy, and lymph node assessment is typically the first recommended option.[5,28–30] As many patients will get postoperative radiation therapy, removal or transposition of the ovaries is recommended. Although there may be concern for transposing diseased ovaries out of the radiation field, the risk of isolated metastases to normal appearing ovaries in the absence of grossly metastatic disease elsewhere is low.[21]

Overall, patients with stage IA NEC of the cervix have a 5-year survival of 82% and those with stage IB disease a 5-year survival of 55% (Table 14.1). In one study, patients with early stage disease who forego surgery as part of their primary therapy were found to have a hazard ratio for death of 4.74 when compared to those who do have a surgical procedure.[25] In another study, patients who were able to have a radical hysterectomy for their disease had a 38% decrease in their risk of recurrence compared to those who did not.[12]

However, not all studies support surgery in the treatment of early stage high grade NEC of the cervix. In a study of 146 patients with stages IA–IIB small cell carcinoma of the cervix, Wang et al. reported patients who had surgery as part of their primary therapy for disease showed a trend toward worse disease-free survival (DFS) compared to those who had combination radiation and chemotherapy without surgery (41% vs 61%, $P = 0.09$).[26] In their population, 7 (78%) of 9 patients who underwent chemoradiation followed by additional chemotherapy were alive without evidence of recurrence. In another study, patients with stages I–IIA disease who underwent definitive chemoradiation instead of surgery had a significantly improved median DFS compared to those who had surgery.[18] However, this latter study only had 14 patients. Although there are some who might argue for chemoradiation in place of surgery for early stage disease, consensus among most experts and societies is that radical hysterectomy should be the initial treatment for patients with early stage disease (Table 14.5).

In addition to surgery, postoperative chemotherapy is an integral part of treatment for early stage disease and should be a part of adjuvant therapy for every patient. Patients with early stage disease who recur after surgery will have a distant component 86% of the time.[31] Common sites of recurrence include the lung, liver, and the peritoneal cavity (see "Survival and patterns of recurrence" below). Patients who receive chemotherapy after surgery have a 3-year distant RFS of 83% compared to 0% for those who do not ($P = 0.03$).[31] Three-year overall survival is also higher at 83% for those who received adjuvant chemotherapy as compared to only 20% for those who do not.

TABLE 14.5 Summary of treatment guidelines published to date.

	SGO	GCIG	Italy	MDACC
Stages IA1–IB2, IIA1 (<4 cm)				
Surgery for tumors <4 cm	+	+	+	+
Postoperative chemotherapy	+	+	+	+
Postoperative radiotherapy	+/−	+/−	+/−	+
Stages IB3–IIA2 (≥4 cm)				
Neoadjuvant chemo followed by surgery	+/−	+	+	−
Stages IIB–IVA				
Chemoradiation followed by chemotherapy	+	+	+	+

SGO: Society of Gynecologic Oncology; *GCIG*: Gynecologic Cancer InterGroup; *MDACC*: MD Anderson.

Although no prospective studies have compared chemotherapeutic agents, cisplatin and etoposide are the most commonly utilized based on their known activity in patients with small cell lung cancer. The standard dosing for this regimen is cisplatin is 60 mg/m^2 on day 1 and etoposide 120 mg/m^2 on days 1–3 on a 21-day cycle. For patients receiving postoperative radiation in addition to chemotherapy, the etoposide dosage is reduced to 100 mg/m^2 on days 1–3. Bone marrow support with granulocyte colony-stimulating factor (G-CSF) is recommended.

Many medical oncologists who treat small cell lung cancer are hesitant to give >4 cycles of cisplatin and etoposide to their patients. However, most patients are able to tolerate 6 cycles without difficulty, especially when bone marrow support is utilized. Retrospective studies have shown that patients see a benefit from ≥5 cycles of cisplatin and etoposide. In one study, when ≥5 cycles of cisplatin and etoposide was used as a reference, patients who received ≥5 cycles of postoperative, adjuvant chemotherapy other than cisplatin and etoposide had a hazard ratio for recurrence of 3.4 and those that received no postoperative chemotherapy a hazard ratio for recurrence of 5.4.[27] This study speaks to the importance of (1) postoperative chemotherapy for patients with early stage disease, (2) choosing cisplatin and etoposide as the administered regimen, and (3) giving at least 5 cycles of chemotherapy with a goal of six.

For patients with early stage, high grade NEC of the cervix, radical surgery followed by adjuvant chemotherapy should be considered the standard of care and is the recommendation of all published guidelines (Table 14.5).[5,28–30] The benefits of adding postoperative radiation therapy to surgery and chemotherapy, however, remains less clear. Pelvic radiation after surgery does reduce pelvic recurrence. In one study, only 16% of patients who received postoperative pelvic radiation had a pelvic recurrence compared to 25% who did not.[25] Another study showed a similar decrease in pelvic recurrences with postoperative pelvic radiation (13% vs 31%).[32] However, although postoperative pelvic radiation reduces pelvic recurrences, no studies have shown that it improves survival. This may be because studies are inadequately powered to show such a difference due to small sample sizes in this rare disease or it may be that due to the high risk of distant sites of recurrence (liver/lung), local control of the pelvis does not improve survival. That said, we hypothesize that larger studies would show a benefit of postoperative pelvic radiation and as any recurrence is incurable with survival less than 10 months, we recommend postoperative radiation in addition to chemotherapy as adjuvant therapy for most patients with early stage disease.[33] Chemotherapy with cisplatin and etoposide should be given concurrently with radiation and does not need to be given sequentially. For patients who have undergone a cervical biopsy or small conization for microscopic disease where no residual disease is found on the radical hysterectomy specimen, consideration of postoperative chemotherapy only without radiation may be reasonable.

Locally advanced disease

The role of chemotherapy and radiation is much clearer for patients with locally advanced (stages IB3–IVA) high grade NEC of the cervix. All of the major guidelines recommend chemoradiation followed by chemotherapy for these patients (Table 14.5).[5,28–30] Traditionally oncologists have given weekly cisplatin with radiation and followed that with 4 cycles of cisplatin and etoposide. However, more recently many have switched to concurrent cisplatin and etoposide with radiation followed by additional cisplatin and etoposide. In the seminal study on concurrent cisplatin and etoposide with radiation, Hoskins and colleagues reported a recurrence rate of only 35% in 17 patients.[17] In that study, however, half the patients had stage I disease so they may have done equally well with surgery and adjuvant therapy as described above.

Similar to postoperative chemotherapy, there appears to be a benefit to at least 5 cycles of chemotherapy with during and after radiation. In the Hoskins study, giving 5 cycles along with radiation improved both 5-year DFS (63% vs 13%, $P = 0.025$) and overall survival (75% vs 17%, $P = 0.016$). In another study, 78% of patients who completed concurrent chemoradiation followed by chemotherapy for a total ≥ 5 cycles of chemotherapy were alive without disease at median follow-up of over 4 years for surviving patients.[26]

Administering cisplatin and etoposide with chemotherapy requires both a reduction in starting dose as well as support with G-CSFs. The standard dosing for this regimen is cisplatin is 60 mg/m^2 on day 1 and etoposide 100 mg/m^2 on days 1–3 on a 21-day cycle. Typically, patients will receive 2 cycles of chemotherapy during radiation and then an additional 4 cycles after completing brachytherapy.

For patients with stage IB3 disease, some have advocated for neoadjuvant chemotherapy followed by radical surgery (Table 14.5).[28–30] However, we do not recommend this approach. It is unclear where this approach originated as this treatment is not utilized commonly in small cell lung cancer or squamous or adenocarcinoma cervical cancers. In addition, 30% of patients with all clinical stage I tumors will have metastatic disease on imaging or pathology.[24] These patients will require radiation to control disease anyway. Also, as mentioned above, radiation achieves excellent local control with pelvic recurrences after primary radiation occurring in <20% of patients.[18,32,34] Patients with stage IB3–II disease who received primary radiation have the same survival as patients with stages IA–IB2 disease who receive surgery as primary therapy.[32] When reviewing the published literature since 2000, 19 (79%) of 24 patients who received neoadjuvant chemotherapy followed by radical surgery were noted to have recurrence.[35–38] We would expect significantly better outcomes for patients with stage IB3 tumors with primary chemoradiation followed by chemotherapy.

Metastatic disease

Metastatic disease (stage IVB) is largely incurable and treatment should be considered for life prolongation as opposed to being administered with intent to cure. Administration of chemotherapy with cisplatinum and etoposide will prolong survival and many patients will have a good initial response. The standard dosing for this regimen is cisplatinum is 60 mg/m^2 on day 1 and etoposide 120 mg/m^2 on days 1–3 on a 21-day cycle. Support with G-CSFs should be given with cycle 1 in anticipation of neutropenia. Imaging should be performed after every 3 cycles to assess for response and the regimen should be continued until progression or chemotherapy related toxicity.

Surveillance for recurrent disease

National guidelines for surveillance of NEC of the cervix after completing primary treatment are somewhat vague stating "frequent" clinical evaluations with "periodic" imaging with either CT or PET/CT scans.[29] Guidelines for the more common squamous or adenocarcinoma cancers of the cervix describe pelvic exams every 3–6 months in the first 2 years and then every 6–12 months for an additional 3 years with an annual Papanicolaou test.[39] As the majority of patients who recur will do so within the first 2 years, we recommend more frequent visits in that period with symptom review, physical exam with pelvic exam every 3 months (Fig. 14.7) in the first year and every 4 months in the second year then every 6 months for the next 3 years. In addition, as recurrences may occur both locally and at distant sites and due to the high rates of recurrence, imaging with CT scan or PET/CT at each appointment is also recommended.[5] As the risk of isolated brain recurrence is low, imaging of the brain with an MRI should not be routine and performed only if disease recurrence in the upper abdomen or chest is documented or if the patient is experiencing neurologic symptoms. Some oncologists also follow serum NSE levels to detect recurrence although the utility of this has not been established.

Survival and patterns of failure

Survival for patients staged using the 2008 FIGO staging system which was based on clinical factors is shown in Table 14.1. When utilizing the more recent 2018 FIGO staging system to patients with these tumors, stage I tumors had a 5-year survival of 65% compared to 50% for stage II tumors, 30% for patients with stage III disease, and only 3% for those with stage IV disease.[24] Although there are reports of patients having their first recurrence 5–10 years after completing initial therapy, the majority of patients destined to recur will do so within 2 years. For those patients who eventually recur, the median time

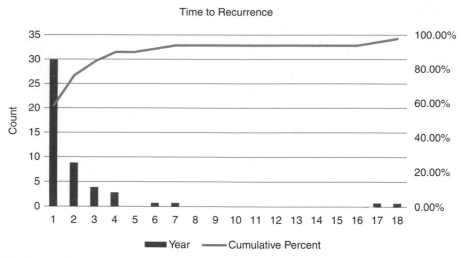

FIG. 14.7 Temporal distribution of first recurrence from time of diagnosis. *Black bars* indicate number of events within each 1-year bin. The *gray line* depicts cumulative recurrence rate (as a percentage of all recurrences) over time. *(From Salvo G, Ramalingam P, Flores Legarreta A, et al. Role of radical hysterectomy in patients with early-stage high-grade neuroendocrine cervical carcinoma: a NeCTuR study. Int J Gynecol Cancer. 2021;31(4):495–501. https://doi.org/10.1136/ijgc-2020-002213. Epub 2021 Feb 9. PMID: 33563641.)*

to recurrence is 9.0 months (range 5–34 months) with 85% of recurrences presenting by 18 months and 94% by 24 months (Fig. 14.7).[18] For patients who recur, the median survival after recurrence is only 10 months.[33]

The most common site for first recurrence is the lymph nodes (46%) followed by liver (38%) with lung closely behind (36%). In addition, patients may experience first recurrence in the brain (11%) or present with carcinomatosis (5%) (unpublished data). For all patients who recur, regardless of stage or treatment, 60% will recur at a distant site(s) only (outside the pelvis), 13% will recur locally only (in the pelvis), and 27% will have both local and distant sites of recurrence. For early stage patients who receive postoperative radiation, about 15% will have a pelvic recurrence compared to 25%–30% for those who did not receive radiation.[25,32] Patients who receive definitive radiation as primary treatment have a pelvic in-field recurrence rate of 21%.[18]

Treatment of recurrent disease

Very few options exist for patients with recurrent NEC of the cervix (Table 14.6). As therapeutic options are limited, patients who recur >6 months from completing primary therapy may be considered for retreatment with cisplatin and etoposide. Other options based on active agents in small cell lung cancer include single agent irinotecan, topotecan, paclitaxel, docetaxel, and temozolomide. Patients with NEC of the GI tract have shown response to combination therapy with temozolomide and capecitabine.[40] There has also been a case report of a complete response of recurrent disease to carboplatin, paclitaxel, and bevacizumab.[41] These are all reasonable options for patients with recurrent cervical disease.

We have had success with the three-drug regimen topotecan, paclitaxel, and bevacizumab and this has become our treatment of choice for recurrent disease.[33] The rationale for this regimen is based on the fact that single agent topotecan and paclitaxel are both effective in treating recurrent small cell lung cancer.[42,43] In addition, high grade neuroendocrine cell cervical cancers express the VEGF receptor 94% of the time making the addition of bevacizumab a reasonable option.[44] Finally, GOG240 demonstrated the three-drug combination is tolerable in women with cervical cancer (squamous and adenocarcinoma) who have been previously treated with concurrent chemotherapy and radiation.[45] Women with recurrent high grade neuroendocrine cervical cancer who receive this regimen were noted to have a progression-free survival (PFS) of 7.8 months compared to only 4.0 months for those who received other chemotherapy regimens (hazard ration for progression 0.21, $P = 0.001$). Women who received this regimen were also more likely to be on treatment for >6 months than those who did not receive it (62% vs 19%, $P = 0.02$).[33] The regimen is given on a 21-day cycles with paclitaxel given at 175 mg/m^2 on day 1, bevacizumab given at 15 mg/kg on day 1, and topotecan given at 0.75 mg/m^2 on days 1–3.

Immunotherapies are commonly utilized in patients with small cell lung cancer. Nivolumab and pembrolizumab as single agents have been approved for the treatment of recurrent small cell lung cancer although responses are very modest at 15%–20%.[46,47] In addition, in patients who received single agent pembrolizumab the overall PFS was only 2.0 months.

TABLE 14.6 Therapeutic options for recurrent high grade neuroendocrine carcinoma of the cervix.

Regimen	Level of support
Cisplatin/etoposide	Case series
Topotecan/paclitaxel/bevacizumab	Case series
Topotecan	Small cell lung cancer
Irinotecan	Small cell lung cancer
Paclitaxel	Small cell lung cancer
Docetaxel	Small cell lung cancer
Temozolomide	Small cell lung cancer
Temozolomide/capecitabine	Gastrointestinal neuroendocrine tumors
PARP inhibitors	Case report
Trametinib	Case report
Nivolumab	Case report
Carboplatin/paclitaxel/bevacizumab	Case report

The addition of ipilimumab to nivolumab for patients with small cell lung cancer increased response rates from 12% to 21% but also added significant toxicity.[46]

Although there is a single case report of a patient with high grade NEC of the cervix having a good response to single agent nivolumab, there are few other reported cases of success with anti-PD-1/PD-L1 therapies.[48] In a phase II basket study of 12 patients with extrapulmonary small cell carcinomas, 6 women had small cell cervical cancer. In the entire cohort there were no responses and the median progression-free interval (PFI) for the 6 patients with small cell cervical cancer was 2.1 months with no patients on treatment past 14 weeks.[49] However, a basket trial of 18 patients with recurrent nonpancreatic high grade NEC treated with ipilimumab and nivolumab showed an overall response rate (ORR) of 44%. In this study there were 3 patients with high grade NEC of the cervix and 1 (33%) woman had a partial response that lasted about 6 months.[50] The lack of response to single agent PD-1/PD-L1 inhibitors may not be surprising as a study looking at immunohistochemistry staining of neuroendocrine cervical cancers showed no specimens as microsatellite instability (MSI) high and only 8% positive for PD-L1 expression.[20]

With few standard therapeutic options available, clinical trials should be considered early in the treatment planning for patients with recurrent disease. Triaging patients to trials based on molecular testing may be a sensible approach for many patients. Although there is not a unifying mutation found in all tumor specimens, multiple targetable mutations are found in these cancers. An actionable mutation can be found in over half the patients with high grade NEC of the cervix including PIK3CA (18%), KRAS (14%), and p53 (11%).[51] Another study using next generation sequencing to detect somatic mutations also found no unifying mutations but a similar distribution of mutations including p53 (40%), PIK3CA (30%), BRCA (20%), and KRAS (10%).[52] Based on molecular testing, there have been reports of disease response to targeted therapies including a patient with a BRCA mutation who had prolonged disease stabilization with a PARP inhibitor and a patient with a KRAS mutation who had a complete response with a MEK inhibitor.[53,54]

Special considerations

As the median age at diagnosis for women with high grade NEC of the cervix is 48 years old, fertility preservation may be a concern for the newly diagnosed patient.[3] When considering fertility sparing options, one must consider uterine and ovary sparing procedures. Due to the highly aggressive nature of NEC of the cervix, radical trachelectomy is not recommended. Although case reports have been published on successful outcomes after radical trachelectomy,[55,56] experts and national guidelines recommend against offering radical trachelectomy to patients with these tumors.[57,58] In addition, many of these patients will get postoperative radiation therapy making the uterine fundus unable to maintain an intrauterine pregnancy.

For patients with negative metastatic workup and normal appearing ovaries at the time of radical hysterectomy, ovarian sparing surgery may be considered. However, as most patients with grossly visible disease will require postoperative radiation therapy, transposition of the ovaries out of the radiation field may be necessary to maintain ovarian function. Patients should be counseled that >35% of patients will still have ovarian failure if postoperative radiation therapy is prescribed.[59]

Case resolution

This 34-year-old patient was counseled for radical hysterectomy, bilateral salpingectomy, and ovarian transposition if the ovaries appeared normal and there was no evidence of metastatic disease at surgery. She underwent a successful open radical hysterectomy, bilateral salpingectomy, lymphatic mapping with sentinel lymph node biopsies, and transposition of the right ovary. Pathology revealed a 1 cm small cell carcinoma of the cervix with lymphovascular space invasion and negative margins and lymph nodes. Postoperatively she underwent pelvic radiation with concurrent cisplatin and etoposide and then additional chemotherapy with cisplatin and etoposide to complete 6 cycles. She is now 3 years disease free and maintains ovarian function based on lack of menopausal symptoms and laboratory testing.

References

1. Papatsimpas G, Samaras I, Theodosiou P, et al. A case of cervical carcinoid and review of the literature. *Case Rep Oncol.* 2017;10(2):737–742.
2. American Cancer Society Cancer Facts & Figures 2020 2020 Available from http://cancerstatisticscenter.cancer.org.
3. Gibbs J, Mei S, Economos K, Lee YC, Kanis MJ. Clinicopathologic features, incidence, and survival trends of gynecologic neuroendocrine tumors: a SEER database analysis. *Am J Obstet Gynecol.* 2019;221(1). 53.e1–53.e6.
4. Margolis B, Tergas AI, Chen L, et al. Natural history and outcome of neuroendocrine carcinoma of the cervix. *Gynecol Oncol.* 2016;141(2): 247–254.
5. Salvo G, Gonzalez Martin A, Gonzales NR, Frumovitz M. Updates and management algorithm for neuroendocrine tumors of the uterine cervix. *Int J Gynecol Cancer.* 2019;29(6):986–995.
6. Hillman RT, Cardnell R, Fujimoto J, et al. Comparative genomics of high grade neuroendocrine carcinoma of the cervix. *PLoS One.* 2020;15(6), e0234505.
7. Castle PE, Pierz A, Stoler MH. A systematic review and meta-analysis on the attribution of human papillomavirus (HPV) in neuroendocrine cancers of the cervix. *Gynecol Oncol.* 2018;148(2):422–429.
8. Alvarado-Cabreo I, Euscher ED, Ganesan R, et al. Small cell neuroendocrine carcinoma. In: WHO Classification of Tumors Editorial Board, ed. *Female Genital Tumors.* World Health Organization Classification of Tumors. Lyon: IARC Press; 2020:455–456.
9. Alvarado-Cabreo I, Euscher ED, Ganesan R, et al. Large cell neuroendocrine carcinoma. In: WHO Classification of Tumors Editorial Board, ed. *Female Genital Tumors.* World Health Organization Classification of Tumors. Lyon: IARC Press; 2020:457–458.
10. Xing D, Zheng G, Schoolmeester JK, et al. Next-generation sequencing reveals recurrent somatic mutations in small cell neuroendocrine carcinoma of the uterine cervix. *Am J Surg Pathol.* 2018;42(6):750–760.
11. Frumovitz M, Burzawa JK, Byers LA, et al. Sequencing of mutational hotspots in cancer-related genes in small cell neuroendocrine cervical cancer. *Gynecol Oncol.* 2016;141(3):588–591.
12. Cohen JG, Kapp DS, Shin JY, et al. Small cell carcinoma of the cervix: treatment and survival outcomes of 188 patients. *Am J Obstet Gynecol.* 2010;203(4). 347.e1–6.
13. Chen CA, Wu CC, Juang GT, Wang JF, Chen TM, Hsieh CY. Serum neuron-specific enolase levels in patients with small cell carcinoma of the uterine cervix. *J Formos Med Assoc.* 1994;93(1):81–83.
14. Tian Z, Liang C, Zhang Z, et al. Prognostic value of neuron-specific enolase for small cell lung cancer: a systematic review and meta-analysis. *World J Surg Oncol.* 2020;18(1):116.
15. Hricak H, Gatsonis C, Chi DS, et al. Role of imaging in pretreatment evaluation of early invasive cervical cancer: results of the intergroup study American College of Radiology Imaging Network 6651-Gynecologic Oncology Group 183. *J Clin Oncol.* 2005;23(36):9329–9337.
16. Fischerova D, Cibula D, Stenhova H, et al. Transrectal ultrasound and magnetic resonance imaging in staging of early cervical cancer. *Int J Gynecol Cancer.* 2008;18(4):766–772.
17. Hoskins PJ, Swenerton KD, Pike JA, et al. Small-cell carcinoma of the cervix: fourteen years of experience at a single institution using a combined-modality regimen of involved-field irradiation and platinum-based combination chemotherapy. *J Clin Oncol.* 2003;21(18):3495–3501.
18. Stecklein SR, Jhingran A, Burzawa J, et al. Patterns of recurrence and survival in neuroendocrine cervical cancer. *Gynecol Oncol.* 2016;143(3): 552–557.
19. Gabriel M, Decristoforo C, Kendler D, et al. 68Ga-DOTA-Tyr3-octreotide PET in neuroendocrine tumors: comparison with somatostatin receptor scintigraphy and CT. *J Nucl Med.* 2007;48(4):508–518.
20. Carroll MR, Ramalingam P, Salvo G, et al. Evaluation of PARP and PDL-1 as potential therapeutic targets for women with high-grade neuroendocrine carcinomas of the cervix. *Int J Gynecol Cancer.* 2020;30(9):1303–1307.

21. Salvo G, Ramalingam P, Legarreta A, et al. Role of radical hysterectomy in patients with early-stage high-grade neuroendocrine cervical carcinoma: a NeCTuR study. *Int J Gynecol Cancer.* 2021 Apr;31(4):495–501. https://doi.org/ 10.1136/ijgc-2020-002213. Epub 2021 Feb 9. Erratum in: Int J Gynecol Cancer. 2021 Dec;31(12):1625. PMID: 33563641.

22. Boruta 2nd DM, Schorge JO, Duska LA, Crum CP, Castrillon DH, Sheets EE. Multimodality therapy in early-stage neuroendocrine carcinoma of the uterine cervix. *Gynecol Oncol.* 2001;81(1):82–87.

23. Chan JK, Loizzi V, Burger RA, Rutgers J, Monk BJ. Prognostic factors in neuroendocrine small cell cervical carcinoma: a multivariate analysis. *Cancer.* 2003;97(3):568–574.

24. Ishikawa M, Kasamatsu T, Tsuda H, et al. A multi-center retrospective study of neuroendocrine tumors of the uterine cervix: prognosis according to the new 2018 staging system, comparing outcomes for different chemotherapeutic regimens and histopathological subtypes. *Gynecol Oncol.* 2019;155(3):444–451.

25. Ishikawa M, Kasamatsu T, Tsuda H, et al. Prognostic factors and optimal therapy for stages I-II neuroendocrine carcinomas of the uterine cervix: a multi-center retrospective study. *Gynecol Oncol.* 2018;148(1):139–146.

26. Wang KL, Chang TC, Jung SM, et al. Primary treatment and prognostic factors of small cell neuroendocrine carcinoma of the uterine cervix: a Taiwanese Gynecologic Oncology Group study. *Eur J Cancer.* 2012;48(10):1484–1494.

27. Pei X, Xiang L, Ye S, et al. Cycles of cisplatin and etoposide affect treatment outcomes in patients with FIGO stage I-II small cell neuroendocrine carcinoma of the cervix. *Gynecol Oncol.* 2017;147(3):589–596.

28. Gadducci A, Carinelli S, Aletti G. Neuroendocrine tumors of the uterine cervix: a therapeutic challenge for gynecologic oncologists. *Gynecol Oncol.* 2017;144(3):637–646.

29. Gardner GJ, Reidy-Lagunes D, Gehrig PA. Neuroendocrine tumors of the gynecologic tract: a Society of Gynecologic Oncology (SGO) clinical document. *Gynecol Oncol.* 2011;122(1):190–198.

30. Satoh T, Takei Y, Treilleux I, et al. Gynecologic Cancer InterGroup (GCIG) consensus review for small cell carcinoma of the cervix. *Int J Gynecol Cancer.* 2014;24(9 suppl. 3):S102–S108.

31. Zivanovic O, Leitao Jr MM, Park KJ, et al. Small cell neuroendocrine carcinoma of the cervix: analysis of outcome, recurrence pattern and the impact of platinum-based combination chemotherapy. *Gynecol Oncol.* 2009;112(3):590–593.

32. Chen TC, Huang HJ, Wang TY, et al. Primary surgery versus primary radiation therapy for FIGO stages I-II small cell carcinoma of the uterine cervix: a retrospective Taiwanese Gynecologic Oncology Group study. *Gynecol Oncol.* 2015;137(3):468–473.

33. Frumovitz M, Munsell MF, Burzawa JK, et al. Combination therapy with topotecan, paclitaxel, and bevacizumab improves progression-free survival in recurrent small cell neuroendocrine carcinoma of the cervix. *Gynecol Oncol.* 2017;144(1):46–50.

34. Viswanathan AN, Deavers MT, Jhingran A, Ramirez PT, Levenback C, Eifel PJ. Small cell neuroendocrine carcinoma of the cervix: outcome and patterns of recurrence. *Gynecol Oncol.* 2004;93(1):27–33.

35. Bermudez A, Vighi S, Garcia A, Sardi J. Neuroendocrine cervical carcinoma: a diagnostic and therapeutic challenge. *Gynecol Oncol.* 2001;82(1): 32–39.

36. Lee JM, Lee KB, Nam JH, et al. Prognostic factors in FIGO stage IB-IIA small cell neuroendocrine carcinoma of the uterine cervix treated surgically: results of a multi-center retrospective Korean study. *Ann Oncol.* 2008;19(2):321–326.

37. Nasu K, Hirakawa T, Okamoto M, et al. Advanced small cell carcinoma of the uterine cervix treated by neoadjuvant chemotherapy with irinotecan and cisplatin followed by radical surgery. *Rare Tumors.* 2011;3(1), e6.

38. Dongol S, Tai Y, Shao Y, Jiang J, Kong B. A retrospective clinicopathological analysis of small-cell carcinoma of the uterine cervix. *Mol Clin Oncol.* 2014;2(1):71–75.

39. Salani R, Backes FJ, Fung MF, et al. Posttreatment surveillance and diagnosis of recurrence in women with gynecologic malignancies: Society of Gynecologic Oncologists recommendations. *Am J Obstet Gynecol.* 2011;204(6):466–478.

40. Kunz PL, Catalano PJ, Nimeiri H, et al. A randomized study of temozolomide or temozolomide and capecitabine in patients with advanced pancreatic neuroendocrine tumors: a trial of the ECOG-ACRIN Cancer Research Group (E2211). *J Clin Oncol.* 2018;36(15 suppl):4004.

41. Nakao Y, Tamauchi S, Yoshikawa N, Suzuki S, Kajiyama H, Kikkawa F. Complete response of recurrent small cell carcinoma of the uterine cervix to paclitaxel, carboplatin, and bevacizumab combination therapy. *Case Rep Oncol.* 2020;13(1):373–378.

42. O'Brien ME, Ciuleanu TE, Tsekov H, et al. Phase III trial comparing supportive care alone with supportive care with oral topotecan in patients with relapsed small-cell lung cancer. *J Clin Oncol.* 2006;24(34):5441–5447.

43. Smit EF, Fokkema E, Biesma B, Groen HJ, Snoek W, Postmus PE. A phase II study of paclitaxel in heavily pretreated patients with small-cell lung cancer. *Br J Cancer.* 1998;77(2):347–351.

44. Tangjitgamol S, Ramirez PT, Sun CC, et al. Expression of HER-2/neu, epidermal growth factor receptor, vascular endothelial growth factor, cyclooxygenase-2, estrogen receptor, and progesterone receptor in small cell and large cell neuroendocrine carcinoma of the uterine cervix: a clinicopathologic and prognostic study. *Int J Gynecol Cancer.* 2005;15(4):646–656.

45. Tewari KS, Sill MW, Long 3rd HJ, et al. Improved survival with bevacizumab in advanced cervical cancer. *N Engl J Med.* 2014;370(8):734–743.

46. Antonia SJ, Lopez-Martin JA, Bendell J, et al. Nivolumab alone and nivolumab plus ipilimumab in recurrent small-cell lung cancer (CheckMate 032): a multicentre, open-label, phase 1/2 trial. *Lancet Oncol.* 2016;17(7):883–895.

47. Chung HC, Lopez-Martin JA, Kao SC-H, et al. Phase 2 study of pembrolizumab in advanced small-cell lung cancer (SCLC): KEYNOTE-158. *J Clin Oncol.* 2018;36(15 suppl):8506.

48. Paraghamian SE, Longoria TC, Eskander RN. Metastatic small cell neuroendocrine carcinoma of the cervix treated with the PD-1 inhibitor, nivolumab: a case report. *Gynecol Oncol Res Pract.* 2017;4:3.

49. Frumovitz M, Westin SN, Salvo G, et al. Phase II study of pembrolizumab efficacy and safety in women with recurrent small cell neuroendocrine carcinoma of the lower genital tract. *Gynecol Oncol.* 2020;158(3):570–575.

50. Patel SP, Othus M, Chae YK, et al. A phase II basket trial of dual anti-CTLA-4 and anti-PD-1 blockade in rare tumors (DART SWOG 1609) in patients with nonpancreatic neuroendocrine tumors. *Clin Cancer Res.* 2020;26(10):2290–2296.

51. Frumovitz M, Burzawa JK, Byers LA, et al. Sequencing of mutational hotspots in cancer-related genes in small cell neuroendocrine cervical cancer. *Gynecol Oncol.* 2016;141(3):588–591.

52. Xing D, Zheng G, Schoolmeester JK, et al. Next-generation sequencing reveals recurrent somatic mutations in small cell neuroendocrine carcinoma of the uterine cervix. *Am J Surg Pathol.* 2018;42(6):750–760.

53. Rose PG, Sierk A. Treatment of neuroendocrine carcinoma of the cervix with a PARP inhibitor based on next generation sequencing. *Gynecol Oncol Rep.* 2019;30:100499.

54. Lyons YA, Frumovitz M, Soliman PT. Response to MEK inhibitor in small cell neuroendocrine carcinoma of the cervix with a KRAS mutation. *Gynecol Oncol Rep.* 2014;10:28–29.

55. Singh S, Redline R, Resnick KE. Fertility-sparing management of a stage IB1 small cell neuroendocrine cervical carcinoma with radical abdominal trachelectomy and adjuvant chemotherapy. *Gynecol Oncol Rep.* 2015;13:5–7.

56. Rajkumar S, Iyer R, Culora G, Lane G. Fertility sparing management of large cell neuroendocrine tumour of cervix: a case report & review of literature. *Gynecol Oncol Rep.* 2016;18:15–17.

57. National Comprehensive Cancer Network. Cervical Cancer (Version 2.2020) 2020 Available from https://www.nccn.org/professionals/physician_gls/pdf/cervical.pdf.

58. Plante M, Gregoire J, Renaud MC, Roy M. The vaginal radical trachelectomy: an update of a series of 125 cases and 106 pregnancies. *Gynecol Oncol.* 2011;121(2):290–297.

59. Gubbala K, Laios A, Gallos I, Pathiraja P, Haldar K, Ind T. Outcomes of ovarian transposition in gynaecological cancers; a systematic review and meta-analysis. *J Ovarian Res.* 2014;7:69.

Chapter 15

Other rare cervical cancers: cervical rhabdomyosarcoma, adenoid cystic carcinoma, verrucous carcinoma

Michael Frumovitz and Preetha Ramalingam

Introduction

The overwhelming majority of cervical cancer cases will be either squamous cell or adenocarcinoma. In a National Cancer Database (NCDB) study of cervical cancer in the United States, 79.5% of cervical cancer cases consisted of the squamous cell subtype, 19.0% were adenocarcinoma, and 1.5% were high-grade neuroendocrine carcinoma.[1] These estimates round to 100% meaning that there are very few cervical cancer cases of the ultra-rare subtypes such as rhabdomyosarcoma, clear cell carcinoma, adenoid cystic carcinoma, or verrucous carcinoma. In fact, the majority of the literature for these subtypes comes from case reports of single patients, small case series that span decades, and population database studies whose data sources lack the details necessary to make any specific treatment recommendations. In this chapter, we will review these ultra-rare subtypes and attempt to make recommendations for treatment based on the current literature as well as drawing from similar histologic subtypes from other primary tumor sites (for clear cell cervical cancer, see Chapter 16 on clear cell vaginal cancer).

Cervical rhabdomyoscarcoma

Rhabdomyosarcoma is a malignancy of the skeletal muscle phenotype with incomplete myogenesis. It is the most common pediatric soft tissue tumor accounting for 50% of the soft tissue malignancies and 3%–4% of all childhood cancers.[2] In children, these tumors are most commonly found in the head and neck region, specifically within the orbit. The genitourinary tract may be the primary site in 20% of pediatric cases; however, most of these will be seen in the bladder or vagina with the cervix as site of origin exceedingly rare. Rhadbomyosarcoma accounts for only 1% of all malignancies in adults and only 5% of all soft tissue sarcomas.[3] Rhabdomyosarcoma of the cervix most commonly occurs in the second and third decades of life in contrast to the more common vaginal rhabdomyosarcoma that occurs more frequently in the first decade of life.[4] The incidence of these tumors in adults is exceedingly rare. Over a 40-year period at Memorial Sloan Kettering Cancer Center, only 8 cases of adult cervical rhabdomyosarcoma were observed and only 6 cases were seen in a 30-year period at MD Anderson Cancer Center.[3,5] Rhabdomyosarcoma accounts for <0.5% of all cervical cancers.

For rhabdomyosarcoma of the lower genital tract (cervix, vulva, and vagina), the 5-year overall survival rate approaches 70%.[6] Improved overall survival may be seen with younger age, localized disease with no distant or lymph node metastases, and in patients embryonal histology. The Intergroup Rhabdomyosarcoma Study Group (IRSG) classifies rhabdomyosarcoma into three histologic subtypes: embryonal, alveolar, and undifferentiated. The alveolar and undifferentiated subtypes have a much poorer prognosis than the embryonal subtype.[7] Fortunately, three-fourths of cervical rhabdomyosarcoma will be the embryonal subtype.[3,6] The embryonal subtype can be further classified into classic, botyroid, and spindle cell subtypes. The majority of cervical cancer patients with rhabdomyosarcoma will have the botyroid subtype.

The only known risk factors for rhabdomyosarcoma are genetic in nature. For rhabdomyosarcoma at all sites, there are well-known links to familiar hereditary syndromes such as Li–Fraumini syndrome, Neurofibromatosis type 1, Beckwith–Wiedemann syndrome, Costello syndrome, and Noonan syndrome.[8] For patients with cervical rhabdomyosarcoma, DICER1 syndromes have been most frequently reported.[9,10] Other features of DICER1 syndrome include higher rates of pleuropulmonary blastoma, pediatric cystic nephroma, thyroid multinodular goiter, ovarian Sertoli-Leydig tumor, and Wilm's tumor. The relationship between cervical rhabdomyosarcoma and human papilloma virus (HPV) is unknown but thought to be unlikely.

Diagnosis and Treatment of Rare Gynecologic Cancers. https://doi.org/10.1016/B978-0-323-82938-0.00015-X

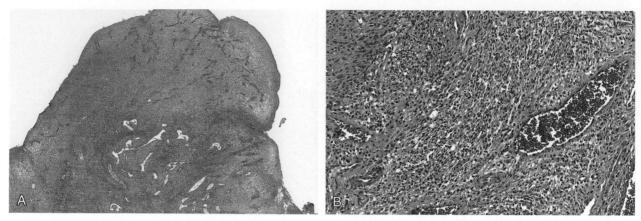

FIG. 15.1 (A) Cervical polyp with rhabdomyosarcoma showing hypo and hypercellular areas. (B) High power examination shows numerous strap cells (rhabdomyoblasts).

Grossly, the tumors are often polypoid with an edematous and fleshy cut surface. In some cases, multiple polyps may be present giving a botryoid/grape-like appearance.[11] The most common histologic subtype of rhabdomyosarcoma in the cervix is of the embryonal-type. Microscopically they have a polypoid appearance lined by squamous or glandular epithelium (Fig. 15.1A). The stroma is edematous with alternating hypocellular and hypercellular areas. The condensation of the spindle cells beneath the surface epithelium results in the so-called cambium layer. The tumor cells are composed of short spindle cells and often surround entrapped endocervical glands. Rhabdomyoblasts/strap cells with cross-striations are variably present (Fig. 15.1B). Brisk mitotic activity and apoptotic bodies are usually present.[12]

The less common alveolar rhabdomyosarcoma is composed of loosely packed cells with high N/C ratio growing in an alveolar pattern, separated by collagenous stroma. The central discohesion with adherence to the periphery of the nests results in the alveolar pattern. The pleomorphic rhabdomyosarcoma subtype is characterized by large multinucleated cells with bizarre atypia and rhabdomyoblasts are variably present. Rhabdomyosarcomas are positive for desmin, myogenin (Fig. 15.2A) and myoD1 (Fig. 15.2B). Alveolar rhabdomyosarcoma can express keratin markers focally.

The differential diagnosis of rhabdomyosarcoma is vast as it can mimic many tumors. The primary differential is an inflamed benign cervical polyp. The inflammation may obscure the rhabdomyoblasts resulting in a benign diagnosis and this is a known pitfall. Distinguishing embryonal rhabdomyosarcoma from adenosarcoma with sarcomatous overgrowth and heterologous rhabdomyoblastic differentiation is particularly challenging, and may not be possible in some cases. The presence of phyllodes-like growth pattern and presence of leaf-like glands with periglandular cuffing will favor a diagnosis of adenosarcoma. Carcinosarcoma with heterologous rhabdomyoblastic differentiation is also in the differential but the presence of malignant glandular component will facilitate the diagnosis. Other sarcomas such as leiomyosarcoma and undifferentiated sarcoma can be differentiated from rhabdomyosarcoma by doing immunohistochemical stains to confirm skeletal muscle differentiation in the latter. Also to be considered in the differential diagnosis is SMARCA4-deficient undifferentiated sarcoma. For these cases, demonstrating loss of SMARCA4 by immunohistochemistry is necessary.

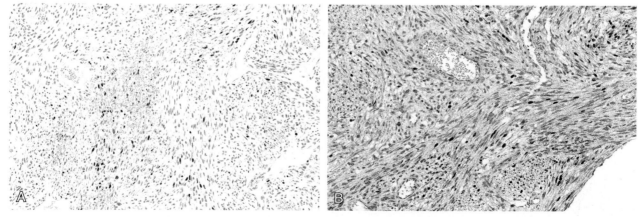

FIG. 15.2 Rhabdomyosarcoma showing patchy positive staining for myogenin (A) and myoD1 (B).

Embryonal rhabdomyosarcoma may show both somatic and germline mutations of *DICER1*.[13] These mutations are less common in adenosarcoma; hence absence makes embryonal rhabdomyosarcoma less likely. Alveolar rhabdomyosarcoma shows recurring translocation in t(2;13)(q35;q14) and less commonly t(1;13)(q36;q14) which fuse the *FOXO1* gene on chromosome 13 with either *PAX3* on chromosome 2 or *PAX7* on chromosome 1, respectively.[14]

The classic description of cervical rhabdomyosarcoma is a friable, polypoid tumor with a "bunch of grapes" appearance. In fact, the term "botyroid" comes from the similar Greek word meaning "bunch of grapes." Most patients will present with vaginal bleeding or discharge. Other patients may experience vaginal mass or protruding cervical polyps.[15]

For all abnormal cervical masses, a biopsy of the tumor should be performed using biopsy forceps. For pediatric and adolescent patients, there should be a high suspicion for a rare type of cervical tumor as the more common HPV-associated cervical cancers (squamous, adeno, and adenosquamous carcinomas) are almost never seen in women under the age of 18 years old. For adult women, the differential diagnosis includes the more common HPV-associated cervical cancers as well as other benign lesions and rare malignancies.

After a pathologic diagnosis has been established, all patients should undergo imaging. We recommend computed tomography (CT) scan of the chest, abdomen, and pelvis or positron emission tomography (PET) scan to evaluate for metastatic disease and magnetic resonance imaging (MRI) of the pelvis to evaluate extent of the primary cervical tumor. A prospective study showed PET scan increases detection of lymph node and bone metastases. However, the same study showed CT scan is better for detection of lung metastases.[16]

There are multiple staging systems that may be considered for patients with cervical rhabdomyosarcoma. For gynecologic oncologists, the most well-known and commonly utilized system will be from the International Federation of Gynecology and Obstetrics (FIGO). The 2018 staging system allows for clinical, pathologic, and radiologic factors to be considered when assigning stage (Table 15.1). Outside of gynecology, the most frequently used surgico-pathologic staging schema is the Clinical Group (CG) system developed by the IRSG. This system incorporates degree of tumor spread at diagnosis and the amount of disease remaining after initial surgery (Table 15.2). More recently, the IRSG developed a TNM-type system that accounts for other important prognostic factors (Table 15.3).

For rhabdomyosarcoma at all sites, pediatric patients have the lowest mortality rates followed by young adults (ages 20–44 years old, HR for death 1.9), middle aged adults (ages 45–64 years old, HR for death 2.6), aged adults (ages 65–84 years old, HR for death 4.0), and geriatric patients (age ≥85 years old, HR for death 8.3).[17] Patients with embryonal subtypes have a better prognosis than alveolar (HR for death 1.5) or pleomorphic (HR for death 1.9) subtypes and those with localized/early stage disease have lower mortality than those with regional (HR for death 1.8) or distant disease (HR for death 4.8). For girls and women with rhabdomyosarcoma of the lower genital tract (cervix, vulva, and vagina), factors predicting improved overall survival were similar to those for rhabdomyosarcoma at all sites and include young age, localized disease, and embryonal histology.[6] Due to the rarity of this disease and small number of patients, there are no publications with sufficient sample size to evaluate prognostic factors for females with cervical rhabdomyosarcoma only.

Treatment for women with localized disease (IRSG Clinical Group I) who have completed child-bearing should begin with a radical hysterectomy and pelvic lymph node assessment (sentinel lymph node biopsy or complete lymphadenectomy) (Fig. 15.3). The risk of lymph node involvement in women with cervical rhabdomyosarcoma is as high as 20% so lymph node assessment is critical.[6] Some have argued that a simple hysterectomy for small tumors may be adequate; however, most would consider the standard to be a radical hysterectomy.[15] For patients with disease limited to the cervix on pathologic exam, we recommend adjuvant chemotherapy with vincristine, actinomycin-D, and cyclophosphamide (VAC). Other regimens with ifosfamide or doxorubicin may be considered as alternatives. For patients with residual or metastatic disease noted after surgery, combination chemotherapy with VAC and radiation therapy should be considered.

For girls or women desiring fertility sparing therapy, cone biopsy or radical trachelectomy followed by chemotherapy with VAC may be offered for small Clinical Group I tumors and imaging negative for metastatic disease. In one such study of women <20 years old, all 5 patients who underwent either cone biopsy or simple polypectomy followed by VAC were without evidence of disease with a median follow-up of 19 months.[3] Another study of 3 adult women (age ≥20) who underwent local excision followed by chemotherapy (various regimens) reported no recurrences at a median follow-up of 22 years.[15]

Women and girls with metastatic disease at diagnosis should have individualized treatment plans that may involve radiation and/or chemotherapy with surgery considered less frequently. Neoadjuvant chemotherapy followed by surgery has been successfully utilized for unresectable or locally advanced disease for rhabdomyosarcoma at other sites such as the orbit, vagina, and bladder. For patients with cervical cancer, one case report of a patient with a large (> 4 cm) tumor of the cervix who received chemotherapy with VAC prior to simple hysterectomy was noted to be disease free 10 years later.[3] However, other oncologists reported recurrence or progression in patients undergoing neoadjuvant chemotherapy.[15]

TABLE 15.1 FIGO staging for cervical cancer.

Stage	Description
I	The carcinoma is strictly confined to the cervix (extension to the uterine corpus should be disregarded)
IA	Invasive carcinoma that can be diagnosed only by microscopy, with maximum depth of invasion <5mm[a]
IA1	Measured stromal invasion ≤3 mm in depth
IA2	Measured stromal invasion >3 mm and ≤5 mm in depth
IB	Invasive carcinoma with measured deepest invasion >5 mm (greater than Stage IA), lesion limited to the cervix uteri
IB1	Invasive carcinoma >5 mm depth of stromal invasion, and ≤2 cm in greatest dimension
IB2	Invasive carcinoma >2 cm and ≤4 cm in greatest dimension
IB3	Invasive carcinoma >4 cm in greatest dimension
II	The carcinoma invades beyond the uterus, but has not extended onto the lower third of the vagina or to the pelvic wall
IIA	Involvement limited to the upper two-thirds of the vagina without parametrial involvement
IIA1	Invasive carcinoma ≤4 cm in greatest dimension
IIA2	Invasive carcinoma >4 cm in greatest dimension
IIB	With parametrial involvement but not up to the pelvic wall
III	The carcinoma involves the lower third of the vagina and/or involves pelvic and/or para-aortic lymph nodes[b]
IIIA	The carcinoma involves the lower third of the vagina, with no extension to the pelvic wall
IIIB	Extension to the pelvic wall and/or hydronephrosis or nonfunctioning kidney (unless known to be due to another cause)
IIIC	Involvement of pelvic and/or para-aortic lymph nodes (including micrometastases), irrespective of tumor size and extent (with r and p notations)[b]
IIIC1	Pelvic lymph node metastasis only
IIIC2	Para-aortic lymph node metastasis
IV	The carcinoma has extended beyond the true pelvis or has involved (biopsy proven) the mucosa of the bladder or rectum. (A bullous edema, as such, does not permit a case to be allotted to Stage IV.)
IVA	Spread to adjacent pelvic organs
IVB	Spread to distant organs
International Federation of Gynecology and Obstetrics (FIGO) staging of cancer of the cervix uteri (2018).	
When in doubt, the lower staging should be assigned.	

[a]*Imaging and pathology can be used, where available, to supplement clinical findings with respect to tumor size and extent, in all stages.*
[b]*Adding notation of r (imaging) and p (pathology) to indicate the findings that are used to allocate the case to Stage IIIC. Example: If imaging indicates pelvic lymph node metastasis, the stage allocation would be Stage IIIC1r, and if confirmed by pathologic findings, it would be Stage IIIC1p. The type of imaging modality or pathology technique used should always be documents.*
The involvement of vascular/lymphatic spaces does not change the staging. The lateral extent of the lesion is no longer considered.
From: N. Bhatla, D. Aoki, D.N. Sharma, Sankaranarayanan R. Cancer of the cervix uteri. Int J Gynaecol Obstet 143 (2018) S2:22. Available at: https:/obgyn.onlinelibrary.wiley.com/doi/full/10.1002/igo.12611. Reproduced under the terms of the Creative Commons License 4.0. Updated with information from: Corrigendum to "Revised FIGO Staging for Carcinoma of the Cervix Uteri." Int J Gynaecol Obstet 147 (2019) 279.

Surveillance for rhabdomyosarcoma should include monitoring for symptoms of recurrence such as vaginal bleeding or discharge as well as physical exam with pelvic exam every 3–4 months for the first 2 years after completing therapy and then every 6 months for an additional three years. For patients with retroperitoneal and intraabdominal soft tissue sarcomas the National Comprehensive Cancer Network (NCCN) recommends routine imaging with CT scan or MRI every 3–6 months for 2–3 years and then every 6–12 months thereafter.[18] Although the NCCN Guidelines do not make any specific recommendations for surveillance imaging for patients with rhabdomyosarcoma at all sites, let alone for those women with cervical rhabdomyosarcoma, we recommend following a similar schedule of imaging for women with cervical rhabdomyosarcoma.

TABLE 15.2 Clinical grouping of rhabdomyosarcoma by the Intergroup Rhabdomyosarcoma Study Group.

Clinical group	Extent of disease/surgical result
I	A: Localized tumor, confined to site of origin, completely resected
	B: Localized tumor, infiltrating beyond site of origin, completely resected
II	A: Localized tumor, gross total resection, but with microscopic residual disease
	B: Locally extensive tumor (spread to regional lymph nodes), completely resected
	C: Locally extensive tumor (spread to regional lymph nodes), gross total resection, but microscopic residual disease
III	A: Localized or locally extensive tumor, gross residual disease after major resection ($\geq$50% debulking)
IV[a]	Any size primary tumor, with or without regional lymph node involvement, with distant metastases, irrespective of surgical approach to primary tumor

[a]Although current Children's Oncology Group (COG) trials include all patients with metastatic disease in the high-risk category, selected patients with favorable site, histology/molecular features (embryonal or alveolar, and FOXO1 fusion-negative), and age (under age 10) with limited metastases may have better outcomes with VAC therapy (vincristine, actinomysin D, and cyclophosphamide) or intensified treatments such as those in the completed ARST0431 protocol. Modified from W. Crist, E.A. Gehan, A.H. Ragab, et al. The third intergroup thabdomyosarcoma study. J Clin Oncol 13 (1995) 610; and W. Crist, L. Garnsey, M. Beltangady, et al. Prognosis in children with rhabdomyosarcoma: A report of the intergroup rhabdomyosarcoma studies I and II. Intergroup Rhabdomyosarcoma Committee. J Clin Oncol 8 (1990) 443.

TABLE 15.3 TNM staging system for rhabdomyosarcoma.

Stage	Sites	Tumor	Size	N	M
1	Orbit Head and neck[a] Genitourinary[b] Biliary tract	T1 or T2	A or B	Any N	M0
2	Bladder/prostate Extremity Cranial Paramenindeal Other[c]	T1 or T2	A	N0 or Nx	M0
3	Bladder/prostate Extremity Cranial Parameningeal Other[c]	T1 or T2	A or B	N0 or N1	M1

T: Tumor stage	N: Regional nodes	M: Metastases
T1: Confined to anatomic site of origin	N0: Not clinically involved	M0: No distant metastases
T2: Extension	N1: Clinically involved	M1: Distant metastases present
A: $\leq$5 cm in diameter B: >5 cm in diameter	Nx: Clinical status unknown	

[a]Excluding parameningeal.
[b]Nonbladder/nonprostrate.
[c]Includes trunk, retroperitoneum, etc., excluding biliary tract.
Adapted from W. Lawrence, E.A. Gehan, D.M. Hays, et al. Prognostic significance of staging factors of the UICC staging system in childhood rhabdomyosarcoma: a report from the Intergroup Rhabdomyosarcoma Study (IRS-II). J Clin Oncol 5 (1987) 46; and W. Lawrence, J.R. Anderson, E.A. Gehan, et al. Pretreatment TNM staging of childhood rhabdomyosarcoma: a report of the Intergroup Rhabdomyosarcoma Study Group. Ancer 80 (1997) 1165.

In the largest series of patients with rhabdomyosarcoma of the lower genital tract ($n = 144$), the 5-year overall survival for all patients was 68%; however, this study did not provide separate survival rates for those women with cervical disease ($n = 70$) as opposed to those with primary disease of the vagina or vulva ($n = 74$).[6] In a smaller paper of 15 patients with cervical rhabdomyosarcoma, Ricciardi et al.[15] reported a 5-year overall survival of 78% with a progression-free survival (PFS) of 58%. In their experience, none of the patients with IRSG Clinical Group I disease had died of their disease while all

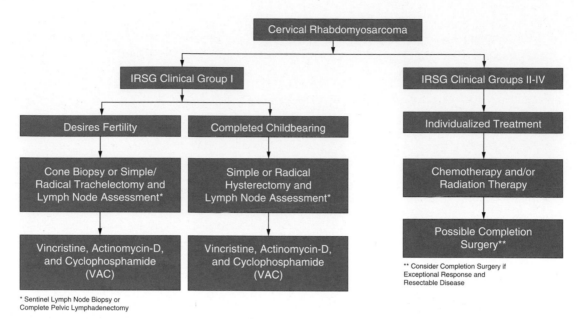

FIG. 15.3 Treatment algorithm for newly diagnosed rhabdomyosarcoma of the cervix. *ISRG*: Intergroup Rhabdomyosarcoma Study Group.

4 patients with IRSG Clinical Group II-III disease having recurred with 3 of those patients having died of their disease. The fourth patient was alive with disease but lost to follow-up. As many patients with cervical rhabdomyosarcoma will have familial syndromes or germline mutations such as *DICER1*, they are at risk for death from other malignancies in addition to rhabdomyosarcoma. For example, Kriseman et al.[3] noted 4 deaths in 11 patients with cervical rhabdomyosaroma but 1 of those patients died of a parotid adenocarcinoma and two of the pediatric patients had Sertoli-Leydig tumors and pinealoblastoma in addition to their cervical rhabdomyosarcoma and ultimately died from the brain cancers.

Treatment for recurrence typically employs those strategies utilized for rhabdomyosarcomas at other sites. If a patient has an isolated recurrence, surgical resection may be considered if feasible. For patients with unresectable disease or multisite recurrence, retreatment with VAC is an option if previously the patient only received VA or a short course of VAC. Other regimens include doxorubicin and ifosfamide with either etoposide or dacarbazine as well as vincristine and irinotecan with or without temozolomide (VI[T]). Salvage therapy with carboplatin, epirubicin, vincristine-ifosfamide, vincristine, etoposide (CEV/IVE) has also been utilized. Overall response rates (ORRs) to these regimens may be as high as 39%.[19] As many of these regimens will not be familiar to the gynecologic oncologist, patients would benefit greatly from consultation with a medical oncologist, particularly one who specializes in the treatment of sarcoma. Salvage chemotherapy may be given neoadjuvantly with the goal of delayed local treatment with surgery and/or radiation after reduction in tumor burden.

Adenoid cystic carcinoma

Adenoid cystic carcinoma is a malignant neoplasm consisting of epithelial and myoepithelial cells most commonly found in the salivary gland, accounting for 10%–15% of primary malignancies at that site. In the cervix, these tumors are extremely rare with an age adjusted-incidence of 0.025 per million women.[20] This tumor was first described as a head and neck cancer in 1856 with the first report of a primary cervical adenoid cystic carcinoma (originally called a "cylindroma") in 1949.[21] This subtype has also been described arising from other sites such as breast, lung, prostate, and vulva. In gynecologic oncology, these malignancies are most frequently seen in the cervix followed by the Bartholin's gland. These tumors are highly aggressive with hallmarks of early metastases and frequent local recurrence.

Adenoid cystic carcinoma of the cervix is most commonly seen in postmenopausal women peaking in the seventh and eight decades (median age 72 years).[20] However, cases in younger women (age <40 years) have also been reported.[22] The age of onset is 20 years later than the average age for squamous cell carcinoma of the cervix.[23] In addition to age, race seems to be a risk factor for developing the disease with black women 4.4 times more likely to develop the disease than their white counterparts.[20]

The role of HPV in the etiology of adenoid cystic carcinoma of the cervix remains unclear. Older reports detail the presence of HPV in adenoid cystic carcinomas of the cervix. For example, Grayson et al.[24] examined 11 specimens of which 8 were found to harbor high-risk HPV. Of these 8, 7 had integrated HPV-16 with HPV-31 in the remaining specimen. It is unclear if these 8 cancers were pure adenoid cystic carcinomas or admixed tumors. More recently, Xing et al.[25] investigated the presence of HPV in adenoid cystic carcinomas of the cervix and vulva. In 6 mixed specimens from the cervix, high-risk HPV was found in 5 with diffuse expression of p16. In 7 specimens of pure adenoid cystic carcinoma (6 from vulvar primaries and 1 from cervical), there was no high-risk HPV detected and variable, nondiffuse p16 expression. Perhaps the presence or absence of HPV depends on other admixed malignant cell types such that are known to be HPV dependent as squamous or adenocarcinoma.

Grossly, these tumors may present with either a mass or microscopic disease. Adenoid cystic carcinoma in the cervix is histologically identical to the salivary gland tumors and is thought to arise from the "reserve cells" that have features of progenitor cells.[25] They can be either pure or mixed with other tumors such as adenoid basal carcinoma, squamous carcinoma, or neuroendocrine carcinoma. Histologically they are characterized by the presence of solid tumor nests, frequently with cribriform pattern and interspersed basement membrane-like material.[26] The cells have scant cytoplasm, have a basaloid appearance, hyperchromatic nuclei with variable degree of atypia. Mitosis and necrosis are frequently identified.

Adenoid cystic tumor cells are usually positive for pankeratin, epithelial membrane antigen (EMA), myoepithelial markers such as p63 and S100. The basement membrane-like material is positive for type IV collagen and laminin. Adenoid cystic carcinomas that are mixed with other carcinomas are usually positive for p16 (diffuse) and high-risk HPV while the pure tumors are negative for these markers.[26]

The characteristic punched out, cribriform pattern can mimic adenocarcinoma; however, the presence of basement membrane-like material should facilitate the correct diagnosis. The solid pattern of adenoid cystic carcinoma can mimic both squamous carcinoma and neuroendocrine carcinoma, and immunostains as mentioned previously maybe used to facilitate the correct diagnosis. Another important differential is adenoid basal carcinoma (ABC), which was previously known as adenoid basal epithelioma. These tumors are usually identified incidentally and are frequently associated with either HSIL or other tumors such as squamous cell carcinoma. The majority are HPV-related. ABC is characterized by basaloid tumor nests with squamous and or glandular differentiation. The nuclei are bland, no basement membrane material is identified, and mitoses are infrequent, unlike in adenoid cystic carcinoma. When it occurs in the pure form, ABC has no metastatic potential.

Clinically, patients with adenoid cystic carcinoma often present with pain and abnormal bleeding. On exam, a hard mass in frequently seen on the cervix which may be friable and/or ulcerated. A biopsy is necessary to confirm the diagnosis and can be performed in the office or clinic utilizing a gold handled (Kevorkian) biopsy forceps. If there is any question about the diagnosis, additional tissue should be procured with more office biopsies, a loop electroexcisional procedure (LEEP), or cone biopsy.

It is important for the pathologist to differentiate between adenoid cystic carcinoma and adenoid basal carcinoma (ABC), also known as adenoid basal epithelioma. Adenoid cystic carcinoma and ABC were previously regarded as a single entity; however, they are now considered separate tumors due to the mostly benign course of the latter. Unlike adenoid cystic carcinoma, ABC lack infiltrative growth and rarely metastasize. They are usually detected as an incidental finding in LEEP or cone biopsy specimen performed for high-grade dysplasia.

After diagnosis, all patients should undergo imaging of the chest, abdomen, and pelvis with PET scan, CT scan, or MRI. On examination, 59% of patients will have disease clinically limited to the cervix with 37% having regional disease and 4% with distant metastases (Table 15.4).[20] However, imaging and/or surgery will ultimately show that 74% of clinical

TABLE 15.4 Distribution by FIGO stage for adenoid cystic carcinoma of the cervix.

Stage	Percent
I	59%
II	25%
III	11%
IV	5%

Adapted from D. Xing, J. Lu. Distinctive clinicopathological features and diseasespecific survival of adenoid cystic carcinoma and adenoid basal carcinoma in the lower female genital tract, Oncol Rep 41 (2019) 1769–1778.

stage I disease will have lymph node involvement.[27] This highlights the importance of radiologic/surgical staging in this disease (Table 15.1).

In a SEER database review, age, race and stage were noted to be prognostic factors for survival on univariate analyses. On multivariate analysis only stage remained significant as a prognostic factor for overall survival with a hazard ratio for death of 3.8.[20] Other prognostic factors include those identified by GOG-92 ("Sedlis criteria") such as tumor size, deep stromal invasion, and the presence of lymphovascular space invasion.[28] Oncologists should have a low threshold for consideration of postoperative radiation therapy if these prognostic factors are present.

Treatment for newly diagnosed adenoid cystic carcinoma follows the well-established guidelines for squamous cell or adenocarcinoma of the cervix. For early-stage disease, this typically entails radical hysterectomy with lymph node assessment. Due to the rarity of the disease, the role of sentinel lymph node biopsy has not been explored however if imaging shows no suspicious nodes sentinel lymph node biopsy in lieu of complete lymphadenectomy is likely adequate. As mentioned, oncologists should consider postoperative adjuvant radiation therapy based on pathologic risk factors including tumor size, deep stromal invasion, and the presence of lymphovascular space invasion. Adenoid cystic carcinomas are thought to be radiosensitive so women with locally advanced disease, concurrent chemoradiation with cisplatin should be undertaken with intent to cure.

For all patients with newly diagnosed adenoid cystic carcinoma of the cervix, the 5-year cancer specific survival rate is 69%.[20] Recurrence may be local and /or distant with the most common distant site being lung. In one study, 23% of recurrences were local only, 38% were distant only, and 38% had both distant and local components.[20] For those patients who have a distant component to their recurrence (with or without a local recurrence), over 50% had lung disease as part of that recurrence.[23]

Local recurrences should be treated with radiation if the patient has not been previously irradiated. For previously irradiated patients with an isolated, local recurrence, surgical resection is the only potential curative option. This may require a pelvic exenteration but should be undertaken with great caution and only after complete workup (including extensive imaging) assures no evidence of multifocal disease.

For patients with unresectable or multifocal disease, chemotherapy may be considered. In this setting, there are no systemic therapies that would offer any hope for cure and patients should be counseled that any treatment would be palliative with life prolongation as the goal of care. There are no standard regimens for recurrent adenoid cystic carcinoma of the cervix. For adenoid cystic carcinomas originating in the salivary gland, most oncologists utilize either adriamycin and cisplatin (AP) or cyclphosphamide, adriamycin, and cisplatin (CAP). Patients can expect response rates of approximately 25% with these regimens.[29] Cisplatin seems to be more active than carboplatin as studies that replace carboplatin for cisplatin show much lower response rates. Single agent paclitaxel lacks any activity in head and neck adenoid cystic carcinomas and most do not use that drug either alone or in combination.[30]

Molecularly, 90% of head and neck adenoid cystic will show high expression of c-kit.[31] However, first-generation tyrosine kinase inhibitors (TKIs) have shown minimal activity. For example, in 6 studies totaling 71 patients with recurrent head and neck adenoid cystic carcinoma, less than 5% showed any response to imatanib.[29] In contrast, the newer multi-receptor TKI lenvatanib does show acceptable activity in this disease. In a phase II study of 32 patients with recurrent head & neck adenoid cystic carcinoma, 16% of patients had a partial response with another 75% having stable disease (overall clinical benefit rate: 91%) with a median PFS of 17.5 months.[32]

Verrucous carcinoma

Verrucous carcinoma of the cervix is an exceedingly rare tumor with less than 50 cases reported in the literature. This tumor type was first described in an oral cavity malignancy in 1948.[33] These tumors are felt to be well-differentiated subtypes of squamous cell carcinoma and generally show a slow growth pattern with a propensity for local aggressiveness but rarely present with metastatic disease. Verrucous carcinomas are most frequently seen in the oral cavity, larynx, and esophagus but cases have been reported in the bladder and rectum as well as in the female genital tract. In the oral cavity, verrucous carcinomas make up 2%–8% of all squamous cell carcinomas where as in cervical cancer verrucous carcinomas are seen <0.01% of the time. In gynecologic oncology, these tumors are more likely to be encountered on the vulva than in the cervix however neither are seen with any true frequency.[34]

HPV has been implicated in the etiology of verrucous carcinoma. Due to the rarity of the disease at all gynecologic sites, definitive studies have not been (and likely will not be) performed. Case reports have more frequently shown HPV present in verrucous carcinoma specimens from the vulva and vagina and less commonly in those from the cervix however one case series of 3 patients with verrucous carcinoma of the cervix had HPV detected in all specimens examined.[35] Small studies have frequently detected HPV-6 in verrucous carcinoma specimens from the vagina but larger studies have not shown this consistently in tumors originating in the cervix.[36] Although HPV may be found in tumor specimens from patients with verrucous carcinoma, it is unknown whether it is causative or a co-factor, or if the virus may simply be a "bystander" that is detected alongside the malignancy on the cervix.

Grossly, verrucous carcinomas present with large exophytic warty masses, resembling a giant condyloma.[37] Histologically the lesion shows an exophytic growth of well-differentiated/mature squamous epithelium without prominent fibrovascular cores. There is minimal to no nuclear atypia or changes associated with HPV cytopathic effect (i.e., koilocytosis). The invasive front of the tumor is of pushing type, without infiltration. This pattern of invasion results in a challenge to make a definitive diagnosis, especially in small biopsies. Sampling the base of the lesion is essential for the diagnosis. p16 is frequently patchy and HPV testing is negative, as these are HPV independent tumors.

The differential diagnosis includes verruca vulgaris and condyloma. In the former, the rete are more pointed and not pushing as seen in verrucous carcinoma. Condylomas have more prominent fibrovascular cores and usually show changes associated with HPV effect.

Primary verrucous carcinoma of the cervix is typically seen in postmenopausal women and displays the classic symptoms of cervical cancer—irregular bleeding, particularly postcoital bleeding, and vaginal discharge. On exam these tumors are typically exophytic with a cauliflower-like appearance. Grossly they resemble large condyloma acuminata.

Diagnosis is made with a biopsy and as these can be frequently misdiagnosed as epithelial hyperplasia or condyloma acuminata, a generous biopsy must be procured. It is important to capture the junction between the tumor and the basement membrane to differentiate verruscous carcinoma from other etiologies such as condyloma acuminata, giant condyloma acuminata (Buschke–Loewenstein tumor), and invasive squamous cell cervical cancer. Frequently this may require a LEEP or cone biopsy. A definitive diagnosis may sometimes be made on final pathologic inspection of a hysterectomy specimen which was performed for what was thought to be a benign process.

The FIGO staging system for cervical cancer is most commonly utilized for this disease (Table 15.1). As mentioned, verrucous carcinoma grow by direct extension as opposed to metastasizing to lymph nodes or distant sites. In a review of the literature summarizing staging of 26 patients from multiple case reports and case series, Degefu et al.[38] found that all but one presented with cervix-confined or locally-extending disease with the lone outlier a patient with metastatic disease to the lungs. Stage-for-stage, patients with verrucous carcinoma seem to have a worse prognosis than comparable patients with squamous cell carcinoma of the cervix.[34]

When disease is limited to the cervix, surgical resection would be considered the most effective treatment for newly diagnosed verrucous carcinoma of the cervix. Due to propensity for local extension, most would perform a radical hysterectomy although there have been reports of successful treatment with simple hysterectomy. Patients who undergo surgery alone have an overall survival of 50% compared to only 38% for those who undergo surgery and radiation or radiation alone.[34] However, patients who had radiation as part of their treatment were more likely to have persistent or recurrent disease after surgery.

Similar results have been reported with the more common verrucous carcinoma of the oral cavity. In that disease, patients who receive radiation have worse outcomes than those who undergo surgery alone even when controlling for tumor stage at diagnosis.[39] That said, some of the patients who received adjuvant radiation after surgical resection may have had positive margins or persistent disease even though clinical stage was similar at diagnosis.

There is good rationale for why radiation may be ineffective in this disease. Radiation therapy targets rapidly dividing cells by causing DNA damage during cell replication. As verrucous carcinomas typically have very low mitotic rate, radiation therapy may not have the opportunity to affect many cells as most will not be actively replicating during treatment. More interestingly, early publications of oral cavity verrucous carcinoma reported an anaplastic transformation rate of 30% after radiation therapy; however, larger studies show a rate closer to 7%.[40] Anaplastic transformation seems to unleash widespread metastatic disease in this malignancy whose hallmark is local extension only. Reports of anaplastic transformation have been published for patients with cervical verrucous carcinoma after treatment with radiation.[41] For oral cavity verrucous carcinoma some recommend re-resection of disease if a margin is positive to avoid radiation therapy.[39] The applicability of re-resecting for positive margins in women with cervical verrucous carcinoma are probably a bit more limited.

As most disease will be cervix-confined or locally-advanced at diagnosis, most patients will undergo surgery and/or radiation with little role for chemotherapy. For patients with recurrent disease there is no standard therapy. One might consider carboplatinum, paclitaxel, and bevacizumab as this regimen is standard of care for squamous carcinomas of the cervix and due to the fact that some have reported strong expression of VEGF in these tumors.[42] There seems to be a lack of consensus on the best systemic therapy even for verrucous carcinoma of the oral cavity. There has been reports of standard chemotherapy, immunotherapy, and retinoid therapy. Tegafur and uracil have been used neoadjuvantly, concomitantly with radiation, and for recurrence with some effect. Oral fluoropyrimidine (capecitabine) has been reported to provide a good response in two patients with oral verrucous carcinoma who had inoperable disease.[43] Other investigators have shown continuous intraarterial methotrexate as extremely active for patients with oral verrucous carcinoma. In their case series, Wu et al.[44] showed complete response to this therapy in 15 patients with inoperable oral verrucous carcinoma at a median of 2.5 months after starting therapy with no patient recurring at a median follow-up of 42 months.

References

1. Margolis B, Tergas AI, Chen L, et al. Natural history and outcome of neuroendocrine carcinoma of the cervix. *Gynecol Oncol.* 2016;141:247–254.
2. Amer KM, Thomson JE, Congiusta D, et al. Epidemiology, incidence, and survival of rhabdomyosarcoma subtypes: SEER and ICES database analysis. *J Orthop Res.* 2019;37:2226–2230.
3. Kriseman ML, Wang WL, Sullinger J, et al. Rhabdomyosarcoma of the cervix in adult women and younger patients. *Gynecol Oncol.* 2012;126:351–356.
4. McClean GE, Kurian S, Walter N, Kekre A, McCluggage WG. Cervical embryonal rhabdomyosarcoma and ovarian Sertoli-Leydig cell tumour: a more than coincidental association of two rare neoplasms? *J Clin Pathol.* 2007;60:326–328.
5. Ferguson SE, Gerald W, Barakat RR, Chi DS, Soslow RA. Clinicopathologic features of rhabdomyosarcoma of gynecologic origin in adults. *Am J Surg Pathol.* 2007;31:382–389.
6. Nasioudis D, Alevizakos M, Chapman-Davis E, Witkin SS, Holcomb K. Rhabdomyosarcoma of the lower female genital tract: an analysis of 144 cases. *Arch Gynecol Obstet.* 2017;296:327–334.
7. Ibrahim U, Saqib A, Mohammad F, et al. Embryonal rhabdomyosarcoma of the cervix: a rare disease at an uncommon age. *Cureus.* 2017;9, e1864.
8. Coffin CM, Davis JL, Borinstein SC. Syndrome-associated soft tissue tumours. *Histopathology.* 2014;64:68–87.
9. Yoon JY, Apellaniz-Ruiz M, Chong AL, et al. The value of DICER1 mutation analysis in "Subtle" diagnostically challenging embryonal rhabdomyosarcomas of the uterine cervix. *Int J Gynecol Pathol.* 2021 Sep 1;40(5):435–440.
10. Merideth MA, Harney LA, Vyas N, et al. Gynecologic and reproductive health in patients with pathogenic germline variants in DICER1. *Gynecol Oncol.* 2020;156:647–653.
11. Li RF, Gupta M, McCluggage WG, et al. Embryonal rhabdomyosarcoma (botryoid type) of the uterine corpus and cervix in adult women: report of a case series and review of the literature. *Am J Surg Pathol.* 2013;37(3):344–355.
12. Dehner LP, Jarzembowski JA, Hill DA. Embryonal rhabdomyosarcoma of the uterine cervix: a report of 14 cases and a discussion of its unusual clinicopathological associations. *Mod Pathol.* 2012;25(4):602–614.
13. Apellaniz-Ruiz M, McCluggage WG, Foulkes WD. DICER1-associated embryonal rhabdomyosarcoma and adenosarcoma of the gynecologic tract: pathology, molecular genetics, and indications for molecular testing. *Genes Chromosomes Cancer.* 2021;60(3):217–233.
14. Arnold MA, Barr FG. Molecular diagnostics in the management of rhabdomyosarcoma. *Expert Rev Mol Diagn.* 2017 Feb;17(2):189–194. PMID: 28058850.
15. Ricciardi E, Plett H, Sangiorgio V, et al. Adult primary cervical rhabdomyosarcomas: a multicentric cross-national case series. *Int J Gynecol Cancer.* 2020;30:21–28.
16. Volker T, Denecke T, Steffen I, et al. Positron emission tomography for staging of pediatric sarcoma patients: results of a prospective multicenter trial. *J Clin Oncol.* 2007;25:5435–5441.
17. Sultan I, Qaddoumi I, Yaser S, Rodriguez-Galindo C, Ferrari A. Comparing adult and pediatric rhabdomyosarcoma in the surveillance, epidemiology and end results program, 1973 to 2005: an analysis of 2,600 patients. *J Clin Oncol.* 2009;27:3391–3397.
18. Network NCC. *Soft Tissue Sarcoma Version 1.2021.* Accessed November 29 https://www.nccn.org/professionals/physician_gls/pdf/sarcoma.pdf.
19. Winter S, Fasola S, Brisse H, Mosseri V, Orbach D. Relapse after localized rhabdomyosarcoma: evaluation of the efficacy of second-line chemotherapy. *Pediatr Blood Cancer.* 2015;62:1935–1941.
20. Xing D, Lu J. Distinctive clinicopathological features and diseasespecific survival of adenoid cystic carcinoma and adenoid basal carcinoma in the lower female genital tract. *Oncol Rep.* 2019;41:1769–1778.
21. Paalman RJ, Counseller VS. Clyindroma of the cervix with procidentia. *Am J Obstet Gynecol.* 1949;58:184–187.
22. Koyfman SA, Abidi A, Ravichandran P, Higgins SA, Azodi M. Adenoid cystic carcinoma of the cervix. *Gynecol Oncol.* 2005;99:477–480.
23. Dixit S, Singhal S, Vyas R, Murthy A, Baboo HA. Adenoid cystic carcinoma of the cervix. *J Postgrad Med.* 1993;39:211–215.
24. Grayson W, Taylor L, Cooper K. Detection of integrated high risk human papillomavirus in adenoid cystic carcinoma of the uterine cervix. *J Clin Pathol.* 1996;49:805–809.
25. Xing D, Schoolmeester JK, Ren Z, Isacson C, Ronnett BM. Lower female genital tract tumors with adenoid cystic differentiation: P16 expression and high-risk HPV detection. *Am J Surg Pathol.* 2016;40:529–536.
26. Mazur MT, Battifora HA. Adenoid cystic carcinoma of the uterine cervix: ultrastructure, immunofluorescence, and criteria for diagnosis. *Am J Clin Pathol.* 1982;77(4):494–500.
27. van Dinh T, Woodruff JD. Adenoid cystic and adenoid basal carcinomas of the cervix. *Obstet Gynecol.* 1985;65:705–709.
28. Sedlis A, Bundy BN, Rotman MZ, Lentz SS, Muderspach LI, Zaino RJ. A randomized trial of pelvic radiation therapy versus no further therapy in selected patients with stage IB carcinoma of the cervix after radical hysterectomy and pelvic lymphadenectomy: a gynecologic oncology group study. *Gynecol Oncol.* 1999;73:177–183.
29. Laurie SA, Ho AL, Fury MG, Sherman E, Pfister DG. Systemic therapy in the management of metastatic or locally recurrent adenoid cystic carcinoma of the salivary glands: a systematic review. *Lancet Oncol.* 2011;12:815–824.

30. Gilbert J, Li Y, Pinto HA, et al. Phase II trial of taxol in salivary gland malignancies (E1394): a trial of the eastern cooperative oncology group. *Head Neck.* 2006;28:197–204.

31. Holst VA, Marshall CE, Moskaluk CA, Frierson Jr HF. KIT protein expression and analysis of c-KIT gene mutation in adenoid cystic carcinoma. *Mod Pathol.* 1999;12:956–960.

32. Tchekmedyian V, Sherman EJ, Dunn L, et al. Phase II study of Lenvatinib in patients with progressive, recurrent or metastatic adenoid cystic carcinoma. *J Clin Oncol.* 2019;37:1529–1537.

33. Ackerman LV. Verrucous carcinoma of the oral cavity. *Surgery.* 1948;23:670–678.

34. Curtis MG, Strong S, Vang R. Pelvic abscess with fistula to the abdominal wall due to verrucous carcinoma. *Gynecol Oncol.* 1999;74:115–117.

35. Frega A, Lukic A, Nobili F, et al. Verrucous carcinoma of the cervix: detection of carcinogenetic human papillomavirus types and their role during follow-up. *Anticancer Res.* 2007;27:4491–4494.

36. Pilotti S, Donghi R, D'Amato L, et al. HPV detection and p53 alteration in squamous cell verrucous malignancies of the lower genital tract. *Diagn Mol Pathol.* 1993;2:248–256.

37. Dane B, Dane C, Erginbas M, et al. Verrucous carcinoma of the cervix in a case with uterine prolapse. *Ann Diagn Pathol.* 2009;13(5):344–346.

38. Degefu S, O'Quinn AG, Lacey CG, Merkel M, Barnard DE. Verrucous carcinoma of the cervix: a report of two cases and literature review. *Gynecol Oncol.* 1986;25:37–47.

39. Mohan S, Pai SI, Bhattacharyya N. Adjuvant radiotherapy is not supported in patients with verrucous carcinoma of the oral cavity. *Laryngoscope.* 2017;127:1334–1338.

40. McDonald JS, Crissman JD, Gluckman JL. Verrucous carcinoma of the oral cavity. *Head Neck Surg.* 1982;5:22–28.

41. Anghel RM, Trifanescu OG, Mitrica RI, et al. Good prognosis went badly: fulminant evolution of a 29-year-old patient with verrucous carcinoma of the cervix. *J Adolesc Young Adult Oncol.* 2017;6:499–502.

42. Matsumoto Y, Ishiko O, Nishimura S, et al. Angiogenesis in metastatic verrucous carcinoma of the uterine cervix. *Oncol Rep.* 2000;7:1079–1082.

43. Salesiotis A, Soong R, Diasio RB, Frost A, Cullen KJ. Capecitabine induces rapid, sustained response in two patients with extensive oral verrucous carcinoma. *Clin Cancer Res.* 2003;9:580–585.

44. Wu CF, Chen CM, Shen YS, et al. Effective eradication of oral verrucous carcinoma with continuous intraarterial infusion chemotherapy. *Head Neck.* 2008;30:611–617.

Chapter 16

Clear cell carcinoma of the vagina and cervix

Katherine C. Kurnit, Barrett Lawson, S. Diane Yamada, and Arthur Herbst

Clinical case

A 29-year-old G2P2 woman with a known bicornuate uterus presents to the office with irregular vaginal bleeding. A pelvic exam demonstrates a 2 cm friable lesion on the proximal vagina adjacent to the cervix (Fig. 16.1). A biopsy is consistent with clear cell carcinoma of the vagina. An MRI shows no parametrial involvement or invasion into nearby structures, and a PET scan demonstrates no distant metastases. How do you proceed?

Epidemiology

Etiology and risk factors

The most well-established risk factor for clear cell carcinomas of the vagina and cervix is in utero exposure to diethylstilbestrol (DES). DES is a synthetic estrogen that is administered orally. Beginning in the late 1940s, physicians in the United States began prescribing DES as a means to decrease adverse pregnancy outcomes, including preterm delivery, recurrent pregnancy loss, and hypertensive disorders of pregnancy.[1] It was prescribed most commonly between 1947 and 1971. In1970, the first case series of six women with clear cell carcinoma of the vagina was published.[2] In 1971, a subsequent case control study showed an increased odds of having been exposed to DES in utero in the women with clear cell carcinoma compared with the control group.[3] At this point, the Food and Drug Administration (FDA) changed the label for DES to no longer include prevention of miscarriage, and added pregnancy as a contraindication.[1] Use of DES during pregnancy declined significantly following.

In the Registry established to study these tumors, 695 women diagnosed with clear cell carcinoma of the vagina and cervix were reported, and 416 of these patients had known in utero exposure to DES.[4] Because of its rarity, the exact quantification of increased odds of developing clear cell carcinomas of the vagina and cervix attributable to DES exposure is uncertain, but the majority of cases have been associated with in utero DES. However, the significant proportion of women in the Registry without a known in utero DES exposure implies that there are probably other mechanisms by which these clear cell carcinomas may develop. In a study using the Central Netherlands Registry, a similar proportion of women developed clear cell carcinomas of the vagina and cervix without having had in utero exposure to DES as compared with the United States registry.[5]

Less is known about the relationship between clear cell carcinoma of the cervix or vagina and race and ethnicity. Only a small number of women in the United States registry were Black women (7%). A smaller proportion of Black women in the Registry had known DES exposure in utero, but this may have been due at least in part to decreased availability of maternal pregnancy histories compared with the white women included in the Registry.[6]

Mullerian abnormalities also have been associated with clear cell carcinomas of the vagina and cervix. Some anomalies are related to DES exposure and abnormal Mullerian embryological development.[7–10] Common anomalies include small, T-shaped uteri and abnormal appearing cervixes (cockscomb) and upper vaginas, which can be associated with infertility. However, non-DES-related anomalies have also been linked to clear cell carcinomas of the vagina and cervix, including Mullerian anomalies (bicornuate uterus, vaginal septum)[11–15] and urinary tract abnormalities such as renal agenesis.[10–12,15] Chromosomal abnormalities have also been linked to development of these rare cancers,[14] as have endometriotic implants in the vagina and cervix which have undergone malignant transformation into clear cell carcinomas.[17] Many cases are likely to be sporadic.[15,18]

Diagnosis and Treatment of Rare Gynecologic Cancers. https://doi.org/10.1016/B978-0-323-82938-0.00016-1

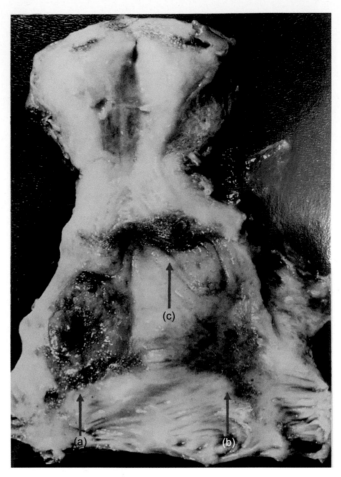

FIG. 16.1 Pathologic specimen showing an adenocarcinoma on the proximal vagina (a) adjacent to the cervix. There are nearby regions of adenosis present on the vagina (b) and cervix (c) as well.[2]

Incidence and mortality

After the association with DES was demonstrated, registries were established to follow women with known diagnoses of clear cell carcinoma arising in the vagina or cervix. Women were included regardless of their DES exposure status. Through these registries, more accurate risk estimates could be made. In women who had DES exposure in utero, the risk of developing clear cell carcinoma of the vagina or cervix by the age of 34 was estimated to be about 1 in 1000.[19] Of the 720 women with clear cell carcinoma who were included in the Registry, 400 (56%) patients had vaginal cancer, 182 (25%) had cervical cancer, and 138 (19%) had cancer involving both the vagina and cervix.[1] After the FDA listed pregnancy as a contraindication for the use of DES, the incidence of clear cell carcinoma of the vagina and cervix declined. However, it is estimated that approximately 50 cases each year are still diagnosed.[20]

The mean age at diagnosis is 22 years old, and 80% of patients are diagnosed between the ages of 15 and 30.[4] Survival outcomes are different for women exposed to DES in utero compared with those who were not exposed, likely due to differences in tumor biology.[4,21] A bimodal age distribution of incidence, one peak centered around 20 years of age and one around 60–80 years of age, has been described for non-DES-exposed women.[5] In 2018, updated survival data were published using the United States Registry. For DES-exposed women, the 5-year survival was slightly better at 86%, compared with 81% for those without exposures. The 20-year survival is approximately 69%, and was similar for both groups.[4] However, given the rarity of vaginal and cervical clear cell carcinomas, it is possible that some number of the women who were considered unexposed actually did have exposure to DES in utero. This theory of possible DES exposure is supported by the similar age distributions in registry patients with clear cell carcinomas of the vagina or cervix who were and were not exposed.[1] When looking at the evolution of overall survival over time, it is thought that an increase in deaths at age 35–49 is related to late recurrences of disease.[4]

Pathology

Adenocarcinoma makes up approximately 10% of all primary vaginal carcinomas and it is more common to have metastasis or extension of tumor from uterus, cervix, or vulva.[22] Clear cell carcinoma of the vagina is of particular interest, due to the known association with DES.[1] The median age of diagnosis for DES-related clear cell carcinoma was 20 years, with 80% of cases between the age of 15 and 31, though they have also been reported up to age 55.[1] Cases of clear cell carcinoma have also been reported to arise from vaginal adenosis without history of prenatal DES exposure and frequently occur in older women. Half of high grade primary vaginal adenocarcinomas may show clear cell differentiation.[23,24] Primary vulvar clear cell carcinoma is extremely rare, and usually arises in association with vulvar endometriosis.[25]

Gross description

Lesions can be more exophytic with polypoid, nodular or papillary appearance or may be flat or ulcerated.[26]

Microscopic description

Clear cell carcinoma can have a variety of architectural patterns, including tubulocystic/glandular, papillary, and solid, and frequently show a mixture of patterns in a given tumor.[26] The tumor cells have a varied appearance from flattened to polyhedral or cuboidal cells to "hobnail" cells with bulbous nuclei that protrude into a gland lumen or surface (Fig. 16.2). Nuclear atypia is moderate to marked, though the mitotic count is usually discordant with the atypia and is often low (approximately 3–4 mitosis per 10 HPF). While the tumors typically have clear cytoplasm, sometimes it can be eosinophilic.

Immunohistochemistry

Clear cell carcinoma is typically positive for cytokeratin 7, PAX-8, HNF1-b, and Napsin, while negative or weakly positive for hormone receptors ER and PR (Figs. 16.3–16.5). However, these markers are frequently not helpful in confirming the diagnosis. HNF1-b is not very specific and Napsin is not sensitive, hence negative staining for the latter does not exclude a diagnosis of clear cell carcinoma.

Differential diagnosis

Benign mimics may include vaginal adenosis or mesonephric remnants, though these would lack typical nuclear atypia of clear cell carcinoma.[26]

The differential diagnosis includes endometrioid adenocarcinoma and serous carcinoma, both of which can show clear cell change. Endometrioid carcinoma is usually diffusely positive for hormone receptors while clear cell carcinoma is negative. In some cases, distinguishing serous carcinoma from clear cell carcinoma may not be possible as both can overexpress p53 and, as mentioned earlier, the clear cell markers may not be helpful.

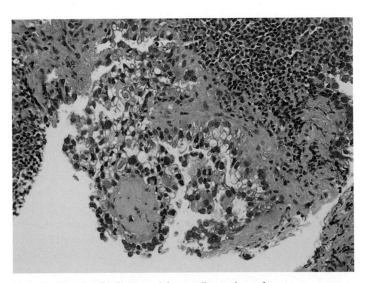

FIG. 16.2   Clear cell carcinoma with "hobnail" cells of bulbous nuclei protruding to the surface.

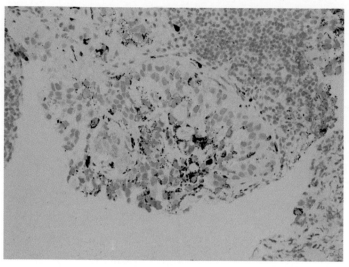

FIG. 16.3   Clear cell carcinoma with immunohistochemical positivity for Napsin.

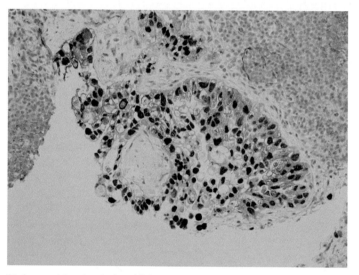

FIG. 16.4   Clear cell carcinoma with immunohistochemical positivity for HNF1-b.

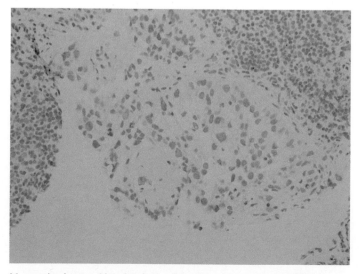

FIG. 16.5   Clear cell carcinoma with negative immunohistochemical staining for estrogen receptor (ER).

Extragonadal yolk sac tumors (YSTs) can be difficult to distinguish by morphology, though typically displaying Schiller–Duval bodies (papillae with central blood vessels), elevated alpha-fetoprotein (AFP) and usually a more reticular morphology.[24] Immunohistochemical stains help, as clear cell carcinoma will be CK7 and EMA positive, while negative in YSTs. SALL4, CDX2 and villin are expressed in most cases of YST and are usually negative in clear cell carcinoma. HNF1-b is positive in both and is not a useful distinguishing marker in this differential.

Molecular findings

Clear cell carcinomas associated with DES have genetic instability by mechanism of somatic mutations of microsatellite repeat sequences, which suggests that genes encoding DNA repair proteins may represent mutational targets of DES-induced mutagenesis.[18] Non-DES vaginal clear cell carcinoma has been reported to harbor chromosomal imbalances, such as chromosomal gain at 20q and loss of heterozygosity at 9p along with *PIK3CA* mutation, which are also seen in ovarian clear cell carcinomas.[27]

Diagnosis and workup

Signs and symptoms

Signs and symptoms may mirror those related to other vaginal and cervical cancers. Vaginal bleeding and discharge are both common presenting complaints, or patients may report bleeding after intercourse. Patients may also note a vaginal mass or nodule, and some girls/women reported changes in urinary symptoms.[2,28]

Physical exam findings

Physical exam may reveal a mass in the vagina or on the cervix. Vaginal adenosis is known to be a precursor lesion,[29,30] and these red, polypoid lesions may be visible prior to or identified concurrently with vaginal clear cell adenocarcinomas.[31] Given the young age at presentation associated with DES-related clear cell carcinomas, gynecologic exams may be more difficult to perform. For both DES and non-DES-exposed cases, an association with Mullerian tract abnormalities has been identified. Patients may have a small or T-shaped uterus,[9,32] or urinary tract abnormalities seen on imaging.[12,13,16,33,27]

Differential diagnosis

The differential diagnosis for clear cell carcinomas should include other histologic subtypes of vaginal and cervical cancers, including squamous cell and other adenocarcinomas. Other benign causes of vaginal and cervical masses should be considered, including polyps, leiomyomas, and cysts. Complaints of vaginal discharge or abnormal bleeding could also be associated with infectious or traumatic etiologies.

Tumor markers

There are no known tumor markers for clear cell carcinoma of the vagina. There are reports of CA-125 correlating with disease burden.[34] In the cases of malignant transformation of endometriotic lesions, it is also plausible that CA-125 levels may be elevated. However, we do not recommend tumor markers be routinely ordered during the diagnostic work-up of a vaginal or cervical clear cell carcinoma.

Imaging studies

In women with a new diagnosis of clear cell carcinoma of the vagina or cervix, we follow imaging guidelines similar to those recommended for new diagnoses of cervical cancer. Pelvic MRI can be useful to determine the extent of local disease. PET/CT or CT with contrast can be useful for evaluation of distant disease.

Diagnostic testing

Screening for women with a history of in utero DES exposure is discussed in the Special Considerations section. As is the case for cytologic abnormalities found on pap tests in other settings, colposcopy and colposcopic-guided biopsies are recommended in concordance with current lower genital tract screening and diagnostic guidelines.

For girls and women in whom a vaginal or cervical mass is identified, a tissue biopsy should be performed. For women and some girls who are comfortable with pelvic exams this may be achieved in the office. For girls or women in whom a pelvic examination may be more uncomfortable or difficult, examination with biopsies may need to be performed under anesthesia.

Staging system

Although historically cervical cancer was clinically staged, in 2018 the FIGO cervical cancer staging guidelines were updated (Table 16.1). Use of pathology and imaging studies are now included to help determine the stage of disease.

TABLE 16.1 FIGO staging for cervical cancer.

Stage	Description
I	The carcinoma is strictly confined to the cervix (extension to the uterine corpus should be disregarded)
IA	Invasive carcinoma that can be diagnosed only by microscopy, with maximum depth of invasion <5mm[a]
IA1	Measured stromal invasion ≤3 mm in depth
IA2	Measured stromal invasion >3 mm and ≤5 mm in depth
IB	Invasive carcinoma with measured deepest invasion >5 mm (greater than Stage IA), lesion limited to the cervix uteri
IB1	Invasive carcinoma >5 mm depth of stromal invasion, and ≤2 cm in greatest dimension
IB2	Invasive carcinoma >2 cm and ≤4 cm in greatest dimension
IB3	Invasive carcinoma >4 cm in greatest dimension
II	The carcinoma invades beyond the uterus, but has not extended onto the lower third of the vagina or to the pelvic wall
IIA	Involvement limited to the upper two-thirds of the vagina without parametrial involvement
IIA1	Invasive carcinoma ≤4 cm in greatest dimension
IIA2	Invasive carcinoma >4 cm in greatest dimension
IIB	With parametrial involvement but not up to the pelvic wall
III	The carcinoma involves the lower third of the vagina and/or involves pelvic and/or para-aortic lymph nodes[b]
IIIA	The carcinoma involves the lower third of the vagina, with no extension to the pelvic wall
IIIB	Extension to the pelvic wall and/or hydronephrosis or nonfunctioning kidney (unless known to be due to another cause)
IIIC	Involvement of pelvic and/or para-aortic lymph nodes (including micrometastases), irrespective of tumor size and extent (with r and p notations)[b]
IIIC1	Pelvic lymph node metastasis only
IIIC2	Para-aortic lymph node metastasis
IV	The carcinoma has extended beyond the true pelvis or has involved (biopsy proven) the mucosa of the bladder or rectum. (A bullous edema, as such, does not permit a case to be allotted to Stage IV.)
IVA	Spread to adjacent pelvic organs
IVB	Spread to distant organs

International Federation of Gynecology and Obstetrics (FIGO) staging of cancer of the cervix uteri (2018).

When in doubt, the lower staging should be assigned.

[a]*Imaging and pathology can be used, where available, to supplement clinical findings with respect to tumor size and extent, in all stages.*
[b]*Adding notation of r (imaging) and p (pathology) to indicate the findings that are used to allocate the case to Stage IIIC. Example: If imaging indicates pelvic lymph node metastasis, the stage allocation would be Stage IIIC1r, and if confirmed by pathologic findings, it would be Stage IIIC1p. The type of imaging modality or pathology technique used should always be documents.*
The involvement of vascular/lymphatic spaces does not change the staging. The lateral extent of the lesion is no longer considered.
From: N. Bhatla, D. Aoki, D.N. Sharma, Sankaranarayanan R. Cancer of the cervix uteri. Int J Gynaecol Obstet 143 (2018) S2:22. Available at: https://obgyn. onlinelibrary.wiley.com/doi/full/10.1002/igo.12611. Reproduced under the terms of the Creative Commons License 4.0. Updated with information from: Corrigendum to "Revised FIGO Staging for Carcinoma of the Cervix Uteri." Int J Gynaecol Obstet 147 (2019) 279.

TABLE 16.2 FIGO staging for carcinoma of the vagina (2009).

FIGO Stage	Description
IA	Tumor confined to the vagina, measuring ≤2.0 cm
IB	Tumor confined to the vagina, measuring >2.0 cm
IIA	Tumor invading paravaginal tissues but not to pelvic wall, measuring ≤2.0 cm
IIB	Tumor invading paravaginal tissues but not to pelvic wall, measuring >2.0 cm
III	Tumor extending to the pelvic sidewall and/or causing hydronephrosis or nonfunctioning kidney OR Pelvic or inguinal lymph node metastasis
IVA	Tumor invading the mucosa of the bladder or rectum and/or extending beyond the true pelvis (bullous edema is not sufficient evidence to classify a tumor as T4)
IVB	Distant metastasis

For vaginal cancer, the 2009 FIGO guidelines are frequently used in the United States (Table 16.2). Similar to new cervical cancer diagnoses, we use a combination of imaging, pathology (biopsies or surgical resection), and clinical findings to determine the extent of disease and stage.

Prognostic factors

Stage remains an important prognostic factor.[21,34,35] Other characteristics that have been associated with worse outcomes include younger age (below 15 years), a nontubulocystic histologic subtype, and nuclear atypia.[20,29–31]

Treatment of primary disease

Early stage disease

Vaginal

Early stage disease is often managed primarily with surgery (Fig. 16.6). In the original case control study published in 1971, seven of the eight patients with vaginal adenocarcinoma were managed with local resection.[3] The eighth underwent

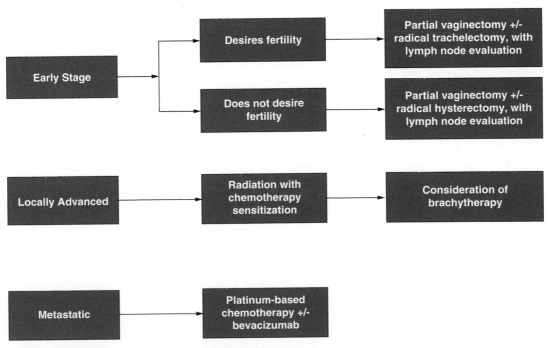

FIG. 16.6 Treatment Algorithm for Clear Cell Carcinoma of the Vagina.

exploratory laparotomy, and presumably was found to have metastatic disease. Of those managed with local resection, surgical approaches ranged from wide local excision to radical hysterectomy and vaginectomy, to anterior or posterior exenterations with vaginectomies. Several patients underwent vaginal reconstruction following the surgical resection. Aside from the patient with distant disease who had died, the other seven patients were alive and well at the time of the publication.[3] Other series have presented similar surgical approaches.[28,37,38] One cohort study of 219 stage I vaginal clear cell carcinoma patients showed that women who underwent less radical resections had improved outcomes when adjuvant radiation was also administered.[39] Furthermore, there are case reports of women with clear cell carcinoma of the upper vagina who have been successfully managed with a radical trachelectomy and upper vaginectomy with pelvic lymphadenectomy.[40,41]

In general, treatment for vaginal clear cell carcinoma can be guided by recommendations similar to those for cervical carcinomas. Tumors that do not have parametrial involvement and can be resected with adequate margins should undergo surgical resection. For vaginal primary tumors, sentinel lymph node mapping has not been evaluated, and thus lymphadenectomy should be performed. Use of pelvic and inguinal lymph node dissections should be guided by the location of the vaginal tumor (proximal two-thirds versus distal one-third of the vagina) and findings on imaging.

Cervical

Similar to other histologic subtypes of cervical cancer, early stage clear cell carcinoma of the cervix is often managed surgically with a simple or radical hysterectomy depending on the clinical features (Fig. 16.7). Additionally, there are case reports of approaches allowing for fertility preservation. One case series of two girls (both under age 10) diagnosed with Stage IB1 clear cell carcinoma of the cervix reported that both were successfully managed with abdominal radical trachelectomy and bilateral pelvic lymphadenectomy.[42] Although long-term survival and fertility outcomes are largely unknown for girls with vaginal or cervical clear cell primary tumors, a fertility-sparing approach is a reasonable option for appropriately selected prepubertal girls and women desiring fertility preservation.

For cervical clear cell adenocarcinomas, we would recommend following guidelines whereby FIGO (2018) stages IA1–IB2 tumors are surgically managed, as well as some FIGO (2018) stage IIA1 tumors. Lymph node assessment can be guided by imaging, but for all cervical cancers being surgically managed except for stage IA1 without lymphatic/vascular space invasion, either sentinel lymph node mapping or pelvic lymphadenectomy should be performed.

Locally advanced disease

Vaginal

One series of 76 stage II vaginal clear cell carcinoma patients showed wide variation in treatment approach, including the use of surgery alone (22 patients), radiation alone (38), a combination of surgery and radiation (12), and a small number of

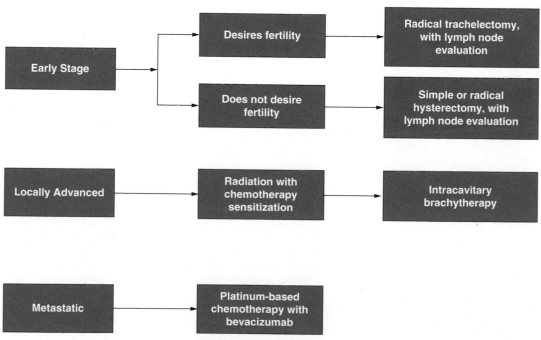

FIG. 16.7 Treatment Algorithm for Clear Cell Carcinoma of the Cervix.

patients (3) treated with chemotherapy with or without radiation therapy.[43] There were no differences in survival by treatment group, although this study was limited by the small numbers. Depending on the size of the primary vaginal tumor and baseline imaging findings, a combination of external beam radiation therapy and subsequent vaginal brachytherapy should be considered. In our practice, the initial treatment plans for these patients are created using a multidisciplinary approach that includes our radiation oncology colleagues, and almost always includes image-guided interstitial brachy-therapy. Similarly, for FIGO stages IIA–IVA clear cell carcinomas of the vagina, treatment frequently includes chemoradiation.

Cervical

Similar to locally advanced cervical cancers of more common histologic subtypes, FIGO (2018) stages IB3–IVA clear cell carcinomas of the cervix are often treated with chemoradiation.[44] Adding brachytherapy for locally advanced cervical cancers remains standard of care.

Metastatic disease

For metastatic clear cell carcinomas of the cervix, we treat with the same regimens used with the more common histologic subtypes. Specifically, we would recommend the combination of cisplatin, paclitaxel, and bevacizumab as utilized in Gynecologic Oncology Group (GOG) 240.[45] In general, fewer data are available for vaginal primary tumors, and thus we would extrapolate from metastatic vulvar or cervical cancers and recommend a platinum-based doublet (frequently carboplatin or cisplatin with paclitaxel) and, possibly, bevacizumab.

Surveillance for recurrent disease

For surveillance, we mirror recommendations for cervical cancers of other histologies.[46] We recommend clinical examinations including pelvic exams every 3 months for 2 years, every 6 months for 3 years, and then yearly thereafter. Examinations should include yearly pap tests and consideration of chest X-rays since the lungs are a frequent site of distant metastases. In patients with early stage disease at diagnosis who have undergone a fertility sparing surgery, an MRI at 6 months and then yearly for 3 years is recommended based on recommendations for patients with cervical cancer who have undergone fertility sparing approaches. For those who had nonfertility–sparing surgery but did not require adjuvant therapy, imaging can be guided by patients' symptoms and exam findings. For patients with more advanced disease or those who underwent adjuvant therapy, repeat imaging 3–6 months after completion of treatment may be useful. Subsequent imaging should be guided by signs and symptoms.

Survival and patterns of failure

Overall survival appears to be slightly better for patients with in utero DES exposure compared with those who did not have in utero exposure.[4] As expected, patients diagnosed at more advanced stages tend to have shorter overall survivals.[21] A summary of survival by stage and DES exposure is summarized in Table 16.3.

Recurrences of clear cell carcinomas of the vagina and cervix most often occur within the first 3 years.[36] However, late recurrences of clear cell carcinomas have also been observed.[34,36,37,47,48] In a series of patients with early recurrences, the majority occurred in the pelvis, with 44% in the vagina, 9% at the pelvic wall, 8% in the bladder, and 3% in the rectum.

TABLE 16.3 Distribution of stage at diagnosis and the associated 5-year and 10-year overall survivals.

	DES exposed			Not DES exposed		
	Proportion	5-year survival	10-year survival	Proportion	5-year survival	10-year survival
Stage I	59%	89%	83%	54%	76%	68%
Stage II	32%			33%		
Stage III	7%	41%	33%	11%	19%	0%
Stage IV	2%			2%		

Adapted from Waggoner, S.E., et al., *Influence of in utero diethylstilbestrol exposure on the prognosis and biologic behavior of vaginal clear-cell adenocarcinoma.* Gynecol Oncol, 1994. **55**(2): p. 238-44.

The remainder occurred at distant locations. In that series, those patients who experienced a pelvic recurrence had a 5-year overall survival of 40%.[36]

Treatment of recurrent disease

Locally recurrent clear cell carcinomas of the vagina can often be treated with surgery,[35] as can some patients with isolated distant recurrences.[47,48] Pelvic exenteration has been shown to be effective for select women with isolated central recurrences of clear cell carcinoma of both vaginal and cervical primary tumors.[49] For locally recurrent clear cell carcinoma of the cervix, we follow the same algorithms to determine appropriateness of surgery (most frequently, exenterative procedures) as for other histologic subtypes of cervical cancer. Adjuvant radiation or chemotherapy, or primary radiation with or without chemotherapy may also be used.[34,35] Preoperative evaluations can mirror the work-up done at the time of an initial diagnosis, with imaging to evaluate for local extent of disease and to ensure no metastatic disease is present. Metastatic recurrences are more often treated with systemic therapy.

Standard or commonly used regimens

There is no standard treatment regimen that has been established. Extrapolating from other vaginal and cervical carcinoma histologies, first-line therapy in chemotherapy naïve women would likely include a platinum agent (either cisplatin or carboplatin) in combination with paclitaxel. There are no prospective studies comparing the use of cisplatin and carboplatin specifically in women with clear cell histologies, but, in the case of cervical clear cell carcinomas, extrapolation from trials of squamous cell carcinomas of the cervix suggest that cisplatin may be first-line treatment if it can be tolerated. There are also no studies evaluating the use of bevacizumab in combination with cytotoxic chemotherapy for women with clear cell carcinomas of the vagina or cervix. However, extrapolation from studies of other cervical cancer histologies as well as clear cell carcinomas of the ovary suggests that bevacizumab may have some efficacy in this setting. In our practice, second and third line cytotoxic therapy is frequently topotecan, or occasionally navelbine or pemetrexed.

Potential therapeutic targets/molecular testing/mutations

As with other rare tumor types, we obtain molecular testing for somatic mutations when possible. There are few data addressing somatic alterations present in clear cell carcinomas of the vagina and cervix. However, clear cell carcinomas of the uterus and ovary frequently have *ARID1A* mutations,[50] and it is possible that this mutation may be seen in vaginal and cervical clear cell tumors as well. A case series of patients diagnosed with clear cell carcinoma of the cervix not thought to be associated with DES found that these tumors were intermittently positive for p53 or estrogen receptor (ER) on immunohistochemistry.[18,51] Another study identified a *PIK3CA* mutation.[27] Of note, these tumors are not commonly associated with the human papillomavirus (HPV).

Immunotherapy targets

Although the role of immunotherapy is unknown in clear cell carcinomas of the vagina and cervix, extrapolation of effectiveness from other tumor types suggests that this may be an effective treatment approach. Evaluation for mismatch repair deficiency (MMR-D) or microsatellite instability (MSI) may be beneficial, given that as many as 13% of ovarian[52,53] and 19% of endometrial clear cell carcinomas[52,54] have these findings. One study of clear cell carcinomas of the vagina found evidence of MSI among many of these tumors.[18] Additionally, during our molecular testing, we routinely evaluate for PD-L1 expression by immunohistochemistry as this has been a useful biomarker in other histologic subtypes. In general, for women with advanced or metastatic tumors of rare histologies, we strongly encourage clinical trial enrollment, particularly those including new immunotherapy agents.

Special considerations

Women and girls with in utero exposure to DES should follow specialized screening algorithms for cervical and vaginal dysplasia. Pap tests for cytology should include sampling of the entire circumference of the upper third of the vagina as well as the cervix.[55] Adenosis is a precursor to DES-related vaginal clear cell carcinoma,[29,30] and may appear as red, polypoid lesions.[31] In contrast to other cervical cancer screening recommendations, there is no recommended age at which screening should be discontinued in women with in utero exposure to DES. Colposcopy as a screening tool is not currently recommended.

Because of the rarity of these tumors, registries throughout the country have been developed. We strongly encourage the continued use of registries for women diagnosed with clear cell carcinomas of the vagina and cervix as a means to improve our understanding of the unique clinical patterns and potential molecular changes associated with these rare tumor types.

Case resolution

This 29-year-old woman was recommended for surgical management. As she did not desire future fertility, she underwent an abdominal radical hysterectomy with proximal vaginectomy, bilateral salpingectomy, and bilateral pelvic lymphadenectomy. Surgical margins were negative, but she had two positive pelvic lymph nodes. She was recommended for pelvic radiation with cisplatin sensitization. Following completion of adjuvant therapy, she entered into surveillance and remains without evidence of disease at 2 years posttreatment.

References

1. Huo D, et al. Incidence rates and risks of diethylstilbestrol-related clear-cell adenocarcinoma of the vagina and cervix: update after 40-year follow-up. *Gynecol Oncol.* 2017;146(3):566–571.
2. Herbst AL, Scully RE. Adenocarcinoma of the vagina in adolescence. A report of 7 cases including 6 clear-cell carcinomas (so-called mesonephromas). *Cancer.* 1970;25(4):745–757.
3. Herbst AL, Ulfelder H, Poskanzer DC. Adenocarcinoma of the vagina. Association of maternal stilbestrol therapy with tumor appearance in young women. *N Engl J Med.* 1971;284(15):878–881.
4. Huo D, Anderson D, Herbst AL. Follow-up of patients with clear-cell adenocarcinoma of the vagina and cervix. *N Engl J Med.* 2018;378(18): 1746–1748.
5. Hanselaar A, et al. Clear cell adenocarcinoma of the vagina and cervix. An update of the Central Netherlands registry showing twin age incidence peaks. *Cancer.* 1997;79(11):2229–2236.
6. Johnston Jr GA, et al. Clear cell adenocarcinoma of the vagina and cervix in black females. *J Natl Med Assoc.* 1982;74(7):639–643.
7. Jefferies JA, et al. Structural anomalies of the cervix and vagina in women enrolled in the diethylstilbestrol Adenosis (DESAD) project. *Am J Obstet Gynecol.* 1984;148(1):59–66.
8. Verloop J, et al. Risk of cervical intra-epithelial neoplasia and invasive cancer of the cervix in DES daughters. *Gynecol Oncol.* 2017;144(2):305–311.
9. Goodman A, Schorge J, Greene MF. The long-term effects of in utero exposures–the DES story. *N Engl J Med.* 2011;364(22):2083–2084.
10. Ben-Baruch G, et al. Uterine anomalies in diethylstilbestrol-exposed women with fertility disorders. *Acta Obstet Gynecol Scand.* 1981;60(4):395–397.
11. Spörri S, et al. Clear cell adenocarcinoma of the cervix associated with a rare genitourinary malformation. *Obstet Gynecol.* 2000;96(5 Pt 2):834–836.
12. Uehara T, et al. A case of vaginal clear cell adenocarcinoma complicated with congenital anomalies of the genitourinary tract and metanephric remnant without prenatal diethylstilbestrol exposure. *J Obstet Gynaecol Res.* 2010;36(3):681–685.
13. Zeeshan-ud-din, Ahsan A. Vaginal clear cell adenocarcinoma with associated Müllerian duct anomalies, renal agenesis and situs inversus: report of a case with no known in-utero exposure with diethyl stilboestrol. *J Pak Med Assoc.* 2009;59(8):568–570.
14. Tanaka H, et al. Clear cell adenocarcinoma of the vagina in a young female, treated by combination chemotherapy (local and systemic chemotherapy), complicated with chromosomal abnormality. *Gynecol Oncol.* 1994;55(2):259–264.
15. Watanabe Y, Etoh T, Nakai H. Adenocarcinoma of the lower female genital tract in patients with Herlyn-Werner-Wunderlich syndrome. *Am J Obstet Gynecol.* 2012;207(6):e5–e6.
16. Plesinac-Karapandzic V, et al. Non-diethylstilbestrol exposed vaginal adenocarcinoma in young patients associated with unilateral renal agenesis: two case reports and literature review. *Eur J Gynaecol Oncol.* 2017;38(1):157–161.
17. Shah C, et al. Clear cell adenocarcinoma of the vagina in a patient with vaginal endometriosis. *Gynecol Oncol.* 2006;103(3):1130–1132.
18. Boyd J, et al. Molecular genetic analysis of clear cell adenocarcinomas of the vagina and cervix associated and unassociated with diethylstilbestrol exposure in utero. *Cancer.* 1996;77(3):507–513.
19. Melnick S, et al. Rates and risks of diethylstilbestrol-related clear-cell adenocarcinoma of the vagina and cervix. An update. *N Engl J Med.* 1987;316 (9):514–516.
20. Trimble EL, et al. Vaginal clear cell adenocarcinoma in the United States. *Gynecol Oncol.* 1996;61(1):113–115.
21. Waggoner SE, et al. Influence of in utero diethylstilbestrol exposure on the prognosis and biologic behavior of vaginal clear-cell adenocarcinoma. *Gynecol Oncol.* 1994;55(2):238–244.
22. Adams TS, Cuello MA. Cancer of the vagina. *Int J Gynecol Obstet.* 2018;143:14–21.
23. Frank SJ, Deavers MT, Jhingran A, et al. Primary adenocarcinoma of the vagina not associated with diethylstilbestrol (DES) exposure. *Gynecol Oncol.* 2007;105:470–474.
24. Pang L, Li L, Zhu L, et al. Malignant transformation of vaginal adenosis to clear cell carcinoma without prenatal diethylstilbestrol exposure: a case report and literature review. *BMC Cancer.* 2019;19:798.

25. Kojima N, Yoshida H, Uehara T, et al. Primary clear cell adenocarcinoma of the vulva: a case study with mutation analysis and literature review. *Int J Surg Pathol.* 2019;27(7):792–797.

26. Offman SL, Longacre TA. Clear cell carcinoma of the female genital tract (not everything is as clear as it seems). *Adv Anat Pathol.* 2019;19:296–312.

27. Ikeda Y, et al. Non-diethylstilbestrol exposed vaginal clear cell adenocarcinoma has a common molecular profile with ovarian clear cell adenocarcinoma: a case report. *Gynecol Oncol Rep.* 2014;10:49–52.

28. Hasanzadeh M, Jafarian AH, Mousavi Seresht L. Primary clear cell carcinoma with no diethylstilbestrol exposure; case series. *Iran J Med Sci.* 2019;44(2):163–167.

29. Sherman AI, et al. Cervical-vaginal adenosis after in utero exposure to synthetic estrogens. *Obstet Gynecol.* 1974;44(4):531–545.

30. Laronda MM, et al. Diethylstilbestrol induces vaginal adenosis by disrupting SMAD/RUNX1-mediated cell fate decision in the Müllerian duct epithelium. *Dev Biol.* 2013;381(1):5–16.

31. Vooijs PG, Ng AB, Wentz WB. The detection of vaginal adenosis and clear cell carcinoma. *Acta Cytol.* 1973;17(1):59–63.

32. Kaufman RH, Adam E. Genital tract anomalies associated with in utero exposure to diethylstilbestrol. *Isr J Med Sci.* 1978;14(3):353–362.

33. Ott MM, et al. Vaginal clear cell carcinoma in a young patient with ectopic termination of the left ureter in the vagina. *Virchows Arch.* 1994;425(4):445–448.

34. Fishman DA, et al. Late recurrences of vaginal clear cell adenocarcinoma. *Gynecol Oncol.* 1996;62(1):128–132.

35. Jones WB, Tan LK, Lewis Jr JL. Late recurrence of clear cell adenocarcinoma of the vagina and cervix: a report of three cases. *Gynecol Oncol.* 1993;51(2):266–271.

36. Herbst AL, et al. Epidemiologic aspects and factors related to survival in 384 registry cases of clear cell adenocarcinoma of the vagina and cervix. *Am J Obstet Gynecol.* 1979;135(7):876–886.

37. Hall WB, et al. Endobronchial clear cell adenocarcinoma occurring in a patient 15 years after treatment for DES-associated vaginal clear cell adenocarcinoma. *Gynecol Oncol.* 2004;93(3):708–710.

38. Thomas MB, et al. Clear cell carcinoma of the cervix: a multi-institutional review in the post-DES era. *Gynecol Oncol.* 2008;109(3):335–339.

39. Senekjian EK, et al. Local therapy in stage I clear cell adenocarcinoma of the vagina. *Cancer.* 1987;60(6):1319–1324.

40. Matthews KS, et al. Fertility-sparing radical abdominal trachelectomy for clear cell adenocarcinoma of the upper vagina: a case report. *Gynecol Oncol.* 2007;105(3):820–822.

41. Shepherd ES, Lowe DA, Shepherd JH. Targeted selective trachelo-colpectomy for preservation of fertility in a young woman with vaginal clear cell carcinoma. *J Obstet Gynaecol.* 2010;30(4):420–421.

42. Abu-Rustum NR, et al. Pediatric radical abdominal trachelectomy for cervical clear cell carcinoma: a novel surgical approach. *Gynecol Oncol.* 2005;97(1):296–300.

43. Senekjian EK, et al. An evaluation of stage II vaginal clear cell adenocarcinoma according to substages. *Gynecol Oncol.* 1988;31(1):56–64.

44. Ansari DO, et al. Successful treatment of an adolescent with locally advanced cervicovaginal clear cell adenocarcinoma using definitive chemotherapy and radiotherapy. *J Pediatr Hematol Oncol.* 2012;34(5):e174–e176.

45. Tewari KS, et al. Improved survival with bevacizumab in advanced cervical cancer. *N Engl J Med.* 2014;370(8):734–743.

46. Salani R, et al. An update on post-treatment surveillance and diagnosis of recurrence in women with gynecologic malignancies: Society of Gynecologic Oncology (SGO) recommendations. *Gynecol Oncol.* 2017;146(1):3–10.

47. Lin LM, et al. Diethylstilbestrol (DES)-induced clear cell adenocarcinoma of the vagina metastasizing to the brain. *Gynecol Oncol.* 2007;105(1):273–276.

48. Herbst AL, et al. An analysis of 346 cases of clear cell adenocarcinoma of the vagina and cervix with emphasis on recurrence and survival. *Gynecol Oncol.* 1979;7(2):111–122.

49. Senekjian EK, Frey K, Herbst AL. Pelvic exenteration in clear cell adenocarcinoma of the vagina and cervix. *Gynecol Oncol.* 1989;34(3):413–416.

50. Wiegand KC, et al. ARID1A mutations in endometriosis-associated ovarian carcinomas. *N Engl J Med.* 2010;363(16):1532–1543.

51. Wang D, et al. Primary clear cell adenocarcinoma of the cervix: a clinical analysis of 18 cases without exposure to diethylstilbestrol. *Obstet Gynecol Int.* 2019;2019:9465375.

52. Willis BC, et al. Mismatch repair status and PD-L1 expression in clear cell carcinomas of the ovary and endometrium. *Mod Pathol.* 2017;30(11):1622–1632.

53. Bennett JA, et al. Mismatch repair protein expression in clear cell carcinoma of the ovary: incidence and morphologic associations in 109 cases. *Am J Surg Pathol.* 2016;40(5):656–663.

54. DeLair DF, et al. The genetic landscape of endometrial clear cell carcinomas. *J Pathol.* 2017;243(2):230–241.

55. Hanselaar AG, et al. Cytologic examination to detect clear cell adenocarcinoma of the vagina or cervix. *Gynecol Oncol.* 1999;75(3):338–344.

Section D

Vulvovaginal cancers

Chapter 17

Vulvovaginal melanoma

Mario M. Leitao, Jr. and Priyadharsini Nagarajan

Clinical case

A 44-year-old nulliparous female presents with vaginal discharge. A vaginal tumor is biopsied, revealing invasive melanoma. On physical exam, there is a 5 cm polypoid and mostly hypopigmented lesion with a broad base arising from the right lateral vaginal wall starting at 3 cm from the vaginal introitus and extending approximately 4 cm along the lateral vaginal wall. A positron emissions tomography (PET) scan notes a F-18-fluorodeoxyglucose (FDG)-avid vaginal mass but no other evidence of metastasis. Magnetic resonance imaging (MRI) of the brain is normal. MRI of the pelvis reveals a circumscribed 3.5 cm × 3 cm × 4.7 cm intermediate T2 signal tumor in the upper to mid vagina spanning the entire thickness of vaginal wall (Fig. 17.1). How do you treat this patient?

Epidemiology

Incidence and mortality

Vulvovaginal (vulvar/vaginal) melanomas are often treated as one entity, but the incidence and mortality of each differs. Although we consider them "mucosal" melanomas, it is unclear whether vulvar and vaginal melanomas are true "mucosal" melanomas. In 2020, an estimated 6120 vulvar cancers were diagnosed in the United States[1]; and on average, 1350 vaginal cancers are diagnosed each year.[2] Melanoma accounts for only 6% of vulvar cancers and 9% of vaginal cancers in the Unites States,[3,4] totaling approximately 500 newly diagnosed cases of vulvovaginal melanoma per year. The median age at diagnosis for vulvovaginal melanoma is 68 years.[5] The median age at diagnosis for vulvar melanoma is slightly younger than that for vaginal melanoma.[6] The range of ages is much wider for vulvar melanomas, with cases reported in girls as young as 10 years old and women as old as 99 years of age.[7] At least 85% of women with vulvar melanoma are white, 4%–12% are Hispanic, and approximately 1%–4% each are African-America, Asian, or of other races.[6–9] It is more difficult to precisely ascertain race distribution for vaginal melanomas[10]; however, a large SEER dataset analysis noted that approximately 9.5% of women with vaginal melanoma are African-American, compared to 3.5% of those with vulvar melanoma.[6] The age-adjusted annual incidence rates for vulvovaginal melanomas are 1.9 for whites and 1.0 for non-whites per million women.[5]

Vulvovaginal melanoma is associated with a worse overall survival (OS) compared to other vulvar cancers, as well as compared to cutaneous melanomas.[3–5] The 5-year OS rate for vulvar melanoma is 59% compared to 76% for squamous cell carcinoma and 92% for adenocarcinoma.[2] Survival appears to vary based on race, as well as whether the primary site is the vulva or vagina (Table 17.1).[5] It is unclear, however, why African-American women have worse survival. Vulvovaginal melanomas seem to be diagnosed at more advanced stages compared to other vulvar cancers, as well as cutaneous melanomas, which may explain the differences in survival as a group overall.[3,5] Individually, vaginal melanomas present at more advanced stages compared to vulvar melanomas, likely due to anatomic location, leading to delayed diagnoses and worse survival.[5,6] For vulvar melanomas, survival seems to be worse stage-for-stage compared to squamous cell carcinomas and adenocarcinomas.[3] It also seems that stage-for-stage, women with vaginal melanoma have a worse survival compared to those with vulvar melanoma.[6]

Etiology/risk factors

Vulvovaginal melanomas are not associated with chronic sun damage (CSD) as are acral and other non-CSD skin melanomas and are generally categorized as mucosal melanomas. There are no known etiologic or well-established risk factors for vulvovaginal melanomas. There are a few reported inherited genetic mutations that increase the lifetime risk of

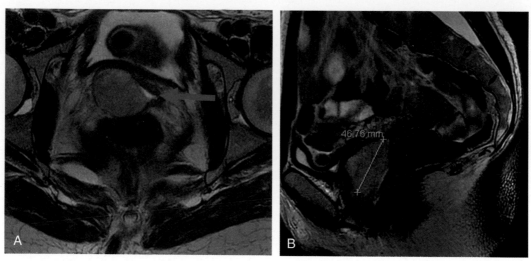

FIG. 17.1 MRI of the pelvis at original presentation. (A) Axial view. (B) Sagittal view.

TABLE 17.1 Median overall survival (OS) for vulvovaginal melanomas compared to cutaneous melanomas by site and race using SEER data, 1973–2008.

	Vulvovaginal melanoma combined	Cutaneous melanoma	P-value
Black	16 months	124 months	<0.0001
Non-black	39 months	319 months	<0.0001
	Vulvar melanoma alone	*Cutaneous melanoma*	
Black	33 months	124 months	0.0057
Non-black	58 months	319 months	<0.0001
	Vaginal melanoma alone	*Cutaneous melanoma*	
Black	8.5 months	124 months	<0.0001
Non-black	19 months	319 months	<0.0001
	Vulvar melanoma	*Vaginal melanoma*	
Black	33 months	8.5 months	0.0135
Non-black	58 months	19 months	<0.0001

Data from Mert I, Semaan A, Winer I, Morris RT, Ali-Fehmi R. Vulvar/vaginal melanoma: an updated Surveillance Epidemiology and End Results Database review, comparison with cutaneous melanoma and significance of racial disparities. Int J Gynecol Cancer 2013;23:1118–1125.

cutaneous and uveal melanomas.[11] These include *CDKN2A, CDK4, POT1, TERT, BRCA1&2, BAP1, MITF, XPC, XPD, XPA, PTEN, and TP53*.[11] There are no reports, however, on the association of risk of vulvovaginal, or mucosal melanomas in general with these specific hereditary syndromes. A maxillary mucosal melanoma in a 21-year-old with Li–Fraumeni syndrome has been reported.[12]

A retrospective analysis of 81 genital or anorectal mucosal melanomas (GAMMs) over a 33-year period compared to 293 cutaneous melanomas attempted to address the familial/hereditary risk of these mucosal melanomas.[13] The majority of the GAMM cases were women (88%) and were vulvar/vaginal melanomas (68%). Other cases included anorectal, penile, and cervical melanomas.[13] The rate of cases with multiple other primary melanomas was similar (6% for GAMM and 5.3% for cutaneous melanoma).[13] A family history of any-type melanoma was noted in 18% of the GAMM cases compared to 7.5% of the cutaneous cases.[13] Germline testing for CDKN2A was performed in 17 of the GAMM cases, and none of these patients had a germline mutation.[13] Although a germline mutation was not identified, the authors suggested that GAMMs are part of familial/hereditary syndromes based on the increased family history of melanoma in GAMM patients. This very small retrospective series is far from conclusive or definitive. However, careful vulvovaginal examination along with the recommended whole-body skin examinations is prudent in patients with known germline mutations and strong familial history of any type of melanoma. Biopsy of any new or concerning (or even if not too concerning) vulvovaginal lesions should be performed in patients with these hereditary syndromes.

Pathology

Primary melanomas of the vulva are characterized by conspicuous histopathologic overlap with primary cutaneous melanomas. However, the exact nature, i.e., whether a vulvar melanoma is mucosal or cutaneous remains one of the most challenging questions for the following reasons: (i) although some may be confined to the cutaneous or mucosal epithelia of the various parts of vulva, the mucocutaneous junction may also be the site of origin for vulvar melanomas; (ii) many of the vulvar melanomas are large with broad lentiginous or nodular patterns of growth at the time of presentation and therefore, may extend across the mucocutaneous junction, irrespective of initial cutaneous or mucosal origin; (iii) mucosal melanomas are frequently multifocal and thus, may involve various parts of the vulva; for instance, both the ipsilateral labium majus and labium minus, or across the midline; (iv) although most are pigmented, approximately 25% of vulvar melanomas may be amelanotic, thus, precluding determination of gross extent of tumor; (v) since pruritus is one of the most common presenting symptoms, chronic scratching-related low-grade trauma can lead to prominent lichenification of squamous mucosa with acquisition of granular and thick cornified layers; therefore, the histologic distinction of mucosa from skin is further muddled.[9,14,15] Therefore, collaborative efforts of gynecologists and oncologists documenting the precise anatomic location(s) of grossly visible lesion and histopathologic evaluation detailing the extent of melanoma along cutaneous and mucosal epithelia by pathologists is essential to determine whether a given vulvar melanoma is principally mucosal or cutaneous in nature.

Gross features

In majority of the cases, primary vulvar melanomas are characterized by a lesion, which is frequently ulcerated. At least focal pigmentation is noted in majority of the cases. However, some cases may lack pigmentation. In those arising from preexisting melanosis or melanocytic lesion, a recent change in color, size, and shape is a clue to malignant transformation.

Microscopic features

Primary melanomas of the vulva display histopathologic features akin to their cutaneous counterparts, and the American Joint Committee on Cancer (AJCC) recommends vulvar melanomas to be analyzed and staged according to the criteria established for primary cutaneous melanomas. The histopathologic features to be assessed and reported in vulvar melanomas are summarized in Table 17.2. Majority of the primary vulvar melanomas are invasive. However, in rare instances, the patient may have long-standing melanoma in-situ before developing invasive disease. Multifocal disease and skip lesions are common in vulvar melanomas.

Primary vulvar melanomas are characterized by architectural and cytopathologic abnormalities. The growth pattern of primary vulvar melanomas is most commonly lentiginous: contiguous proliferation of atypical single melanocytes along the basal layer of stratified squamous epithelium interspersed by a few nests (Fig. 17.2), or nodular: absence of a radial growth phase, in which the intraepithelial component is either absent or does not extend beyond the invasive component (Fig. 17.3). Rare cases of superficial spreading type, characterized by proliferation of predominantly nests of varying sizes and shapes with pagetoid scatter of atypical melanocytes within the suprabasal layers of stratified squamous epithelium (Fig. 17.4) may also be seen, particularly among those that arise from cutaneous surfaces. The in-situ/ intraepithelial component is typically characterized by poor circumscription as well as asymmetry (Fig. 17.5) and often involves the adnexal structures such as vaginal glands and folliculo-sebaceous units extensively.

The extent of dermal/submucosal involvement by melanoma may be evaluated using various methods including (i) Breslow/tumor thickness, (ii) Clark/anatomic level and (iii) Chung level (Fig. 17.6, Table 17.3).[16–18] Of these, the AJCC has incorporated the Breslow/ tumor thickness in staging of primary melanomas.[19] In view of the lack of well-defined papillary dermis in mucosae, Clark level is not applicable to primary vulvar melanomas; the term "anatomic" level is recommended instead (Table 17.2). The invasive component is characterized by irregular proliferation of melanocytes within the dermis and/or submucosa with varying degrees of cytologic atypia, absence of maturation of melanocytes with deeper descent and mitotic activity, including atypical forms (Fig. 17.7).

TABLE 17.2 Primary tumor features recommended for histopathologic assessment of primary vulvar melanomas.

Histopathologic feature	AJCC recommended	CAP recommended
Histologic type		Yes
Clark[a]/anatomic[b] level		
Breslow[a]/tumor[b] thickness	Yes	Yes
Radial (non-tumorigenic) growth phase		
Vertical (tumorigenic) growth phase		
Mitotic rate (number/mm^2)	Yes	Yes
Ulceration	Yes	Yes
Regression		
Lymphovascular invasion		Yes
Perineural invasion		
Microscopic satellitosis	Yes	Yes
Tumor-infiltrating lymphocytes		
Associated precursor melanocytic nevus		
Predominant cytology		
Margins		Yes

[a]Used in evaluation of primary melanomas of cutaneous origin.
[b]Used in evaluation of primary melanomas of mucosal origin.

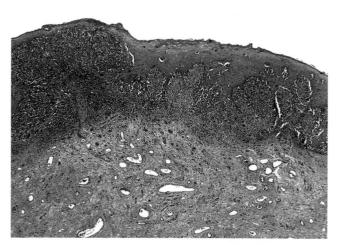

FIG. 17.2 Primary vulvar melanoma with lentiginous pattern of growth, characterized by contiguous proliferation of atypical single melanocytes along the basal layer of stratified squamous epithelium.

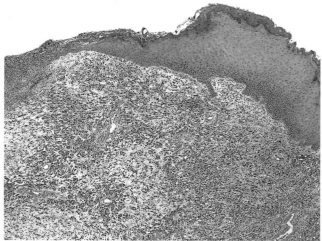

FIG. 17.3 Primary vulvar melanoma, nodular type. The intraepithelial component or in-situ melanoma is either absent or does not extend beyond the invasive component; i.e., there is no radial component.

The maximum depth of invasive tumor, referred to as Breslow thickness in primary melanomas of cutaneous origin and tumor thickness in melanomas of mucosal origin is the parameter of most prognostic importance. It is typically measured from the (i) top of granular layer in keratinized stratified squamous epithelium, (ii) top of nucleated layer in nonkeratinized stratified squamous epithelium or (iii) base of ulcer to the deepest extent of tumor. In particular, tumor thickness >2 mm and mitotic rate of ≥2/mm^2 of the invasive component correlated with poor disease-specific survival (DSS) in a retrospective analysis of 100 cases of primary vulvar melanomas.[15]

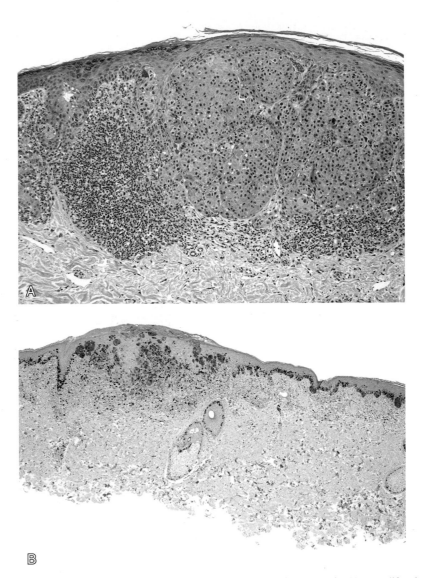

FIG. 17.4 Primary vulvar melanoma, superficial spreading type. (A) The in situ component is characterized by a proliferation of predominantly nests of varying sizes and shapes with pagetoid scatter of atypical melanocytes within the suprabasal layers of stratified squamous epithelium. (B) MART1/Ki67 cocktail immunohistochemical stain highlights the broad radial component, i.e., the in situ component extending beyond the invasive melanoma.

Melanoma-associated ulceration (Fig. 17.8) is more frequent in primary vulvar melanomas (in up to 50%) compared to primary cutaneous melanomas. Even though ulceration correlated with overall and DSS by univariate analysis, it did not emerge as an independent prognostic parameter of overall and disease-specific survival after multivariable analysis. Lymphovascular invasion (LVI) (Fig. 17.9), neurotropism or perineural invasion (PNI) (Fig. 17.10) and microscopic satellitosis may also be present.[15]

The melanoma cells may be of epithelioid or spindled cytology and are typically characterized by varying amounts of pale amphophilic or eosinophilic cytoplasm, fine-dusty pigmentation, ovoid nuclei, vesicular chromatin and prominent nucleoli. In some cases, cytoplasmic pigmentation may be completely absent. Infrequently, the melanoma cells may be of nevoid cytology in which the cytologic atypia is subtle with small ovoid hyperchromatic nuclei, condensed chromatin and inconspicuous nucleoli.

In limited biopsies or when the cytoplasmic pigmentation is minimal, melanocytic origin may be difficult to appreciate; thus, requiring use of immunohistochemical studies. Employing a panel of immunohistochemical markers, including

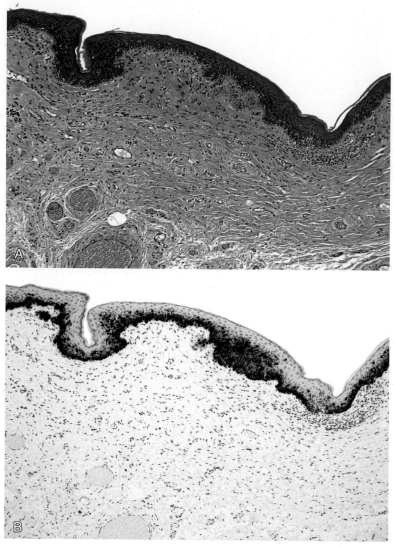

FIG. 17.5 Vulvar melanoma-in situ. (A) Subtle proliferation of small single melanocytes along the basal layer of stratified squamous epithelium with poor circumscription. (B) Melanocytic cocktail (HMB45 and anti-tyrosinase) immunohistochemistry highlights the in situ melanoma.

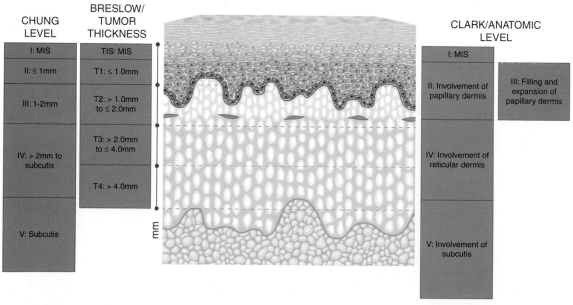

FIG. 17.6 Methods for evaluating extent of dermal/subdermal involvement.

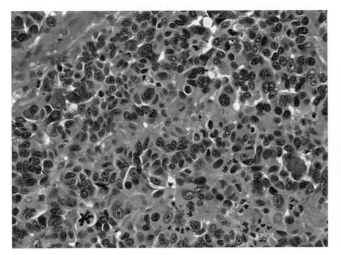

FIG. 17.7 Invasive melanoma with epithelioid cytology, patchy cytoplasmic pigmentation and atypical mitotic figure with multipolar spindle (left lower).

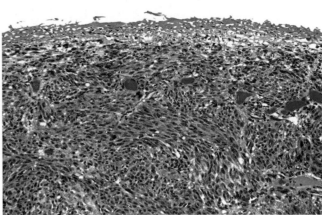

FIG. 17.8 Primary vulvar melanoma with spindled cytology and extensive ulceration.

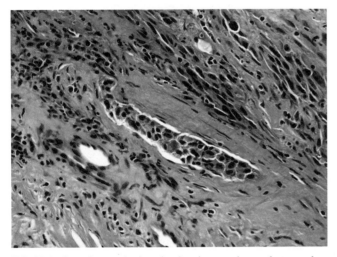

FIG. 17.9 Lymphovascular invasion in primary vulvar melanoma, characterized by presence of atypical cells within lumina lined by flattened endothelial cells.

melanocytic markers such as MelanA, HMB45, tyrosinase, MITF, S100 and SOX10; keratinocytic markers including cytokeratin cocktail(s), p63 and p40; as well as vascular markers including CD34, CD31, and ERG. Typically, primary melanomas of the vulva tend to be MelanA+ HMB45-patchy+ tyrosinase+ MITF+ S100+ SOX10+ cytokeratin cocktail(s)- p63- p40- CD34- CD31- ERG-. In some advanced cases, the tumors may have undergone de-differentiation resulting in loss of expression of melanocytic markers with acquisition of keratinocytic markers such as cytokeratin and less likely, p63. In such scenarios, SOX10 remains the most sensitive marker to demonstrate melanocytic differentiation. SOX10 may also be used as an ancillary test to determine margin status. Presence of LVI may be highlighted using endothelial markers such as D2-40 or CD31 as well as cocktails such as SOX10/CD31 and MITF/D2-40.[20]

Differential diagnoses

Majority of vulvar melanomas are pigmented; therefore, the clinical differential diagnoses include all pigmented or dark lesions of the vulva of reactive and neoplastic origin (Fig. 17.11). Pigmented vulvar lesions may be present in up to 12% of white women,[10] of which 10%–19% may be melanocytic in origin.[21–24] Documentation of the following features is important for optimal diagnosis, management and follow-up: type: rash vs. lesion and palpability; relationship with surrounding skin: well-defined vs. merging; the precise anatomic location(s); color: dark, reddish/ violaceous, brown-black and intralesional variability; multiplicity; size; shape; evidence of associated disease such as lichen sclerosus; nature of specimen submitted: excisional biopsy (recommended for small lesions to include a rim of normal skin) vs. partial biopsy and location of biopsy site (in large lesions). It is also imperative to document any underlying diseases such as lichen sclerosus, diabetes, systemic lupus erythematosus, lichen planus, etc.

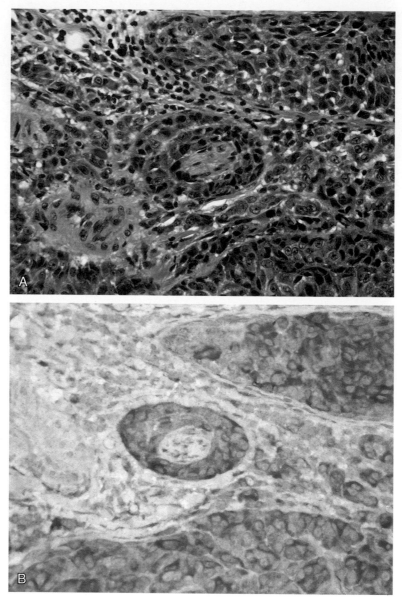

FIG. 17.10   Perineural invasion in primary vulvar melanomas. (A) Small caliber nerve fiber completely encircled by melanoma cells. (B) MART1 immunohistochemical study highlights the melanoma cells and perineural invasion.

Molecular findings

When compared to primary cutaneous melanomas, genomic instability is more frequent in mucosal melanomas, manifesting in the form of copy number changes and structural variations, whereas point mutation burden is overall lower.[25,26] Structural variations targeting *TERT*, *CDK4*, and *MDM2* genes are common. Whole-genome sequencing of mucosal melanomas has revealed almost 10-fold increased frequency of single nucleotide variants when compared to primary cutaneous melanomas.[25] Commonly mutated genes include *SF3B1*, *NRAS*, *NF1*, *KIT*, *TP53*, *SPRED1*, *BRAF*, *ATRX*, *HLA-A*, and *CHD8*[27–29] of which *NF1* and *KIT* co-mutations can also occur.[26,30–32] Preferential mutations of *TERT* and *ATRX* correlated with shorter telomere lengths.[26] *BRAF* mutations are more frequent in primary vulvar melanomas compared to other types of anogenital melanomas, likely due to cutaneous origin.[33]

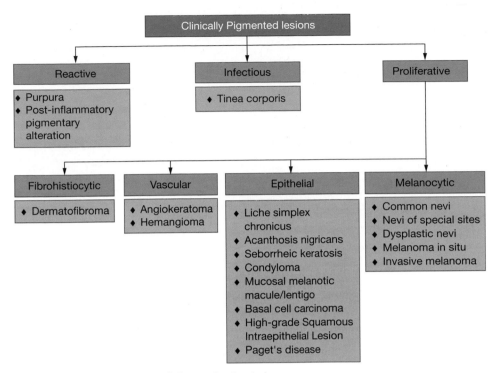

FIG. 17.11   Clinicopathologic differential diagnoses of pigmented vulvar lesions.

Diagnosis and workup

Signs and symptoms

The presenting signs and symptoms differ for women with vulvar compared to vaginal melanomas due to anatomic location. The most common presenting symptoms for vulvar melanomas are the presence of a vulvar mass or nevus/"mole" in 16%–25% of cases, pain in 5%–30%, bleeding in 17%–24%, and pruritis and/or irritation in 16%–24%.[9,27,34] Many patients will have more than one "presenting" sign or symptom. The labia majora or minora alone will be the primary site in 40%–70% of cases.[9,27,34] These masses can also be located primarily on the clitoris or perineum.[8,27] Multiple sites are often involved,[9,27] and the majority of cases are localized (51%–77%).[6,7,9,27] Inguinofemoral nodal involvement occurs in 9%–34% of cases, but only 2%–3% are clinically suspicious.[6,7,9,27]

Vaginal melanomas most commonly present with vaginal bleeding in 60%–100% of cases with vaginal masses, as well as pain or discharge.[10,28,29,35] Approximately 10% of patients will have no symptoms, and the malignancy is discovered on physical exam.[10,35] The anterior vaginal wall is the primary location in 45% of cases, the posterior wall in 32%, and the lateral walls in 24%, with larger tumors occupying greater aspects.[10,28,29,35] The majority of cases (60%) are located in the lower third of the vagina.[10,28,29,35] Pelvic and/or inguinal nodal involvement occurs in 25%–50% of cases.[10,35] The majority of lesions are hyperpigmented.

Physical exam findings

The vast majority of vulvovaginal melanomas are hyperpigmented. There are, however, amelanotic cases. Any new hyperpigmented lesion or tumor-forming lesion on the vulva or vagina should be biopsied. Any preexisting nevi that have changed in appearance should also be biopsied. A careful inspection of the vulva, vagina, and cervix is critical. An assessment of the mobility of lesions should be performed, as well as involvement of the urethra and/or anus. The assessment of vaginal masses is more difficult. Careful palpation of inguinofemoral nodal regions should be performed. A full-body skin examination by a dermatologist is also recommended. Routine cystoscopy or proctoscopy is unnecessary unless there are symptoms that may warrant such examinations or if there is obvious involvement on physical examination.

Tumor markers

There are no known validated serum tumor markers in the diagnosis and/or surveillance of melanomas, including vulvovaginal melanomas.

Imaging

Routine imaging is not recommended for patients diagnosed with clinical stage I or II cutaneous melanoma in the absence of symptoms.[36] Vulvovaginal melanomas are slightly different than cutaneous melanomas and present with regional or distant spread in 40%–60% of patients.[6] Pelvic MRI may provide important information regarding the local extent of disease. However, this is not essential for smaller mobile vulvar melanomas that are unifocal and limited to the labia and/or clitoris. Pelvic MRI should be performed for vulvar melanomas that are large, are encroaching on other structures such as urethra and/or anus, are multifocal, or are fixed. Pelvic MRI should be performed for all vaginal melanomas, as physical examination is limited, and is possibly the best method to follow treatment responses.

Evaluation for distant metastasis can be accomplished with either multidetector computed tomography (CT) or PET/CT imaging in cutaneous melanoma and is recommended for stage III/IV cases or to assess symptoms.[36] It is unclear whether the addition of PET scanning offers a greater value over good-quality CT imaging. CT +/− PET imaging is likely of low yield in melanomas confined the labia and/or clitoris that are unifocal. However, CT (+/−PET) imaging should be performed in all patients with vaginal melanomas, as they are associated with higher risk of distant metastasis at presentation. CT (+/−PET) imaging should also be performed in vulvar melanomas that are larger, fixed, involve other structures, or involve documented nodal metastases. Brain MRI should also be performed in patients with evidence of nodal metastases, other distant metastases, or symptoms.

Diagnostic tests

The key to proper diagnosis is biopsy with pathologic assessment by a dermatopathologists with expertise in melanoma. The following are important features to note in pathology reports for cutaneous melanomas: clinicopathologic type of melanoma, tumor thickness using Breslow depth (mm), presence or absence of ulceration, number of mitoses per square millimeters (mm^2), presence of microsatellites, and the status of all margins.[37] The significance of other features is less clear. Immunohistochemical testing may offer guidance in cases that are not clear-cut, as described in the "Pathology" section above.

Different melanoma subtypes harbor different molecular alterations. Acral melanomas, mucosal melanomas, and those associated with CSD have different molecular profiles than those arising from skin without CSD.[38] *BRAF* and *NRAS* mutations are much more frequent in non-CSD melanomas and less common in the other melanomas, including mucosal melanomas.[39,40] KIT alterations are seen more frequently in CSD-associated, acral, and mucosal melanomas (Table 17.3). Curtin and colleagues noted *BRAF* mutations in 56% of non-CSD melanomas, and no *KIT* alterations were found in any of these melanomas.[39] In contrast, *BRAF* mutations were seen in 3% of mucosal melanomas, with 39% having a *KIT* alteration, either mutation or amplification.[39] In a phase 2 study, KIT alterations were seen in 25% of mucosal melanomas.[40] Mutations in *BRAF, NRAS,* and *GNAQ* were detected in 9%, 12%, and 0% of mucosal melanomas, respectively.[40] Hou and

TABLE 17.3 Assessment of the extent of dermal/ submucosal involvement by melanoma.

Breslow/ tumor thickness	Clark/ anatomic level	Chung level
T0: Melanoma in situ	I: Melanoma in situ	I: Melanoma in situ
T1: Tumor thickness ≤ 1.0 mm	II: Invasive melanoma involves the papillary dermis	II: Invasion ≤1 mm
T2: Tumor thickness > 1.0 mm to ≤2.0 mm	III: Invasive melanoma fills and expands the papillary dermis	III: Invasion 1–2 mm
T3: Tumor thickness > 2.0 mm to ≤4.0 mm	IV: Invasive melanoma involves the reticular dermis	IV: Invasion >2 mm
T4: Tumor thickness > 4.0 mm	V: Invasive melanoma involves the subcutis	V: Invasion into subcutis

colleagues compared the molecular profiles of 51 vulvovaginal melanomas to 2253 nongynecologic melanomas and found *BRAF* mutations in 26% of the vulvovaginal melanomas, which is the highest reported rate[41] *KIT* alterations were found in 22% of the vulvovaginal melanomas.[41] Additional mutations were found in *NRAS* (4%) and *APC* (15%) and in other genes.[41]

Molecular profiling is unlikely to assist in the management of patients with stage I or II melanomas. The National Comprehensive Cancer Network (NCCN) does not recommend routine molecular profiling for stages I and II resected melanomas but does recommended it for stage III/IV, unresectable, and/or recurrent melanoma to help guide treatment.[36] This principle would apply to vulvovaginal melanomas, but considering the rarity of these tumors, it is reasonable to at least perform molecular analysis for *KIT, BRAF,* and *NRAS* in all cases. Broader genomic analysis when obtaining molecular testing, if possible, may provide a better understanding of this disease and also identify other potentially targetable mutations and/or triage cases for select clinical trials. The value of routine testing for programmed death-ligand 1 (PD-L1) expression in melanoma is unclear and not recommended by the NCCN.[36]

The initial workup for newly diagnosed vulvovaginal melanoma is summarized in Table 17.4.

Staging system

The majority of gynecologic malignancies are staged using the International Federation of Gynecology and Obstetrics (FIGO) staging system. Vulvar and vaginal cancers are staged differently within the FIGO staging system (Tables 17.5 and 17.6).[42,43] The FIGO systems are validated in carcinomas of the vulva and vagina, but it is not clear how specific FIGO criteria can be applied in staging of vulvovaginal melanomas. It is also unclear as to whether it is best to use staging systems for other melanomas. In 1970, Ballantyne proposed a staging system for melanomas of the skin of the head and neck.[44] The Ballantyne system grouped cases into three stages and applied it to both newly diagnosed and recurrent cases. Ballantyne

TABLE 17.4 Rates of select genetic mutations among melanoma types.[38–41]

	BRAF	NRAS	KIT
Non-CSD cutaneous	59%	22%	0%
CSD cutaneous	15%–22%	0%–10%	16%–28%
Mucosal (all types)	4%–15%	5%–13%	18%–39%
Acral	20%–23%	7%–16%	21%–36%
Vulvovaginal	4%	13%	26%

CSD = chronic sun-induced.

TABLE 17.5 Initial workup of newly diagnosed vulvovaginal melanoma.

Physical Exam	• Complete physical examination with pelvic and rectovaginal examinations • Inspection of the primary lesion as it relates to urethra and anus as well as to mobility of lesion • Inspection of the inguinofemoral nodal basins • Full body skin examination by experienced dermatologist
Imaging	• Routine imaging not recommended for smaller, unifocal, mobile vulvar lesions without concern for metastases based on symptoms and physical examination • Pelvic MRI and CT (+/−PET) for larger vulvar lesions, lesions encroaching on urethra and/or anus, multifocal lesions, non-mobile/fixed lesions, and/or clinical concern for metastases • Pelvic MRI and CT (+/− PET) should be performed for all vaginal melanomas due to difficulty in accurate assessment based on physical exam alone • MRI of brain in cases with evidence of metastatic disease on the above imaging or if neurologic symptoms present
Laboratory tests	• None recommended routinely for AJCC stage I or II lesions, which are resectable • For stage III/IV and/or unresectable disease and/or recurrent disease, molecular testing for *KIT, NRAS,* and *BRAF* alterations at a minimum • Consider multigene panel testing, if possible, in addition to the above

MRI, magnetic resonance imaging; CT, computed tomography; PET, positron emission tomography; AJCC, American Joint Committee on Cancer.

TABLE 17.6 TNM and FIGO staging systems for vulvar cancer.

The definitions of the T categories correspond to the stages accepted by the International Federation of Gynecology and Obstetrics (FIGO). Both systems are included for comparison

Primary tumor (T)		

T category	FIGO stage	T criteria
TX		Primary tumor cannot be assessed
T0		No evidence of primary tumor
T1	I	Tumor confined to the vulva and/or perineum. Multifocal lesions should be designated as such. The largest lesion or the lesion with the greatest depth of invasion will be the target lesion identified to address the highest pT stage. Depth of invasion is defined as the measurement of the tumor from the epithelial-stromal junction of the adjacent most superficial dermal papilla to the deepest point of invasion.
T1a	IA	Lesions more than 2 cm, or any size with stromal invasion of more than 1 mm, confined to the vulva and/or perineum
T1b	IB	Lesions more than 2 cm, or any size with stromal invasion of more than 1 mm, confined to the vulva
T2	II	Tumor of any size with extension to adjacent perineal structures (lower/distal third of the urethra, lower/distal third of the vagina, anal involvement)
T3	IVA	Tumor of any size with extension to any of the following-upper/proximal two-thirds of the urethra, upper/proximal two-thirds of the vagina, bladder mucosa, or rectal mucosa-or fixed to the pelvic bone
T3a	IIIA	Tumor involving the serosa and/or adnexa (direct extension or metastasis)

Regional lymph nodes (N)		

N category	FIGO stage	N criteria
NX		Regional lymph nodes cannot be assessed
N0		No regional lymph node metastasis
N0(i+)		Isolated tumor cells in regional lymph node(s) no greater than 0.2 mm
N1	III	Regional lymph node metastasis with one or two lymph node metastases each less than 5 mm, or one lymph node metastasis greater than or equal to 5 mm
N1a*	IIIA	One or two lymph node metastases each less than 5 mm
N1b	IIIA	One lymph node metastasis greater than or equal to 5 mm
N2		Regional lymph node metastasis with three or more lymph node metastases each less than 5 mm, or two or more lymph node metastases greater than or equal to 5 mm, or lymph node(s) with extranodal extension
N2a*	IIIB	Three or more lymph node metastases each less than 5 mm
N2b	IIIB	Three or more lymph node metastases each less than 5 mm
N2c	IIIC	Lymph node(s) with extranodal extension
N3	IVA	Fixed or ulcerated regional lymph node metastasis

Note: The site, size, and laterally of lymph node metastases should be recorded.
*Includes micrometastasis, N1mi and N2mi.

Distant metastasis (M)		

M category	FIGO stage	M criteria
M0		No distant metastasis (no pathological M0; use clinical M to complete stage group)
M1	IVB	Distant metastasis (including pelvic lymph node metastasis)

TABLE 17.6 TNM and FIGO staging systems for vulvar cancer—cont'd

Prognostic stage groups			
When T is...	And N is...	And M is...	Then FIGO stage is...
T1	N0	M0	I
T1a	N0	M0	IA
T1b	N0	M0	IB
T2	N0	M0	II
T1-T2	N1-N2c	M0	III
T1-T2	N1	M0	IIIA
T1-T2	N2a, N2b	M0	IIIB
T1-T2	N2c	M0	IIIC
T1-T3	N3	M0-M1	IV
T1-T2	N3	M0	IVA
T3	Any N	M0	IVA
Any T	Any N	M1	IVB

Vulvar melanoma is not included in this staging system; it is staged with the melanoma staging system.
Classification of p16 status will be included if obtained but is not required.
TNM: Tumor, Node, Metastasis, AJCC: American Joint Committee on Cancer; UICC: Union for International Cancer Control.
Used with permission of the American College of Surgeons, Chicago, Illinois. The original source for this information is the AJCC Cancer Staging Manual, Eighth Edition (2017) published by Springer International Publishing. Corrected at 4th printing, 2018.

stage I disease is local, stage II involves regional metastases, and stage III involves distant metastasis.[44] This system was used for melanomas from multiple sites for some time but is no longer favored in the staging of melanoma.

Melanomas are primarily staged using the AJCC staging system.[45] AJCC provides classifications for staging cutaneous melanoma, conjunctival melanoma, uveal melanoma, and mucosal melanoma of the head and neck.[45] However, there is no AJCC staging system for mucosal melanoma of the urethra, vagina, rectum, and anus. Using SEER data, Wohlmuth and colleagues noted good discrimination for outcomes in vulvar melanoma using the AJCC system but were not able to assign AJCC stage to vaginal melanomas.[6] The 5-year DSS for vulvar melanoma based on AJCC stage was as follows: 83.6% for stage I, 51.8% for stage II, 24.9% for stage III, and 6.4% for stage IV disease ($P < 0.001$) (Fig. 17.12).[6] In a prospective trial (GOG73), AJCC staging using available criteria at the time (1992) was the most discriminatory for recurrence-free interval where FIGO stage was not significant on multivariate analysis.[27] An analysis from the Melanoma Institute Australia also suggested that AJCC staging for cutaneous melanoma was appropriate, but the analysis combined vulvar, vaginal, and cervical melanomas.[46] Many consider vulvar melanoma as a "cutaneous" process and will use AJCC staging, and it is preferred for vulvar melanomas (Table 17.7). The AJCC TNM system includes both a clinical stage, which requires a biopsy and used clinical and radiologic information, and a pathologic stage, which includes wide excision of primary site and pathological information about regional nodes after either sentinel lymph node (SLN) biopsy or lymphadenectomy.[45] The best staging system for vaginal melanomas is undetermined, and stage is often difficult to ascertain, as many simply do not undergo adequate biopsy to assess tumor thickness or undergo wide surgical resection with surgical nodal assessment. However, it may suffice to use the AJCC clinical TNM (cTNM) staging system for vaginal melanomas.

Prognostic factors

There are multiple established prognostic factors for cutaneous melanomas; however, prognostic factors are not well established in vulvovaginal melanomas. Published reports to assess various risk factors, for prognosis specifically, in vulvovaginal melanomas are limited due to small cohorts, and the majority of studies only included vulvar melanomas. Many of the studies specific to vulvovaginal melanomas cannot account for confounding when assessing prognostic factors due to the small cohorts included. Additionally, the specific prognostic factors and the number of factors assessed among the studies vary tremendously.

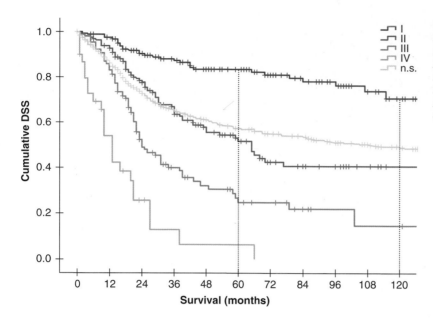

FIG. 17.12 Disease-specific survival by American Joint Committee on Cancer (AJCC) stage in vulvar melanoma. *Reprinted from Wohlmuth C, Wohlmuth-Wieser I, May T, Vicus D, Gien LT, Laframboise S. Malignant melanoma of the vulva and vagina: a US population-based study of 1863 patients. Am J Clin Dermatol 2020;21:285–295. Courtesy of Springer Creative Commons usage.*

TABLE 17.7 FIGO staging of carcinoma of the vagina.

FIGO stage	Stage description
I	The cancer is only in the vagina and is no longer than 2.0 cm (4/5 in.) (T1a) It has not spread to nearby lymph nodes (N0) or to distant sites (M0)
I	The cancer is only in the vagina and is larger than 2.0 cm (4/5 in.) (T1b) It has not spread to nearby lymph nodes (N0) or to distant sites (M0)
II	The cancer has grown through the vaginal wall, but nor as far as the pelvic wall and is no larger than 2.0 cm (4/5 in.) (T2a) It has not spread to nearby lymph nodes (N0) or to distant sites (M0)
II	The cancer has grown through the vaginal wall, but nor as far as the pelvic wall and is no larger than 2.0 cm (4/5 in.) (T2b) It has not spread to nearby lymph nodes (N0) or to distant sites (M0)
III	The cancer can be any size and might be growing into the pelvic wall, and/or growing into the lower one-third of the vagina and/or has blocked the flow of urine (hydronephrosis), which is causing kidney problems (T1 to T3) It has also spread to nearby lymph nodes in the pelvis or groin (inguinal) area (N1) but not distant sites (M0)
III	The cancer is growing into the pelvic wall, and/or growing into the lower one-third of the vagina and/or has blocked the flow of urine (hydronephrosis), which is causing kidney problems (T3) It has not spread to nearby lymph nodes (N0) or to distant sites (M0)
IVA	The cancer is growing into the bladder or rectum or growing out of pelvis (T4) It might or might not have spread to lymph nodes in the pelvis or groin (inguinal area) (Any N). It has not spread to distant sites (M0)
IVB	The cancer has spread to distant organs such as the lungs or bones (M1). It can be any size and might or might not have grown into nearby structures or organs (Any T) It might or might not have spread to nearby lymph nodes (Any N)

Breslow tumor thickness, nodal status, and stage appear to be the most consistent prognostic factors among the studies specific to vulvovaginal melanomas.[5–10,15,27,34,46] For the largest retrospective cohort of 1400 vulvar and 463 vaginal melanomas from the SEER database, the 5-year DSS rate based on Breslow tumor thickness was 74.5% for thickness ≤ 1.0 mm, 61.7% for thickness 1.01–2.0 mm, 58.7% for thickness 2.01–4.0, and 32.5% for thickness > 4.0 mm.[6] Chung level of invasion was reported in only one study, and it was associated with survival on univariate but not on multivariate analysis.[8] Clark levels were assessed in two studies,[9,27] and it was associated with outcome in both studies but not on multivariate modeling.[9,27] There does not seem to be much utility in using the Chung or Clark level of invasion criteria. Breslow tumor thickness is most useful in deciding on surgical nodal assessment (discussed in more detail in Treatment of Primary Disease section) and loses significance when adjusted for presence of nodal metastases and final surgical stage (Table 17.8).[6,27]

The presence of nodal metastases has been shown to be a highly significant prognostic factor in all studies that have assessed it.[5–8,10,27,34] In the aforementioned SEER study, the 5-year DSS rate for vulvar melanomas with no nodal metastases was 70.8%, compared to 29% if one node had metastatic disease and 20.8% if there were two or more positive nodes ($P < 0.001$).[6] For vaginal melanomas, the 5-year DSS rate for node-negative cases was 27.1%, compared to 10.7% for cases with one positive node and 0% for cases with two or more positive nodes ($P = 0.003$).[6] The presence of nodal metastases remained an independently associated prognostic factor on multivariate analysis.[6]

Stage is also a consistent prognostic factor across multiple studies.[5–7,9,27] Stage has been assessed using AJCC criteria as well as SEER criteria (localized, regional, or distant), and both have been associated with outcome. Five-year DSS based on AJCC stage for vulvar melanomas is mentioned above. Stage and presence of nodal disease are highly related variables, as final surgical AJCC staging uses nodal status as an important criterion.[45]

Many other factors that have been validated in cutaneous melanomas have also been assessed for their association with outcome, with varying and inconsistent results. Clinically, these factors are not as important in the treatment decisions for vulvovaginal melanomas compared to Breslow thickness, nodal status, and stage. The presence of ulceration is a significant and routinely used factor in cutaneous melanoma. It was not found to be significant in a series of 89 vulvar melanomas from multiple centers in Germany.[34] Tumor ulceration was associated with outcome in a series of 85 vulvar, vaginal, and cervical melanomas from the Australia Melanoma Institute.[46] However, the study did not assess either nodal status or stage as prognostic factors, and multivariate analysis was also not performed.[46] Ulceration was associated with outcome in a series of 100 vulvar melanomas from MD Anderson Cancer Center; however, the study also did not include nodal status or stage for analyses.[15] Despite this, ulceration was not independently associated with outcome on multivariate analysis. In the large SEER-based analysis by Wohlmuth and colleagues, ulceration was associated with outcome on univariate but not multivariate analysis.[6] Histologic subtype, age, race, mitotic rates, presence of lympho-vascular invasion (LVSI), satellitosis, tumor location, and tumor size have not been consistently associated with outcome across studies.[5–10,15,27,34,46]

Treatment of primary disease

Surgery

Surgery is the preferred primary treatment of newly diagnosed vulvovaginal melanoma if it is feasible and does not require an exenterative procedure (Fig. 17.13). Surgery should address both the primary tumor and the regional nodal basins. Surgical cytoreduction of metastatic and/or extra-nodal disease can be considered in highly selected cases of cutaneous melanoma, but there are no data to guide such an approach in vulvovaginal melanoma.[37] Mostly Breslow thickness, but also other factors, should be considered for surgical decisions. Cutaneous melanomas are generally grouped into either thin (Breslow thickness ≤ 1 mm), intermediate (1.01–4 mm), or thick (>4 mm).[15]

Primary tumor site

Wide local excision of the primary tumor should be performed if a negative margin resection is possible without an exenterative procedure. Historically, wide surgical margins of up to 5 cm were recommended for cutaneous melanomas. The need for such a wide margin was addressed in a randomized trial comparing 2- to 4-cm margins in intermediate-thickness cutaneous melanomas.[15] The local recurrence rate was similar for those with a 2-cm margin (0.8%) and those with a 4-cm margin (1.7%).[15] There was also no difference in 5-year OS rates (79.5% vs 83.7%, respectively).[15] The 2-cm margin also resulted in lower rates of split thickness skin grafting and length of hospital stay.

There have not been any randomized trials for thin or thick melanomas. Margin status and outcome using a histopathologic margin of 1.6 cm as the cutoff, which roughly equates to a 2-cm surgical margin, were assessed in a retrospective analysis of 632 cases of thick melanoma.[47] Tumor margin was independently associated with local and locoregional control.[47,48] However, disease-free survival (DFS) and OS were not impacted by tumor margin status.[47] This suggests that locoregional recurrence can be salvaged or that distant recurrence is of greater concern.

The NCCN guidelines for cutaneous melanoma recommend a clinical surgical margin of 0.5–1.0 cm for in situ disease; 1 cm for invasive disease with tumor thickness ≤ 1 mm; 1–2 cm for thickness of 1–2 mm; and 2 cm for thickness > 2 mm.[36] European consensus guidelines for surgical margin are as follows: 0.5 cm for in situ disease; 1 cm for tumor thickness < 2 mm; and 2 cm for thickness > 2 mm.[49] Taken together, it appears a clinical margin of 1 cm is

TABLE 17.8 AJCC TNM staging system for cutaneous melanomas.[45]

T Category	Thickness	Ulceration status
TX: primary tumor thickness cannot be assessed (e.g., diagnosis by curettage)	Not applicable	Not applicable
T0: no evidence of primary tumor (e.g., unknown primary or completely regressed melanoma)	Not applicable	Not applicable
Tis (melanoma in situ)	Not applicable	Not applicable
T1	≤1.0 mm	Unknown or unspecified
T1a	<0.8 mm	Without ulceration
T1b	<0.8 mm 0.8–1.0 mm	With ulceration With or without ulceration
T2	>1.0–2.0 mm	Unknown or unspecified
T2a	>1.0–2.0 mm	Unknown or unspecified
T2b	>1.0–2.0 mm	With ulceration
T3	>2.0–4.0 mm	Unknown or unspecified
T3a	>2.0–4.0 mm	Without ulceration
T3b	>2.0–4.0 mm	With ulceration
T4	>4.0 mm	Unknown or unspecified
T4a	>4.0 mm	Without ulceration
T4b	>4.0 mm	With ulceration

	Extent of regional lymph node and/or lymphatic metastases	
N Category	**Number of tumor-involved regional lymph node**	**Presence of in-transit, satellite, and/or microsatellite metastases**
NX	Regional nodes not assessed (e.g., SLN biopsy not performed, regional nodes previously removed for another reason)	No
	Exception: pathological N category is not required for T1 melanomas, use cN	
N0	No regional metastases detected	No
N1	One tumor-involved node or in-transit, satellite, and/or microsatellite metastases with no tumor-involved nodes	
N1a	One clinically occult (i.e., detected by SLN biopsy)	No
N1b	One clinically detected	No
N1c	No regional lymph node disease	Yes
N2	Two or three tumor-involved nodes or in-transit, satellite, and/or microsatellite metastases with one tumor-involved node	
N2a	Two or three clinically occult (i.e., detected by SLN biopsy)	No
N2b	Two or three, at least one of which was clinically detected	No
N2c	One clinically occult or clinically detected	Yes

TABLE 17.8 AJCC TNM staging system for cutaneous melanomas—cont'd

N Category	Extent of regional lymph node and/or lymphatic metastases	
	Number of tumor-involved regional lymph node	**Presence of in-transit, satellite, and/or microsatellite metastases**
N3	Four or more tumor-involved nodes or in-transit, satellite, and/or microsatellite metastases with two or more tumor-involved nodes, or any number of matted nodes without or with in-transit, satellite, and/or microsatellite metastases	
N3a	Four or more clinically occult (i.e., detected by SLN biopsy)	No
N3b	Four or more, at least one of which was clinically detected, or presence of any number of matted nodes	No
N3c	Two or more clinically occult or clinically detected and/or presence of any number of matted nodes	Yes

M Category	Extent of regional lymph node and/or lymphatic metastases	
	Anatomic site	**LDH level**
M0	No evidence of distant metastasis	Not applicable
M1	Evidence of distant metastasis	See below
M1a	Distant metastasis to skin, soft tissue including muscle, and/or nonregional lymph node	Not recorded or unspecified
M1a(0)		Not elevated
M1a(1)		Elevated
M1b	Distant metasis to lung with or without M1a sites of disease	Not recorded or unspecified
M1b(0)		Not elevated
M1b(1)		Elevated
M1c	Distant metastasis to non-CNS visceral sites with or without M1a or M1b sites of disease	Not recorded or unspecified
M1c(0)		Not elevated
M1c(1)		Elevated
M1d	Distant metastasis to CNS with or without M1a, M1b, or M1c sites of disease	Not recorded or unspecified
M1d(0)		Normal
M1d(1)		Elevated

Suffixes for M category: (0) LDH elevated. No suffix is used if LDH is not recorded or is unspecified.

When T is...	And N is...	And M is...	Then the clinical stage group is...
Tis	N0	M0	0
T1a	N0	M0	IA
T1b	N0	M0	IB
T2a	N0	M0	IB
T2b	N0	M0	IIA
T3a	N0	M0	IIA
T4a	N0	M0	IIB
T4a	N0	M0	IIB
T4b	N0	M0	IIC
Any T, Tis	≥N1	M0	III
Any T	Any T	M1	IV

Continued

TABLE 17.8 AJCC TNM staging system for cutaneous melanomas—cont'd

When T is...	And N is...	And M is...	Then the pathological stage group is...
Tis	N0	M0	0
T1a	N0	M0	IA
T1b	N0	M0	IB
T2a	N0	M0	IIA
T2b	N0	M0	IIA
T3a	N0	M0	IIB
T3b	N0	M0	IIB
T4a	N0	M0	IIC
T4b	N0	M0	IIIB
T0	N1b, N1c	M0	IIIC
T0	N2b/c, N3b/c	M0	IIIB
T1a/b, T2a	N1a, N2a	M0	IIIC
T1a/b, T2a	N1b/c, N2b	M0	IIIA
T2b, T3a	N1a/b/c, N2a/b	M0	IIIB
T1a/b, T2a/b, T3a	N2c, N3a/b/c	M0	IIIB
T3b, T4a	Any N ≥ N1	M0	IIIC
T4b	N1a/b/c, N2a/b/c	M0	IIIC
T4b	N3a/b/c	M0	IIID
Any T, Tis	Any N	M1	IV

Pathological Stage 0 (melanoma in situ) and T1 do not require pathological evaluation of lymph nodes to complete pathological staging; use cN information to assign their pathological stage.

sufficient for invasive melanoma with tumor thickness ≤ 2 mm. A 2-cm clinical margin is the goal for those with tumor thickness of >2 mm.

The appropriate margins for vulvovaginal melanomas are not established. It is unclear whether or not the recommended margins for cutaneous melanomas should apply to vulvovaginal melanomas, even though we do so in practice. In a small group of vulvovaginal melanomas analyzed retrospectively, a final margin of 1 mm was associated with DFS and melanoma-specific survival (MSS).[46] The 5-year DFS was 53.8% for cases with a pathologic margin of ≥1 mm compared to only 8.3% for those with a margin of <1 mm.[46] MSS was 78.8% compared to 38.1%, respectively.[46] A negative-margin resection of the primary tumor is the goal of vulvovaginal melanoma surgery. The amount of clinical margin should be the same as that for cutaneous melanomas, if possible. It may also be acceptable to resect with a smaller clinical margin. Primary tumor excision should not be attempted if a negative margin is not feasible without the need for resection of critical structures, which would lead to excessive morbidity and/or require an exenterative resection.

Surgical nodal assessment

Elective complete regional lymphadenectomy is not therapeutic in all patients presenting with cutaneous melanoma. In one study, the 10-year OS was similar for all patients with intermediate-thickness cutaneous melanoma with a negative-margin resection and randomized to either observation or an elective lymphadenectomy.[50] There were, however, some subgroups that benefited from a lymphadenectomy.[50] Inguinofemoral lymphadenectomy is a morbid procedure and should be avoided in most patients with vulvovaginal melanoma.

SLN biopsy is now considered standard for patients with cutaneous melanoma.[36,49] The multicenter selective lymphadenectomy trial-I (MSLT-I) randomized patients with biopsy-proven invasive melanoma at time of wide excision to

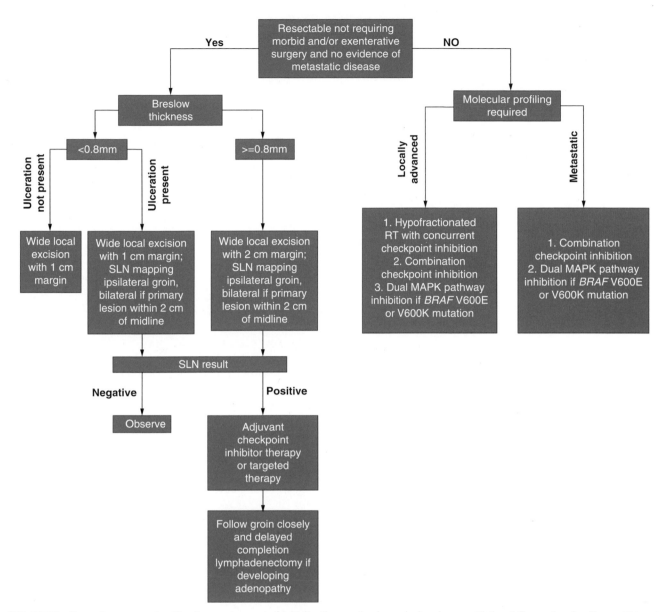

FIG. 17.13 General summary algorithm for management of initially diagnosed vulvovaginal melanoma. National Comprehensive Cancer Network (NCCN) guidelines should also be referred for additional details and to remain current.[36] Surgical resection in select cases of locally advanced and/or metastatic cases is a consideration.

either nodal observation or SLN mapping.[50,51] In the SLN mapping arm, no further intervention was attempted if the SLNs were normal, whereas an immediate completion lymphadenectomy was performed if the SLN had metastatic disease.[50] The SLN mapping arm had a significantly improved 10-year DFS for both intermediate and thick melanomas.[51] However, the 10-year MSS was the same for both the nodal observation and SLN mapping cohorts.[51] These results suggest that the DFS difference was due to the undetected nodal disease that was then salvaged in those who were observed.

MSLT-II subsequently randomized localized cutaneous melanomas with metastatic disease in the SLNs to either an immediate completion lymphadenectomy or close observation with serial nodal ultrasound of the SLN basin and delayed completion lymphadenectomy in those noted to have developing adenopathy.[52] The primary endpoint of MSS was the same in both arms (86% and 86%, respectively [$P = 0.42$]).[52] DFS was improved in those who underwent immediate completion lymphadenectomy due to an improvement in nodal recurrence-free survival (RFS) only.[52] The final results of the DeCOG-SLT randomized trial also showed that an immediate completion lymphadenectomy did not improve RFS or

OS.[53] The 7-year OS rate was 65.9% in those who underwent nodal observation compared to 67.9% in those who underwent an immediate lymphadenectomy ($P = 0.94$).[53]

The NCCN recommends SLN mapping for all cutaneous melanomas with a Breslow thickness ≥ 0.8 mm, as well as for melanomas <0.8 mm if ulceration is present.[36] Thin cutaneous melanomas (<0.8 mm) without ulceration have a very low risk of lymph node metastasis, and SLN biopsy can be omitted in these cases.[36] The correlation between Breslow thickness and risk of groin node metastasis is very limited but also appears to be correlated.[27,34] The decision to pursue SLN mapping of the groin for vulvar melanoma should follow the same guidelines as those for cutaneous melanomas, and bilateral SLN mapping should be performed in those with lesions within 2 cm of the midline. SLN mapping for vaginal melanoma is not understood, as most of these cases do not undergo a surgical nodal evaluation and independent drainage to either the pelvic or inguinofemoral nodal basins is possible. Also, the majority of vaginal melanomas are best treated with a non-surgical approach, and nodal assessment of normal-appearing nodes is not likely to offer additional value. In select cases of vaginal melanoma in which a primary negative resection is possible, both the pelvic and inguinal nodal basins should be assessed, but the best technique is unknown.

Completion lymphadenectomy is unnecessary in cases with metastatic disease in the SLN. These cases should be followed with serial assessment of the groins by ultrasound every 3 months. Based on recent trials, these patients now receive adjuvant therapy (described in a later section). A delayed completion inguinofemoral lymphadenectomy should be performed if there is concern for adenopathy, even if the patient is receiving adjuvant therapy. In a practical sense, many practitioners perform routine CT (+/−PET) scanning every 6 months in node-positive cases. We alternate imaging with groin ultrasound (US) and CT (+/− PET) every 3 months to limit imaging tests, but this is not based on prospective evaluation and a groin US every 3 months can be performed.

Lymphadenectomy is considered in cutaneous melanomas with clinically apparent nodal disease.[36,49] Wide excision of the primary tumor can also be performed.[36,49] Vulvovaginal melanomas with clinically involved inguinofemoral and/or pelvic adenopathy should be considered for regional lymphadenectomy with or without excision of the primary tumor.

Adjuvant treatment in surgically resected disease

Published trials of adjuvant radiation therapy, chemotherapy, or older immunotherapies (e.g., interferon-alpha) do not support the routine use of any of these agents in the adjuvant setting. Randomized trials specific to adjuvant therapy in mucosal melanomas of any type are sparse to non-existent. Patients with nodal disease (stage III) and completely resected stage IV melanomas should undergo at minimum molecular profiling for the presence of a *BRAF* mutation, but ideally they would undergo multigene panel testing.

Adjuvant therapy specifically for mucosal melanomas has only been assessed in a single randomized, phase 2 trial.[54] Patients with completely resected AJCC stage II or III mucosal melanomas of various sites were randomized to one of three treatment arms: (1) observation; (2) high-dose interferon (HDI) given as interferon-alpha2b 15×10^6 U/m^2/d intravenous on days 1–5 each week for 4 weeks followed by subcutaneous injection of 9×10^6 U three times per week for 48 weeks; or (3) (CHEMO): temozolomide 200 mg/m^2 daily orally on days 1–5 plus cisplatin 75 mg/m^2 intravenous divided into 3 days, and repeated every 3 weeks for 6 cycles.[54] This trial randomized 189 patients (63 per arm) and included 21 vulvar, 19 vaginal, and 1 cervical melanoma. RFS was significantly improved with HDI or CHEMO compared to observation. The median OS was 21.2 months with observation, 40.4 months with HDI, and 48.7 months with CHEMO.[54] CHEMO was also significantly better than HDI ($P = 0.009$).[54] This is the only randomized clinical trial to show such an OS advantage for either HDI or CHEMO in any melanoma. Adjuvant CHEMO with temozolomide and cisplatin can be discussed with patients who have stage II/III vulvovaginal melanoma; however, strong recommendations cannot be made based on one single-center phase 2 trial.

Adjuvant ipilimumab, a monoclonal antibody of cytotoxic T-lymphocyte-associated protein 4 (CTLA-4), was shown to significantly improve median RFS and 5-year OS compared to placebo in a randomized trial of completely resected stage III cutaneous melanomas.[55] The median RFS was 17.1 months in the placebo arm compared to 27.6 months in the ipilimumab arm (HR 0.76; 95% CI: 0.64–0.89; $P < 0.001$), with 5-year RFS rates of 30.3% and 40.8%, respectively.[55] Ipilimumab was given as 10 mg/kg IV every 3 weeks for 4 doses and then every 3 months for up to 3 years.[55] In another randomized trial, ipilimumab at 3 mg/kg given every 3 weeks for 4 doses and then every 12 weeks for 4 additional doses also resulted in significantly improved OS compared to HDI.[56] This trial included stage IIIB, IIIC, and IV completely resected cutaneous melanomas. The 5-year OS rates were 72% with ipilimumab compared to 67% with HDI (HR 0.78; 95% CI: 0.61–0.99; $P = 0.04$).[56] Ipilimumab at 3 mg/kg was less toxic and seemed to be as effective as, if not better, than the 10 mg/kg dose in the trial.[56]

Nivolumab, a programmed cell death protein 1 (PD-1) inhibitor, significantly improved RFS compared to ipilimumab in another randomized trial of completely resected stage IIIB, IIIC, and IV cutaneous melanomas.[57] Nivolumab was given as 3 mg/kg IV every 2 weeks for 1 year, and ipilimumab was given as 10 mg/kg every 3 weeks for 4 doses and then every 3 months for up to 1 year.[57] The 1-year RFS rate was 70.5% for nivolumab compared to 60.8% for ipilimumab (HR 0.65; 97.56% CI: 0.51–0.83; $P < 0.001$).[57] Ipilimumab was associated with more adverse events compared to nivolumab.[57] The CheckMate 238 trial confirmed the superiority of adjuvant nivolumab compared to ipilimumab in completely resected stage IIIB, IIIC, and IV cutaneous melanoma.[58] In the EORTC 1325-MG/Keynote-054 trial, adjuvant pembrolizumab at 200 mg IV given every 3 weeks for 18 doses led to a significantly improved RFS compared to placebo in stage III cutaneous melanoma.[59,60]

Adjuvant dabrafenib and trametinib should be administered in patients with melanomas harboring V600E or V600K mutations. The COMBI-AD trial randomized patients with completely resected stage IIIA-C *BRAF* V600E/V600K-mutated cutaneous melanoma to either dabrafenib 150 mg orally twice daily or trametinib 2 mg orally once daily versus placebo for 12 months.[61] The 5-year RFS rate was 52% for the combination therapy compared to 36% with placebo (HR 0.51; 95% CI: 0.42–0.61).[61] Interestingly, there was no significant difference between the combination therapy and placebo with regard to the incidence or severity of serious adverse events.[61] These regimens are summarized in Table 17.9.[55–61]

Adjuvant pembrolizumab or nivolumab for up to 1 year should be given to patients with completely resected stages III–IV vulvovaginal melanomas based on the above trial results. Adjuvant dabrafenib and trametinib should be given for *BRAF* V600E- or V600K-mutated vulvovaginal melanoma. One must consider that none of the above trials, except the cisplatin/temozolomide trial, included mucosal melanomas. Furthermore, there were not enough vulvovaginal melanomas in any trial to definitively apply the trial results to these melanomas. All SLN-positive cases required a completion lymphadenectomy as they were conducted prior to the completion and publication of MSLT-II. It is not definitively proven that these results would apply to a SLN-positive case that does not undergo a completion lymphadenectomy. Serial groin imaging should be performed, as discussed above, and a delayed completion lymphadenectomy should be performed if any concerning lymphadenopathy develops while the patient is receiving adjuvant therapy or thereafter. Lastly, the optimal length of continued adjuvant therapy is unclear, as the duration of therapy varied among the trials.

Locally advanced disease

Radical and exenterative resections for vulvar melanomas are highly morbid and disfiguring. Radical excisions compared to wide excisions with 1–2 cm margins do not result in improved oncologic outcomes.[7–9,34] Pelvic exenterations should not be routinely considered in patients with locally advanced disease. Nonsurgical approaches using concurrent immunotherapy with hypofractionated radiation therapy should be considered in patients with vulvovaginal melanomas requiring primary exenterative resections. Our preliminary experience with neoadjuvant hypofractionated external beam radiotherapy (3000 cGy in 5 fractions) with concurrent ipilimumab led to promising results in the first 4 patients with vaginal and cervical melanomas who would have required exenterative surgery.[62] After completing neoadjuvant ration and immunotherapy, 3 patients underwent a much less extensive local excision, and 1 of the 3 patients had a complete pathologic response. All 4 patients achieved a complete radiologic response after therapy and surgery.[62] Distant recurrence developed in 2 patients at 9 and 10 months, and the other 2 patients were disease free at 20 and 38 months.

TABLE 17.9 Adjuvant therapy regimens tested in recent, select phase 3 trials for AJCC stage III (node positive) and resected stage IV cutaneous melanoma.

Agent	Dose	Treatment duration
Ipilimimumab[55]	10 mg/kg IV every 3 weeks for 4 doses, then every 3 months	Up to 3 years
Ipilimumab[56]	3 and 10 mg/kg IV every 3 weeks for 4 doses, then every 3 months*	Up to 60 weeks
Nivolumab[57,58]	3 mg/kg IV every 2 weeks	Up to 1 year
Pembrolizumab[59,60]	200 mg IV every 3 weeks	Up to a total of 18 doses
Dabrafenib and Trametinib[a] [61]	150 mg orally twice daily 2 mg orally once daily	Up to 12 months

[a]For BRAF *V600E/V600K-mutated cases.*
[b]Higher dose more toxic and not more efficacious.

The combination of radiation therapy and ipilimumab was prospectively assessed in a single-arm study of 10 patients with locally advanced melanoma, of which only one had mucosal melanoma.[63] A radiographic complete response was achieved in 4 of the 10 patients. Three patients achieved a partial response. These 3 patients all underwent a surgical resection for what was considered residual disease. Two of these 3 patients achieved a pathologic complete response.

We currently offer concurrent hypofractionated radiation therapy to patients with locally advanced vulvovaginal melanomas, along with either pembrolizumab or nivolumab. After 4 doses of immunotherapy, patients are assessed for residual disease and whether a local excision is warranted. We then continue with immunotherapy. This approach has not been prospectively assessed in mucosal melanomas, and there is a serious need to test this approach and seek other regimens. The use of hypofractionated radiation therapy is controversial and debatable. Some may prefer to use combination immunotherapy or dabrafenib/trametinib without radiation. The decisions for these locally advanced cases or recurrent/metastatic cases (discussed in subsequent sections) must be individualized within a multidisciplinary team setting of gynecologic oncologists, medical oncologists, and radiation oncologists, and treatment should be conducted by specialists who have expertise in the management of melanoma.

Metastatic disease

Metastatic vulvovaginal melanoma (AJCC stage IV) is associated with a 5-year survival rate of less than 10%.[6] These patients are best served by medical oncologists with expertise in the management of melanoma, and more specifically, mucosal melanomas. Almost all available data come from metastatic cutaneous melanoma, and management should be based on guidelines and algorithms provided by the NCCN and other groups.[36,49] Molecular profiling, preferably with multigene panels, should be performed in all of these cases. It is beyond the scope of this chapter to provide an in-depth review of all published data and available therapeutic options for metastatic and/or recurrent disease. We will present a brief and pertinent overview.

Dacarbazine (DTIC) was FDA approved for stage IV melanoma in 1975 and remained the standard for many years. In the 1990s, interferon and interleukin-2 (IL2) were also approved. In 2011, ipilimumab, a monoclonal antibody of CTLA-4, received FDA approval after a randomized trial demonstrated improved survival with ipilimumab over gp100, a melanoma specific antibody, alone.[64] The median OS with ipilimumab was 10.1 months compared to 6.4 months with gp100 ($P = 0.003$).[64] The combination of ipilimumab and dacarbazine led to a median OS of 11.2 months compared to 9.1 months with dacarbazine alone ($P < 0.001$).[65] The median duration of response was 19.3 months with the ipilimumab and dacarbazine combination compared to only 8.1 months with dacarbazine in those who responded to therapy ($P = 0.03$).[65] Combination ipilimumab and dacarbazine is not recommended, as the effect was likely due to ipilimumab.

Nivolumab and pembrolizumab, anti-PD-1 monoclonal antibodies, as well as other more recently developed anti-PD1 and PD-L1 agents, are preferred over ipilimumab. The antitumor activity of these agents is not affected by the presence of *BRAF* mutations. The regimen of nivolumab 1 mg/kg with ipilimumab 3 mg/kg given every 3 weeks for 4 doses followed by maintenance nivolumab 3 mg/kg every 2 weeks compared to ipilimumab 3 mg/kg every 3 weeks for 4 doses followed by placebo was tested in a randomized trial.[66] The median PFS was not reached in the combination group, compared to 4.4 months in the ipilimumab group (HR 0.40; 95% CI: 0.23–0.68; $P < 0.001$).[66] KEYNOTE-006 randomized patients to pembrolizumab 10 mg/kg every 2 or 3 weeks (2 arms) given for up to 24 months (an additional 17 cycles allowed in certain cases) or ipilimumab 3 mg/kg every 3 weeks for 4 doses.[67] The median OS was 32.7 months for the two groups that single-agent pembrolizumab combined (either every 2 weeks or every 3 weeks) compared to 15.9 months in the ipilimumab group (HR 0.73; 95% CI: 0.61–0.88; $P < 0.001$).[67] Nivolumab alone or in combination with ipilimumab resulted in improved PFS and OS compared to ipilimumab alone in the CheckMate 067 trial.[68] Toxicities are higher with CTLA-4 and PD-1 combination therapies, and monotherapy is preferred, although combinations are acceptable.

Patients with *BRAF* V600E or V600K mutations will benefit from targeted therapy. In a phase 3 trial, patients with these mutations were randomized to the BRAF inhibitor vemurafenib 960 mg twice daily orally or dacarbazine 1000 mg/m² IV every 3 weeks.[69] Response rates were 48% for vemurafenib compared to 5% for dacarbazine.[69] The 6-month OS rate was 84% for the vemurafenib group compared to 64% for the dacarbazine group (HR 0.37; 95% CI: 0.26–0.55; $P < 0.001$).[69] Dual MAPK pathway inhibition with a BRAF inhibitor and a MEK inhibitor have been tested and shown to be superior to vemurafenib alone.[70–72] In the most recent randomized clinical trial (COLUMBUS), encorafenib 950 mg orally once a day plus biminetinib 45 mg orally twice a day was compared to encorafenib 300 mg orally once a day or vemurafenib 960 orally twice a day.[72] The combination resulted in a median OS of 33.6 months compared to 23.5 months for encorafenib alone and 16.9 months for vemurafenib alone.[72] The OS difference was significant for the combination compared to vemurafenib alone (HR 0.61; 95% CI: 0.47–0.79; $P < 0.0001$).[72] The difference between the combination and encorafenib did not meet statistical significance (HR 0.81; 95% CI: 0.61–1.06; $P = 0.12$).[72] The overall response rates (ORRs) were 65% for the combination, 52% for encorafenib alone, and 41% for vemurafnib.[72] Dual MAPK pathway inhibition is preferred over single-agent BRAF inhibition.

Mucosal melanomas, and more specifically, vulvovaginal melanomas, generally have not been included in the many published trials, including the ones described above. It is, however, generally accepted to treat vulvovaginal melanomas as one would cutaneous melanomas. In a multi-institutional retrospective study that included 14 vulvovaginal melanomas, the ORR to either pembrolizumab or nivolumab was 23% for patients with advanced mucosal melanomas who had received prior therapy, similar to response rates seen in pretreated cutaneous melanomas.[73] Response and outcomes with checkpoint inhibition for vulvar ($n = 28$) and vaginal ($n = 4$) melanomas of various stages were similar to those of published reports for cutaneous melanomas in a single-center retrospective study.[74] The largest pooled analysis of mucosal melanomas ($N = 121$) demonstrated that nivolumab alone or in combination with ipilimumab was superior to ipilimumab alone[75]; however, nivolumab was not as efficacious in mucosal compared to cutaneous melanomas.[75]

Imatinib mesylate, a KIT inhibitor, has been looked at in mucosal, acral, and chronically sun-damaged skin. In a phase 2 study, the best ORR was 29%–54% in those with a *KIT* mutation compared to 0% in those with a *KIT* amplification.[76] The median time to progression (TTP) was 3.7 months, and the median OS was 12.5 months.[76] Neither TTP nor OS was affected by *KIT* mutation or amplification.[76] Dasatinib, a multityrosine kinase inhibitor, demonstrated an overall 18% response rate, all partial responses, in *KIT*-mutated mucosal, acral, and vulvovaginal melanomas.[77] There were no responses in the eight vulvovaginal melanomas.[77] KIT inhibition with imatinib is an option in select cases but not as a first choice.

Immunotherapy and targeted therapy are the preferred first options for patients with mucosal melanomas, but these agents are not readily available worldwide. Carboplatin, paclitaxel, plus bevacizumab was tested in a randomized phase 2 trial of patients with previously untreated advanced mucosal melanoma, which included 40 cases from "genitourinary" sites.[78] All patients were treated with carboplation area under the curve (AUC) 5 plus paclitaxel 175 mg/m^2 every 4 weeks either alone or with bevacizumab 5 mg/kg biweekly.[78] The response rates were not statistically different, but the addition of bevacizumab resulted in an improved median PFS (3.0 vs 4.8 months; $P < 0.001$) and OS (9.0 vs 13.6 months; $P = 0.017$).[78] This regimen may be an option when targeted or immunotherapies are not readily available.

Surgical resection of metastatic lesions in patients who present with stage IV disease may be a consideration in select cases. Metastatectomy was associated with an improved survival in patients with stage IV melanoma in a SEER analysis of 4229 patients with cutaneous melanoma.[79] The median OS was 5 months for those who did not undergo metastatectomy compared to 12 months for those who did ($P < 0.001$).[79] While still not associated with optimal outcomes, surgical resection may be an option in those in whom a negative-margin resection may be possible without extensive morbidity. Adjuvant therapy should be given postoperatively in such cases. Neoadjuvant therapy followed by surgical resection may also be a consideration.[49] However, surgical debulking (cytoreduction) of multisite disease, as is often considered in patients with ovarian carcinoma, should be considered cautiously in patients with melanoma, as the overall prognosis is poor.

Surveillance for recurrence

There are little to no level I data to establish best recommendations for the optimal surveillance of patients with melanomas of any type, as is the case with many other cancers. Surveillance for recurrence should follow the general NCCN guidelines.[36] Generally, in patients with resected and node-negative vulvovaginal melanoma, a physical examination every 6 months for 5 years is reasonable. Patients should be instructed to perform self-inspection of the vulva and all skin as often as possible. Routine imaging is not recommended but should be performed for any concerning signs or symptoms. More intense surveillance is recommended for those with stage IIB or higher disease.[36] Generally, physical examination every 3 months for 2 years and then every 6 months for another 3 years is reasonable for patients with locally resected but SLN-positive disease. Imaging with CT (+/−PET) every 6 months for 5 years and alternating with groin US every 6 months is a reasonable approach. In the MSLT-II and DeCOG trials, however, US of the nodal basin in SLN-positive cases was performed every 4 months for 2 years and then every 6 months for an additional 3 years.[52,53] Physical examination and imaging (CT+/−PET) every 3 months should be considered in patients with locally advanced, unresectable melanoma or stage IV disease and then modified based on response. There is no routine blood work indicated in the surveillance of these patients.

Treatment of recurrent disease

The management of recurrent disease does not vary much from the approaches described above. The majority of trials mentioned above included both newly diagnosed, untreated melanomas as well as metastatic and recurrent cases. It is beyond scope of this chapter to cover all additional available literature on the management of recurrent disease.

Wide local excision is preferred in women who develop a local recurrence that is still amenable to a nonexenterative resection. SLN mapping, as described in prior sections, should also be considered. SLN mapping of a previously fully dissected groin is difficult, and we would not consider it in these cases. Completion lymphadenectomy of a groin that develops suspicious lymphadenopathy should be performed, as described in prior sections. The use of adjuvant therapy should be based on previously mentioned factors.

Resection of metastatic melanoma may also be an option in select patients who develop recurrence and in whom a negative-margin, limited-morbidity procedure is possible.[36,79] Systemic therapy for those who develop unresectable vulvovaginal melanoma includes immunotherapy and targeted therapies, as described above. There is an extensive body of literature on treatment options for recurrent and metastatic melanoma that includes chemotherapeutics, radiation therapy, and other available and novel agents. We recommend following published guidelines, such as those provided by the NCCN.[36]

Special considerations

Vulvovaginal melanomas are exceedingly rare. Management strategy is extrapolated from the data and management of cutaneous melanomas. We do not know for certain whether this is the best approach or whether these and other mucosal melanomas should be treated differently. Clinical trials specific to mucosal and vulvovaginal melanomas are lacking. Patients with vulvovaginal melanomas should be strongly encouraged to participate in clinical trials. These patients are also best managed, when possible, within a multidisciplinary team of experts from gynecologic oncology, medical oncology, and radiation oncology who have knowledge of this disease.

Case resolution

This 44-year-old patient underwent hypofractionated external beam radiation therapy with 3000 cGy delivered over 5 fractions once a day. The patient was also given concurrent ipilimumab 3 mg/kg IV every 3 weeks for 4 doses. An MRI after the fourth dose of ipilimumab revealed a residual mass measuring $2.1 \times 2.0 \times 3.8$ cm. CT of the chest, abdomen, and pelvis did not reveal any new metastatic lesions. The patient underwent a wide local excision, with a complete pathologic response, and only granulation tissue and a mixed inflammatory infiltrate containing rare atypical epithelioid cells were noted. Postoperatively, she was placed on maintenance ipilimumab 3 mg/kg IV every 3 months for 2 years. She remains disease free, without recurrence, 100 months (8+ years) since her initial diagnosis.

References

1. Siegel RL, Miller KD, Jemal A. Cancer statistics, 2020. *CA Cancer J Clin.* 2020;70:7–30.
2. U.S. Cancer Statistics Working Group. *U.S. Cancer Statistics Data Visualizations Tool, Based on 2019 Submission Data (1998–2017).* U.S. Department of Health and Human Services, Centers for Disease Control and Prevention and National Cancer Institute; 2021. www.cdc.gov/cancer/dataviz, released in June 2020.
3. Kosary CL. Cancer of the vulva. In: Ries LA, Young JL, Keel GE, Eisner MP, Lin YD, Jorner MJ, eds. *SEER Survival Monograph: Cancer Survival among Adults: US SEER Program 1988–2001, Patient and Tumor Characteristics.* Bethesda, MD: National Cancer Institute; 2007. SEER Program, NIH Pub. No. 07-6215.
4. Kosary CL. Cancer of the vagina. In: Ries LA, Young JL, Keel GE, Eisner MP, Lin YD, Jorner MJ, eds. *SEER Survival Monograph: Cancer Survival among Adults: US SEER Program 1988–2001, Patient and Tumor Characteristics.* Bethesda, MD: National Cancer Institute; 2007. SEER Program, NIH Pub. No. 07-6215.
5. Mert I, Semaan A, Winer I, Morris RT, Ali-Fehmi R. Vulvar/vaginal melanoma: an updated surveillance epidemiology and end results database review, comparison with cutaneous melanoma and significance of racial disparities. *Int J Gynecol Cancer.* 2013;23:1118–1125.
6. Wohlmuth C, Wohlmuth-Wieser I, May T, Vicus D, Gien LT, Laframboise S. Malignant melanoma of the vulva and vagina: a US population-based study of 1863 patients. *Am J Clin Dermatol.* 2020;21:285–295.
7. Sugiyama VE, Chan JK, Shin YJ, Berek JS, Osann K, Kapp DS. Vulvar melanoma: a multivariable analysis of 644 patients. *Obstet Gynecol.* 2007;110:296–301.
8. Trimble ER, Lewis Jr JL, Williams LL, et al. Management of vulvar melanoma. *Gynecol Oncol.* 1992;45:254–258.
9. Verschraegen CF, Benjapibal M, Supakarapongkul W, et al. Vulvar melanoma at the M.D. Anderson cancer center: 25 years later. *Int J Gynecol Cancer.* 2001;11:359–364.
10. Frumovitz M, Etchepareborda M, Sun CC, et al. Primary malignant melanoma of the vagina. *Obstet Gynecol.* 2010;116:1358–1365.
11. Abdo JF, Sharma A, Sharma R. Role of heredity in melanoma susceptibility: a primer for the practicing surgeon. *Surg Clin N Am.* 2020;100:13–28.
12. Klein JD, Kupferman ME. Li-Fraumeni syndrome presenting as mucosal melanoma: case report and treatment considerations. *Head Neck.* 2017;39:E20–E22.

13. Cazenave H, Maubec E, Mohamdi H, et al. Genital and anorectal mucosal melanoma is associated with cutaneous melanoma in patients and in families. *Br J Dermatol.* 2013;169:594–599.

14. Moxley KM, Fader AN, Rose PG, et al. Malignant melanoma of the vulva: an extension of cutaneous melanoma? *Gynecol Oncol.* 2011;122:612–617.

15. Nagarajan P, Curry JL, Ning J, et al. Tumor thickness and mitotic rate robustly predict melanoma-specific survival in patients with primary vulvar melanomas: a restrospective review of 100 cases. *Clin Cancer Res.* 2017;23(8):2093–2104.

16. Breslow A. Prognosis in cutaneous melanoma: tumor thickness as a guide to treatment. *Pathol Annu.* 1980;15:1–22.

17. Clark Jr WH, Elder DE, Guerry 4th D, et al. Model predicting survival in stage I melanoma based on tumor progression. *J Natl Cancer Inst.* 1989;81:1893–1904.

18. Chung AF, Woodruff JM, Lewis Jr JL. Malignant melanoma of the vulva: a report of 44 cases. *Obstet Gynecol.* 1975;45:638–646.

19. Moreno MA, Roberts DB, Kupferman ME, et al. Mucosal melanoma of the nose and paranasal sinuses, a contemporary experience from the M. D Anderson Cancer Center. *Cancer.* 2010;116:2215–2223.

20. Feldmeyer L, Tetzlaff M, Fox P, et al. Prognostic implication of lymphovascular invasion detected by double immunostaining for D2-40 and MITF1 in primary cutaneous melanoma. *Am J Dermatopathol.* 2016;38:484–491.

21. Rock B. Pigmented lesions of the vulva. *Dermatol Clin.* 1992;10:361–370.

22. Rock B, Hood AF, Rock JA. Prospective study of vulvar nevi. *J Am Acad Dermatol.* 1990;22:104–106.

23. Murzaku EC, Penn LA, Hale CS, et al. Vulvar nevi, melanosis, and melanoma: an epidemiologic, clinical, and histopathologic review. *J Am Acad Dermatol.* 2014;71:1241–1249.

24. Venkatesan A. Pigmented lesions of the vulva. *Dermatol Clin.* 2010;28:795–805.

25. Furney SJ, Turajlic S, Stamp G, et al. Genome sequencing of mucosal melanomas reveals that they are driven by distinct mechanisms from cutaneous melanoma. *J Pathol.* 2013;230:261–269.

26. Newell F, Kong Y, Wilmott JS, et al. Whole-genome landscape of mucosal melanoma reveals diverse drivers and therapeutic targets. *Nat Commun.* 2019;10:3163.

27. Phillips GL, Bundy BN, Okagaki T, Kucera PR, Stehman FB. Malignant melanoma of the vulva treated by radical hemivulvectomy: a prospective study of the gynecologic oncology group. *Cancer.* 1994;73:2626–2632.

28. Petru E, Nagele F, Czerwenka K, et al. Primary malignant melanoma of the vagina: long-term remission following radiation therapy. *Gynecol Oncol.* 1998;70:23–26.

29. Tjalma WA, Monaghan JM, de Barros LA, Naik R, Nordin A. Primary vaginal melanoma and long-term survivors. *Eur J Gynaecol Oncol.* 2001;22:20–22.

30. Zhou R, Shi C, Tao W, et al. Analysis of mucosal melanoma whole-genome landscapes reveals clinically relevant genomic aberrations. *Clin Cancer Res.* 2019;25:3548–3560.

31. Nassar KW, Tan AC. The mutational landscape of mucosal melanoma. *Semin Cancer Biol.* 2020;61:139–148.

32. Hintzsche JD, Gorden NT, Amato CM, et al. Whole-exome sequencing identifies recurrent SF3B1 R625 mutation and comutation of NF1 and KIT in mucosal melanoma. *Melanoma Res.* 2017;27:189–199.

33. Wylomanski S, Denis MG, Theoleyre S, et al. BRAF mutations might be more common than supposed in vulvar melanomas. *Exp Dermatol.* 2018;27:210–213.

34. Raber G, Mempel V, Jackisch C, et al. Malignant melanoma of the vulva: report of 89 patients. *Cancer.* 1996;78:2353–2358.

35. Cobellis L, Calabrese E, Stefanon B, Raspagliesi F. Malignant melanoma of the vagina: a report of 15 cases. *Eur J Gynaecol Oncol.* 2000;21:295–297.

36. National Comprehensive Cancer Network. *Melanoma: cutaneous (Version 1.2021)*; 2021. https:/www.nccn.org/professionals/physician_gls/pdf/cutaneous_melanoma.pdf. [Accessed December 14, 2020].

37. Garbe C, Amaral T, Peris K, et al. European consensus-based interdisciplinary guideline for melanoma. Part I: diagnostics – update 2019. *Eur J Cancer.* 2020;126:141–158.

38. Curtin JA, Fridlyand J, Kageshita T, et al. Distinct sets of genetic alterations in melanoma. *N Engl J Med.* 2005;353:2135–2147.

39. Curtin JA, Busam K, Pinkel D, Bastian BC. Somatic activation of KIT in distinct sybtypes of melanoma. *J Clin Oncol.* 2006;24:4340–4346.

40. Carvajal RD, Antonescu CR, Wolchok JD, et al. KIT as a therapeutic target in metastatic melanoma. *JAMA.* 2011;305:2327–2334.

41. Hou JY, Baptiste C, Hombalegowda RB, et al. Vulvar and vaginal melanoma: a unique subclass of mucosal melanoma based on comprehensive molecular analysis of 51 cases compared to 2253 cases of nongynecologic melanoma. *Cancer.* 2012;123:1333–1344.

42. Rogers LJ, Cuello MA. Cancer of the vulva. *Int J Gynecol Obstet.* 2018;143(Suppl 2):4–13.

43. Adams TS, Cuello MA. Cancer of the vagina. *Int J Gynecol Obstet.* 2018;143(Suppl 2):14–21.

44. Ballantyne AJ. Malignant melanoma of the skin of the head and neck. An analysis of 405 cases. *Am J Surg.* 1970;120:425–431.

45. Gershenwald JE, Scolyer RA, Hess KR, et al. Melanoma of the skin. In: Amin MB, Edge SB, Fl G, et al., eds. *AJCC Cancer Staging Manual.* 8th edition. Springer; 2017.

46. Seifried S, Haydu LE, Quinn MJ, et al. Melanoma of the vulva and vagina: principles of staging and their relevance to management based on a clinicopathologic analysis of 85 cases. *Ann Surg Oncol.* 2015;22:1959–1966.

47. Balch CM, Urist MM, Karakousis CP, et al. Efficacy of 2-cm surgical margins for intermediate-thickness melanomas (1 to 4 mm). *Ann Surg.* 1993;218:262–269.

48. Pasquali S, Haydu LE, Scolyer RA, et al. The importance of adequate primary tumor excision margins and sentinel node biopsy in achieving optimal locoregional control for patients with thick primary melanomas. *Ann Surg.* 2013;258:152–157.

49. Garbe C, Amaral T, Peris K, et al. European consensus-based interdisciplinary guideline for melanoma. Part 2: treatment – update 2019. *Eur J Cancer.* 2020;126:169–177.

50. Morton DL, Thompson JF, Cochran AJ, et al. Sentinel-node biopsy or nodal observation in melanoma. *N Engl J Med.* 2006;355:1307–1317.

51. Morton DL, Thompson JF, Cochran AJ, et al. Final trial report of sentinel-node biopsy versus nodal observation in melanoma. *N Engl J Med.* 2014;370:599–609.

52. Faries MB, Thompson JF, Cochran AJ, et al. Completion dissection or observation for sentinel-node metastasis in melanoma. *New Engl J Med.* 2017;376:2211–2222.

53. Leiter U, Stadler R, Mauch C, et al. Final analysis of DeCOG-SLT trial: no survival benefit for complete lymph node dissection in patients with melanoma with positive sentinel node. *J Clin Oncol.* 2019;37:3000–3008.

54. Lian B, Si L, Cui C, et al. Phase II randomized trial comparing high-dose IFN-α2b with temozolomide pus cisplatin as systemic adjuvant therapy for resected mucosal melanoma. *Clin Cancer Res.* 2013;19:4488–4498.

55. Eggermont AMM, Chiarion-Sileni V, Grob JJ, et al. Prolonged survival in stage III melanoma with ipilimumab adjuvant therapy. *N Engl J Med.* 2016;375:1845–1855.

56. Tarhini AA, Lee SJ, Hodi S, et al. Phase III study of adjuvant ipilimumab (3 or 10 mg/kg) versus high-dose interferon alfa-2b for resected high-risk melanoma: north American intergroup E1609. *J Clin Oncol.* 2020;38:567–575.

57. Weber J, Mandala M, Del Vecchio M, et al. Adjuvant nivolumab versus ipilimumab in resected stage III or IV melanoma. *N Engl J Med.* 2017;377:1824–1835.

58. Ascierto PA, Del Vecchio M, Mandala M, et al. Adjuvant nivolumab versus ipilimumab in resected stage IIIB-IIIC and stage IV melanoma (CheckMate 238): 4-year results from a multicenter, double-blind, randomized controlled, phase III trial. *Lancet Oncol.* 2020;21:1465–1477.

59. Eggermont AMM, Blank CU, Mandala M, et al. Adjuvant pembrolizumab versus placebo in resected stage III melanoma. *N Engl J Med.* 2018;378:1789–1801.

60. Eggermont AMM, Blank CU, Mandala M, et al. Longer follow-up confirms recurrence-free survival benefit of adjuvant pembrolizumab in high-risk stage III melanoma: updated results from the EORTC 1325-MG/KEYNOTE-054 trial. *J Clin Oncol.* 2020;38:3925–3936.

61. Dummer R, Hauschild A, Santinami M, et al. Five-year analysis of adjuvant dabrafenib plus trametinib in stage III melanoma. *N Engl J Med.* 2020;383:1139–1148.

62. Schiavone MB, Broach V, Shoushtari AN, et al. Combined immunotherapy and radiation for treatment of mucosal melanomas of the lower genital tract. *Gynecol Oncol Rep.* 2016;16:42–46.

63. Salama AKS, Palta M, Rushing CN, et al. Ipilimumab and radiation in patients with high risk resected or regionally advanced melanoma. *Clin Cancer Res.* 2020; [Online ahead of print].

64. Hodi FS, O'Day SJ, Mcdermott DF, et al. Improved survival with ipilimumab in patients with metastatic melanoma. *N Engl J Med.* 2010;363:711–723.

65. Robert C, Thomas L, Bondarenko I, et al. Ipilimumab plus dacarbazine for previously untreated metastatic melanoma. *N Engl J Med.* 2011;364:2517–2526.

66. Postow MA, Chesney J, Pavlick AC, et al. Nivolumab and ipilimumab versus ipilimumab in untreated melanoma. *N Engl J Med.* 2015;372:2006–2017.

67. Robert C, Ribas A, Schachter J, et al. Pembrolizumab versus ipilimumab in advanced melanoma (KEYNOTE-006): post-hoc 5-year results form an open-label, multicenter, randomized, controlled, phase 3 study. *Lancet Oncol.* 2019;20:1239–1251.

68. Hodi FS, Chiarion-Sileni V, Gonzalez R, et al. Nivolumab plus ipilimumab or nivolumab alone versus ipilimumab alone in advanced melanoma (CheckMate 067): 4-year outcomes of a multicenter, randomized, phase 3 trial. *Lancet Oncol.* 2018;19:1480–1492.

69. Chapman PB, Hauschild A, Robert C, et al. Improved survival with vemurafenib in melanoma with BRAF V600E mutation. *N Engl J Med.* 2011;364:2507–2516.

70. Larkin J, Ascierto PA, Dreno B, et al. Combined vemurafenib and cobimetinib in BRAF-mutated melanoma. *N Engl J Med.* 2014;371:1867–1876.

71. Robert C, Karaszewska B, Schachter J, et al. Improved overall survival in melanoma with combined dabrafenib and trametinib. *N Engl J Med.* 2015;372:30–39.

72. Dummer R, Ascierto PA, Gogas HJ, et al. Overall survival in patients with BRAF-mutant melanoma receiving encorafenib plus binimetinib versus vemurafenib or encorafenib (COLUMBUS): a multicenter, open-label, randomized, phase 3 trial. *Lancet Oncol.* 2018;19:1315–1327.

73. Shoushtari AN, Munhoz RR, Kuk D, et al. Efficacy of anti-PD-1 agents in acral and mucosal melanoma. *Cancer.* 2016;122:3354–3362.

74. Wohlmuth C, Wohlmuth-Wieser I, Laframboise S. Clinical characteristics and treatment response with checkpoint inhibitors in malignant melanoma of the vulva and vagina. *J Low Genit Tract Dis.* 2021;25(2):146–151.

75. D'Angelo SP, Larkin J, Sosman JA, et al. Efficacy and safety of nivolumab alone or in combination with ipilimumab in patients with mucosal melanoma: a pooled analysis. *J Clin Oncol.* 2016;35:226–235.

76. Hodi FS, Corless CL, Giobbie-Hurder A, et al. Imatinib for melanomas harboring mutationally activated or amplified *KIT* arising in mucosal, acral, and chronically sun-damaged skin. *J Clin Oncol.* 2013;31:3182–3190.

77. Kalinsky K, Lee S, Rubin KM, et al. A phase 2 trial in patients with locally advanced or stage IV mucosal, acral, or vulvovaginal melanoma: a trial of the ECOG-ACRIN cancer research group (E2607). *Cancer.* 2017;123:2688–2697.

78. Yan X, Sheng X, Chi Z, et al. Randomized phase II study of bevacizumab in combination with carboplatin plus paclitaxel in patients with previously untreated advanced mucosal melanoma. *J Clin Oncol.* 2021;35(8):881–889.

79. Wasif N, Bagaria SP, Ray P, et al. Does metastatectomy improve survival in patients with stage IV melanoma? A cancer registry analysis of outcomes. *J Surg Oncol.* 2011;104:111–115.

Chapter 18

Bartholin gland carcinomas

Vance Broach and Barrett Lawson

Clinical case

A 62-year-old woman presents to her general gynecologist with a complaint of right-sided vulvar itching and discomfort over the past 2 months. She is an otherwise healthy person who receives age-appropriate, routine health maintenance, and screening. She notes the vulvar discomfort is pronounced with vaginal intercourse. The patient does have a history of a right-sided Bartholin gland infection in her 40s, which was treated with incision and drainage and Word catheter placement (Fig. 18.1). On exam, the gynecologist notes a 2 cm firm, indurated nodule located at 8 o'clock in the labia minora, just cranial to the introitus. The mass is tender to palpation. The remainder of the exam is unremarkable. The clinician does not appreciate any palpable lymphadenopathy in the groins bilaterally. The clinician diagnoses a Bartholin gland abscess, and a plan for Bartholin gland marsupialization is made. In the OR, the surgeon incises the overlying epithelium. Minimal fluid is expressed. A firm, whitish nodule measuring approximately 3 cm is appreciated in the area of the suspected abscess. This nodule bleeds easily to minimal palpation, and a biopsy is taken. The procedure is aborted, given the unexpected intraoperative findings. Pathology demonstrates a Bartholin gland adenocarcinoma. What are the next steps in management? How might the treatment approach to Bartholin gland carcinoma differ from treatment of more common vulvar carcinomas?

Epidemiology

Vulvar cancer is a rare disease which accounts for 5% of all gynecologic malignancies. Approximately 6000 women are diagnosed with vulvar cancer annually.[1] Among vulvar cancers, Bartholin gland carcinomas are rarer still, accounting for 1%–7% of all vulvar tumors[2–5] and less than 1% of all gynecologic cancers. The Bartholin gland (also known as Bartholin's gland, or greater vestibular gland) was first described by the Danish anatomist Caspar Bartholin in 1675[6] and has the normal function of providing vulvovaginal lubrication. The Bartholin glands and ducts are located bilaterally at approximately the 4 and 8 o'clock positions in the labia minora, with duct openings just proximal to the introitus, and with an approximate size of 0.5–1 cm. Bartholin gland carcinomas occur in women with a median age of 53 years. The average tumor size at diagnosis is 39 mm.[7]

Approximately 17% of all patients are diagnosed with stage I disease, and 28% are diagnosed with stage II disease. Another 32% of patients are found to have stage III disease, in which disease has reached the inguinofemoral lymph nodes and 23% of patients are diagnosed with stage IV disease. Among patients who undergo primary surgical treatment, 5-year survival ranges from 70% to 93%.[2,4,8]

There are no known etiologies or risk factors for Bartholin gland carcinomas. Prior history of a Bartholin gland abscess or cyst does not seem to be a risk factor for Bartholin gland carcinoma. HPV has been isolated at the site of some Bartholin gland carcinomas, and, in the case of squamous cell carcinomas HPV infection may have an etiological role.[9]

Pathology

Bartholin gland carcinomas encompass a broad variety of histologic patterns, best conceptualized by knowing the histology of the Bartholin gland. The gland is composed of mucinous epithelial lined glands that drain via ducts lined by squamous and transitional cell epithelium. As such, different histotypes may arise from their respective cell lineage, including: squamous cell carcinoma, adenocarcinoma, adenosquamous carcinoma, adenoid cystic carcinoma, transitional cell carcinoma, small cell neuroendocrine carcinoma, Merkel cell carcinoma (MCC), epithelial-myoepithelial carcinoma, and lymphoepithelioma-like carcinoma.[7]

Diagnosis and Treatment of Rare Gynecologic Cancers. https://doi.org/10.1016/B978-0-323-82938-0.00018-5

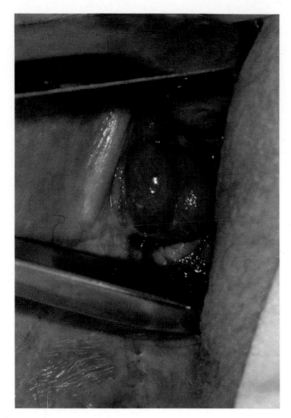

FIG. 18.1 Bartholin gland cyst.

Gross description

The mean size is 3.8 cm, with a reported standard deviation of approximately 2 cm. The tumors may either have an ulcerated surface or be deep seated with smooth overlying surface.

Microscopic description

As these are rare tumors and the Bartholin gland may be secondarily involved by vulvar tumors, histologic criteria for diagnosis must be met to determine if the carcinoma is a primary from the Bartholin gland. These criteria are: (1) histology of the tumor is compatible with a Bartholin gland origin, (2) there is a transition from normal Bartholin gland elements to tumor and (3) no evidence of other primary tumor in the adjacent structures.[6] In practice, not all criteria are met in a given case and sometimes distinction of a primary tumor from secondary involvement may be challenging. Squamous cell carcinoma is the most predominant histology, comprising approximately 50% of all Bartholin gland carcinomas, followed by adenocarcinoma (Fig. 18.2) and adenoid cystic carcinoma.[10]

All carcinomas that arise in the Bartholin gland show similar morphology to their counterparts elsewhere in the body. Squamous cell carcinomas, for example, show similar histology to that of squamous cell carcinomas from other sites, varying in keratinization and cytologic atypia.

Adenoid cystic carcinomas show similar histology to that in the salivary gland, with uniform small cells arranged in cords and nests with an overall cribriform and cystic appearance, filled with an acellular basement membrane-like material (Fig. 18.3).[11] Perineural and lymphovascular invasion are characteristic findings.[12] Immunohistochemistry shows positivity for c-kit (CD117) and p63, with the latter showing staining in the myoepithelial component.

Neuroendocrine carcinomas involving the Bartholin gland are either small cell carcinomas or Merkel cell carcinoma. Small cell carcinoma has monotonous small cells, ovoid hyperchromatic nuclei with scant cytoplasm (Fig. 18.4), and brisk

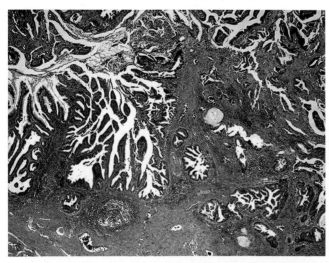

FIG. 18.2 Bartholin gland adenocarcinoma showing papillary and glandular patterns.

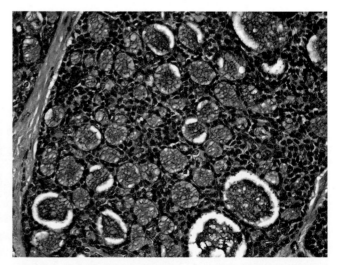

FIG. 18.3 Adenoid cystic carcinoma with uniform small cells in a cribriform and cystic pattern, filled with acellular basement membrane-like material.

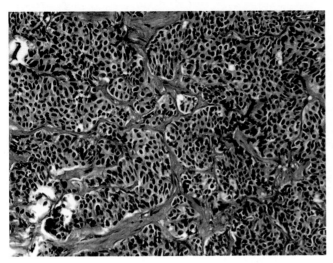

FIG. 18.4 Neuroendocrine carcinoma with monotonous small cells and ovoid, hyperchromatic nuclei.

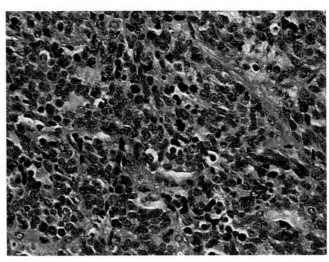

FIG. 18.5 Merkel cell carcinoma with hyperchromatic nuclei, scant cytoplasm and brisk mitotic/apoptotic activity.

mitotic/apoptotic activity with foci of necrosis.[13] Some small cell carcinomas of the Bartholin gland have exhibited distinct lobular architecture and/or Flexner–Wintersteiner rosette-like structures. These findings may represent a characteristic histology for small cell carcinomas arising in this area. MCC has a similar morphologic appearance to small cell neuroendocrine carcinoma (Fig. 18.5) but has a different immunophenotype from the latter.

Ancillary testing

As some Bartholin gland carcinomas are HPV associated, they are diffusely positive for p16 immunostain, as well as for HPV by in-situ hybridization. Adenoid cystic carcinoma shows *NFIB* rearrangement in approximately two-thirds of cases.[11] Merkel cell carcinomas express CK20, CAM5.2 and neurofilament in a paranuclear dot-like or ring-like pattern. MCC are positive for Merkel cell virus polyoma virus, which can be tested for by immunohistochemistry. Small cell carcinomas are typically negative for CK20 and neurofilament. MCC are also distinguished by differing driving viral infections, as previously mentioned.

Differential diagnosis

The differential diagnosis includes benign cysts, abscess, and endometriosis, all of which can be readily distinguished from malignant tumors. Glandular mimics may include hyperplasia or adenoma, but as these are benign lesions, there is no accompanying atypia or mitotic activity. Once a neoplasm has been diagnosed, it needs to be determined if the neoplasm represents metastasis or extension to the vulva from another primary site. Following the previously mentioned histologic criteria for will help rule in or rule out the tumor as a primary Bartholin gland neoplasm.

Diagnosis and work-up

The differential diagnosis of Bartholin gland carcinomas includes benign etiologies, such as Bartholin gland abscess, cyst or vulvar endometriosis; infectious etiologies such as syphilis and chancroid; and other vulvar cancers such as vulvar melanoma, sarcoma and squamous cell carcinoma of the overlying skin.[14] Given the numerous benign etiologies on differential diagnosis and the rarity of these tumors, diagnosis of Bartholin gland carcinoma is often delayed. Frequently patients experience vague or modest symptoms for months, only seeking care when symptoms become more severe or when they are evaluated during routine health maintenance visits.[2,7] The most common symptom at presentation is a vulvar mass, in 54% of women, followed by pain (9%), bleeding (3%), and burning sensation (2%).[7] As mentioned, prior history of a Bartholin gland abscess or cyst does not seem to be a risk factor for Bartholin gland carcinoma; however, it may add to the diagnostic complexity, as a Bartholin gland carcinoma is often confused with a cyst or abscess, which may be the leading differential in a patient with this history.

Physical exam findings frequently include a palpable, firm mass which may be fixed to the underlying tissue (Table 18.1). Bartholin gland carcinoma may bleed easily when palpated, a finding that may help distinguish it from other, benign etiologies.[15,16]

TABLE 18.1 Initial work-up for Bartholin gland carcinoma.

Physical exam	Complete physical exam with pelvic and rectovaginal examinations
Laboratories	CBC Liver function tests Renal function tests HIV testing
Imaging	PET or CT scan to evaluate for metastatic disease MRI pelvis for surgical or radiation planning
Additional testing	Biopsy of primary lesion HPV testing and cervical cytology as indicated

When a Bartholin gland carcinoma is suspected, careful physical exam is the most important first step in evaluation. Care should be taken to evaluate the size of the mass and its involvement of adjacent structures such as the vagina, urethra, and anus or rectum. Lesions which are fixed and immobile may involve surrounding structures. Groins should be evaluated bilaterally for signs of inguinofemoral adenopathy.

Imaging may be utilized on an individual basis, depending on the tumor's characteristics on physical exam and the concern for nodal metastasis or extension to surrounding structures. This is particularly helpful when counseling patients on the anticipated extent of surgical resection. Imaging is recommended for patients who present with larger tumors (>4 cm), have palpably enlarged lymph nodes, have symptoms which suggest metastatic involvement of the lower urinary tract or bowel, or who are not otherwise surgical candidates and for whom non-surgical management is planned.[17] Imaging modality may be selected depending on the clinical scenario. Magnetic resonance imaging (MRI) is most helpful in determining local lymph node metastasis, as well as tumor extension into surrounding structures.[18] Imaging outside of the pelvis with computed tomography (CT) is also useful in evaluating for distant metastases. Positron emitting tomography is utilized by some clinicians, though the clinical benefit over CT is debatable. Finally, exam under anesthesia with or without cystourethroscopy and proctoscopy may be required to evaluate for involvement of the lower urinary tract, bowel, and in cases where patient discomfort obviates adequate examination. Advances in imaging, particularly the use of MRI, to characterize extent of disease has obviated this practice in most cases, however.

While a Bartholin gland carcinoma may be suspected on presurgical evaluation, the diagnosis requires pathologic evaluation. The first diagnostic criteria for Bartholin gland carcinomas was proposed in 1897 by Honan and required that the following be met: the tumor is located in the area of the Bartholin gland, the tumor is located deep to the labia majora, the overlying skin is intact, the histologic type of tumor is consistent with that seen in Bartholin gland carcinoma, there is a transition from normal to invasive carcinoma in the specimen, and there is no evidence of a primary tumor at another site (i.e., the Bartholin gland carcinoma does not represent a metastasis). Given the burdensome extent of these criteria, they were simplified in 1971 by Chamlian and Taylor to include the following: the tumor invades the area histologically matching the Bartholin gland, it has areas which transition from tumor to normal in the sample, and there is no evidence of a primary tumor elsewhere in the vulva.[6]

Staging system

Bartholin gland carcinomas are classified as vulvar cancers, and their staging follows FIGO and AJCC staging systems for cancers of the vulva (Table 18.2). Staging involves a combination of clinical and surgical factors. Clinical factors include tumor size, local extension, gross lymph node involvement, and distant metastases detected by imaging. Surgical factors may include microscopic lymph node metastases, and depth of invasion. The staging system is summarized in the table below.

Prognostic factors

Given the rarity of Bartholin gland carcinomas, prognostic factors for squamous cell and adenocarcinomas of the Bartholin glands are extrapolated from vulvar carcinomas which do not arise from the Bartholin gland. Size of the tumor and lymph node involvement are the most important predictors of outcome. Among patients with positive nodes, the number and size of lymph node metastases affects survival. The size of the lymph node metastasis is an important prognostic factor in vulvar

TABLE 18.2 TNM and FIGO staging systems for vulvar cancer.

The definitions of the T categories correspond to the stages accepted by the International Federation of Gynecology and Obstetrics (FIGO). Both systems are included for comparison

Primary tumor (T)		
T category	FIGO stage	T criteria
TX		Primary tumor cannot be assessed
T0		No evidence of primary tumor
T1	I	Tumor confined to the vulva and/or perineum. Multifocal lesions should be designated as such. The largest lesion or the lesion with the greatest depth of invasion will be the target lesion identified to address the highest pT stage. Depth of invasion is defined as the measurement of the tumor from the epithelial-stromal junction of the adjacent most superficial dermal papilla to the deepest point of invasion.
T1a	IA	Lesions more than 2 cm, or any size with stromal invasion of more than 1 mm, confined to the vulva and/or perineum
T1b	IB	Lesions more than 2 cm, or any size with stromal invasion of more than 1 mm, confined to the vulva
T2	II	Tumor of any size with extension to adjacent perineal structures (lower/distal third of the urethra, lower/distal third of the vagina, anal involvement)
T3	IVA	Tumor of any size with extension to any of the following-upper/proximal two-thirds of the urethra, upper/proximal two-thirds of the vagina, bladder mucosa, or rectal mucosa-or fixed to the pelvic bone
T3a	IIIA	Tumor involving the serosa and/or adnexa (direct extension or metastasis)

Regional lymph nodes (N)		
N category	FIGO stage	N criteria
NX		Regional lymph nodes cannot be assessed
N0		No regional lymph node metastasis
N0(i+)		Isolated tumor cells in regional lymph node(s) no greater than 0.2 mm
N1	III	Regional lymph node metastasis with one or two lymph node metastases each less than 5 mm, or one lymph node metastasis greater than or equal to 5 mm
N1a*	IIIA	One or two lymph node metastases each less than 5 mm
N1b	IIIA	One lymph node metastasis greater than or equal to 5 mm
N2		Regional lymph node metastasis with three or more lymph node metastases each less than 5 mm, or two or more lymph node metastases greater than or equal to 5 mm, or lymph node(s) with extranodal extension
N2a*	IIIB	Three or more lymph node metastases each less than 5 mm
N2b	IIIB	Three or more lymph node metastases each less than 5 mm
N2c	IIIC	Lymph node(s) with extranodal extension
N3	IVA	Fixed or ulcerated regional lymph node metastasis

Note: The site, size, and laterally of lymph node metastases should be recorded.
*Includes micrometastasis, N1mi and N2mi.

Distant metastasis (M)		
M category	FIGO stage	M criteria
M0		No distant metastasis (no pathological M0; use clinical M to complete stage group)
M1	IVB	Distant metastasis (including pelvic lymph node metastasis)

Continued

TABLE 18.2 TNM and FIGO staging systems for vulvar cancer—cont'd

Prognostic stage groups			
When T is...	And N is...	And M is...	Then FIGO stage is...
T1	N0	M0	I
T1a	N0	M0	IA
T1b	N0	M0	IB
T2	N0	M0	II
T1-T2	N1-N2c	M0	III
T1-T2	N1	M0	IIIA
T1-T2	N2a, N2b	M0	IIIB
T1-T2	N2c	M0	IIIC
T1-T3	N3	M0-M1	IV
T1-T2	N3	M0	IVA
T3	Any N	M0	IVA
Any T	Any N	M1	IVB

Vulvar melanoma is not included in this staging system; it is staged with the melanoma staging system.
Classification of p16 status will be included if obtained but is not required.
TNM: Tumor, Node, Metastasis, AJCC: American Joint Committee on Cancer; UICC: Union for International Cancer Control.
Used with permission of the American College of Surgeons, Chicago, Illinois. The original source for this information is the AJCC Cancer Staging Manual, Eighth Edition (2017) published by Springer International Publishing. Corrected at 4th printing, 2018.

cancer. In patients with lymph node metastasis of less than 5 mm in size, 5-year overall survival of 90% has been reported; however, this drops to 42% and 21% when lymph node metastasis is between 5 and 15 mm and >15 mm respectively.[19] The presence of extracapsular spread is also negatively correlated with outcome.[20,21] The ratio of the number of positive lymph nodes to the number of lymph nodes removed has also been shown to correlate with outcome: overall survival was 90%, 65%, and 42% among patients with lymph node positive ratio of 0%, <20% and ≥20%, respectively.[22] Tumor size and presence of lymph-vascular space involvement also negatively correlate with survival.[21] Adenoid cystic carcinoma of the Bartholin gland, as described previously, may have a higher propensity to metastasize to the bone and lung, and may have a higher propensity to both local and distant recurrence than other histologic subtypes.[23–25]

Treatment of primary disease

The mainstay of treatment for early-stage Bartholin gland carcinoma, as with other vulvar cancers, is surgical resection (Table 18.3). Surgical management includes radical resection of the primary lesion with lymph node evaluation (discussed below). The Bartholin gland carcinoma should be resected in its entirety, with the goal of a 1 cm gross margin. This typically involves resection to the level of the urogenital diaphragm. Not infrequently, patients inadvertently undergo primary surgical management with a general gynecologist when a Bartholin gland carcinoma is not suspected, and the tumor is excised with positive margins. Reexcision of the margin is the preferred treatment in such cases where surgically feasible. Given the potential morbidity of this reexcision, this is not always possible, and postsurgical radiation therapy may be used in cases of positive or narrow margins.

Given the location of the Bartholin gland and the vascular supply to this area, surgical resection may be more complex and challenging than in other vulvar carcinomas. The robust blood supply often leads to higher blood loss, and the proximity to the anus, rectum, vagina, and bladder may necessitate more radical surgical resection. Resection of the anus and rectum, the bladder and even the bony structures of the pelvis, in order to obtain adequate margin, have been described.[8,26] Following a thorough discussion of the risks of extensive surgery with the patient, when feasible surgical resection is preferred for these patients over primary radiotherapy. There is often ample surrounding tissue to allow for primary closure of surgical defects. However, advancement and rotational flaps and even myocutaneous flaps in the case of large defects, may be considered for primary closure of the surgical wound.

TABLE 18.3 Treatment of newly diagnosed disease.

Stage at presentation	Treatment
I/II	If depth of invasion <1 mm, resection of the primary lesion with no lymph node assessment In patients with depth of invasion >1 mm, resection of primary lesion including entire Bartholin Gland to urogenital diaphragm with tumor free margin of 1 cm and bilateral lymph node sampling, either with SLN or full inguinofemoral lymph node dissection If sentinel LN positive, <2 mm, postoperative RT to the groins, if >2 mm, full side specific lymph node dissection followed by RT
III	Surgical resection with full lymph node dissection and radiation therapy For large tumors or tumors involving the urethra, clitoris or anus, exenterative procedures may be required for primary resection, or primary radiation therapy or chemoradiation may be considered to shrink the primary tumor, followed by resection
IV	Chemotherapy

Adenoid cystic carcinoma of the Bartholin gland may benefit from less radical surgery because margin status is not as strong a predictor of outcome as in other histologies. In one retrospective review, 29% of patients were found to have positive margins following resection of adenoid cystic Bartholin gland carcinoma; however, the rate of recurrence in the patients with positive margins (52.9%) was no different than in those who had more radical resection with negative margins (52.1%).[27]

Lymph node sampling

The radicality of surgery for vulvar cancer of all types has become more modest over the past 75 years. Radical surgery for vulvar cancer is associated with considerable morbidity including infection, wound breakdown, and lymphedema.[28,29] Strategies to minimize the radicality and potential morbidity of surgical resection have been investigated.

When considering the role of node sampling in these patients, again we draw our experience from other vulvar carcinoma which does not derive from the Bartholin gland. In women with carcinomas with <1 mm of invasion, the chance of nodal positivity is less than 1%, and lymph node sampling may be omitted in these patients.[30,31] In patients with clinical stage I or II tumors and depth of invasion >1 mm, lymph node excision should be performed. The lymphatic drainage of the vulva is the inguinofemoral lymphatics, but the lymphatic drainage of the Bartholin gland may not always follow this paradigm; the lymphatic drainage may be to the inguinofemoral lymph nodes, pelvic nodes or gluteal or rectal lymph nodes[32] (Fig. 18.6). This underscores the importance of preoperative imaging, particularly in patients who have increased risk of lymph node spread, including those with larger tumors and delayed diagnosis.

Sentinel lymph node (SLN) biopsy in patients with vulvar cancer has been established as a safe and effective method of lymph node evaluation in well-selected patients. Two prospective, multiinstitutional studies evaluating the oncologic safety of this technique have established it as the standard of care in patients with vulvar tumors of <4 cm in size and no lymphadenopathy on exam or imaging.[33–35] SLN detection may be performed with a combination of radiocolloid lymphoscintigraphy and blue dye or, more recently, with near infrared imaging and indocyanine green.[36] The use of SLN mapping and biopsy has been described in women with Bartholin gland carcinomas in case reports.[32,37] In patients for whom SLN mapping and biopsy are considered, preoperative imaging and radiocolloid lymphoscintigraphy or SPECT/CT is recommended to evaluate for abnormal nodes in the inguinofemoral chains as well as the pelvis, and to determine the individual lymphatic drainage on a patient-by-patient basis.

Again extrapolating treatment from patients with vulvar carcinomas not arising from the Bartholin gland, patients

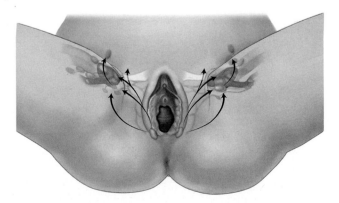

FIG. 18.6 Bartholin Gland anatomy including lymphatic drainage.

who are found to have positive SLNs and who have lymph node metastasis of >2 mm should undergo completion lymphadenectomy followed by radiation therapy (discussed below). In women with lymph node metastasis <2 mm, the option of radiation without completion lymphadenectomy is reasonable and associated with similar rates of nodal recurrence.[38]

In the case of adenoid cystic carcinomas of the Bartholin gland, there is ongoing controversy as to the role of lymph node evaluation. In some series, clinicians have reported a very low rate of nodal metastases and advocated for omitting this as part of surgical management of patients this histologic type.[39,40] Further investigation of this rare disease is needed before lymph node evaluation should be omitted entirely, and the authors recommend continued lymph node evaluation as part of the surgical management of this disease.

Stage III or IV disease

Patients who have palpably enlarged lymph nodes at the time of diagnosis should undergo full inguinofemoral lymphadenectomy. As noted above, in patients who have large tumors or local extension to surrounding structures such as the bladder or rectum, exenterative procedures may be required. In patients who are unwilling to undergo a more radical procedure or for whom radical surgery is not feasible, primary radiation therapy or chemotherapy may be utilized.[41,42] When used in the neoadjuvant setting, the extent of surgery may be lessened with robust response to chemoradiation.[43–45]

Surveillance for recurrence

Following primary treatment, surveillance consists of history, physical exam, and imaging in select patients. History and physical should be performed every 3–6 months for 2 years, then every 6–12 months for 2–5 years, and then annually. Routine health maintenance including cervical cytology should be performed per guidelines. Imaging may be utilized based on symptoms or concerning physical exam findings. Imaging of the groin with ultrasound is an effective strategy for evaluating for inguinofemoral lymph node recurrence in high-risk patients, including those with previously positive nodes.

In patients with adenoid cystic carcinoma of the vulva, the risk of distant metastasis is higher than in other histologies, particularly in cases of extensive perineural involvement. For this reason, imaging of distant sites should be considered in these patients as part of surveillance.[25]

Survival and patterns of failure

Among all patients with Bartholin gland carcinoma, 5-year overall survival is approximately 85%.[4] The most important prognostic factors are stage, size of the primary tumor, and lymph node involvement. In patients with node negative disease, 5-year overall survival is approximately 93%.[46] In patients with lymph node metastasis, 5-year survival ranges from 25% to 71%[2,19,33]; though, as described earlier, the number and size of lymph node metastases are negatively associated with outcome. Despite the reduction in radicality of primary treatment, outcomes among patients with vulvar cancer have been improving in recent years. This may be due to the improvement in postsurgical treatment and treatment of recurrence.[47]

In patients with local recurrent disease, surgical excision is the preferred treatment (Table 18.4). In some patients, local excision is possible with lymph node dissection. However, in patients with central recurrences, total pelvic exenteration may be required, and may be curative in some.[48] Lymph node recurrences are treated with excision of the involved lymph nodes, followed by radiation therapy.[49]

TABLE 18.4 Treatment of recurrent disease.

Surgical treatment	Non-surgical treatment
Consider in patients with local or central recurrences	Consider in patients with distant metastasis or in whom surgery is not medically feasible
Surgical excision of the recurrent vulvar tumor, and/or involved lymph nodes Exenteration may be required in patients with central recurrences involving the lower urinary tract or rectum and anus	Radiation therapy with concurrent cisplatin may be utilized for pelvic and lymph node recurrences Liposomal Doxorubicin and weekly paclitaxel can be considered in cases of distant recurrence

In patients for whom surgery is not feasible, treatment with chemoradiation or chemotherapy alone, as in cases of advanced primary Bartholin gland carcinoma, is the most appropriate treatment. Chemotherapeutic options include single agent pegylated liposomal doxorubicin (PLD), paclitaxel, and cisplatin.[45,50]

Case resolution

Biopsy of this patient reveals a Bartholin gland adenocarcinoma. The surgeon counsels the patient and obtains imaging with pelvic MRI, which demonstrates no evidence of involvement of the rectum, anus, vagina or lower urinary tract and reveals no abnormal inguinofemoral or pelvic lymph nodes. The surgeon recommends radical vulvectomy with bilateral SLN evaluation. Lymphoscintigraphy is performed preoperatively and identifies primary lymphatic drainage to the bilateral superficial inguinofemoral lymph nodes. Bilateral inguinofemoral lymph nodes are identified intraoperatively with a gamma counter and near infrared imaging with indocyanine green. Final pathologic assessment demonstrates a 2.5 cm Bartholin gland adenocarcinoma with negative margins and negative lymph nodes. The patient does not receive postsurgical treatment and is followed in surveillance every 6 months for 2 years, then annually.

References

1. Siegel RL, et al. Cancer statistics, 2021. *CA Cancer J Clin.* 2021;71(1):7–33.
2. Ouldamer L, et al. Bartholin's gland carcinoma: Epidemiology and therapeutic management. *Surg Oncol.* 2013;22(2):117–122.
3. Masterson JG, Goss AS. Carcinoma of Bartholin gland; review of the literature and report of a new case in an elderly patient treated by radical operation. *Am J Obstet Gynecol.* 1955;69(6):1323–1332.
4. Copeland LJ, et al. Bartholin gland carcinoma. *Obstet Gynecol.* 1986;67(6):794–801.
5. Nasu K, et al. Adenoid cystic carcinoma of Bartholin's gland. Case report with review of the literature. *Gynecol Obstet Invest.* 2005;59(1):54–58.
6. Chamlian DL, Taylor HB. Primary carcinoma of Bartholin's gland. A report of 24 patients. *Obstet Gynecol.* 1972;39(4):489–494.
7. Di Donato V, et al. Bartholin gland cancer. *Crit Rev Oncol Hematol.* 2017;117:1–11.
8. Cardosi RJ, et al. Bartholin's gland carcinoma: a 15-year experience. *Gynecol Oncol.* 2001;82(2):247–251.
9. Felix JC, et al. Carcinomas of Bartholin's gland. Histogenesis and the etiological role of human papillomavirus. *Am J Pathol.* 1993;142(3):925–933.
10. Bhalwal AB, Nick AM, dos Reis R, et al. Carcinoma of the Bartholin's gland: a review of 33 cases. *Int J Gynecol Cancer.* 2016;26(4):785–789.
11. Xing D, Bakhsh S, Melnyk N, et al. Frequent *NFIB*-associated gene rearrangement in adenoid cystic carcinoma of the vulva. *Int J Gynecol Pathol.* 2017;36:289–293.
12. Woida FM, Ribeiro-Silva A. Adenoid cystic carcinoma of the Bartholin gland. *Arch Pathol Lab Med.* 2007;131:796–798.
13. Chen PP, Ramalingam P, Alvarado-Cabrero I, et al. High-grade neuroendocrine carcinomas of the vulva: a clinicopathologic study of 16 cases. *Am J Surg Pathol.* 2020;45:304–316.
14. Heller DS, Bean S. Lesions of the Bartholin gland: a review. *J Low Genit Tract Dis.* 2014;18(4):351–357.
15. Wheelock JB, et al. Primary carcinoma of the Bartholin gland: a report of ten cases. *Obstet Gynecol.* 1984;63(6):820–824.
16. Finan MA, Barre G. Bartholin's gland carcinoma, malignant melanoma and other rare tumours of the vulva. *Best Pract Res Clin Obstet Gynaecol.* 2003;17(4):609–633.
17. Homesley HD, et al. Prognostic factors for groin node metastasis in squamous cell carcinoma of the vulva (a Gynecologic Oncology Group study). *Gynecol Oncol.* 1993;49(3):279–283.
18. Kataoka MY, et al. The accuracy of magnetic resonance imaging in staging of vulvar cancer: a retrospective multi-centre study. *Gynecol Oncol.* 2010;117(1):82–87.
19. Origoni M, et al. Prognostic value of pathological patterns of lymph node positivity in squamous cell carcinoma of the vulva stage III and IVA FIGO. *Gynecol Oncol.* 1992;45(3):313–316.
20. van der Velden J, et al. Extracapsular growth of lymph node metastases in squamous cell carcinoma of the vulva. The impact on recurrence and survival. *Cancer.* 1995;75(12):2885–2890.
21. Paladini D, et al. Prognostic significance of lymph node variables in squamous cell carcinoma of the vulva. *Cancer.* 1994;74(9):2491–2496.
22. Polterauer S, et al. Lymph node ratio in inguinal lymphadenectomy for squamous cell vulvar cancer: results from the AGO-CaRE-1 study. *Gynecol Oncol.* 2019;153(2):286–291.
23. Barcellini A, et al. Adenoid cystic carcinoma of Bartholin's gland: what is the best approach? *Oncology.* 2020;98(8):513–519.
24. Segarra Vidal B, et al. Adenoid cystic carcinoma of the Bartholin's gland. *Int J Gynecol Cancer.* 2021;31(2):292–298.
25. Chang Y, Wu W, Chen H. Adenoid cystic carcinoma of the Bartholin's gland: a case report and literature review. *J Int Med Res.* 2020;48(2). 300060519863540.
26. Nomura H, et al. Resection of the inferior pubic ramus to completely remove locally advance adenoid cystic carcinoma of Bartholin's gland. *Gynecol Oncol.* 2017;147(3):723–724.
27. Yang SY, et al. Adenoid cystic carcinoma of the Bartholin's gland: report of two cases and review of the literature. *Gynecol Oncol.* 2006;100(2):422–425.

28. Barton DP. The prevention and management of treatment related morbidity in vulval cancer. *Best Pract Res Clin Obstet Gynaecol.* 2003;17(4): 683–701.

29. Magrina JF, et al. Primary squamous cell cancer of the vulva: radical versus modified radical vulvar surgery. *Gynecol Oncol.* 1998;71(1):116–121.

30. Farias-Eisner R, et al. Conservative and individualized surgery for early squamous carcinoma of the vulva: the treatment of choice for stage I and II (T1-2N0-1M0) disease. *Gynecol Oncol.* 1994;53(1):55–58.

31. Magrina JF, et al. Squamous cell carcinoma of the vulva stage IA: long-term results. *Gynecol Oncol.* 2000;76(1):24–27.

32. Kraemer B, et al. Stage I carcinoma of the Bartholin's gland managed with the detection of inguinal and pelvic sentinel lymph node. *Gynecol Oncol.* 2009;114(2):373–374.

33. Van der Zee AG, et al. Sentinel node dissection is safe in the treatment of early-stage vulvar cancer. *J Clin Oncol.* 2008;26(6):884–889.

34. Levenback CF, et al. Lymphatic mapping and sentinel lymph node biopsy in women with squamous cell carcinoma of the vulva: a gynecologic oncology group study. *J Clin Oncol.* 2012;30(31):3786–3791.

35. Moore RG, et al. Sentinel node identification and the ability to detect metastatic tumor to inguinal lymph nodes in squamous cell cancer of the vulva. *Gynecol Oncol.* 2003;89(3):475–479.

36. Broach V, et al. Evolution and outcomes of sentinel lymph node mapping in vulvar cancer. *Int J Gynecol Cancer.* 2020;30(3):383–386.

37. Balepa L, et al. First detection of sentinel node in adenocarcinoma of Bartholin's gland. *J Gynecol Obstet Biol Reprod (Paris).* 2004;33(7):649–651.

38. Oonk M, et al. Radiotherapy instead of inguinofemoral lymphadenectomy in vulvar cancer patients with a metastatic sentinel node: results of GROINSS-V II. *Int J Gynecol Cancer.* 2019;29(suppl. 4):A14.

39. Anaf V, et al. Adenoid cystic carcinoma of Bartholin's gland: what is the optimal approach? *Eur J Surg Oncol.* 1999;25(4):406–409.

40. Hatiboglu MA, et al. Brain metastasis from an adenoid cystic carcinoma of the Bartholin gland. Case report. *J Neurosurg.* 2005;102(3):543–546.

41. Hacker NF, et al. Preoperative radiation therapy for locally advanced vulvar cancer. *Cancer.* 1984;54(10):2056–2061.

42. Moore DH, et al. A phase II trial of radiation therapy and weekly cisplatin chemotherapy for the treatment of locally-advanced squamous cell carcinoma of the vulva: a gynecologic oncology group study. *Gynecol Oncol.* 2012;124(3):529–533.

43. Massad LS, De Geest K. Multimodality therapy for carcinoma of the Bartholin gland. *Gynecol Oncol.* 1999;75(2):305–307.

44. Downs LS, et al. Stage IV carcinoma of the Bartholin gland managed with primary chemoradiation. *Gynecol Oncol.* 2002;87(2):210–212.

45. Tanaka H, et al. Adenocarcinoma of mammary-like glands in the vulva successfully treated by weekly paclitaxel. *Int J Gynecol Cancer.* 2005; 15(3):568–571.

46. Maggino T, et al. Patterns of recurrence in patients with squamous cell carcinoma of the vulva. A multicenter CTF Study. *Cancer.* 2000;89(1): 116–122.

47. Landrum LM, et al. Gynecologic Oncology Group risk groups for vulvar carcinoma: improvement in survival in the modern era. *Gynecol Oncol.* 2007;106(3):521–525.

48. Miller B, et al. Pelvic exenteration for primary and recurrent vulvar cancer. *Gynecol Oncol.* 1995;58(2):202–205.

49. Salom EM, Penalver M. Recurrent vulvar cancer. *Curr Treat Options Oncol.* 2002;3(2):143–153.

50. Huang GS, et al. Liposomal doxorubicin for treatment of metastatic chemorefractory vulvar adenocarcinoma. *Gynecol Oncol.* 2002;87(3):313–318.

Chapter 19

Vulvar extramammary Paget disease

Beverly Long, Lora Hedrick Ellenson, and William Cliby

Clinical case

A 72-year-old patient presents with a 6-month history of vulvar pruritus and irritation. She has tried multiple antifungal medications with no improvement. On physical examination, she has an erythematous plaque-like rash involving the perineum and bilateral labia majora (Fig. 19.1). You perform a biopsy, which reveals extramammary Paget disease. What additional testing is indicated? How would you treat this patient?

Epidemiology

Incidence and mortality

Extramammary Paget disease is a rare intraepithelial neoplasm that presents as eczematous, pruritic plaques of the perineal, perianal, inguinal, and/or axillary regions of both men and women. In Europe, the incidence of extramammary Paget disease is 0.7 per 100,000 persons per year, and women make up approximately 80% of cases. Conversely, a male predominance is noted in Asian populations.[1] Vulvar extramammary Paget disease most commonly occurs in postmenopausal Caucasian women with a mean age at presentation of 65 years.[2] However approximately 15% of cases of vulvar extramammary Paget disease in the United States occur in non-Hispanic Asians or Pacific Islanders.[3] While most vulvar extramammary Paget disease is intraepithelial/noninvasive, invasive disease is identified in 15%–20% of cases and accounts for 1%–2% of vulvar malignancies.[1,4]

Local recurrence is common in patients with extramammary Paget disease, but mortality is rare. Most series report 95%–100% survival among patients with noninvasive or microinvasive extramammary Paget disease, and the risk of developing invasive or metastatic extramammary Paget disease after treatment for noninvasive extramammary Paget disease is extremely low.[1] Five-year survival in most series of invasive extramammary Paget disease is 40%–80%. However, patients who present with metastatic disease have worse prognosis, with 5-year overall survival as low as 0%–15% in small series.[1,3,5–8]

Etiology and risk factors

The etiology of extramammary Paget disease is poorly understood; however, several origin theories exist including that Paget cells (1) arise from apocrine glands or stem cells in the epidermal basal layer of the skin or hair follicle, (2) originate from mammary-like glands, or (3) originate from Toker cells. Toker cells are CK7 positive cells that normally occur in the nipple, areola, and vulva. They can become hyperplastic and atypical, which gives a similar appearance to that of Paget cells.[1,9] Clinically, vulvar extramammary Paget disease is often classified as either primary or secondary extramammary Paget disease based on Wilkinson criteria (Table 19.1). Primary vulvar extramammary Paget disease is a cutaneous neoplasm, which is either comprised solely of Paget cells or is associated with a contiguous cutaneous malignancy (i.e., direct extension from an adjacent malignancy). Secondary extramammary Paget disease is associated with noncutaneous, non contiguous malignancy (i.e., malignancy diagnosed at a distant site without direct extension).

Rates of secondary malignancies associated with extramammary Paget disease vary in the literature, ranging from 4% to 58% in published series. This discrepancy is likely due to varying definitions of "associated" malignancies, as some series include contiguous cutaneous malignancies and others include only occult or distant cancers. Chronology of "associated" malignancies also varies, as some studies only include cancers diagnosed within 1–2 years of extramammary Paget disease, while others include remote malignancies. Most of these studies lack comparison groups (specifically, true age-associated rates of specific cancers), so the true association between extramammary Paget disease and distant or contiguous cancers is

Diagnosis and Treatment of Rare Gynecologic Cancers. https://doi.org/10.1016/B978-0-323-82938-0.00019-7

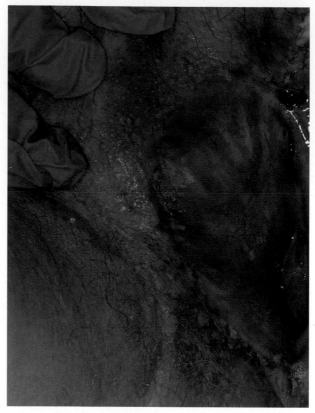

FIG. 19.1 Vulvar extramammary Paget disease with cake-icing appearance.

TABLE 19.1 Wilkinson criteria for vulvar EMPD.

Classification	Subtype
Primary (cutaneous)	1a Cutaneous vulvar noninvasive EMPD
	1b Cutaneous vulvar invasive EMPD (dermal invasion)
	1c Cutaneous vulvar EMPD contiguous with underlying vulvar adenocarcinoma
Secondary (noncutaneous)	2 Vulvar EMPD originating from rectal or anal adenocarcinoma
	3 Vulvar EMPD originating from urogenital neoplasia

not clear. Using SEER data, Kilts et al. observed a rate of synchronous cancer of only 2.8%, and the majority were breast, gastrointestinal (GI), or skin. Additionally, the risk of developing a subsequent secondary cancer compared to age and gender-based population controls was elevated (standardized incidence ratio (SIR) 3.9 (95% CI 2.2–4.7)).[3]

Schmitt et al. defined associated malignancies as "contiguous" if direct extension from an adjacent malignancy was noted on histology and as "noncontiguous" if cancer was diagnosed at a distant site without direct cytologic extension. Associated noncontiguous cancers were deemed "synchronous" if identified within 1 year of extramammary Paget disease diagnosis. In their series of male and female patients diagnosed with extramammary Paget disease at Mayo Clinic, synchronous, noncontiguous malignancies were diagnosed in 8% of patients with vulvar extramammary Paget disease, and contiguous malignancies were found in 18%.[10] Other series report somewhat higher rates of synchronous, noncutaneous malignancies (11%–46%) in vulvar extramammary Paget disease, specifically, though definitions were not standardized in these studies.[11–15]

Risk factors for vulvar extramammary Paget disease include advanced age and Caucasian race. While several genomic alterations have been noted on somatic testing (HER2 amplification, ERBB2, TP53, PIK3CA, and PTEN mutations,

FOXA1 overexpression), there are no known germline mutations associated with increased risk of extramammary Paget disease.[16] Environmental risk factors are also unknown.

Pathology

Gross appearance

Paget disease is usually a red to pink lesion that is slightly raised and may be focal but can also diffusely involve the vulva with extension into the vagina, cervix, and anus. These features overlap with more common dermatoses and high grade squamous intraepithelial lesion (VIN 3).

Microscopic features

Primary Paget disease is most often an entirely intraepithelial process (Fig. 19.2A). Paget disease is characterized by the presence of large, atypical cells with abundant, pale cytoplasm and large nuclei with prominent nucleoli (Fig. 19.2B). The cells can form clusters or be distributed as single cells and are most often located in the basal or parabasal portion of the epithelium, but can extend into the more superficial layers. It is commonly associated with a superficial dermal inflammatory response. This form of Paget disease is thought of as an in situ adenocarcinoma of the vulva. In resection specimens the margin status should be carefully evaluated and reported.

However, Paget disease can progress resulting in invasion of the dermis by the neoplastic cells. The invasion can be subtle with single cells extending into the superficial dermis or more readily appreciated if small groups of invasive cells are present. If invasive Paget disease is identified, the depth of invasion should be reported in addition to the presence or absence of invasive disease at the surgical margins.

Differential diagnosis and immunohistochemical

Paget disease must be distinguished from other intraepithelial processes such as high grade squamous intraepithelial lesions and melanoma. Although it is usually possible to distinguish Paget disease from these entities, ancillary studies can be helpful in difficult cases. Paget disease cells diffusely express CK7, which is negative in both squamous intraepithelial lesions and melanoma. p16 can be positive in Paget disease so it is not useful in the differential with HPV-associated squamous intraepithelial lesions, however it will be negative for HPV by in situ hybridization. Melanoma is not only negative for CK7, but its presence can be verified using S100, HMB-45, and Melan-A which are all negative in Paget disease.

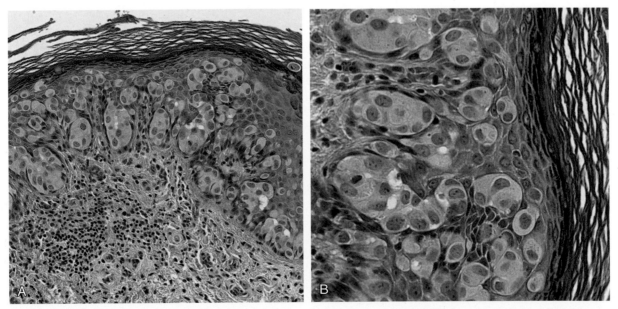

FIG. 19.2 Paget disease cells in nests and clusters involving squamous mucosa (A), Paget cells showing abundant cytoplasm, enlarged nuclei, and prominent nucleoli (B).

In addition, Paget disease must not be confused with the intraepithelial involvement of the vulva by invasive urothelial or rectal adenocarcinoma (referred to as secondary Paget disease). Uroplakin-3, CDX2, and CK20 can be used in this case as Paget disease is usually negative for all three markers (CK20 can be focally positive in Paget disease). CK7 can also be helpful in assessing the margin status of resections for Paget disease as well as for identifying invasive Paget disease if it is indefinite on H&E stained slides.

Molecular findings

Primary vulvar Paget disease (as discussed above) is thought to arise from stem cells in the skin adnexal structures or the epidermis. A recent study found alterations in the following genes: *PIK3CA* (35%), *ERBB2* (27%), and *TP53* (27%).[17] Amplification and deletion of specific regions of the genome as well as hypermethylation of *CDH1* have also been identified. The presence of *ERBB2* alterations (amplification and mutations) suggest that patient's with HER2 positive Paget disease by IHC may be candidates for targeted therapy and the presence of *PIK3CA* mutations may render patients sensitive to inhibitors of the PI3K pathway.

Diagnosis and work-up

Signs and symptoms

Vulvar extramammary Paget disease typically presents as a violaceous rash with intense pruritus and vulvar irritation, though 10%–15% of patients present with an asymptomatic rash. The diagnosis is often delayed, as signs and symptoms are attributed to candidiasis, lichen sclerosis, intertrigo, or contact dermatitis. In one series, patients experienced a median of 2 years of pruritus before their diagnosis of vulvar extramammary Paget disease.[18]

Physical exam findings

On physical exam, patients with extramammary Paget disease have a unifocal or multifocal, well-demarcated, eczematous rash with a plaque-like appearance and an irregular border. Raised white areas of hyperkeratosis can exist on an erythematous background, giving a "cake-icing" or "strawberries and cream" appearance (Fig. 19.1). This rash may extend beyond the perineum to involve the distal vagina, perianal and anal areas, and groin. Physical exam should include inspection of the entire genitalia and groins, as well as palpation of inguinal nodes. A breast exam, pelvic exam, and rectal exam should also be performed to assess for underlying malignancy. Given the data above regarding contiguous malignancies, more detailed focused examinations should be performed in cases with lesions contiguous with the urethra and anus in particular.

Differential diagnosis

The differential diagnosis of vulvar extramammary Paget disease includes benign conditions such as vulvovaginal candidiasis, lichenoid sclerosis, lichenoid simplex chronicus, psoriasis, contact dermatitis, Pagetoid reticulosis, and Pagetoid vulvar intraepithelial neoplasia as well as malignant conditions including superficial spreading malignant melanoma and vulvar squamous cell carcinoma. Histologically, the differential diagnosis for Paget cells includes melanoma, pagetoid spitz nevus, clear cell papulosis, sebaceous carcinoma, cutaneous T-cell lymphoma, eccrine porocarcinoma, and Langerhans cell microabscess.[1]

Tumor markers

There are no validated tumor markers for vulvar extramammary Paget disease. However, tumor cells typically express carcinoembryonic antigen (CEA), and serum CEA may be elevated in patients with metastatic or invasive extramammary Paget disease. Elevated CEA levels have been associated with poor prognosis.[6] In a study of patients undergoing chemotherapy for stage IV extramammary Paget disease, increasing CEA during chemotherapy was associated with progressive disease.[19]

Imaging studies

For patients with noninvasive extramammary Paget disease, imaging studies are typically performed only as necessary to screen for underlying malignancies and to ensure all patients have up to date, age-appropriate cancer screening. There are no national guidelines to inform screening recommendations in the setting of extramammary Paget disease. Based on their case series from Mayo Clinic, Schmitt et al. recommended updated screening mammography in women with newly diagnosed extramammary Paget disease.[10] Some experts recommend pelvic ultrasound, though this is low yield in the setting of a normal pelvic exam.

In patients with invasive extramammary Paget disease and lymphadenopathy, further imaging should be performed to assess for distant metastases. Image-guided biopsy of enlarged lymph nodes can also be performed when indicated. The optimal imaging modality for metastatic extramammary Paget disease is not defined, though computer tomography (CT) scan or positron emission tomography (PET) scan is reasonable. Case reports of metastatic invasive extramammary Paget disease confirm fluorodeoxyglucose (FDG)-avidity of metastatic lesions.[20,21]

Diagnostic testing

The diagnosis of extramammary Paget disease is confirmed by vulvar biopsy (Table 19.2). Punch biopsy is usually performed near the periphery of the lesion, as central necrosis can result in a nondiagnostic sample, especially in the case of a contiguous squamous cell carcinoma or other malignancy. Punch biopsy or excisional biopsy should include both the epidermal and dermal layers. Multiple scouting biopsies may be performed to map the extent of the lesion.

As with imaging, additional diagnostic testing after diagnosis of extramammary Paget disease is performed primarily for screening for secondary malignancy. Urine cytology should be performed to rule out associated urothelial malignancy, and cystoscopy can be considered, usually at the time of tumor resection in cases where extramammary Paget disease is contiguous with the periurethral tissues. Similarly, anoscopy or sigmoidoscopy in cases with anal skin involvement is reasonable. Up to date age-appropriate colonoscopy, cervical cancer screening, and mammography should be confirmed or performed. All patients with extramammary Paget disease should have age-appropriate cancer screening according to American Cancer Society or US Preventative Services Task Force guidelines.[10] Table 19.3 provides a summary of recommendations for secondary malignancy screening.

HER2/neu amplification testing may be considered in cases of advanced extramammary Paget disease. Approximately 30%–60% of extramammary Paget disease specimens will overexpress HER2/neu. This may provide potential therapeutic options when systemic therapy is necessary for metastatic or recurrent disease or to attempt to preserve critical organs (e.g., anus, urethra); however, its ability to predict response to trastuzumab is not well described.

Staging system

Most vulvar extramammary Paget disease is noninvasive and does not require staging. While there is no standard TNM staging system for invasive vulvar extramammary Paget disease, specifically, a TNM system for invasive extramammary Paget disease, in general, was proposed by Ohara et al. in 2016 (Table 19.4). This system is based on their analysis of 301 patients with extramammary Paget disease. A statistically significant decrease in survival was confirmed at each increasing stage of disease. Local tumor ≤4 mm in thickness without lymphovascular invasion is classified as stage I (T1). Locally

---

TABLE 19.2 Diagnostic work-up for patients with newly diagnosed extramammary Paget disease of the vulva.

Diagnosis and treatment planning
• History and physical examination
○ Cervical/vaginal/vulvar
○ Digital rectal exam
○ Breast examination
○ Nodal assessment
• Biopsy
○ Consider mapping biopsies to guide excision
• Imaging
○ CT or PET/CT if metastatic disease is suspected based on history and/or examination

TABLE 19.3 Summary of cancer screening recommendations for women diagnosed with vulvar EMPD.

Type	Screening recommendation
Any	Age-appropriate guideline screening or as appropriate based on full review of symptoms
Urologic (applies to lesions in close proximity to urethra)	Urine cytology Consider cystoscopy at time of resection
Gynecologic	Vulvar/vaginal exam Bimanual exam Cervical cancer screening (age 25–65 or history of CIN2+ within 25 years)
Gastrointestinal (applies to lesions with close proximity to anus)	Digital rectal exam Colonoscopy Consider anoscopy at time of resection
Breast	Clinical breast exam Mammogram
Lung	Low dose chest CT (age 55–80 with 30-pack year history within the last 15 years)

CIN, cervical intraepithelial neoplasia; *CT*, computed tomography.
Based on Schmitt et al.,[10] United States Preventative Task Force guidelines, and American Cancer Society guidelines.

TABLE 19.4 Proposed TNM staging system for EMPD.

	Stage	Description
Primary tumor (T)		
T0		Tumor in situ (noninvasive)
T1	I	Tumor thickness ≤4 mm **and** no lymphovascular space invasion
T2	II	Tumor thickness >4 mm **or** lymphovascular space invasion
Regional lymph nodes (N)		
N0		No lymph node metastasis
N1	IIIa	One lymph node metastasis
N2	IIIb	Two or more lymph node metastases
Distant metastases (M)		
M0		No distant metastases
M1	IV	Any distant metastases

advanced disease (tumor thickness >4 mm or lymphovascular invasion, T2) is classified as stage II. Cases with lymph node metastases are assigned to stage III (N1 or N2), and distant metastases constitute stage IV disease (M1). While patients with higher stage disease demonstrated worse progression free and overall survival in this study, biopsy of metastatic lesions was not required for staging. Since the rate of contiguous malignancies in this cohort was not reported, some metastases may have represented spread of a contiguous malignancy rather than metastatic Paget disease.[22] AJCC or FIGO staging for vulvar cancer may not be prognostic for vulvar extramammary Paget disease since these systems rely heavily on tumor size and involvement of surrounding structures, like the vagina and anus. Local spread is common in extramammary Paget disease, but lesion size is not consistently associated with prognosis.[6]

Prognostic factors

While extramammary Paget disease is noninvasive in the majority of cases, deeply invasive and widely metastatic disease does occur and, the latter in particular, is associated with poor prognosis. Metastatic extramammary Paget disease is near universally fatal. In a series by Ohara et al., patients with distant metastases exhibited a median overall survival of 1.5 years and 5-year survival of only 7% compared to 84% among patients with localized invasive extramammary Paget disease.[22] Similarly, Kilts et al. reported 5-year survival of 83% in cases with regional metastases and 13% among those with distant metastases.[3] Inguinal lymph node metastases also portend poor prognosis, though some series report worse survival only among those with multiple lymph node metastases or clinically enlarged nodes.[5,23] Data on the impact of regional lymph node metastases is limited: in a recent SEER study only 4.6% of patients with invasive vulvar extramammary Paget disease underwent lymphadenectomy.[3]

For clinically localized invasive tumors, deep invasion (>1 mm) is associated with poor prognosis with overall survival ranging from 40% to 80% in small series.[1,5,7,8] In contrast, disease-specific survival for noninvasive or microinvasive (≤1 mm) extramammary Paget disease approaches 100%.[1] When extramammary Paget disease is associated with an underlying malignancy, prognosis is variable based on the site, histologic subtype, and stage of the associated cancer.

While noninvasive extramammary Paget disease is rarely fatal, it is associated with high rates of local recurrence and almost always the recurrences are noninvasive as well. Lesion size, disease site, synchronous malignancy, and treatment type have been variably associated with recurrence risk in published literature. The role of margin status in extramammary Paget disease is controversial. Data from small case series are conflicting. For instance, Tebes et al. observed no difference in recurrence risk among patients with positive vs negative resection margins (37.6% vs 28.6, $P = 0.53$) in a series of 23 patients.[24] Parker et al. reported similar findings in a series of 76 patients with 31% and 33% recurrence rates for patients with positive and negative margins, respectively.[13] However, other series report lower recurrence rates after resection with negative margins.[25,26] Many of the series that associate negative margins with lower recurrence risk include patients treated with Mohs micrographic surgery (MMS), an advanced surgical technique that allows intraoperative examination of 100% of the surgical margin. For instance, Pierie et al. reported no recurrences among 33 male and female patients with negative margins compared to a 72% recurrence rate among those with microscopically positive margins among patients undergoing either wide local excision (WLE) or MMS.[26] In a Mayo Clinic series of 154 male and female patients, positive margin status was associated with a 3.5-fold increased risk of recurrence compared to negative margins ($P < 0.001$). Positive margins were significantly more common after WLE compared to MMS. Though statistical significance was limited by small sample size, there were trends toward lower recurrence risk in patients treated with MMS and in patients with negative margins after MMS, compared to those with negative margins after WLE.[27] Together, these findings suggest that margin status may be an important predictor of recurrence when margins are adequately examined. Use of MMS typically results in larger excisions, often requiring more complex reconstructive procedures. More data are needed to determine the risk/benefits ratio of a more complex resection and whether MMS is superior to WLE to prevent local recurrence of extramammary Paget disease.

Treatment of primary disease

Early stage disease: Extramammary Paget disease

Over 80% of vulvar extramammary Paget disease is noninvasive and confined to the vulva. Treatment of primary, localized disease is surgical, typically consisting of vulvar WLE. Surgery is both therapeutic and diagnostic, as the pathologic specimen is assessed for deep invasion or contiguous carcinoma. Most surgeons aim for complete gross resection (CGR) with 1–2 cm margins, though approximately 30% of grossly negative margins will be pathologically positive. Margins are difficult to evaluate grossly or with use of traditional frozen section due to the irregular borders and multifocal nature of extramammary Paget disease. Frozen section can be utilized but has a high false negative rate.[28,29] Scouting biopsies may also be performed to map the extent of a lesion prior to surgery, but this method is also fraught with false negatives when compared to assessment of final surgical margins. Many studies suggest that margin guided surgery (e.g., Moh's) is associated with lowest rate of pathologically involved margins and lower rates of recurrence, though additional time and observational data will be important to confirm this. (Fig. 19.3). The compromise of achieving negative margins and the cost in terms of size and complexity of resection must be individualized. Though the role of extensive resection for extramammary Paget disease is debated, reconstruction is required when large vulvovaginal resections are performed. Local cutaneous flaps, gluteal flaps, and gracilis flaps are the most common reconstructive techniques. Plastic surgery consultation should be obtained when necessary. Nonsurgical options or observation may be preferred for large lesions.

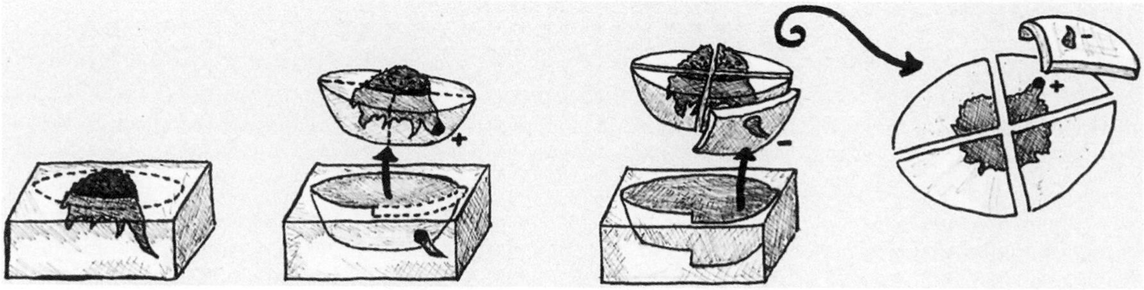

FIG. 19.3 Mohs micrographic surgery procedure. *Source: Illustration by Brandon Goodwin, MD, Department of Dermatology, University of Texas Medical Branch, Galveston.*

MMS is performed at specialized centers in both men and women with extramammary Paget disease, based mostly on single-institution, retrospective series, which show lower recurrence rates after MMS compared to WLE. This approach is often favored by dermatologists and has been more frequently used in male perineal extramammary Paget disease. MMS utilizes a beveled or oblique incision that allows for examination of the entire surgical margin.[30,31] Immediate, intraoperative pathologic assessment is performed by the Mohs surgeon, typically in the office setting with local anesthetic. Reexcision is performed until negative circumferential margins are obtained. A moat technique is used to remove a rim of tissue along the circumferential margin of the lesion; once circumferential margins are cleared by the Mohs surgeon, a WLE can be performed by the gynecologist to remove the central lesion. This technique ensures accurate, negative margins, while maximally sparing normal tissue. Gynecologic oncologists have often favored WLE with grossly free margins. In our experience, the use of MMS in extramammary Paget disease is associated with larger excisions. The risk of these extended procedures should be weighed against the higher local recurrence risk associated with WLE, especially in noninvasive extramammary Paget disease, which can typically be managed with subsequent excisions at the time of recurrence.

Nodal assessment is not recommended for women with noninvasive or microinvasive extramammary Paget disease with clinically normal inguinal lymph nodes. This applies to complete inguinal femoral dissection and sentinel lymph node (SLN) assessment. When invasion >1 mm is present, nodal assessment is rarely performed, and evidence supporting its routine use is lacking, particularly in patients with clinically negative lymph nodes.[1] Specifically regarding SLN the evidence is limited in vulvar extramammary Paget disease. In one study of 107 patients, the rate of SLN metastasis was 15%. However, positive sentinel lymph node metastases were not associated with worse survival.[32] While smaller series have found higher recurrence risk in the setting of positive sentinel lymph nodes, the value of surgical lymph node assessment (including SLN) of clinically normal nodes is not clear.[33] Summarizing, lymph node assessment for staging of Paget disease is not currently recommended. In cases of invasive Paget disease, imaging of regional lymphatics is reasonable (PET/CT scan) followed by individualized multidisciplinary care team decision-making to develop a comprehensive treatment plan.

Nonsurgical management of extramammary Paget disease is typically reserved for patients with recurrent disease, poor surgical candidates, or to preserve critical structures in the setting of extensive disease. Nonsurgical treatment options are reviewed below (see Section "Treatment of recurrent disease").

Locally advanced disease

There is no standard management for invasive vulvar extramammary Paget disease with regional lymph node involvement. Several case series report the use of radiation for patients with inguinal lymph node metastases. However, the efficacy of this treatment is unclear. Some series also report surgical resection of microscopic or clinically evident inguinal lymph node metastases. Patients with locoregional disease are at high risk of distant recurrence, and systemic therapies have been used to treat patients with locoregional metastases in case reports and small series.[34,35] However, prognosis is poor for patients with regional lymph node metastases, and survival ranges from 0% to 20% for patients with clinically enlarged nodes or multiple involved lymph nodes regardless of treatment.

Distant metastatic disease

Treatment of metastatic disease is not curative. Multiple chemotherapy agents, including combination 5-fluorouracil, epirubicin, carboplatin, vincristine, and mitomycin C (FECOM); 5-fluorouracil, epirubicin, and cyclophosphamide; and docetaxel have demonstrated initial response rates in case reports and small series, but responses are not typically durable.[1]

Targeted therapy has also been used to treat metastatic extramammary Paget disease when HER2/neu amplification is present. HER2/neu amplification occurs in approximately 30%–60% of vulvar extramammary Paget disease, with the highest incidence in invasive and metastatic disease. Trastuzumab has been used alone and in combination with cytotoxic chemotherapy, with responses reported between 6 and 36 months.[36] Responses to other targeted therapies based on next generation sequencing have also been reported. PIK3CA, ERBB2, and TP53 mutations are most common, and a durable response to a PI3K-inhibitor was reported in one series.[37] Next generation sequencing should be considered in metastatic or recurrent disease. Palliative resection or radiation can be considered for symptomatic vulvar extramammary Paget disease in the setting of distant metastases.

Surveillance for recurrent disease

Because most vulvar extramammary Paget disease is noninvasive and localized, surveillance is focused on detection of genital recurrence. Most experts recommend physical exam, with attention to the perineum and groins, every 6 months. Surveillance for locoregional or metastatic disease should be individualized, with consideration of the treatment options and goals of care, given the high risk of distant recurrence and mortality.

Survival and patterns of failure

For patients with noninvasive vulvar extramammary Paget disease, disease-specific survival approaches 100%. Microinvasive extramammary Paget disease is also associated with good prognosis, ranging from 88% to 100% in published series.[5,6] However, local recurrence occurs in 30%–50% of cases of intraepithelial or minimally invasive disease, and patients may undergo multiple resections or courses of topical therapy, radiation, or systemic treatment. Invasive or metastatic recurrence after initially noninvasive or minimally invasive extramammary Paget disease is extremely rare (less than 3% of cases). In a 2016 review of the literature, Van der Linden et al. found only four cases of metastatic disease after initial presentations of noninvasive vulvar extramammary Paget disease.[1]

Invasive vulvar extramammary Paget disease is present in 15%–20% of cases and has a significantly higher risk of recurrence and metastasis. In a 2012 SEER database study of over 1400 patients with invasive extramammary Paget disease, 80% of patients presented with localized disease, while 17% and 3% had locoregional or distant metastases, respectively. While small series report survival rates ranging from 0% to 15% for patients with invasive extramammary Paget disease,[5,6] 5-year disease-specific survival among these SEER database patients was 95% (localized disease), 85% (locoregional metastases), and 53% (distant metastases), suggesting better outcomes than those reported in small series.[4] This discrepancy may be due to varying definitions of invasive extramammary Paget disease, coexisting contiguous or occult malignancies, small sample sizes, or disparate treatment methods.

Treatment of recurrent disease

Despite high recurrence rates of vulvar extramammary Paget disease, optimal treatment for recurrent disease is not well defined. Management should be individualized after consideration of patient and tumor factors, including time to recurrence, previous treatments, surgical morbidity, and severity of symptoms at the time of recurrence. Efficacy data for non-surgical management is based mostly on small case series (Table 19.5).

Surgical resection

Surgery is the most common treatment for recurrent extramammary Paget disease. In one series, 73% of patients underwent repeat surgical resection for recurrent vulvar extramammary Paget disease. Most patients had multiple recurrences, and 40% underwent 2 or more surgical procedures, while almost 20% underwent 3 or more procedures.[38] Principles of surgery are similar for primary and recurrent disease. As in primary disease, the impact of margin status after resection for recurrent disease is controversial. MMS has been proposed to treat recurrent extramammary Paget disease, in order to prevent morbidity from multiple vulvar resections. In a series by Hendi et al., the rate of subsequent recurrence after MMS for recurrent

TABLE 19.5 Treatment options for recurrent extramammary Paget disease.

- Surgical resection
- Carbon dioxide laser ablation
- Topical therapy
  - Imiquimod
  - 5-Fluorouracil
  - Rapamycin
  - Bleomycin
- Photodynamic therapy
- Systemic therapy
  - Chemotherapy
  - Trastuzumab
  - Other targeted agents based on tumor profiling
- Radiation

extramammary Paget disease was 50%; however, all patients were salvaged by a second MMS procedure. No additional recurrences were noted among six patients who underwent Mohs micrographic salvage surgery at a median follow-up of 76 months.[30]

Topical treatment

Imiquimod

Imiquimod is a topical immune modulator, which works as a toll-like receptor-7 agonist to trigger the production of cyto-kines and activate skin Langerhans cells. Imiquimod is Food and Drug Administration (FDA)-approved to treat genital warts, actinic keratosis, and basal cell carcinoma. It is also used to treat vulvar and anal carcinoma in situ. Its effectiveness in the treatment of noninvasive vulvar extramammary Paget disease has been demonstrated in multiple observational series and case reports. In their review of the literature, Van der Linden et al. reported an objective clinical response in 56 of 64 (88%) women treated for noninvasive vulvar extramammary Paget disease. Complete response was noted in 43 women (67%).[1] Published treatment regimens and durations vary. Topical 5% imiquimod applied three times per week for 16 weeks was recently evaluated in the Paget Trial, a multicenter observational cohort study of 24 patients with vulvar extramammary Paget disease. Twenty-three patients were evaluable. Complete response was noted in 12 patients (52.2%), and 7 patients (30.4%) had a partial response. Long term follow-up for this study is pending.[39] A similar regimen was used in a pilot study by Cowan et al., which included eight patients with noninvasive extramammary Paget disease. A complete response was noted in six (75%) patients at 12 weeks following therapy; however, four of these patients (67%) recurred at intervals ranging from 4 to 10 months.[40]

The use of topical imiquimod is limited mostly by pain and local reaction at the application site. In the Paget Trial, 80% of patients required pain medications, three patients stopped imiquimod, and eight patients adjusted the regimen to two applications per week due to side effects. Topical lidocaine and/or Vaseline ointment or other skin barrier creams can be used to coat adjacent normal tissue to limit skin exposure to imiquimod and reduce application-site pain. Less common reactions include flu-like symptoms, fatigue, and headaches.

Bleomycin

Bleomycin is an antineoplastic agent, which is most commonly used as systemic chemotherapy. Its primary mechanism of action is to affect double- and single-stranded DNA breaks via oxidative damage by metalloproteinase complexes. One series describes the use of topical bleomycin therapy in seven patients with recurrent vulvar extramammary Paget disease. Four patients (57%) achieved complete response after treatment with up to four 2-week courses of topical bleomycin (3.5% ointment consisting of 105 mg bleomycin sulfate in 1 mL of sterile water, suspended in 2 g of Aquaphor base) applied twice daily with 4–6-week interruptions between courses to allow for healing and evaluation of response. One patient (14%) had a partial response but declined further therapy. Among four patients with complete response, three had no evidence of disease at 8–10 months of follow-up. Recurrence was noted in one patient at 30 months; retreatment resulted in complete response after only one additional cycle.[41]

Local pain and moist desquamation were the most common side effects. No other side effects were noted in the above study. Series reporting the use of topical bleomycin for other indications (squamous cell carcinoma, cutaneous warts) do not report systemic reactions.[42,43]

5-Fluorouracil

5-Fluorouracil is an antimetabolite chemotherapy that is used as a topical treatment for multiple types of skin cancer. It has been used with calcipotriene for the treatment of recurrent extramammary Paget disease, refractory to imiquimod. In a series of three patients, topical 5-FU and calcipotriene was applied one to two times per week every 2–4 weeks. All women experienced symptomatic improvement and clinical reduction in disease burden, two of which were pathologically proven.[44] Side effects are similar to other topical therapies including skin irritation and local pain.

Rapamycin

Topical rapamycin has been described in a small series ($n = 4$) and appeared to improve symptoms of refractory extramammary Paget disease. Rapamycin (0.4%) was applied twice daily for 2 weeks. All four patients achieved a positive clinical response, and a reduction in Pagetoid cells was seen on histologic examination. Molecular profiling was not used to select for alterations in the mTOR pathway in this series; however, based on the incidence of mTOR and PIK3CA mutations in extramammary Paget disease, more studies are warranted to determine the efficacy of rapamycin in both mTOR-mutated and unselected patients.[45] Future research, and tumor testing as described above, will facilitate participation of Paget disease in clinical trials based on proven molecular/genetic alterations.

Photodynamic therapy

Photodynamic therapy (PDT) is a type of radiation used to treat superficial nonmelanoma skin cancers or precancers. When used to treat vulvar extramammary Paget disease, a topical photosensitizer such as 5-aminolevulinic acid (5-ALA) is applied to the vulva and absorbed by Paget cells. The photosensitizer is allowed to incubate for several hours before it is washed off, and the lesion is irradiated with red light. This sequence destroys any proliferating tumor cells that have absorbed the photosensitizing ointment. Several small series report 50%–100% complete clinical response rates in recurrent genital extramammary Paget disease with follow-up periods of 3–6 months.[1] One series including 16 men and women with both primary and recurrent genital extramammary Paget disease reported a 50% rate of complete response; however, 37.5% of responders recurred by 10 months posttherapy.[46] Better responses have been reported with combination therapy (see below).

PDT is well tolerated but can be associated with pain and swelling at the lesion site, skin blistering, erythema, and urticaria. PDT is also associated with increased risk of subsequent skin cancers in some studies, though it is not clear whether there is a causative association between PDT and skin cancer.[47]

Laser ablation

Carbon dioxide (CO_2) laser ablation is typically used in the setting of recurrent or unresectable intraepithelial vulvar extramammary Paget disease. Laser ablation is performed to a depth of 1 mm in nonhair baring skin and 2–3 mm in hair baring skin. If laser ablation alone is used in the primary setting, extensive biopsies should be performed to rule out invasive disease. Frozen section or mapping biopsies can be performed to ensure ablation of the entire lesion. CO_2 laser ablation may be used alone or in combination with other modalities including surgery of PDT.

One series by Ewing et al. reported six cases of vulvar extramammary Paget disease, which were treated with WLE followed by CO_2 laser ablation of unresectable areas, positive margins, or recurrent disease occurring within months of initial excision. Though some patients required multiple laser procedures, long term recurrence free intervals were noted after laser ablation of the entire lesion was confirmed (4 months to 4.5 years).[48]

CO_2 laser ablation has also been used in combination with PDT. In a series by Fuikui et al., five patients (four vulvar, one penile extramammary Paget disease) underwent CO_2 laser ablation followed by 3 h of occlusive application of aminolevulinic acid (ALA) and 100 J/cm^2 irradiation with a 630-nm excimer dye laser for recurrent disease or for primary disease with positive margins after initial resection. Treatment was administered every 2 weeks for three sessions. There were no recurrences after 12 months of follow-up in this small series, though one patient died of unrelated causes.[49]

CO$_2$ laser ablation can be performed as an outpatient procedure, and serious complications, such as infection, are rare. However, the recovery can be uncomfortable and prolonged. Scarring can occur after extensive ablation, but vulvar anatomy is typically preserved.

Systemic therapy

Trastuzumab

Trastuzumab is a monoclonal antibody that binds the HER2/neu, a transmembrane tyrosine kinase receptor, to prevent HER2/neu receptor activation, increase apoptosis, and impair DNA damage repair and neovascularization. It is most commonly used in breast and serous uterine cancers that overexpress HER2/neu. Approximately 30%–60% of Paget cases overexpress HER2/neu. There are several case reports demonstrating improvement in lesion size and extramammary Paget disease symptoms with the use of trastuzumab for HER2/neu-overexpressing extramammary Paget disease. Karam et al. reported clinical response to trastuzumab in a 54-year-old patient with multiple recurrent vulvar extramammary Paget disease with strong HER2/neu overexpression (IHC with 3+ staining). The patient noted decreased pain and pruritus with a corresponding decrease in lesion size and erythema, which was sustained during 12 cycles of monthly trastuzumab. No pathologic testing was performed to assess response.[50] Hsieh et al. reported a complete radiologic response to carboplatin/paclitaxel/trastuzumab followed by trastuzumab maintenance in a patient with metastatic, recurrent HER2/neu-overexpressing vulvar extramammary Paget disease. Progression-free survival (PFS) was 7 months.[36] Ichiyama et al. reported an initial response and 2 years of stable disease in a similar patient with recurrent, HER2/neu-amplified vulvar extramammary Paget disease treated with paclitaxel and trastuzumab.[51] Based on these case reports, trastuzumab can be considered for HER2/neu-overexpressing, recurrent or metastatic extramammary Paget disease when a patient has failed traditional treatments or is not a candidate for surgery.

Cytotoxic chemotherapy

Chemotherapy has been used to treat metastatic primary or recurrent extramammary Paget disease in small series of both male and female patients. Oashi et al. reported eight cases of metastatic extramammary Paget disease, of which four had a partial response or stable disease in response to combination therapy with 5-fluorouracil, epirubicin, carboplatin, FECOM.[52] Another study of eight male patients with metastatic extramammary Paget disease, reported a 50% rate of partial response and 37.5% rate of stable disease after four or more cycles of cisplatin and docetaxel. Mean PFS was 9.9 months with overall survival of 28.9 months.[53] Similar results have been noted in other small series, with most studies demonstrating short-term response to chemotherapy in at least half of patients with metastatic extramammary Paget disease.[54,55]

Radiation therapy

Radiation can be used to treat noninvasive or invasive extramammary Paget disease in several scenarios, including recurrent disease, primary treatment in nonsurgical candidates, or as postoperative therapy after incomplete resection or nodal metastases. Hata et al. published a series 22 patients (18 women) with genital extramammary Paget disease. Twelve patients had invasive extramammary Paget disease, and nine had inguinal lymph node metastases. Ten patients received primary radiation, four patients received radiation for recurrence after initial surgical excision, and eight patients received adjuvant radiation immediately following primary surgery. Radiation was given to the local tumor site ± regional lymph nodes (inguinal and pelvic) with doses ranging from 45 to 70.2 Gy. All patients had an initial complete response, but 59% (n = 13) had recurrent disease after 3–43 months of follow-up. Three of the 13 recurrences occurred within the radiation field, while 10 had regional or distant metastases outside of the radiation field.[56] A smaller series of both intraepithelial (n = 2) and invasive (n = 1) vulvar extramammary Paget disease, reported complete clinical response in all three patients. After 0.6–11 years of follow-up, only one recurrence was noted. It occurred at the margins of the radiation field and did not require further treatment due to tolerable symptoms.[57] In a SEER database study by Karam and Dorigo, only 6.4% of patients with primary, invasive extramammary Paget disease underwent radiation therapy, and receipt of radiation therapy was independently associated with lower disease-specific survival compared to other treatment methods.[4] Therefore, the role of radiation therapy in extramammary Paget disease is controversial. However, radiation therapy can be considered in patients with local or regional extramammary Paget disease who have failed traditional treatments or those who cannot undergo surgery.

Special considerations

Due to high rates of local recurrence, most women with vulvar extramammary Paget disease undergo repeated excisions, which can have unrecognized and under reported impact. There is a paucity of data regarding long term surgical morbidity, sexual function, and other patient reported outcomes after treatment for vulvar extramammary Paget disease.

Case resolution

This patient was counseled regarding treatment options for primary vulvar extramammary Paget disease including WLE and MMS. Dermatology was consulted to perform MMS. She underwent multiple mapping biopsies to determine the extent of her lesion. She then underwent MMS to obtain negative peripheral margins followed by next-day vulvectomy to remove the central lesion. Plastic surgery was consulted to perform left medial thigh keystone flap for reconstruction. Final pathology confirmed intraepithelial vulvar extramammary Paget disease with negative margins. Postoperative recovery was complicated by focal superficial wound breakdown, but the incision completely healed by secondary intention after localized wound care. She is currently without evidence of disease after 3 months of follow-up.

References

1. Van der Linden M, Meeuwis KAP, Buiten J, Bosse T, van Poelgreest MIE, de Hullu JA. Paget disease of the vulva. *Crit Rev Oncol Hematol.* 2016;101 (5):60–74.
2. Delport ES. Extramammary Paget's disease of the vulva: an annotated review of the current literature. *Australas J Dermatol.* 2013;54(1):9–21.
3. Kilts TP, et al. Invasive vulvar extramammary Paget's disease in the United States. *Gynecol Oncol.* 2020;157(3):649–655.
4. Karam A, Dorigo O. Treatment outcomes in a large cohort of patients with invasive extramammary Paget's disease. *Gynecol Oncol.* 2012;125 (2):346–351.
5. Ito Y, et al. Prognostic indicators in 35 patients with extramammary Paget's disease. *Dermatol Surg.* 2012;38(12):1938–1944.
6. Hatta N, et al. Extramammary Paget's disease: treatment, prognostic factors, and outcome in 76 patients. *Br J Dermatol.* 2008;158(2):313–318.
7. Creasman WT, et al. Paget's disease of the vulva. *Gynecol Oncol.* 1975;3(2):133–148.
8. Jones I, Crandon A, Sanday K. Paget's disease of the vulva: diagnosis and follow-up key to management; a retrospective study of 50 cases from Queensland. *Gynecol Oncol.* 2011;122(1):42–44.
9. Asel M, LeBoeuf N. Extramammary Paget's disease: the clinics. *Hematol Oncol Clin North Am.* 2019;33:73 85.
10. Schmitt AR, et al. Evidence-based screening recommendations for occult cancers in the setting of newly diagnosed extramammary Paget's disease. *Mayo Clin Proc.* 2018;93(7):877–883.
11. Feuer GA, Shevchuck M, Calanog A. Vulvar Paget's disease: the need to exclude an invasive lesion. *Gynecol Oncol.* 1990;38(1):81–89.
12. Fanning J, et al. Paget's disease of the vulva: prevalence of associated vulvar adenocarcinoma, invasive Paget's disease, and recurrence after surgical excision. *Am J Obstet Gynecol.* 1999;180(1):24–27.
13. Parker L, et al. Paget's disease of the vulva: pathology, pattern of involvement, and prognosis. *Gynecol Oncol.* 2000;77(1):183–189.
14. Onaiwu CO, et al. Paget's disease of the vulva: a review of 89 cases. *Gynecol Oncol Rep.* 2016;30(19):46–49.
15. Parashurama R, Nama V, Hutson R. Paget's disease of the vulva: a review of 20 years' experience. *Int J Gynecol Cancer.* 2017;27(4):791–793.
16. Kilts T, et al. Identification of unique genomic alterations in extramammary Paget's disease. In: *Poster Presentation at the Society of Gynecologic Oncology Annual Meeting March 17, 2019*; 2019.
17. Kang Z, Xu F, Zhang QA, et al. Oncogenic mutations in extramammary Paget's disease and their clinical relevance. *Int J Cancer.* 2013;132 (4):824–831. https://doi.org/10.1002/ijc.27738. Epub 2012 Aug 7. PMID: 22821211.
18. Fanning J, et al. Paget's disease of the vulva: prevalence of associated vulvar adenocarcinoma, invasive Paget's disease, and recurrence after surgical excision. *Am J Obstet Gynecol.* 1999;95(3):755–758.
19. Umemura H, et al. Serum carcinoembryonic antigen level as a marker for advanced stage and chemotherapeutic response in extramammary Paget's disease. *Acta Derm Venereol.* 2018;98(7):706–707.
20. Tung K, Nguyen BA. Inguinal and scrotal extramammary Paget's disease: [18]FDG PET/CT imaging. *Radiol Bras.* 2018;51(3):204–205.
21. Li ZG, et al. Extensive invasive extramammary Paget disease evaluated by F-18 FDG PET/CT. *Medicine (Baltimore).* 2015;94(3), e371.
22. Ohara K, et al. A proposal or a TNM staging system for extramammary Paget disease: retrospective analysis of 301 patients with invasive primary tumors. *J Dermatol Sci.* 2016;83(3):234–239.
23. Yoshino K, et al. Lymph node metastasis and sentinel node biopsy in the extramammary Paget's disease. *Jpn J Dermatol.* 2006;116:1473–1477.
24. Tebes S, Cardosi R, Hoffman M. Paget's disease of the vulva. *Am J Obstet Gynecol.* 2002;187(2):281–283.
25. Shaco-Levy R, Bean SM, Vollmer RT, et al. Paget disease of the vulva: a histologic study of 56 cases correlating pathologic features and disease course. *Int J Gynecol Pathol.* 2010;29(1):69–78.
26. Pierie JP, Choudry U, Muzikansky A, Finkelstein DM, Ott MJ. Prognosis and management of extramammary Paget's disease and the association with secondary malignancies. *J Am Coll Surg.* 2003;196(1):45–50.

27. Long B, et al. A matter of margins: surgical and pathologic risk factors for recurrence in extramammary Paget's disease. *Gynecol Oncol.* 2017;147 (2):358–363.

28. Chan J, et al. Extramammary Paget's disease: 20 years of experience in the Chinese population. *Int J Surg Oncol.* 2012;2012, 416418.

29. Zhu Y, et al. Frozen section-guided wide local excision in the treatment of penoscrotal extramammary Paget's disease. *BJU Int.* 2007;100 (6):1282–1287.

30. Hendi A, Brodland DG, Zitelli JA. Extramammary Paget's disease: surgical treatment with Mohs micrographic surgery. *J Am Acad Dermatol.* 2004; 51(5):767–773.

31. Bae JM, Choi YY, Kim H, et al. Mohs micrographic surgery for extramammary Paget disease: a pooled analysis of individual patient data. *J Am Acad Dermatol.* 2013;68:632–637.

32. Fujisawa Y, et al. The role of sentinel lymph node biopsy in the management of invasive extramammary Paget's disease: multi-center, retrospective study of 151 patients. *J Dermatol Sci.* 2015;79(1):38–42.

33. Nakamura Y, et al. Usefulness of sentinel lymph node biopsy for extramammary Paget disease. *Br J Dermatol.* 2012;167:954–956.

34. Cai Y, et al. Primary extramammary Paget disease of the vulva: the clinicopathological features and treatment outcomes in a series of 43 patients. *Gynecol Oncol.* 2013;129:412–416.

35. Voigt H, et al. Cytoreductive combination chemotherapy for regionally advanced unresectable extramammary Paget carcinoma. *Cancer.* 1992; 70(3):704–708.

36. Hsieh GL, et al. Case of metastatic extramammary Paget disease of the vulva treated successfully with trastuzumab emtansine. *JCO Precis Oncol.* 2018;2.

37. Stasenko M, et al. Genomic alterations as potential therapeutic targets in extramammary Paget disease of the vulva. *JCO Precis Oncol.* 2020;15(4). PO.20.00073.

38. Onaiwu C, et al. Paget's disease of the vulva: a review of 89 cases. *Gynecol Oncol Rep.* 2017;19:46–49.

39. Van der Linden M, et al. P191 Paget trial: topical 5% imiquimod for vulvar Paget disease: first results of clinical efficacy. *Int J Gynecol Cancer.* 2019;29(suppl. 4):A170–A171. Presented at ESGO Annual Meeting 2019.

40. Cowan R, et al. A pilot study of topical imiquimod therapy for the treatment of recurrent extramammary Paget's disease. *Gynecol Oncol.* 2016; 142(1):139–143.

41. Watring WG, et al. Treatment of recurrent Paget's disease of the vulva with topical bleomycin. *Cancer.* 1978;41(1):10–11.

42. Al-Naggar MR, et al. Intralesional bleomycin injection vs. microneedling-assisted topical bleomycin spraying in treatment of plantar warts. *J Cosmet Dermatol.* 2019;18:124–128.

43. Kwok CS, et al. Topical treatments for cutaneous warts. *Cochrane Database Syst Rev.* 2006.

44. Molina GE, et al. Topical combination of fluorouracil and calcipotriene as a palliative therapy for refractory extramammary Paget disease. *JAMA Dermatol.* 2019;155(5):599–603.

45. Song Y, et al. The Msi1-mTOR pathway drives the pathogenesis of mammary and extramammary Paget disease. *Cell Res.* 2020;1–19.

46. Shieh S, et al. Photodynamic therapy for the treatment of extramammary Paget disease. *Br J Dermatol.* 2002;146(60):1000–1005.

47. Borgia F, et al. Early and late onset side effects of photodynamic therapy. *Biomedicines.* 2018;6(12):1–16.

48. Ewing TL. Paget's disease of the vulvar treated by combined surgery and laser. *Gynecol Oncol.* 1991;43:137–140.

49. Fuikui T, et al. Photodynamic therapy following carbon dioxide laser enhances efficacy in the treatment of extramammary Paget's disease. *Acta Derm Venereol.* 2009;89:150–154.

50. Karam A, et al. HER-2/neu targeting for recurrent vulvar Paget's disease: a case report and literature review. *Gynecol Oncol.* 2008;111:568–571.

51. Ichiyama T, et al. Successful and long-term response to trastuzumab plus paclitaxel combination therapy in human epidermal growth factor receptor 2-positive extramammary Paget's disease: a case report and review of the literature. *Mol Clin Oncol.* 2017;7(5):763–766.

52. Oashi K, et al. Combination chemotherapy for metastatic extramammary Paget disease. *Br J Dermatol.* 2014;170(6):1354–1357.

53. Cai H, et al. Docetaxel combined with cisplatin for metastatic extramammary Paget disease. *Clin Genitourin Cancer.* 2018;16(4):e899–e901.

54. Yoshino K, et al. Usefulness of docetaxel as first-line chemotherapy for metastatic extramammary Paget's disease. *J Dermatol.* 2016;43:633–637.

55. Zhu Y, et al. Clinicopathological characteristics, management, and outcome of metastatic penoscrotal extramammary Paget's disease. *Br J Dermatol.* 2009;161:577–582.

56. Hata M, et al. Role of radiotherapy as curative treatment of extramammary Paget's disease. *Int J Radiat Oncol Biol Phys.* 2011;80(1):47–54.

57. Son SH, et al. The role of radiation therapy for the extramammary Paget's disease of the vulva: experience of 3 cases. *Cancer Res Treat.* 2005; 37(6):365–369.

Chapter 20

Other rare vulvovaginal cancers: Verrucous carcinoma, aggressive angiomyxoma, vulvar yolk sac tumor

Vance Broach and Lora Hedrick Ellenson

Clinical case

A 38-year-old woman presents to her general gynecologist with a complaint of a vaginal "cyst" at the introitus. She notes some fullness at the opening to the vagina and feels that this interferes with penetrative intercourse. She denies pain or drainage. She is G1P1 with a history of one prior uncomplicated vaginal delivery. She has an otherwise unremarkable medical and surgical history. On exam, the gynecologist notes a 2 cm firm nodule in the midline at the level of the introitus. The mass is minimally fluctuant and mobile and is located just deep to the dermis. The gynecologist counsels the patient, and they agree to perform an excision of the mass, presuming benign etiology. The mass is excised, and the pathology reveals a deep, aggressive angiomyxoma. What are the next steps in management of this patient? How would her treatment differ from treatment of other, more common vulvar cancers? What factors should a clinician keep in mind in order to identify uncommon vulvar cancers at the time of presentation?

Epidemiology

Vulvar cancer is a rare gynecologic malignancy, accounting for approximately 6000 new cases and 1350 deaths annually.[1] This represents approximately 0.3% lifetime risk of vulvar cancer among American women. The rate of vulvar cancer diagnosis has increased steadily over the past 30 years, with incidence of 2.1/100,000 in 1992 to 2.5/100,000 in 2018; however, the death rate has remained stable at approximately 0.5/100,000 women. The median age of vulvar cancer diagnosis is 68 years.[2]

The majority of vulvar cancers, approximately 75%, are squamous cell carcinomas (SCCs). However, numerous other histologic tumor types have been described. Many of these have clinical courses which differ from that of SCC. In this chapter, we will discuss several rare vulvar malignancies—HPV-independent vulvar cancers, verrucous carcinoma, aggressive angiomyxoma, and yolk sac tumors (YSTs)—and describe how their treatment may differ from the treatment of other, more common vulvar cancers (Table 20.1).

HPV-independent vulvar cancers and verrucous carcinoma

Vulvar squamous cell carcinoma (SCC) is the most common vulvar cancer. Recent investigation into the pathogenesis of this disease has identified two distinct entities; carcinomas which arise in the presence of HPV; and carcinomas which arise in the absence of HPV. Sixteen to 40% of vulvar SCC is caused by HPV infection, whereas approximately 60% are HPV-independent.[3–5] HPV-associated vulvar carcinomas are typically diagnosed in women who are younger (in their 30s–50s), have a precursor high-grade squamous intraepithelial lesion, and express p16 histopathologically. By contrast, HPV-independent tumors are diagnosed in older women, (age 40–60 years), are associated with chronic inflammatory conditions of the vulva such as lichen sclerosis, have a precursor lesion of differentiated vulvar intraepithelial neoplasia (VIN) (discussed in the pathology section of this chapter), and are associated with p53 alterations pathologically.[6–8] Importantly, HPV-independent SCCs have a worse prognosis compared with HPV-associated tumors. McAlpine and colleagues published their experience evaluating the survival outcomes of nearly 200 women with vulvar SCC[9] and found that HPV-independent tumors were associated with worse overall, progression-free and disease-specific survival compared with similarly matched HPV-associated disease.

TABLE 20.1 Comparison of HPV- and non-HPV–associated vulvar cancers.

Characteristic	HPV associated vulvar squamous cell carcinoma	Non-HPV–associated vulvar squamous cell carcinoma
Age of diagnosis	30–50 years	40–60 years
Precursor Lesion	High grade squamous intraepithelial lesion	Differentiated vulvar intraepithelial neoplasia (dVIN)
Immunohistochemical characteristics	P16 abnormalities	P53 abnormalities
Prognosis	Favorable compared to non-HPV associated vulvar carcinomas	Poor compared to HPV-associated carcinomas

Verrucous carcinomas are another rare type of SCC. While HPV infection has been demonstrated in patients with vulvar verrucous carcinoma,[10,11] the pathogenesis of this entity is not clearly established. Verrucous carcinomas tend to grow into large tumors, but rarely metastasize to the lymph nodes. For this reason, they may be associated with improved survival compared with other SCCs. Nodal or distant recurrence rates are very rare, and local recurrence rates of 12%–17% have been reported.[11]

Aggressive angiomyxoma

Aggressive angiomyxomas are very rare vulvar tumors that tend to occur in young women (in their mid-30s–40s). No known precursor lesions or risk factors have been identified. Patients have a high rate of local recurrence, ranging from 36% to 72%, though the rate of lymph node and distant metastasis is very low.[12–14]

Vulvar yolk sac tumors

YSTs represent a very rare subset of extraovarian germ cell tumors. The incidence of all extragonadal germ cell tumors among males and females is 1.8–3.4 per 1 million.[15] The incidence of vulvar YSTs is rarer still, with fewer than 20 cases reported in the published literature. The median age of diagnosis is 19 years, though cases have been reported in multiple age groups, from infancy to the 50s. Interestingly, though perhaps merely coincidentally, a preponderance of reports describe tumors arising in the right labia majora.[16]

Pathology

The most recent classification of preinvasive and invasive squamous neoplastic lesions of the vulva is now broadly classified as HPV-dependent and HPV-independent. Only the less common HPV-independent category will be discussed below.

Vulvar intraepithelial neoplasia, HPV-independent

This category of vulvar intraepithelial neoplasia (VIN) has been evolving rapidly over the last few years. It was initially thought that differentiated vulvar intraepithelial neoplasia (dVIN) was the sole precursor to HPV-independent SCC but recently two other lesions, now thought to be precursors, have been described. These lesions have been termed differentiated exophytic vulvar intraepithelial lesion (DE-VIL) and vulvar acanthosis with altered differentiation (VAAD). The discussion below will focus predominately on dVIN.

Gross appearance

HPV-independent VIN, often arises in the setting of lichen sclerosus or lichen simplex chronicus and can be uni- or multi-focal. The lesions can be ulcerated and erythematous or can present as a slightly raised, white lesion.

Microscopic features

The lesion is characterized by pleomorphic keratinocytes with ample eosinophilic cytoplasm and large vesicular nuclei with prominent nucleoli confined to the basal and parabasal layers with normally differentiated cells in the superficial layers of the epithelium. For this reason, in the past it was referred to as dVIN which will be used interchangeably with HPV-independent VIN. The epithelium can have range of findings from atrophic or acanthotic; however, it often demonstrates elongation and fusion of the rete pegs (Fig. 20.1A). The squamous epithelium has spongiosis, and the atypical cells often show pronounced intercellular bridges and abrupt keratinization. Dyskeratosis and keratin pearls at the base of the rete ridges i.e. paradoxical maturation is characteristic. The atypical basal and parabasal cells (Fig. 20.1B) frequently demonstrate atypical mitotic figures and may be hyperchromatic.

Differential diagnosis

The identification of this form of VIN is difficult as the findings can be subtle and overlap with other more common entities with which it is often associated, including lichen simplex chronicus and hypertrophic lichen sclerosus. In addition, it can be confused with reactive changes that have associated pseudo-epitheliomatous hyperplasia. In small biopsies distinguishing reactive squamous atypia from dVIN is particularly challenging and in some cases multiple sequential biopsies are necessary prior to making the correct diagnosis. dVIN can also be mistaken for HPV-dependent high grade VIN, when they have a more basaloid appearance, and ancillary studies (see below) can aid in this distinction. Finally, as mentioned above, two other types of HPV-independent VIN have been recently identified, namely DE-VIL and VAAD, which share some features with dVIN; however, they both lack significant basal atypia and *TP53* mutations and are thought to be precursors to the more uncommon form of HPV-independent squamous carcinoma called verrucous carcinoma.

Squamous cell carcinoma, HPV-independent

This category consists of two histologically distinct forms of carcinoma. The most common is referred to as HPV-independent vulvar squamous cell carcinoma (VSCC), while the other less common form is called verrucous carcinoma (VC). The discussion will focus primarily on VSCC. However, the section on molecular findings will cover VC as well.

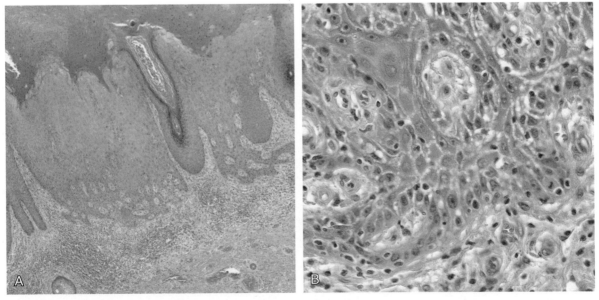

FIG. 20.1   dVIN with acanthosis and elongation and fusion of the rete ridges (A) demonstrating basal and parabasal cytologic atypia (B).

Gross appearance

Invasive squamous carcinoma can present as focal ulcers or hyperkeratotic, exophytic masses. They can be unifocal or multifocal. Unlike HPV dependent SCC, patients can present with rapidly enlarging tumors.

Microscopic features

These tumors are typically well-differentiated and demonstrate prominent keratinization with keratin pearl formation. The invasive front of the tumor is composed of wide-spread infiltrating tongues of neoplastic squamous epithelium (Fig. 20.2A). VSCC can also show a variety of other patterns including a warty or basaloid appearance and can lack keratinization. A note must be made about the challenges with measuring depth of invasion. In exophytic tumors and those that are not well oriented accurately measuring depth of invasion is challenging. As the required depth for distinguishing stage IA from IB is 1 mm, in microscopic lesions, there can be interobserver variability in measuring depth of invasion, i.e., <1 mm versus >1 mm. In a subset of cases, adjacent lichen sclerosus and dVIN may be present. In contrast, verrucous carcinoma is characterized by broad, pushing invasive borders (Fig. 20.2B) and basal atypia is minimal. The diagnosis of verrucous carcinoma and distinction from precursor lesions such as DE-VIL and VAAD is often not possible and conservative excision of the mass is recommended for definite diagnosis.

Differential diagnosis and immunohistochemistry

Because of the wide variety of histologic patterns and their overlap with HPV-dependent SCC, a reliable distinction between the two types of tumors is often not possible based solely on morphology. However, the presence of a precursor lesion or the background changes in the vulva can aid in the distinction, as HPV-independent tumors may have associated dVIN and arise in the background of lichen sclerosus or lichen planus. Immunohistochemical stains can be helpful in the identification of HPV-independent VIN and squamous carcinoma. Since *TP53* mutations are frequently present in dVIN and VSCC, immunohistochemistry for p53 can be used to help in the identification and classification of the lesions. The p53 staining can take on two appearances in dVIN. It can show diffuse, strong staining in the basal and parabasal zone with nearly all of the cells in the regions showing intense staining. A null p53 staining pattern can also be seen where there is a complete lack of staining in the cells of the basal and parabasal zone. In normal or reactive squamous epithelium p53 shows heterogeneous staining with negative and positive cells with varying intensity of staining.[17] The same holds true for SCC which can show either strong, diffuse nuclear staining or a null staining pattern of p53, both indicative for the presence of a mutation. This is helpful in distinguishing the lesions from HPV-dependent SCC. However, if the lesion has definitive features of dVIN or SCC without abnormal p53 then the diagnosis can still be made, as not all dVIN or HPV-independent

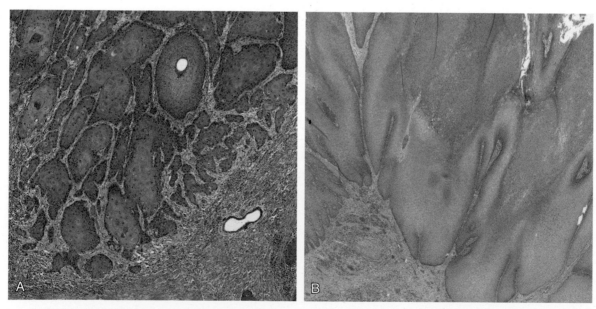

FIG. 20.2 HPV-independent squamous carcinoma showing infiltrative pattern of invasion (A) and verrucous carcinoma with broad pushing invasive border (B).

SCCs harbor *TP53* mutations. For the acanthotic, hyperkeratotic lesions that have overlap with HPV-dependent lesions, p16 immunohistochemistry can be helpful as the latter show diffuse, block-like staining which is not a typical feature of dVIN or HPV-independent SCCs. If HPV RNA in situ hybridization is available, it can also be useful in the distinction of the two types of carcinomas and precursor lesions.

Molecular findings

This is an active area of investigation, but recent studies have provided considerable insight into this once poorly understood aspect of HPV-independent squamous cell neoplasia of the vulva. As mentioned above, there are three types of HPV-independent VIN (dVIN, DE-VIL, and VAAD) and two types of vulvar squamous carcinomas (VSCC and VC). Molecular profiling of these lesions has shown that approximately 73% and 85% of VSCC and dVIN have mutations in *TP53*, respectively. In contrast, DE-VIL, VAAD, and VC lack mutations in *TP53* but have mutations in *PIK3CA* and *HRAS*. However, it is interesting to note that dVIN and VSCC also have mutations in *PIK3CA* and *HRAS*, but at much lower frequency than the other lesions. The numbers of cases with thorough molecular analyses remains small; however, these analyses along with morphologic and immunohistochemical data have suggested that dVIN is the precursor of VSCC while DE-VIL and VAAD may be precursors of VC. It has also been postulated that VC can progress to VSCC and/or that DE-VIL and VAAD may also give rise to VSCC. Mutations in other genes (*PTEN*, *MET*, and *BRAF*) have also been identified in the precursor lesions as well as in VSCC and VC. There are limited data to suggest that tumors with both *TP53* and *PIK3CA* mutations demonstrate the most aggressive behavior.[18] Future studies will continue to shed light on the pathogenesis of these lesions and their relationships to one another.

Yolk sac tumor

Gross appearance

The tumors have a heterogeneous appearance with a soft, grey to white color usually associated with hemorrhage and necrosis.

Microscopic features

Like YSTs arising elsewhere, those arising in the vulva demonstrate a number of morphologic patterns and are composed of large cells with irregular, hyperchromatic nuclei and prominent nucleoli. The cytoplasm shows clearing and may contain PAS positive hyaline globules that can also be present in the extracellular space. The reticular pattern is the most common and shows cystic structures lined by attenuated cells in the background of sheets of tumor cells giving it an appearance similar to the fetal yolk sac (Fig. 20.3). Papillary, glandular and solid patterns can also be present. Schiller-Duvall bodies can be seen which have features similar to fetal glomeruli. Rarely, other primitive types of germ cell tumors can be identified admixed with YST.

Immunohistochemistry

The tumor cells are positive for SALL4, glypican-3, and AFP. In some cases, CDX2 and villin may be positive.

Differential diagnosis

The papillary pattern of YST can mimic clear cell carcinoma (CCC). The above-mentioned germ cell markers are typically negative in CCCs, while the latter are positive for CK7, PAX-8, HNF-1B, and napsin-A, facilitating the correct diagnosis. When the glandular pattern predominates, YST can mimic adenocarcinomas. In this context, the positive staining for CDX2 and villin may result in an erroneous diagnosis of colonic adenocarcinoma.

Deep (aggressive) angiomyxoma

Gross appearance

The tumors are usually large (greater than 10 cm), lobular and poorly circumscribed with a gelatinous, glistening cut surface with a pink or slightly reddish color. They may show hemorrhage and cystic change and adherent normal tissue (fat, muscle, etc.) indicative of its infiltrative behavior.

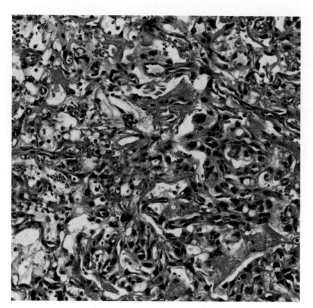

FIG. 20.3 Yolk sac tumor with a reticular pattern.

Microscopic features

Aggressive angiomyxoma has a relatively uniform appearance composed of a small, stellate spindle cells embedded in a myxedematous background, that is overall of low-to-moderate cellularity. Blood vessels of various caliber and wall thickness are irregularly distributed throughout the tumor. Some of the vessels can demonstrate thick walls with prominent hyalinization. The vessel lumens are usually widely patent. The tumor cells show minimal atypia and lack appreciable mitotic activity (Fig. 20.4A and B). The tumor cells may entrap normal fat, nerve and muscle cells as it infiltrates the surrounding normal soft tissue elements. Evaluation of the borders of the tumor and adjacent tissue is important to appreciate the infiltrative nature. Necrosis is usually absent.

Immunohistochemistry

Aggressive angiomyxomas are most commonly positive for desmin, SMA, ER, and PR, with focal CD34 staining. They are negative for S100. In addition, approximately 37%–90% of cases have been shown to have nuclear expression of HMGA2.

Differential diagnosis and immunohistochemistry

The most common tumors in the differential include superficial angiomyxoma and angiomyofibroblastoma. In addition, other soft tissue tumors with myxoid and edematous features (smooth muscle tumors, low grade myxofibrosarcoma, etc.) should be considered. Superficial angiomyxomas (SA), as the name suggests, are not deeply located like aggressive angiomyxoma, and are typically well-circumscribed. The vessels are curvilinear and thin walled with vascular congestion. SA are usually negative for desmin, hormone receptors, and HMGA2. Angiomyofibroblastomas are usually well-circumscribed. The tumor cells are short spindled with admixed thin-walled capillary-like vessels. The spindle cells tend to surround the blood vessels. Both angiomyofibroblastoma and aggressive angiomyxoma have similar desmin and hormone receptor expression, but the former are typically negative for HMGA2.

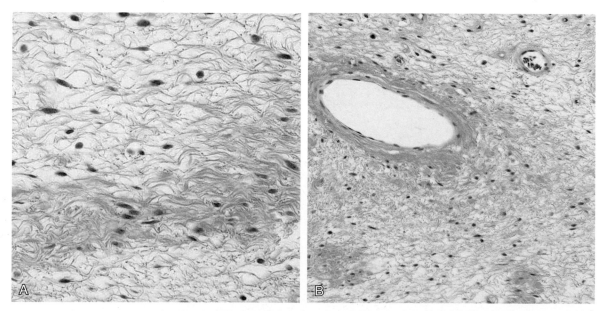

FIG. 20.4 Aggressive angiomyxoma with a homogenous appearance composed of small stellate cells embedded in a myxedematous background (A) and scattered blood vessels of various caliber and wall thickness (B).

Molecular findings

Approximately one-third of cases show rearrangements in the *HMGA2* gene which is involved in transcriptional regulation. *HMGA2* is located at 12q14.3 and the rearrangements involve a number of different chromosomes. However, a novel fusion partner *YAP1* at 11q22.1 has been identified.[19] The role these fusions play in the pathogenesis of the disease is not clear at this time; however, studies have shown the presence of aberrant *HMGA2* transcripts in aggressive angiomyxomas with *HMGA2* rearrangements.

Diagnosis and work-up

Like most vulvar cancers, rare vulvar tumors present as a raised lesion which is palpable on exam or to the patient. However, some clinical differences do exist between these tumors and more common vulvar malignancies. It is important to keep these differences in mind when evaluating patients with vulvar masses (Table 20.2).

Non-HPV-associated squamous cell carcinoma and verrucous carcinoma

The differential diagnosis of non-HPV-associated SCC includes benign etiologies such as Bartholin gland cyst or abscess, as well as other vulvar malignancies including HPV-associated vulvar SCC non-HPV-associated SCCs may be associated with surrounding lichenoid disease. Pruritis is another common presenting symptom.[20] Unfortunately, there is often a delay in diagnosis, with one study suggesting that 88% of women with vulvar cancer had symptoms for at least 6 months prior to initial evaluation. Moreover, these women often received inappropriate treatment at their initial presentation and required evaluation by multiple providers prior to diagnosis.[21]

Physical examination is a critical first step in evaluation, and biopsy of suspicious lesions should be performed. Biopsies should include underlying stroma in order to assess for invasion. Additionally, care should be taken to examine the inguinofemoral nodes bilaterally. While palpation of the lymph nodes is associated with a relatively poor rate of detection of lymph node metastasis, grossly enlarged lymph nodes are often identifiable on exam, and their identification can help guide therapy.[22]

In select patients, radiographic studies may be helpful in evaluating for distant metastases and local invasion of perineal structures such as the anus and lower urinary tract. The risk of metastatic disease at the time of presentation is relatively low, however, occurring in less than 5% of patients.[23] It is reasonable to obtain radiographic evaluation for patients with tumors larger than 4 cm, with depth of invasion >1 mm on biopsy, who have signs or symptoms suggesting metastatic disease, or who are not otherwise candidates for surgical management, or for whom nonsurgical management has been planned. The imaging modality should be selected on a case-by-case basis. Magnetic resonance imaging (MRI) is most helpful when evaluating for inguinofemoral lymph node involvement.[24] Positron emission tomography (PET) and computed tomography (CT) may also be helpful, particularly when evaluating for distant metastasis. We suggest a strategy of utilizing MRI in patients to evaluate the inguinal nodes and extent of tumor invasion. Based on these findings, a CT or PET may be

TABLE 20.2 Initial workup for rare vulvar cancers.

Physical exam	Complete physical exam with pelvic and recotvaginal examinations Exam under anesthesia with cystoscopy and proctoscopy as indicated
Laboratories	CBC LFTs Renal function studies HIV testing
Imaging	PET or CT scan to evaluate for metastatic disease MRI pelvis for surgical or radiation planning
Additional testing	Biopsy of primary lesion HPV testing and cervical cytology as indicated

performed if the risk of metastasis is high or if clinical findings such as enlarged nodes or symptoms warrant imaging outside the pelvis.

Verrucous carcinomas tend to present as large exophytic tumors which may be slow-growing. Verrucous carcinomas are associated with palpably enlarged lymph nodes at time of diagnosis, but these nodes are typically reactive and are very rarely involved by disease[11,25]

Aggressive angiomyxoma

Aggressive angiomyxoma is often misdiagnosed as a benign process. For this reason, initial surgical management is typically undertaken without oncologic goals in mind. Examination prior to resection often reveals a solitary mass, which may vary in size from 1 to 2 cm to larger (>10 cm). Very rarely do these cancers present with multifocal disease in the vulva or with distant metastases.[14] Aggressive angiomyxoma has a propensity to invade deeply into the surrounding tissue, with no definitive border. Physical examination alone is often insufficient to evaluate depth of invasion. Imaging is very helpful in this setting, and MRI can best characterize the full extent of the mass.[26–28] On MRI, a "swirled" internal pattern is characteristic of this tumor type.[29]

Yolk sac tumors

YSTs of the vulva are very uncommon and may vary in appearance. Given that most clinicians will never have seen these tumors, diagnosis on physical exam alone is challenging. Differential diagnosis includes mucinous carcinoma, Bartholin gland cancer and SCC. As noted above, these tumors tend to occur on the right labia and typically occur in women of a comparatively younger age. Alpha-fetoprotein (AFP) is a marker of YSTs of the female genital tract, and may be elevated in patients with vulvar YSTs.[16]

Staging

The staging of rare vulvar cancers follow the staging process for other, more common vulvar cancers. Staging involves a combination of clinical and surgical factors. Clinical factors include tumor size, local extension, gross lymph node involvement, and distant metastases detected on imaging. Surgical factors may include microscopic lymph node metastases and depth of invasion. The staging system are summarized in Table 20.3.

Treatment of primary disease

Non-HPV-associated squamous cell carcinoma

Early-stage disease

The treatment of non-HPV-associated SCC is similar to the treatment of HPV-related SCC (Table 20.4). Surgical resection is the mainstay in early-stage disease and includes radical resection of the primary lesion and lymph node evaluation with sentinel lymph node (SLN) biopsy or full inguinofemoral lymphadenectomy. Classically, the surgical goal is pathologic tumor-free margin of at least 0.8 cm, as a smaller margin has been associated with increased likelihood of local recurrence.[30] However, recent analyses of the AGO-Care-1 study failed to demonstrate that this tumor free margin improved outcomes.[31] Retrospective studies comparing complete radical vulvectomy with local excision demonstrate no oncologic differences between these approaches (Table 20.5).[32,33]

The approach to inguinofemoral lymph node evaluation in patients with vulvar cancer has evolved over the past 30 years. Lymphadenectomy has been associated with improved survival in women with early-stage vulvar cancer, but this procedure is fraught with both short-term and long-term morbidity including infection, wound breakdown and lymphedema.[34–37] Therefore, the virtue of lymph node sampling in various clinical settings has been examined. In carcinomas with <1 mm of invasion, the chance of nodal positivity is very low (<1%); lymph node sampling may be omitted in these patients.[38,39] In women with tumor depth of invasion >1 mm, but with lesions <4 cm and with adenopathy on exam or imaging, SLN biopsy has become standard management. The safety and efficacy of this approach in VSCC has been well established by two prospective studies, GOG-173, and GROINSS-V. These studies noted a false-negative predictive value of sentinel inguinofemoral lymph node dissection of 3.7% and a groin failure rate of approximately 2% in appropriately selected patients who underwent inguinofemoral sentinel node biopsy.[40–42] SLN detection may be performed with a combination of radiocolloid lymphoscintigraphy and blue dye; more recently, near infrared imaging and indocyanine green have been utilized.[43] Following the treatment paradigm outlined in the GROINSS-V2 study, patients found to have positive

TABLE 20.3 TNM and FIGO staging systems for vulvar cancer.

The definitions of the T categories correspond to the stages accepted by the International Federation of Gynecology and Obstetrics (FIGO). Both systems are included for comparison

		Primary tumor (T)
T category	FIGO stage	T criteria
TX		Primary tumor cannot be assessed
T0		No evidence of primary tumor
T1	I	Tumor confined to the vulva and/or perineum. Multifocal lesions should be designated as such. The largest lesion or the lesion with the greatest depth of invasion will be the target lesion identified to address the highest pT stage. Depth of invasion is defined as the measurement of the tumor from the epithelial-stromal junction of the adjacent most superficial dermal papilla to the deepest point of invasion.
T1a	IA	Lesions more than 2 cm, or any size with stromal invasion of more than 1 mm, confined to the vulva and/or perineum
T1b	IB	Lesions more than 2 cm, or any size with stromal invasion of more than 1 mm, confined to the vulva
T2	II	Tumor of any size with extension to adjacent perineal structures (lower/distal third of the urethra, lower/distal third of the vagina, anal involvement)
T3	IVA	Tumor of any size with extension to any of the following-upper/proximal two-thirds of the urethra, upper/proximal two-thirds of the vagina, bladder mucosa, or rectal mucosa-or fixed to the pelvic bone
T3a	IIIA	Tumor involving the serosa and/or adnexa (direct extension or metastasis)

		Regional lymph nodes (N)
N category	FIGO stage	N criteria
NX		Regional lymph nodes cannot be assessed
N0		No regional lymph node metastasis
N0(i+)		Isolated tumor cells in regional lymph node(s) no greater than 0.2 mm
N1	III	Regional lymph node metastasis with one or two lymph node metastases each less than 5 mm, or one lymph node metastasis greater than or equal to 5 mm
N1a*	IIIA	One or two lymph node metastases each less than 5 mm
N1b	IIIA	One lymph node metastasis greater than or equal to 5 mm
N2		Regional lymph node metastasis with three or more lymph node metastases each less than 5 mm, or two or more lymph node metastases greater than or equal to 5 mm, or lymph node(s) with extranodal extension
N2a*	IIIB	Three or more lymph node metastases each less than 5 mm
N2b	IIIB	Three or more lymph node metastases each less than 5 mm
N2c	IIIC	Lymph node(s) with extranodal extension
N3	IVA	Fixed or ulcerated regional lymph node metastasis

Note: The site, size, and laterally of lymph node metastases should be recorded.
*Includes micrometastasis, N1mi and N2mi.

		Distant metastasis (M)
M category	FIGO stage	M criteria
M0		No distant metastasis (no pathological M0; use clinical M to complete stage group)
M1	IVB	Distant metastasis (including pelvic lymph node metastasis)

Continued

TABLE 20.3 TNM and FIGO staging systems for vulvar cancer—cont'd

Prognostic stage groups			
When T is...	And N is...	And M is...	Then FIGO stage is...
T1	N0	M0	I
T1a	N0	M0	IA
T1b	N0	M0	IB
T2	N0	M0	II
T1-T2	N1-N2c	M0	III
T1-T2	N1	M0	IIIA
T1-T2	N2a, N2b	M0	IIIB
T1-T2	N2c	M0	IIIC
T1-T3	N3	M0-M1	IV
T1-T2	N3	M0	IVA
T3	Any N	M0	IVA
Any T	Any N	M1	IVB

Vulvar melanoma is not included in this staging system; it is staged with the melanoma staging system.
Classification of p16 status will be included if obtained but is not required.
TNM: Tumor, Node, Metastasis, AJCC: American Joint Committee on Cancer; UICC: Union for International Cancer Control.
Used with permission of the American College of Surgeons, Chicago, Illinois. The original source for this information is the AJCC Cancer Staging Manual, Eighth Edition (2017) published by Springer International Publishing. Corrected at 4th printing, 2018.

TABLE 20.4 Treatment of newly diagnosed rare vulvar cancers.

Non-HPV–dependent vulvar SCC	
Stage at presentation	Treatment
I/II	If depth of invasion <1 mm, resection of the primary lesion with no lymph node assessment In patients with depth of invasion >1 mm, resection of primary lesion to urogenital diaphragm with tumor free margin of 1 cm and bilateral lymph node sampling, either with SLN or full inguinofemoral lymph node dissection If sentinel LN positive, <2 mm, postoperative RT to the groins, if >2 mm, full side specific lymph node dissection followed by RT
III	Surgical resection with full lymph node dissection and RT For large tumors or tumors involving the urethra, clitoris or anus, exenterative procedures may be required for primary resection or primary RT or chemoradiation may be considered to shrink the primary tumor, followed by resection
IV	Chemotherapy

Aggressive angiomyxoma
Primary Resection of the tumor with negative margins if possible. Exenterative procedure may be required for complete resection Preoperative GnRH agonist or RT may be considered to reduce surgical extent Postoperative GnRH agonist or RT may be considered in the case of positive surgical margins if re-resection is not feasible

Yolk sac tumors
Primary surgical resection with evaluation of the inguinofemoral lymph nodes or SLN Postsurgical chemotherapy with BEP ± RT

TABLE 20.5 Treatment of recurrent disease rare vulvar cancers.

HPV independent SCC	
Surgical treatment	**Nonsurgical treatment**
Consider in patients with local or central recurrences	Consider in patients with distant metastasis or in whom surgery is not medically feasible
Surgical excision of the recurrent vulvar tumor, and/or involved lymph nodes Exenteration may be required in patients with central recurrences involving the lower urinary tract or rectum and anus	Radiation therapy with concurrent cisplatin may be utilized for pelvic and lymph node recurrences
Aggressive angiomyxoma	
Radical resection Exenteration may be required to completely resect recurrences	
Yolk sac tumors	
Resection of recurrent disease when surgically feasible Chemotherapy with BEC of VAC in the case of recurrent distant metastasis Radiation therapy may be considered to the site of recurrence if localized or if surgery is not feasible.	

SLNs and lymph node metastasis of >2 mm should undergo completion lymphadenectomy followed by radiation therapy. In women with lymph node metastasis <2 mm, radiation without completion lymphadenectomy was associated with an isolated groin recurrence rate of 1.6%. In these patients, radiation without full inguinofemoral lymph node dissection is reasonable.[44]

Advanced stage disease

Patients who have suspiciously enlarged lymph nodes at the time of diagnosis should undergo full inguinofemoral lymphadenectomy as initial surgical management. In the setting of large tumors or local extension to surrounding structures such as the bladder or rectum, exenterative procedures may be required.

In patients who are not amenable to radical or exenterative procedures, preoperative combined radiation and chemotherapy has been described. One retrospective series of 18 patients treated with preoperative 5 fluorouracil and cisplatin with radiation therapy to 44.6 Gy to the tumor and nodes demonstrated a complete clinical response in 13 of 18 patients, among whom 12 remained without evidence of disease at 2-year follow-up.[45]

Postsurgical treatment

The role of postoperative radiation for "close" margins has come into question. Traditionally, in cases where the microscopic surgical margin was either close to or involved by tumor (<8 mm) re-resection to obtain a negative margin or adjuvant radiation therapy was considered. However, recent retrospective studies have found this distance may not be as important. In one study, researchers were unable to show a connection between local recurrence and the amount of normal tissue between tumor margin and resection margin using cutoffs of 8, 5, or 3 mm (HR 1.03, 95% CI 0.99–1.06). The presence of dysplasia or lichen sclerosis at the margin, however, did portend a higher risk of recurrence (HR 2.14, 95% CI 1.11–4.12).[46] We recommend re-resection or radiation therapy for a positive margin but the role of additional therapy for patients with close but negative margins remains uncertain.

Aggressive angiomyxoma

Surgical resection is the bedrock of treatment for aggressive angiomyxoma. As these tumors are often large and locally invasive, surgical resection may be quite radical. Intraoperatively, it may be challenging to identify the borders of the tumor; for this reason, margins are commonly involved following resection. Moreover, if the tumor involves pelvic organs, lower urinary tract or bowel, intended subtotal resection may be undertaken.[28]

Unlike in SCC of the vulva, radiation therapy has not been demonstrated to be an effective treatment strategy for aggressive angiomyxoma.[47,48] As these tumors are often hormone receptor-positive, treatment with gonadotropin-releasing hormone agonists have been utilized in the neoadjuvant setting to reduce tumor size and lessen extent of surgery or for definitive treatment.[27,49] In one case report, a patient who refused surgical resection was treated with GnRH agonist for a course of 3 months and had complete radiographic resolution of her disease.[50] In another case, a patient had considerable radiographic evidence of persistent disease following resection. GnRH agonist was initiated and the patient had a complete radiographic response and was maintained on GnRH agonist.[51]

Lymph node metastasis has not been described in patients with aggressive angiomyxoma of the vulva. While the rarity of this tumor may limit the generalizability of recommendations for surgical management, routine sampling or resection of inguinofemoral lymph nodes is not recommended.[52,53]

Metastatic disease

Distant metastases are exceedingly rare in patients with aggressive angiomyxoma. Treatment of metastatic disease in this uncommon setting includes resection, if anatomically possible. Radiation therapy or hormonal blockage may also be considered. There is no established role for cytotoxic chemotherapy.

Vulvar yolk sac tumors

YSTs of the vulva are exceedingly rare and, therefore, treatment is individualized and determined on a case-by-case basis. Metastasis from the ovary or other more common sites of origin is possible. Evaluation for other primary site of disease should be done, and should include abdominopelvic imaging with CT or MRI.

Primary surgical management, when feasible, should adhere to the principles of resection applied to other vulvar cancers, with the goal of achieving negative margins. Lymph node metastasis appears to be an important prognostic factor for patients with vulvar YSTs, and lymph node evaluation should be performed in this setting.[54,55] SLN biopsy—based on anatomic considerations and lymphatic drainage—may be a reasonable approach.[56]

Postoperative management of vulvar YSTs has been based on the experiences reported with YSTs in other primary sites, specifically the ovary. Historically patients were treated with a combination of vincristine, actinomycin and cyclophosphamide,[57] but this regimen has been shown to be inferior to a combination of bleomycin, etoposide and cisplatin.[58] Adjuvant radiotherapy has also been described and may aid in local control or in cases of nodal positivity. For this reason, we recommend surgery followed by chemotherapy with bleomycin, etoposide and cisplatin,[55,59] with or without radiotherapy.

Surveillance for recurrence

Following primary treatment, surveillance consists of history, physical exam, and imaging. History and physical should be performed every 3–6 months for 2 years, then every 6–12 months for 2–5 years, and annually thereafter. Routine health maintenance, including cervical cytology, should be performed per guidelines. Imaging may be utilized based on symptoms or concerning physical exam findings. Imaging of the groin with ultrasound is an effective strategy for evaluating for inguinofemoral lymph node recurrence in high-risk patients, including those with previously positive nodes.

In patients with aggressive angiomyxoma, special care should be taken to evaluate the primary site of resection, given its propensity to recur locally. MRI may be helpful and should be used to evaluate anatomic abnormalities. In patients with YSTs, AFP should be assessed every 3–6 months.

Survival and patterns of failure

As the majority of vulvar SCCs, including verrucous carcinomas, are diagnosed at an early stage, overall survival is excellent. For early-stage and low-risk disease, 5-year survival approaches 100%.

In patients with aggressive angiomyxoma, recurrence rates are very common. The 5-year recurrence rate is 85%; time to recurrence ranges from 2 to 15 months. Recurrent tumors are, however, frequently amenable to retreatment with local excision.[28]

Survival varies in patients with vulvar YSTs, and prognosis is difficult due to the extreme rarity of the disease. Node negativity, and tumor <5 cm, are good prognostic factors. Long-term survival following treatment has been described, with survival reaching 90 months. Patients may recur shortly following diagnosis; however, and in these cases, the prognosis is poor.[60]

Case resolution

Following diagnosis on excisional biopsy of aggressive angiomyxoma, the patient is referred to a gynecologic oncologist. Exam demonstrates a healing vulvar wound, with no evidence of adenopathy. An MRI is obtained, and residual disease is noted extending into the perineal body and close to the anus. A reexcision of the mass is performed to the level of the anal sphincter; again, positive margins are noted. Given the risk of disrupting the anus and rectum with further resection, the patient is started on GnRH. She remains on this postoperative treatment regimen 18 months following surgery.

References

1. Siegel RL, et al. Cancer statistics, 2021. *CA Cancer J Clin.* 2021;71(1):7–33.
2. Saraiya M, et al. Incidence of in situ and invasive vulvar cancer in the US, 1998-2003. *Cancer.* 2008;113(Suppl. 10):2865–2872.
3. Trimble CL, et al. Heterogeneous etiology of squamous carcinoma of the vulva. *Obstet Gynecol.* 1996;87(1):59–64.
4. Singh N, Gilks CB. Vulval squamous cell carcinoma and its precursors. *Histopathology.* 2020;76(1):128–138.
5. van de Nieuwenhof HP, et al. The etiologic role of HPV in vulvar squamous cell carcinoma fine tuned. *Cancer Epidemiol Biomark Prev.* 2009;18(7):2061–2067.
6. McAlpine JN, et al. HPV-independent differentiated vulvar intraepithelial neoplasia (dVIN) is associated with an aggressive clinical course. *Int J Gynecol Pathol.* 2017;36(6):507–516.
7. Cheng AS, et al. p16 immunostaining allows for accurate subclassification of vulvar squamous cell carcinoma into HPV-associated and HPV-independent cases. *Int J Gynecol Pathol.* 2016;35(4):385–393.
8. Dong F, et al. Squamous cell carcinoma of the vulva: a subclassification of 97 cases by clinicopathologic, immunohistochemical, and molecular features (p16, p53, and EGFR). *Am J Surg Pathol.* 2015;39(8):1045–1053.
9. McAlpine JN, et al. Human papillomavirus (HPV)-independent vulvar squamous cell carcinoma has a worse prognosis than HPV-associated disease: a retrospective cohort study. *Histopathology.* 2017;71(2):238–246.
10. Iavazzo C, et al. HPV-related verrucous carcinoma of the vulva. A case report and literature review. *Eur J Gynaecol Oncol.* 2011;32(6):680–681.
11. Liu G, et al. Verrucous carcinoma of the vulva: a 20 year retrospective study and literature review. *J Low Genit Tract Dis.* 2016;20(1):114–118.
12. Sereda D, et al. Aggressive angiomyxoma of the vulva: a case report and review of the literature. *J Low Genit Tract Dis.* 2009;13(1):46–50.
13. Fetsch JF, et al. Aggressive angiomyxoma: a clinicopathologic study of 29 female patients. *Cancer.* 1996;78(1):79–90.
14. Siassi RM, Papadopoulos T, Matzel KE. Metastasizing aggressive angiomyxoma. *N Engl J Med.* 1999;341(23):1772.
15. Ronchi A, et al. Extragonadal germ cell tumors: not just a matter of location. A review about clinical, molecular and pathological features. *Cancer Med.* 2019;8(16):6832–6840.
16. Euscher ED. Unusual presentations of gynecologic tumors: extragonadal yolk sac tumor of the vulva. *Arch Pathol Lab Med.* 2017;141(2):293–297.
17. Tessier-Cloutier B, Kortekaas KE, Thompson E, et al. Major p53 immunohistochemical patterns in in situ and invasive squamous cell carcinomas of the vulva and correlation with TP53 mutation status. *Mod Pathol.* 2020;33(8):1595–1605. https://doi.org/10.1038/s41379-020-0524-1. Epub 2020 Mar 20. PMID: 32203095.
18. Tessier-Cloutier B, Pors J, Thompson E, et al. Molecular characterization of invasive and in situ squamous neoplasia of the vulva and implications for morphologic diagnosis and outcome. *Mod Pathol.* 2021;34(2):508–518. https://doi.org/10.1038/s41379-020-00651-3. Epub 2020 Aug 13. PMID: 32792599.
19. Lee MY, da Silva B, Ramirez DC, et al. Novel *HMGA2-YAP1* fusion gene in aggressive angiomyxoma. *BMJ Case Rep.* 2019;12(5):e227475. https://doi.org/10.1136/bcr-2018-227475. PMID: 31142482; PMCID: PMC6557357.
20. Rosen C, Malmstrom H. Invasive cancer of the vulva. *Gynecol Oncol.* 1997;65(2):213–217.
21. Jones RW, Joura EA. Analyzing prior clinical events at presentation in 102 women with vulvar carcinoma. Evidence of diagnostic delays. *J Reprod Med.* 1999;44(9):766–768.
22. Ansink A. Vulvar squamous cell carcinoma. *Semin Dermatol.* 1996;15(1):51–59.
23. Madsen BS, et al. Risk factors for invasive squamous cell carcinoma of the vulva and vagina—population-based case-control study in Denmark. *Int J Cancer.* 2008;122(12):2827–2834.
24. Kataoka MY, et al. The accuracy of magnetic resonance imaging in staging of vulvar cancer: a retrospective multi-centre study. *Gynecol Oncol.* 2010;117(1):82–87.
25. Haidopoulos D, et al. Coexistence of verrucous and squamous carcinoma of the vulva. *Aust N Z J Obstet Gynaecol.* 2005;45(1):60–63.
26. Chen L, et al. Sonographic findings in superficial angiomyxoma of the vulva in a perimenopausal female. *J Med Ultrasound.* 2019;27(4):202–204.
27. Sutton BJ, Laudadio J. Aggressive angiomyxoma. *Arch Pathol Lab Med.* 2012;136(2):217–221.
28. Brzezinska BN, et al. A persistent mass: a case of aggressive angiomyxoma of the vulva. *Gynecol Oncol Rep.* 2018;24:15–17.
29. Sun NX, Li W. Aggressive angiomyxoma of the vulva: case report and literature review. *J Int Med Res.* 2010;38(4):1547–1552.
30. Messing MJ, Gallup DG. Carcinoma of the vulva in young women. *Obstet Gynecol.* 1995;86(1):51–54.
31. Woelber L, et al. Role of tumour-free margin distance for loco-regional control in vulvar cancer-a subset analysis of the Arbeitsgemeinschaft Gynakologische Onkologie CaRE-1 multicenter study. *Eur J Cancer.* 2016;69:180–188.
32. Ansink A, van der Velden J. Surgical interventions for early squamous cell carcinoma of the vulva. *Cochrane Database Syst Rev.* 2000;2, CD002036.

33. DeSimone CP, et al. The treatment of lateral T1 and T2 squamous cell carcinomas of the vulva confined to the labium majus or minus. *Gynecol Oncol.* 2007;104(2):390–395.

34. Anderson JA, et al. Preoperative prognosis for cancer of the vulva. *Obstet Gynecol.* 1981;58(3):364–367.

35. Barton DP. The prevention and management of treatment related morbidity in vulval cancer. *Best Pract Res Clin Obstet Gynaecol.* 2003;17(4):683–701.

36. Gould N, et al. Predictors of complications after inguinal lymphadenectomy. *Gynecol Oncol.* 2001;82(2):329–332.

37. Burke TW, et al. Radical wide excision and selective inguinal node dissection for squamous cell carcinoma of the vulva. *Gynecol Oncol.* 1990;38(3):328–332.

38. Farias-Eisner R, et al. Conservative and individualized surgery for early squamous carcinoma of the vulva: the treatment of choice for stage I and II (T1-2N0-1M0) disease. *Gynecol Oncol.* 1994;53(1):55–58.

39. Magrina JF, et al. Squamous cell carcinoma of the vulva stage IA: long-term results. *Gynecol Oncol.* 2000;76(1):24–27.

40. Van der Zee AG, et al. Sentinel node dissection is safe in the treatment of early-stage vulvar cancer. *J Clin Oncol.* 2008;26(6):884–889.

41. Levenback CF, et al. Lymphatic mapping and sentinel lymph node biopsy in women with squamous cell carcinoma of the vulva: a gynecologic oncology group study. *J Clin Oncol.* 2012;30(31):3786–3791.

42. Moore RG, et al. Sentinel node identification and the ability to detect metastatic tumor to inguinal lymph nodes in squamous cell cancer of the vulva. *Gynecol Oncol.* 2003;89(3):475–479.

43. Broach V, et al. Evolution and outcomes of sentinel lymph node mapping in vulvar cancer. *Int J Gynecol Cancer.* 2020;30(3):383–386.

44. Maaike HM, Oonk et al. Radiotherapy Versus Inguinofemoral Lymphadenectomy as Treatment for Vulvar Cancer Patients With Micrometastases in the Sentinel Node: Results of GROINSS-V II. *J Clin Oncol.* 2021;39(32):3623–3632.

45. Gerszten K, et al. Preoperative chemoradiation for locally advanced carcinoma of the vulva. *Gynecol Oncol.* 2005;99(3):640–644.

46. Te Grootenhuis NC, et al. Margin status revisited in vulvar squamous cell carcinoma. *Gynecol Oncol.* 2019;154(2):266–275.

47. Magtibay PM, et al. Aggressive angiomyxoma of the female pelvis and perineum: a case series. *Int J Gynecol Cancer.* 2006;16(1):396–401.

48. Dierickx I, et al. Aggressive angiomyxoma of the vulva: a case report and review of literature. *Arch Gynecol Obstet.* 2008;277(6):483–487.

49. Orfanelli T, et al. A case report of aggressive angiomyxoma in pregnancy: do hormones play a role? *Case Rep Obstet Gynecol.* 2016;2016:6810368.

50. Fine BA, et al. Primary medical management of recurrent aggressive angiomyxoma of the vulva with a gonadotropin-releasing hormone agonist. *Gynecol Oncol.* 2001;81(1):120–122.

51. McCluggage WG, et al. Aggressive angiomyxoma of the vulva: dramatic response to gonadotropin-releasing hormone agonist therapy. *Gynecol Oncol.* 2006;100(3):623–625.

52. Bai HM, et al. Individualized managing strategies of aggressive angiomyxoma of female genital tract and pelvis. *Eur J Surg Oncol.* 2013;39(10):1101–1108.

53. Shinohara N, et al. Medical management of recurrent aggressive angiomyxoma with gonadotropin-releasing hormone agonist. *Int J Urol.* 2004;11(6):432–435.

54. Flanagan CW, et al. Primary endodermal sinus tumor of the vulva: a case report and review of the literature. *Gynecol Oncol.* 1997;66(3):515–518.

55. Ungerleider RS, et al. Endodermal sinus tumor: the Stanford experience and the first reported case arising in the vulva. *Cancer.* 1978;41(4):1627–1634.

56. Kim SI, et al. Robot-assisted inguinal sentinel lymph node biopsy in primary yolk sac tumor of the vulva. *Surg Oncol.* 2018;27(3):520.

57. Andersen WA, et al. Endodermal sinus tumor of the vagina. The role of primary chemotherapy. *Cancer.* 1985;56(5):1025–1027.

58. Williams SD, et al. Treatment of disseminated germ-cell tumors with cisplatin, bleomycin, and either vinblastine or etoposide. *N Engl J Med.* 1987;316(23):1435–1440.

59. Dudley AG, et al. Endodermal sinus tumor of the vulva in an infant. *Obstet Gynecol.* 1983;61(Suppl. 3):76S–79S.

60. Khunamornpong S, et al. Yolk sac tumor of the vulva: a case report with long-term disease-free survival. *Gynecol Oncol.* 2005;97(1):238–242.

Section E

Gestational trophoblastic disease

Chapter 21

Gestational trophoblastic disease

Kevin M. Elias, Lora Hedrick Ellenson, Neil S. Horowitz, and Ross S. Berkowitz

Clinical case

A 32-year-old G1P0 at 9 weeks and 3 days gestational age by last menstrual period presents with new onset vaginal bleeding. A transvaginal ultrasound shows no embryo, but notes a complex, echogenic intrauterine mass containing many small cystic spaces (Fig. 21.1). A serum human chorionic gonadotropin (hCG) level is 190,000 IU/L. On physical exam, her chest is clear to auscultation. Speculum exam shows a slightly dilated cervical os with prune-colored bleeding, but no lesions visible on the cervix or in the vagina. Bimanual examination reveals an 11-week size uterus with bilateral adnexal fullness. She undergoes an uneventful ultrasound-guided electric vacuum aspiration of the uterus. The pathology is consistent with complete hydatidiform mole (CHM). A week later, her hCG level is 200,000 IU/L, and the week after that her hCG has climbed to 350,000 IU/L. Chest X-ray shows no metastatic disease. A repeat ultrasound shows a 6 cm heterogeneous and cystic mass with myometrial invasion. The patient desires fertility sparing treatment for her disease. How do you treat this patient?

Epidemiology

Incidence and mortality

Gestational trophoblastic disease (GTD) refers to a category of lesions characterized by abnormal proliferation of placental trophoblasts. Benign forms of GTD include exaggerated placental site, atypical placental site nodule (PSN), and partial and CHM. Malignant forms of GTD are referred to as gestational trophoblastic neoplasia (GTN). GTN includes invasive mole, choriocarcinoma, and the very rare placental site trophoblastic tumor (PSTT) and epithelioid trophoblastic tumor (ETT) (see Section "Pathology" below). Unique among gynecologic cancers, GTN does not require a definitive histopathologic diagnosis. The diagnosis can also be made with laboratory tests alone when there is a persistent elevation of hCG after evacuation of a molar pregnancy.[1]

The precise incidence of GTD is uncertain because data regarding molar pregnancies and trophoblastic neoplasms are not available in most countries. The incidence is thought to be higher in Asia and South America than Western Europe or North America.[2] The most reliable data come from the United Kingdom, were for the past 50 years all GTD cases have been required to undergo registration at one of three national reference centers. From 2000 to 2009, the overall incidence of molar pregnancies in the UK was 1 case per 607 conceptions.[3]

GTN may occur after any gestational event. The histology of postmolar GTN may be invasive mole, choriocarcinoma, PSTT, or ETT. GTN after a non-molar pregnancy is usually choriocarcinoma but may also present as either PSTT or ETT. Approximately 50% of cases of GTN arise from molar pregnancy, 25% from miscarriages or tubal pregnancy, and 25% from term or preterm pregnancy. About 15%–20% of patients after CHM will develop GTN, and 5% will develop metastatic disease. GTN only occurs in 1%–4% of patients after partial hydatidiform mole (PHM) and is rarely metastatic.[4] The incidence of GTN after abortion is estimated at 1 in 15,000 pregnancies, while the incidence after a term pregnancy is estimated at 1 per 150,000 pregnancies. The overall incidence of GTN following all types of pregnancies is estimated at 1 in 40,000 pregnancies.[5]

The International Federation of Gynaecology and Obstetrics (FIGO) and the World Health Organization (WHO) have adopted a prognostic scoring system to risk-stratify patients with GTN (Table 21.1).[1]

Patients with a risk score <7 are considered "low risk" while patients with a risk score ≥7 are considered "high-risk." Patients with PSTT or ETT are automatically considered high-risk. Risk scores of ≥12 are frequently referred to as "ultra high-risk," although this term has not been universally adopted.[6] The "risk" refers to the likelihood of response to single-agent chemotherapy, but also conveys the risk of mortality. Patients with low-risk disease are first treated with single-agent

Diagnosis and Treatment of Rare Gynecologic Cancers. https://doi.org/10.1016/B978-0-323-82938-0.00021-5

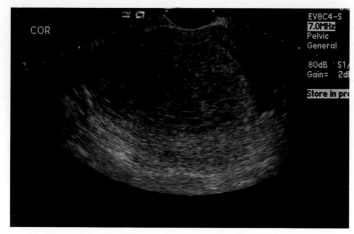

FIG. 21.1 Transvaginal ultrasound showing complex, echogenic uterine mass containing many small cystic spaces.

TABLE 21.1 FIGO/WHO scoring system for gestational trophoblastic neoplasia.

International Federation of Gynaecology and Obstetrics (FIGO)/World Health Organization (WHO) score	0	1	2	4
Age (years)	<40	≥40	-	-
Antecedent pregnancy	Mole	Abortion	Term	-
Interval months from index pregnancy	<4	4–6	7–13	>13
Pretreatment hCG (IU/L)	<1000	1000–10,000	10,000–100,000	>100,000
Largest tumor mass (cm)	<3	3–5	>5	-
Site of metastases	Lung	Spleen, Kidney	Gastro-intestinal	Liver, brain
Number of metastases	-	1–4	5–8	>8
Previous failed chemotherapy	-	-	Monotherapy	Combined therapy

hCG is human chorionic gonadotropin. Score is calculated by the addition of each variable score to gain a total score. Total scores are classified as low risk of resistance if 0–6 and high risk if more than 7.

therapy, usually either methotrexate or actinomycin D, while patients with high-risk disease receive multiagent etoposide-based regimens (more details below). While resistance to first-line chemotherapy in low-risk disease ranges from 20% to 50%, the salvage rate is extremely high, such that overall survival approaches 100%.[7–9] For high-risk disease, overall survival ranges from 90% to 95%, while in ultra high-risk disease overall survival is 60%–70%.[10–12] In addition to the FIGO/WHO risk score, patients with a histologic diagnosis of choriocarcinoma or metastatic disease to the brain or liver are at substantially elevated risk of disease-related death.[13] Underscoring the importance of expert consultation for these diseases, the risk of death is also increased by as much as 28-fold for patients with high-risk disease initiating therapy outside an experienced treatment center.[13–15]

Etiology and risk factors

Molar pregnancies occur due to abnormalities of fertilization causing an excess of paternal chromosomes.[16] CHM are generally diploid (rarely tetraploid), purely androgenetic conceptions, with most (~85%) arising from fertilization of an egg lacking maternal chromosomes by a single sperm that then duplicates its chromosomes (homozygous/monospermic

46,XX). A small subset arises via fertilization by 2 sperm (heterozygous/dispermic 46,XY or 46,XX). PHM are triploid with a single set of maternal and two sets of paternal chromosomes.[17] In both CHM and PHM, mitochondrial DNA remains maternal. The relative imbalance of parental chromosomes is thought to cause an imprinting defect. Genomic imprinting describes an epigenetic phenomenon wherein a gene is expressed only on the maternally or paternally inherited chromosome. Imprinting is a form of gene inactivation. Although a cell may have two copies of a gene, only the copy on the maternal or paternal chromosome is expressed. A classic example is Angelman Syndrome and Prader–Willi Syndrome. Both disorders stem from imprinting on the same region of chromosome 15, but loss of the maternal contribution results in Angelman syndrome while the loss of the paternal contribution leads to Prader–Willi Syndrome. The hypothesis of molar pregnancy as an imprinting defect has been supported by rare cases of biparental moles wherein genome-wide DNA methylation loss in the oocyte produces familial recurrent molar pregnancy.[18,19]

The cause of nonmolar GTN has not been defined but is also likely epigenetic. While changes such as copy number variation, loss of heterozygosity, and abnormal methylation are seen in gestational choriocarcinomas, molecular studies have been striking for the relative lack of common driver mutations.[20,21] Even less is known about the causes of PSTT or ETT. However, small studies have suggested that the tumors do share similar transcriptomic profiles.[22]

The leading risk factor for GTD and GTN is maternal age. The risk of complete molar pregnancy ranges from <1:1000 conceptions for women for ages 18–40, to 1:156 for women aged 45 and above and 1:8 for those aged 50 and above.[3] There is also about a 7-fold increased risk of CHM for adolescents.[23] Risks of PHM do not vary appreciably with maternal age. Interestingly, despite having higher rates of CHM than adults, adolescents have lower rates of postmolar GTN.[24] The risks of both postmolar and nonmolar GTN also increase with advancing maternal age.[25,26]

Patients with a prior history of GTD are at elevated risk of GTD in subsequent pregnancies. After a molar pregnancy, 1%–2% of patients will have GTD in a later gestation.[27,28] This risk rises to about 10% after two previous molar pregnancies.[29] Patients with more than two complete molar pregnancies should be referred for genetic testing for possible familial recurrent hydatidiform mole (FRHM).[30]

FRHM describes a family of exceptionally rare hereditary autosomal recessive disorders with incomplete penetrance characterized by the near-inability of affected women to have a noncomplete molar pregnancy. Affected families have multiple members with multiple complete molar pregnancies. The most commonly affected gene is *NLRP7*, an important immune response activator that responds to microbial acetylated lipopeptides.[19] Other genes implicated in FRHM include *KHDC3L*, *MEI1*, and *c11ORF80*.[18] Unlike sporadic complete moles, which are entirely androgenetic, familial complete moles display chromosomes from both maternal and paternal origins. Women with FRHM can only conceive using an egg donor. While homozygosity is required for the full manifestation of FRHM, carriers have an increased risk of recurrent miscarriage, partial moles, and stillbirth. Penetrance is considered incomplete because rarely normal pregnancies do occur among homozygous carriers.

Pathology

Gestational trophoblastic disease

As described above GTD is defined by abnormal proliferation of trophoblastic tissue and encompasses a spectrum of diseases that can be broadly divided into non-neoplastic and neoplastic diseases. The non-neoplastic diseases include PHM and CHM, in addition to exaggerated implantation site and PSN. The neoplastic diseases, also referred to as GTN, are comprised of choriocarcinoma, PSTT and ETT. Invasive hydatidiform moles are considered a form of GTN because they invade the myometrium and can be found outside of the uterus. However, they are not composed of a clonal proliferation and thus, in the true sense of the word, are not neoplastic.

Although the pathogenesis of the various forms of GTD is not completely understood, recent studies have increased our understanding of some of the entities and their relationship to normal placental trophoblast. There are three types of placental trophoblast: syncytiotrophoblast, cytotrophoblast, and intermediate trophoblast. Syncytiotrophoblast are large, multinucleated, differentiated cells that produce most of the placental hormones. They are located on the surface of the chorionic villi, overlying the cytotrophoblast, and are terminally differentiated cells. Unlike syncytiotrophoblast, cytotrophoblast are smaller, mononuclear cells that have stem cell–like properties and are mitotically active. They form a continuous layer lining the surfaces of the villi. Intermediate trophoblast are large, mononuclear cells that can be further subdivided into three subtypes called implantation site, chorionic type, and villous type intermediate trophoblast. As will be discussed below, these subtypes of intermediate trophoblast give rise to different types of GTD. In addition, immunohistochemical and molecular tests are currently being used as ancillary studies to improve diagnostic accuracy and, thus, patient management.

Given the complexity of the lesions not all of the entities can be discussed in detail in this chapter. Only those entities directly related to the case discussed in this chapter will be presented in detail.

Partial hydatidiform mole

Gross

The gross appearance shows an admixture of enlarged villi and normal appearing villi. The hydropic changes are not so prominent as in complete moles, hence may not be evident grossly.

Microscopic findings

PHM show two villous populations, one that is normal appearing and the other with changes including hydropic change, irregular villous contours, circumferential trophoblastic proliferation, and trophoblastic pseudo-inclusions. Evidence of fetal development is demonstrated by the presence of nucleated red blood cells in the villous capillaries. When the histologic features of PHM are not well-developed they can be easily missed. If there is histologic suspicion, then ancillary testing such as DNA flow cytometry may be performed.

Complete hydatidiform mole

Gross appearance

A well-developed CHM consists of markedly enlarged, edematous chorionic villi that have a translucent appearance. The abnormal villi may vary in size but virtually all of the villi are affected. However, given the identification of abnormal gestations early in the first trimester by ultrasonography, the villi may only demonstrate mild enlargement that may not be readily apparent on gross examination.

Microscopic features

CHM is an abnormal placenta with markedly hydropic chorionic villi with associated trophoblast proliferation due to a purely androgenetic conception. Most CHM (approximately 85%) are due to fertilization of an empty egg by one sperm (monospermic) with reduplication of the genome and are usually diploid (46, XX), however fertilization by 2 sperm (dispermic) can occur and also are usually diploid (46, XX or 46, XY). Due to the purely androgenetic nature of the conceptus there is a lack of embryonic development.

As mentioned above, the chorionic villi of a CHM are enlarged, bulbous and edematous (hydropic) with central cisterns (acellular, empty space) and circumferential proliferation of cytotrophoblast, syncytiotrophoblast, and intermediate villous trophoblast (Fig. 21.2A and B). Although vessels are present in the villous stroma they lack the presence of nucleated red blood cells given the absence of fetal development. These features are well developed in CHM evacuated in the second trimester; however, they can be subtle in the first trimester and are referred to as "early CHM." Consequently, early CHM present diagnostic difficulties especially in the absence of clinical history. The villi do show abnormalities with bulbous, irregularly shaped villi with mild circumferential trophoblast proliferation and stroma with increased cellularity with a myxoid appearance and small vessels with scattered karyorrhectic debris, closely resembling hydropic villi. However, the utilization of immunohistochemistry for p57 is very helpful in recognizing this entity (as discussed below).[31,32]

Invasive hydatidiform mole

Gross appearance

An invasive mole is detected grossly by the presence of enlarged, irregular chorionic villi invading the myometrium.

Microscopic features

An invasive mole has similar features to a CHM however, the molar villi invade the myometrium and/or uterine vessels. In addition, invasive moles can spread to extrauterine sites including lung, vagina, vulva, and ovary/broad ligament, which is why they are considered clinically malignant despite not actually being neoplastic. In the extrauterine sites, the molar villi are largely confined to vascular structures without invasion of surrounding tissue.

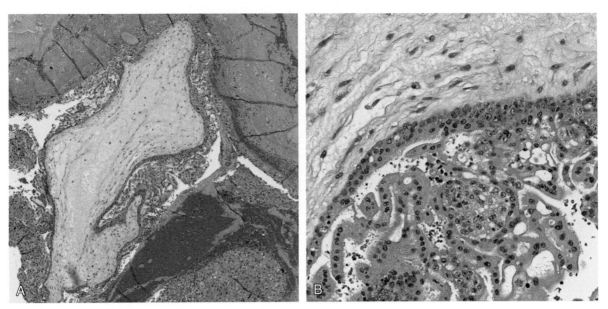

FIG. 21.2   Representative hydropic villous from a complete hydatidiform mole showing circumferential trophoblast proliferation (A) consisting of both cytotrophoblast and syncytiotrophoblast (B).

Choriocarcinoma

Gross appearance

The size of choriocarcinoma varies significantly from microscopic foci to very large tumors with extensive hemorrhage and necrosis. When they are grossly apparent they are usually dark red in color and have irregular surfaces. The metastatic lesions are often well-circumscribed with associated hemorrhage.

Microscopic features

This discussion will be limited to gestational choriocarcinoma which are composed of neoplastic syncytiotrophoblast, cytotrophoblast and intermediate villous trophoblast (Fig. 21.3) with morphological features of primitive trophoblast of the previllous stage of placental development. As such, it is considered the most primitive form of GTN. The tumor cells demonstrate marked cytologic atypia and a high mitotic index and usually show areas of necrosis, hemorrhage, and lymphovascular invasion. Historically, the presence of chorionic villi has precluded a diagnosis of choriocarcinoma; however, it has been recently acknowledged that they can occur in the setting of complete/invasive hydatidiform moles. Of note, this diagnosis should be made with caution since trophoblast proliferation is often exuberant in CHM mimicking choriocarcinoma. Furthermore, intraplacental choriocarcinoma is a well-recognized entity in term placentas and can be mistaken for a placental infarct.

Placental site trophoblastic tumor

Gross appearance

The majority of the tumors are well-circumscribed and can either be situated in the myometrium or project into the endometrial cavity. Upon sectioning the tumors are tan and soft usually with only focal areas of necrosis or hemorrhage.

Microscopic features

This tumor is thought to arise from transformed cytotrophoblast that differentiate to resemble implantation type intermediate trophoblast. It is composed largely of mononuclear cells with ample amphophilic cytoplasm that display considerable nuclear pleomorphism with occasional, scattered multinucleated cells (Fig. 21.4A and B). The tumor cells form sheets that infiltrate the myometrium by separating the smooth muscle bundles and invade vessels often replacing the vessel walls with a fibrinoid deposit similar to what is seen in the normal implantation site. The mitotic index is usually low (approximately

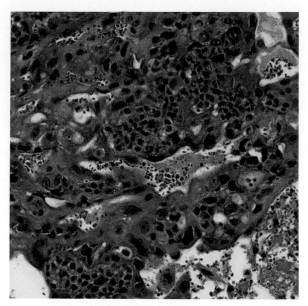

FIG. 21.3 Choriocarcinoma demonstrating its biphasic nature with both syncytiotrophoblast and cytotrophoblast.

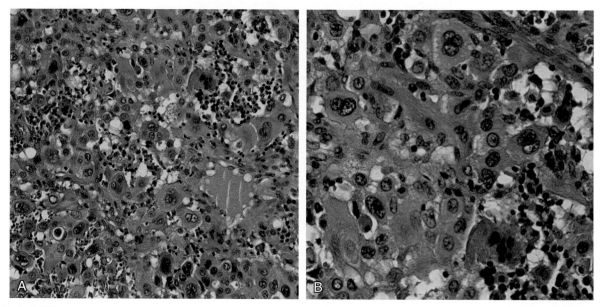

FIG. 21.4 PSTT demonstrating predominately mononuclear cells with scattered multinucleated cells (A and B).

2–4 mitoses/10 hpf). Although the tumor may cause little tissue destruction, some tumors can show considerable necrosis which is a feature that is associated with malignant behavior.

Epithelioid trophoblastic tumor

Gross appearance

Although they can be located in the uterine corpus a substantial number (approximately 50%) are found in the lower uterine segment or endocervix. They can also occur in extrauterine sites. The tumors range in size from 0.5 to 4.0 cm. The tumors form discrete nodules that can be solid or cystic with areas of hemorrhage and necrosis.

Microscopic features

The tumor nodules are composed of medium-sized, mononucleate trophoblastic cells that are fairly uniform and grow in solid masses, nests or cords and have finely granular eosinophilic to clear cytoplasm with round nuclei and moderate atypia. The tumor cells are associated with an eosinophilic, fibrillary, hyaline-like substance that can be admixed between the cells or in the center of tumor nests. The tumor commonly demonstrates extensive necrosis which can have a geographic appearance (Fig. 21.5A and B). The presence of calcification is a unique feature of ETT which is not seen in other GTDs. When the tumor involves the cervix the tumors cells can extend into the cervical epithelium and may be mistaken for a high-grade squamous intraepithelial lesion.

Differential diagnosis

The main differential for CHM is PHM and hydropic villi from nonmolar conceptuses. This is mainly an issue with early CHM as the features characteristic of CHM are not clearly developed.

A p57 immunostain can help in these distinctions as the cytotrophoblast and villous stromal cells of PHM and hydropic villi express p57, while it is lacking in CHM. p57 is a protein encoded by the gene *CDKN1C* that is paternally imprinted and maternally expressed such that expression is lacking in villi resulting from a completely androgenetic conceptus, the feature that defines CHM. This has become a very powerful tool for identifying early CHM and separating them from PHM and hypdropic villi from nonmolar conceptuses with which the microscopic features have considerable overlap. DNA flow cytometry may be used to distinguish early CHM from PHM as the former are diploid while the latter are triploid. In addition, CHM with detached islands of an admixture or cyto- and syncytiotrophoblast can be hard to distinguish from early choriocarcinomas arising in the setting of a CHM. The diagnosis of choriocarcinoma in this setting should be made with caution as this is an uncommon occurrence. In fact, some pathologists don't diagnose choriocarcinoma in the presence of villi.

Given that there can be overlapping morphologic features between choriocarcinomas and both PSTT and ETT, it is important to make these distinctions as the treatment regimens may vary. These distinctions are largely made on morphologic grounds however, immunohistochemical stains can be helpful (see below).

ETT and PSTT must be distinguished from PSN and exaggerated implantation site, respectively, that are currently considered their nonneoplastic, benign counterparts, as discussed below.

Immunohistochemistry and differential diagnosis

As mentioned earlier molecular studies have not only contributed to our understanding of GTD but have also resulted in ancillary studies that have improved diagnostic accuracy. The expression of specific proteins in the different types of trophoblast along with determination of proliferative activity has had a profound impact on the differential diagnosis of GTD.

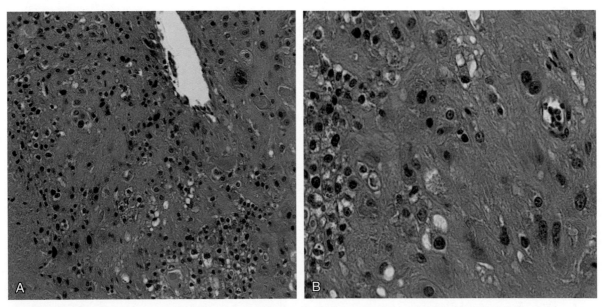

FIG. 21.5 ETT demonstrating uniform mononuclear cells with cytoplasmic clearing embedded in a hyaline-like material (A and B).

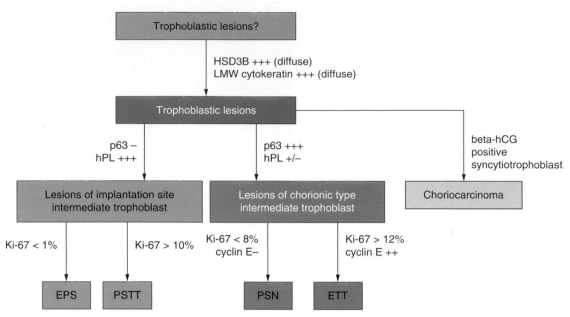

FIG. 21.6 Immunohistochemical algorithm for the diagnosis of GTD.

The first step is to determine that it is a trophoblastic lesion. Trophoblast are positive for low molecular weight keratins and a protein, HSD3B1, that is involved in progesterone biosynthesis in the placenta and this combination of markers in this setting is indicative of trophoblast differentiation.[33] Immunostains for distinguishing CHM from PHM and hydropic villi were discussed above. The main algorithm used for the differential for GTD (ETT, PSTT and choriocarcinoma) includes several antibodies (Fig. 21.6).[33a]

ETT can mimic PSTT, and PSN. ETT is strongly diffusely positive for p63 while only focally positive for hPL and Mel-CAM, whereas PSTT is p63 negative and shows diffuse strong staining with the other two markers. ETT can also mimic squamous cell carcinoma (SCC). Both tumors are positive for p63; however, cervical SCC does not express trophoblastic markers, and is positive for HR HPV, while the opposite is true of ETT.[34]

Like ETT, PSN expresses intermediate trophoblast markers hence, these markers cannot be used in this differential. However, Ki-67 immunostain is extremely useful in separating the two entities, as its expression is typically low (below 10%) in PSN but much higher in ETT (10%–25%). Additionally, cyclin E is positive in ETT while negative in PSN.[34]

Choriocarcinomas are positive for keratin markers such as AE1/AE3. The syncytiotrophoblastic cells are positive for hCG, HSD3B, and inhibin, while the cytotrophoblasts are positive for GATA3 and SALL4.[34] Of note, syncytiotrophoblasts may be seen in some somatic carcinomas; therefore, a diagnosis of choriocarcinoma should not be made if there is only focal hCG staining in the absence of typical histologic findings.

Molecular findings

Very little is known about the underlying molecular pathogenesis of GTD however, genotyping the lesions using short tandem repeats (STRs) is useful in a number of settings in determining the diagnosis of GTDs, when it is not clear from the histopathologic and immunohistochemical findings. Although a complete discussion of the technique is beyond the scope of this chapter a few instances in which it is applied will be presented. STRs are highly polymorphic DNA sequences that can be used to identify maternal and paternal derived alleles.[35] Thus, the analysis of STRs is very useful in distinguishing CHM, PHM and hydropic villi, as CHM are entirely androgenetic and lack maternally derived alleles, unlike PHM and hydropic villi both of which contain maternal alleles.[35] In addition, STRs can be used to distinguish gestational choriocarcinoma from somatic choriocarcinoma as the later will have a biallelic pattern instead of unique parental alleles as seen in gestational choriocarcinomas.[36]

Diagnosis and workup

Signs and symptoms

Classically, molar pregnancy was associated with vaginal bleeding, excessive uterine enlargement, theca lutein cysts, and early onset hyperemesis gravidarum and preeclampsia.[37,38] However, this presentation reflects the second trimester manifestations of GTD. In locations where hCG measurement and ultrasound are readily available, most molar pregnancies are now diagnosed in the first trimester (see Section Imaging studies below).[39,40] Importantly, earlier identification and evacuation of molar pregnancies has not changed the rate of postmolar GTN.[40,41] For example, at the New England Trophoblastic Disease Center, the average gestational age at diagnosis decreased from 16.5 weeks in the 1960s to 9 weeks in the 2000s.[41] However, the rate of postmolar GTN did not change. This strongly suggests that malignant transformation is an inherent biologic property of certain molar pregnancies and not a trait acquired during disease progression. In both classic descriptions and more modern experience, the most common symptom for molar GTD remains abnormal uterine bleeding. Excessive uterine size, hyperemesis, and anemia may still be seen, but are less common in the first trimester.[41] GTD should be in the differential for any woman presenting with bleeding in early pregnancy.

In cases of nonmolar GTN, abnormal uterine bleeding is also the most common symptom. Postterm choriocarcinoma is in the differential diagnosis for postpartum hemorrhage, particularly delayed postpartum hemorrhage, and should be the leading consideration in any postpartum patient presenting with vaginal bleeding and signs of metastatic disease. Women may alternatively present with amenorrhea. This is particularly true for PSTT or ETT.[42]

In both molar and nonmolar GTN, patients may also be symptomatic from metastatic disease. This may present as hemoptysis, respiratory insufficiency, hemoperitoneum, or vaginal lesions.

Physical exam findings

While second-trimester complete molar pregnancies may present with uterine size greater than dates and palpable adnexal masses on bimanual exam, most patients with first-trimester molar pregnancies will not have notable physical exam findings. However, evaluation of any patient with suspected GTD should include a thorough physical exam to exclude metastatic disease. A speculum examination is essential to exclude cervical or vaginal metastases, which can present as pigmented, fleshly lesions on the cervical portio, vaginal walls, or external genitalia (Fig. 21.7). The exam should also include a thorough auscultation of the lungs to evaluate for pulmonary edema or effusions and a basic neurologic exam to exclude focal neurologic deficits. Rarely, metastases may present as pigmented lesions on the skin, oral mucosa, retina, or nail beds. These may be confused for melanoma, underscoring the importance of obtaining an hCG during the diagnostic evaluation of any malignancy of unknown origin.

Differential diagnosis

For a woman presenting with abnormal uterine bleeding, an elevated hCG level, and an intrauterine mass, the differential diagnosis includes abortion, partial or complete molar pregnancy, choriocarcinoma, PSTT, or ETT as well as non-neoplastic

placental abnormalities and primary uterine neoplasms. Nonmolar hydropic abortion and placental mesenchymal dysplasia are frequently mistaken for molar pregnancies, since they can both present with villous edema and dilated cystic spaces on ultrasound. Ancillary testing (see below) is often required for a definitive diagnosis. Ectopic production of hCG, choriocarcinoma, and even trophoblastic differentiation can also be seen in other cancer types. Making the distinction between gestational and non-gestational choriocarcinoma (e.g., ovarian or uterine) is particularly important, as the latter is much less responsive to chemotherapy.

Tumor markers

hCG is the definitive tumor marker for GTD. hCG is a glycoprotein hormone composed of an alpha and beta subunit. Various hCG assays have varying sensitivity for hCG-related molecules including total hCG, hyperglycosylated hCG, nicked hCG, hCG missing the beta-subunit C-terminal peptide, free alpha-subunit, free beta-subunit, nicked free b-subunit and the urine beta-core fragment.[43] Different commercial assays may return markedly different results for hCG values depending on inherent ability to recognize hCG isoforms.[44] Providers should always order a "tumor-specific" hCG test, not a pregnancy hCG test, whenever possible.

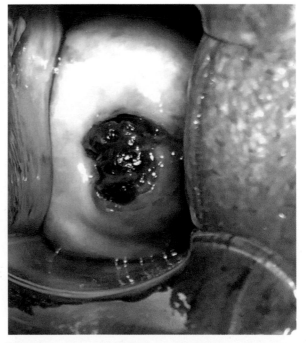

FIG. 21.7 Cervical metastasis of GTN. *(Photo courtesy of Dr. Antonio Braga).*

hCG testing is also prone to both false negative and false positive results. A false-negative hCG may occur when hCG values are extremely high, such as more than 2,000,000 IU/mL. Known as the "hook effect," this occurs in sandwich assays when an overabundance of hCG saturates the capture antibody and prevents formation of the capture and detect antibody complex.[45] A variant can occur if the capture and detection antibodies recognize different variants of hCG.[46] If the hook effect is suspected, one should ask the laboratory to perform a serial dilution assay as well as to consider a second hCG platform. False-positive or "phantom" hCG results may occur with low level hCG. Several well-known causes of false positive hCG results are pituitary hCG (commonly in perimenopausal patients), ectopic production of hCG from other tumor types, and heterophile antibodies (such as anti-mouse antibodies).[47] Placing a patient on high-dose oral contraceptives or GnRH agonists can suppress pituitary hCG. Comparing urine hCG values to serum hCG values can help distinguish heterophile antibodies as these do not cross the glomerulus. Additional laboratory testing at diagnosis should include a complete blood count due to the risk of anemia from vaginal bleeding, blood typing to assess for the need for Rhogam, and a complete metabolic profile. If the hCG is markedly elevated (>100,000 IU/L), thyroid function tests are also indicated due to the risk of cross-reactivity between TSH and hCG.

Imaging studies

Molar pregnancy

A transvaginal pelvic ultrasound is the only required imaging study for cases of presumed molar pregnancies. Ultrasonography has proven to be an accurate and sensitive technique for the diagnosis of complete mole.[48] While the gestational sac appears macroscopically normal at 4 weeks gestation, a polyploid mass emerges between 5 and 7 weeks gestation and by 8 weeks gestation, the characteristic vesicular or "snowstorm" pattern appears due to generalized swelling of the chorionic villi[49] (Fig. 21.8). Partial moles are frequently misdiagnosed as missed abortions, but two sonographic findings significantly associated with the diagnosis of PHM are cystic spaces in the placenta and a ratio of transverse to anteroposterior dimension of the gestational sac >1.5.[50,51] When both criteria are present, the positive predictive value for partial mole is 87%, while when both criteria were absent, the positive predictive value for missed abortion is 90%.

GTN

The transvaginal ultrasound may also suggest GTN. By ultrasound, invasive mole typically appears as one or more poorly defined, highly vascular masses in the uterus with anechoic areas. Invasion into the myometrium may be evident. Choriocarcinoma will appear as a heterogeneous hypervascular lesion with areas of necrosis and hemorrhage. In contrast, PSTT reveals a hyperechoic-intrauterine mass, usually with less hemorrhage than observed with choriocarcinoma, with cystic and solid components.[52] ETT typically shows a well-circumscribed echogenic lesion in the uterine fundus, frequently with no detectable blood flow on Doppler imaging. Whereas ETT appears as a solitary nodule with sharp margins on ultrasound, PSTT shows infiltrative growth interdigitating among myometrial fibers.[53]

In all cases of GTN, a chest radiograph is also ordered because the lungs are the most common site of metastases. For postmolar GTN, a plain film is recommended to evaluate for lung metastases rather than chest computed tomography (CT), since a chest radiograph, not CT, is the basis for International Federation of Gynecology and Obstetrics (FIGO) staging. Patients incorrectly scored by CT may be incorrectly classified as high-risk for chemotherapy resistance and unnecessarily exposed to multiagent chemotherapy. CT does not improve prediction of primary chemotherapy resistance.[54] In addition to metastases, chest X-ray may also reveal clinically relevant pleural effusions or pulmonary edema. For postmolar GTN, if the chest imaging is normal and there are no vaginal metastases on examination, additional imaging is not necessary since other sites of distant metastases are unlikely. For patients with metastases on chest imaging, vaginal metastases, choriocarcinoma, or non-molar GTN, additional imaging should include CT of the abdomen and pelvis and MRI of the brain.

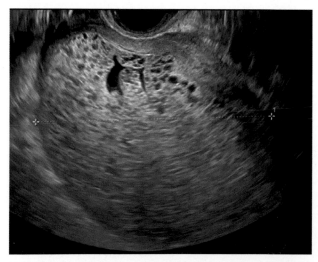

FIG. 21.8 Sonographic appearance of complete molar pregnancy with classic vesicular pattern.

Staging system

Anatomic staging for GTD follows the FIGO staging system (Table 21.2). Stage I disease is confined to the uterus or is based on hCG levels alone. Stage II disease reflects metastases to the vagina or other gynecologic organs. Stage III disease refers specifically to lung metastases, while stage IV disease refers to other visceral spread. The FIGO stage is designated by a Roman numeral and is followed by the modified WHO Prognostic Score (Table 21.1) designated by an Arabic number separated by a colon (e.g., I:4).

Prognostic factors

As noted above, the FIGO/WHO Prognostic scoring system helps triage patients into risk categories based on the likelihood of responding to single agent chemotherapy. In addition to the variables included in the risk score, a histology of chorio-carcinoma has been identified as an independent risk factor for resistance to chemotherapy and death.[13,55] However, in patients with a histologic diagnosis of choriocarcinoma, apparent stage I disease, and a normal hCG following uterine evac-uation, chemotherapy can be withheld in favor of close clinical surveillance.[56]

For PSTT and ETT, specifically, the time from the antecedent pregnancy to diagnosis is particularly important. Patients presenting more than 48 months from the last gestation are at markedly increase risk of treatment failure and death.[57] These patients may benefit from high-dose chemotherapy (HDC) and peripheral blood stem cell support.[58]

Treatment of primary disease

Low-risk disease

Patients with low-risk disease according to the WHO prognostic scoring system should be treated with single-agent che-motherapy in 14-day cycles. At most centers, this will be methotrexate or actinomycin D. Several common regimens have been described (Table 21.3). Pulsed actinomycin D is generally favored over the 5-day regimen due to more convenient dosing and lower cost.[59,60] A phase III Gynecologic Oncology Group (GOG) study of weekly methotrexate versus actinomycin D for patients with low-risk GTN randomized 216 patients to either weekly methotrexate versus pulse actinomycin D and the remission rate was 58% and 73%, respectively.[61] Since weekly IM dosing of methotrexate is no longer recommended, the GOG/NRG attempted a second randomized trial between pulse actinomycin D and 8-day or 5-day methotrexate regimens, but this trial closed prematurely due to poor accrual.[62] The reported response rates in 54 patients, however, was 88% for methotrexate and 79% for actinomycin D. A meta-analysis of low-risk regimens concluded that while actinomycin D might be slightly more effective than methotrexate, this comes at the expense of a slightly higher risk of serious adverse events such as neutropenia, thrombocytopenia, and mucositis.[63] Notably, the 8-day methotrexate regimen is sometimes difficult to employ because of the need for chemotherapy administration on the weekend. A large study of 937 patients comparing standard dosing with weekend administration versus a modified dosing with methotrexate administered on the 8th day rather than 7th to avoid treatment on the weekend showed equivalent response rates.[64]

If the hCG level plateaus with either single agent regimen, about 75% of patients will achieve remission if switched to the alternate single agent.[8] However, the likelihood of requiring multiagent therapy increases with higher prognostic risk scores, even within the "low-risk" category. Approximately 70% of patients with WHO Prognostic Scores of 5 and 6 will ultimately require the use of combination chemotherapy to achieve remission.[65] Even so, an attempt at therapy with the less toxic single-agent regimens is preferred, as virtually all patients can be cured with salvage multiagent therapy.[66]

A second uterine curettage is sometimes pursued prior to the initiation of chemotherapy in patients with apparent stage I disease and may obviate the need for chemotherapy. The decision to repeat the curettage is typically either to treat ongoing

TABLE 21.2 FIGO anatomic staging of GTD.

FIGO anatomic staging
Stage I: Disease is only in the uterus
Stage II: GTD extends outside the uterus but is limited to the genital structures.
Stage III: GTD extends to the lungs and may or may not involve the genital tract.
Stage IV: GTD has extended to other distant sites.

TABLE 21.3 Common single agent chemotherapy regimens.

Agent/regimen	Standard dose	Maximum dose
8-day methotrexate and folinic acid[8]	IM methotrexate 1 mg/kg days 1, 3, 5, and 7 and FA 0.1 mg/kg or 15 mg fixed dose days 2, 4, 6 and 8	
One-day methotrexate infusion and folinic acid[104]	100 mg/m² IV bolus, then 200 mg/m² 12 h infusion and 15 mg PO every 12 h in 4 doses beginning 24 h after start of methotrexate	
5-day methotrexate infusion[105]	0.4 mg/kg intravenously daily for 5 days	
5-day actD[106]	IV 12 µg/kg/day	<1000 µg/day
Pulsed intravenous actD[61]	IV 1.25 mg/m² every 2 weeks	Maximum of 2 mg

vaginal bleeding or out of concern that the first evacuation was incomplete. In one series, 40% of patients undergoing second curettage achieved hCG remission without the need for chemotherapy.[67]

In select patients who do not desire future fertility, primary hysterectomy for treatment of non-metastatic GTN is another option. Open and laparoscopic approaches have similar oncologic outcomes.[68] Following hysterectomy, a single postoperative dose of pulsed actinomycin D is given prior to hospital discharge. Using this approach for 40 patients at the New England Trophoblastic Disease Center, primary hysterectomy with a single dose of adjuvant chemotherapy attained complete remission in all patients with no further therapy.[69] Whether achieving remission with a second curettage or hysterectomy, patients must be counseled that even with surgical management, guidelines for hCG surveillance are unchanged.

High-risk disease

The combination regimen of etoposide, methotrexate, actinomycin D, cyclophosphamide and vincristine (EMACO) is the preferred primary regimen for high-risk metastatic GTN.[70] While this regimen can be given outpatient, usually the EMA portion requires an inpatient stay due to the long infusion time. Dosing follows a 14-day cycle. A typical regimen is as follows:

- Etoposide—100 mg/m² IV over 60 min on days 1 and 2
- MTX—1000 mg/m² IV over 24 h on day 1
- ActD—0.5 mg IV bolus on days 1 and 2
- Leucovorin calcium—30 mg intramuscular (IM) or orally every 12 h for 3 days, starting 32 h after treatment with MTX
- Cyclophosphamide—600 mg/m² IV on day 8
- Vincristine—1.0 mg/m² IV on day 8

The regimen is generally well-tolerated and complete remission rates range between 70% and 94%.[12,71–73] Neutropenia is the primary reason for treatment delays and can be prevented with routine administration of granulocyte colony-stimulating factors (G-CSFs).[74] If patients become resistant to EMACO, typically they are then treated with modification of this regimen by substituting cisplatin (75 mg/m²) and etoposide (150 mg/m²) on day 8 (EMAEP). Approximately 80% of patients with primary resistance to EMACO can achieve remission with EMAEP, sometimes in combination with hysterectomy or resection of isolated sites of metastatic disease (e.g., a solitary lung nodule).[75,76]

Women with ultra-high-risk GTN are at risk for early death due to hemorrhagic conversion of CNS or pulmonary lesions.[77] These patients should receive induction with low-dose etoposide (100 mg/m²) and cisplatin (20 mg/m²) on days 1 and 2 every 7 days prior to the initiation of EMA-CO.[78] Adopting this approach has almost eliminated these early deaths. For patients with brain metastases, a neurosurgical consult should be obtained prior to treatment and a higher dose of methotrexate (1000 mg/m² over 24 h) is recommended.[79] Chemotherapy may be given concurrently with stereotactic or whole brain radiation.

PSTT and ETT

PSTT and ETT require special care because these variants of GTN are relatively resistant to chemotherapy.[42] Unlike choriocarcinoma, these tumors tend to remain localized in the uterus for long periods of time before metastasizing. In cases of non-metastatic disease, the preferred treatment is hysterectomy.[80] The overall survival for patients with metastatic PSTT and ETT is relatively poor. EMACO or EMAEP is recommended for all patients with extrauterine disease. Patients diagnosed more than 4 years from the last pregnancy are an especially poor prognosis group.[81] Because PSTT and ETT produce relatively low levels of hCG, serum monitoring alone may be insufficient for gauging remission, and patients should undergo surveillance CT scans in addition to blood-based monitoring.

Surveillance for recurrent disease

All patients with stages I, II, and III GTN are followed with weekly hCG levels until undetectable for 3 weeks, and then monthly for 12 months. Patients with stage IV disease who enter complete remission are monitored with monthly hCG levels until undetectable for 24 months because they have an increased risk for late relapse. In a population-based cohort study of more than 4000 GTN patients from the United Kingdom, the authors reported the risk of relapse was 4.4% for low-risk patients (154/3507) and 6.3% (44/694) for high-risk patients.[82] The median time to recurrence after chemotherapy completion was 4 months. No relapses were detected after seven years. The overall risk of relapse beyond one year was 1.2% for low-risk patients (42/3507) and 0.9% (6/694) for high-risk patients.[83] The risk of recurrence is reduced by administration of consolidation chemotherapy. For both low-risk and high-risk disease, patients should receive three cycles of chemotherapy beyond the first normal hCG.[84]

For patients retaining fertility, reliable contraception is essential during gonadotropin follow-up. Oral contraceptives are especially useful because in addition to providing contraception, estrogen containing preparations suppress pituitary hCG. Intrauterine devices should not be used until the patient is in gonadotropin remission because of the possibility of infection, bleeding and perforation if viable tumor is present in the uterine wall.

Survival and patterns of failure

For low-risk GTN, overall survival rates approach 100%, but it is important to emphasize that treatment of GTN in a reference center is associated with higher survival. In Brazil, which has a nationwide network of GTN reference centers, the risk of mortality for patients who initiated their treatment outside of a reference center increased in low-risk and high-risk GTN by 12.2- and 28.3-fold, respectively.[13] Similarly, high-risk patients treated inappropriately with single-agent therapy prior to referral are at increased risk of death.[85]

Most patients diagnosed with disease relapse will be identified by a re-elevation of serum hCG.[82] When relapse is diagnosed, physical exam and repeat imaging should be performed, including transvaginal ultrasound (if the uterus remains), CT chest, abdomen, and pelvis, and brain MRI.[7,86,87] If a focus of recurrent disease is identified on imaging, the most common sites are the uterus, lung, or brain.[88]

Treatment of recurrent disease

Even after relapse, most patients will achieve remission with subsequent lines of chemotherapy. In fact, patients treated after relapse actually have slightly better outcomes than patients who develop chemotherapy resistance during primary therapy. Resection of isolated metastases via pulmonary wedge resection, hysterectomy, or in select cases, craniotomy, can be very effective in treating patients with isolated foci of resistance disease.[89–91]

Patients developing resistance to EMACO and EMAEP may still achieve durable remissions with further lines of chemotherapy. One well tolerated option is an alternating doublet of paclitaxel-etoposide and paclitaxel-cisplatin (TE/TP).[11,92,93] Combinations of bleomycin, etoposide, and cisplatin (BEP), vinblastine, cisplatin, and bleomycin (PVB), and ifosfamide, carboplatin, etopside (ICE) have also been used.[94] For patients progressing through cytotoxic chemotherapy, autologous bone marrow transplantation with stem cell rescue is an option with a durable remission rate of 41% in the largest series, although this appears to be most effective in patients with persistent disease but low hCG levels.[58] Antiangiogenic therapy has also been used to achieve remission in individual highly pretreated patients.[95]

Immune checkpoint inhibitors have emerged as another promising option. Of note, the ligand PD-L1 is expressed universally by trophoblast cells.[96] Pembrolizumab has been used successfully as salvage therapy in several heavily pretreated patients.[97–100] Because checkpoint inhibitors are generally well-tolerated, they have also been investigated as an alternative to multiagent chemotherapy for patients with low-risk disease not responsive to single-agent therapy.[101]

Special considerations

Twin molar pregnancy

Rarely, molar pregnancy can occur in twin gestations along with a normal fetus.[102] In these cases, partial mole should first be excluded. Twin molar gestations are at increased risk of life-threatening medical complications such as preeclampsia and vaginal hemorrhage, and the need to treat these conditions may require termination of the pregnancy. Moreover, twin molar gestations are at an approximately 2-fold increased risk of GTN. However, elective termination of pregnancy is not associated with a reduction in GTN risk, and approximately 60% of continued pregnancies result in viable live birth.

Subsequent pregnancies

Women successfully treated for GTN have similar subsequent pregnancy outcomes to age-matched peers.[3] After partial molar pregnancy, patients are advised to wait until 1 month of normal hCG values prior to conception. After complete molar pregnancy, patients are advised to wait until 6 months of normal hCG values. Patients receiving chemotherapy should wait until a full 12 months of documented monthly normal hCG values before conception. The length of surveillance is determined by the relative risk of disease relapse and the fact that an intercurrent pregnancy will confound hCG monitoring. Women who do conceive before the end of recommended surveillance are not at increased risk of relapse, however, there is a higher rate of miscarriage among women who conceive within 6 months of chemotherapy. Other than a slightly increased risk of repeat GTD in subsequent pregnancies, women can be counseled that the incidence of term deliveries is normal. Furthermore, women treated with either single agent or multiagent chemotherapy after the recommended surveillance period do not have a higher incidence of first trimester miscarriage or congenital abnormalities.[27] Despite the recommendation to use contraception during the posttreatment follow-up, patients occasionally do become pregnant during the hCG surveillance period. There is no need to interrupt the pregnancy in these circumstances, but an early ultrasound should be performed (between 8 and weeks' gestation) to document a normal intrauterine pregnancy, and the placenta should be sent for pathologic evaluation after delivery. Interval pregnancy should always be considered with a new rise in hCG. In a cohort of 1204 patients with early pregnancy following chemotherapy for GTN, no increase in fetal malformations was observed.[103] Following delivery, we do recommend checking a serum hCG 6 weeks postpartum to ensure the hCG has normalized.

Case resolution

The patient was diagnosed with postmolar GTN I:6. She received 2 points for the uterine tumor and 4 points for her elevated hCG level. She initiated chemotherapy with 8-day methotrexate, but after 8 cycles, her hCG plateaued at 3,000. She was then switched to pulsed actinomycin D 1.25 m^2. Her hCG fell below 5 IU/mL after 3 cycles of actinomycin D, and she went on to receive 3 consolidation cycles. She completed 12 months of hCG surveillance following chemotherapy. During this time, she used oral contraceptive pills for contraception and adhered to monthly hCG testing. Upon completing hCG surveillance, she conceived spontaneously and went on to have a full-term vaginal delivery of a healthy infant.

References

1. Ngan HYS, et al. Update on the diagnosis and management of gestational trophoblastic disease. *Int J Gynaecol Obstet.* 2018;143(Suppl 2):79–85.
2. Altieri A, et al. Epidemiology and aetiology of gestational trophoblastic diseases. *Lancet Oncol.* 2003;4(11):670–678.
3. Savage PM, et al. The relationship of maternal age to molar pregnancy incidence, risks for chemotherapy and subsequent pregnancy outcome. *J Obstet Gynaecol.* 2013;33(4):406–411.
4. Growdon WB, et al. Postevacuation hCG levels and risk of gestational trophoblastic neoplasia among women with partial molar pregnancies. *J Reprod Med.* 2006;51(11):871–874.
5. Smith HO. Gestational trophoblastic disease epidemiology and trends. *Clin Obstet Gynecol.* 2003;46(3):541–556.
6. Lok C, et al. Practical clinical guidelines of the EOTTD for treatment and referral of gestational trophoblastic disease. *Eur J Cancer.* 2020;130:228–240.
7. Jareemit N, et al. Outcomes for relapsed versus resistant low risk gestational trophoblastic neoplasia following single-agent chemotherapy. *Gynecol Oncol.* 2020;159(3):751–757.
8. Maesta I, et al. Effectiveness and toxicity of first-line methotrexate chemotherapy in low-risk postmolar gestational trophoblastic neoplasia: the New England Trophoblastic Disease Center experience. *Gynecol Oncol.* 2018;148(1):161–167.
9. Chapman-Davis E, et al. Treatment of nonmetastatic and metastatic low-risk gestational trophoblastic neoplasia: factors associated with resistance to single-agent methotrexate chemotherapy. *Gynecol Oncol.* 2012;125(3):572–575.
10. Maesta I, et al. Outcomes in the management of high-risk gestational trophoblastic neoplasia in trophoblastic disease centers in South America. *Int J Gynecol Cancer.* 2020;30(9):1366–1371.
11. Li J, et al. Chemotherapy for gestational trophoblastic neoplasia patients with a FIGO score of 12 or greater: a multistudy analysis. *Eur J Obstet Gynecol Reprod Biol.* 2019;238:164–169.

12. Agarwal R, et al. Management and survival of patients with FIGO high-risk gestational trophoblastic neoplasia: the U.K. experience, 1995-2010. *J Reprod Med.* 2014;59(1-2):7–12.

13. Freitas F, et al. Gestational trophoblastic neoplasia lethality among Brazilian women: a retrospective national cohort study. *Gynecol Oncol.* 2020;158 (2):452–459.

14. Lurain JR, Hoekstra AV, Schink JC. Results of treatment of patients with gestational trophoblastic neoplasia referred to the Brewer Trophoblastic Disease Center after failure of treatment elsewhere (1979-2006). *J Reprod Med.* 2008;53(7):535–540.

15. Diver EJ, et al. Timing of referral to the new england trophoblastic disease center: does referral with molar pregnancy versus postmolar gestational trophoblastic neoplasia affect outcomes? *J Reprod Med.* 2016;61(5-6):187–191.

16. Bynum J, et al. Invasive complete hydatidiform moles: analysis of a case series with genotyping. *Int J Gynecol Pathol.* 2016;35(2):134–141.

17. Khawajkie Y, et al. Comprehensive analysis of 204 sporadic hydatidiform moles: revisiting risk factors and their correlations with the molar genotypes. *Mod Pathol.* 2020;33(5):880–892.

18. Demond H, et al. A KHDC3L mutation resulting in recurrent hydatidiform mole causes genome-wide DNA methylation loss in oocytes and persistent imprinting defects post-fertilisation. *Genome Med.* 2019;11(1):84.

19. Monk D, Sanchez-Delgado M, Fisher R. NLRPs, the subcortical maternal complex and genomic imprinting. *Reproduction.* 2017;154(6):R161–R170.

20. Savage P, et al. A case of intraplacental gestational choriocarcinoma; characterised by the methylation pattern of the early placenta and an absence of driver mutations. *BMC Cancer.* 2019;19(1):744.

21. Jung SH, et al. Distinct genomic profiles of gestational choriocarcinoma, a unique cancer of pregnant tissues. *Exp Mol Med.* 2020.

22. Cho EJ, et al. Whole transcriptome analysis of gestational trophoblastic neoplasms reveals altered PI3K signaling pathway in epithelioid trophoblastic tumor. *Gynecol Oncol.* 2020;157(1):151–160.

23. Gockley AA, et al. The effect of adolescence and advanced maternal age on the incidence of complete and partial molar pregnancy. *Gynecol Oncol.* 2016;140(3):470–473.

24. Braga A, et al. Molar pregnancy in adolescents. *J Reprod Med.* 2012;57(5-6):225–230.

25. Savage P, et al. Demographics, natural history and treatment outcomes of non-molar gestational choriocarcinoma: a UK population study. *BJOG.* 2020;127(9):1102–1107.

26. Elias KM, et al. Complete hydatidiform mole in women aged 40 to 49 years. *J Reprod Med.* 2012;57(5-6):254–258.

27. Vargas R, et al. Subsequent pregnancy outcomes after complete and partial molar pregnancy, recurrent molar pregnancy, and gestational trophoblastic neoplasia: an update from the New England Trophoblastic Disease Center. *J Reprod Med.* 2014;59(5-6):188–194.

28. Eagles N, et al. Risk of recurrent molar pregnancies following complete and partial hydatidiform moles. *Hum Reprod.* 2015;30(9):2055–2063.

29. Gadducci A, Lanfredini N, Cosio S. Reproductive outcomes after hydatiform mole and gestational trophoblastic neoplasia. *Gynecol Endocrinol.* 2015;31(9):673–678.

30. Nguyen NM, Slim R. Genetics and epigenetics of recurrent hydatidiform moles: basic science and genetic counselling. *Curr Obstet Gynecol Rep.* 2014;3:55–64.

31. Ronnett BM, DeScipio C, Murphy, KM. Hydatidiform moles: ancillary techniques to refine diagnosis. *Int J Gynecol Pathol.* 2011;30(2):101–116.

32. Vang R, Gupta M, Wu LS, et al. Diagnostic reproducibility of hydatidiform moles: ancillary techniques (p57 immunohistochemistry and molecular genotyping) improve morphologic diagnosis. *Am J Surg Pathol.* 2012;36(3):443–453.

33. Mao TL, Kurman RJ, Jeng YM, et al. HSD3B1 as a novel trophoblast-associated marker that assists in the differential diagnosis of trophoblastic tumors and tumorlike lesions. *Am J Surg Pathol.* 2008;32(2):236–242.

33a. Shih IM, Ronnett BM, Mazur M, Kurman RJ. Gestational trophoblastic tumors and related tumorlike lesions. In: Kurman R, Hedrick Ellenson L, Ronnett B, eds. *Blaustein's Pathology of the Female Genital Tract.* New York, NY: Springer; 2018. https://doi.org/10.1007/978-1-4614-3165-7_20-2.

34. Buza N, Hui P. Immunohistochemistry and other ancillary techniques in the diagnosis of gestational trophoblastic diseases. *Semin Diagn Pathol.* 2014;31(3):223–232.

35. Murphy KM, McConnell TG, Hafez MJ, et al. Molecular genotyping of hydatidiform moles: analytic validation of a multiplex short tandem repeat assay. *J Mol Diagn.* 2009;11(6):598–605.

36. Aranake-Chrisinger J, Huettner PC, Hagemann AR, et al. Use of short tandem repeat analysis in unusual presentations of trophoblastic tumors and their mimics. *Hum Pathol.* 2016;52:92–100.

37. Curry SL, et al. Hydatidiform mole: diagnosis, management, and long-term followup of 347 patients. *Obstet Gynecol.* 1975;45(1):1–8.

38. Kohorn EI. Molar pregnancy: presentation and diagnosis. *Clin Obstet Gynecol.* 1984;27(1):181–191.

39. Sun SY, et al. Clinical presentation of complete hydatidiform mole and partial hydatidiform mole at a regional trophoblastic disease center in the United States over the past 2 decades. *Int J Gynecol Cancer.* 2016;26(2):367–370.

40. Braga A, et al. Changing trends in the clinical presentation and management of complete hydatidiform mole among Brazilian women. *Int J Gynecol Cancer.* 2016;26(5):984–990.

41. Sun SY, et al. Changing presentation of complete hydatidiform mole at the New England Trophoblastic Disease Center over the past three decades: does early diagnosis alter risk for gestational trophoblastic neoplasia? *Gynecol Oncol.* 2015;138(1):46–49.

42. Moutte A, et al. Placental site and epithelioid trophoblastic tumours: diagnostic pitfalls. *Gynecol Oncol.* 2013;128(3):568–572.

43. Cole LA, Butler S. Detection of hCG in trophoblastic disease. The USA hCG reference service experience. *J Reprod Med.* 2002;47(6):433–444.

44. Harvey RA, et al. Differences in total human chorionic gonadotropin immunoassay analytical specificity and ability to measure human chorionic gonadotropin in gestational trophoblastic disease and germ cell tumors. *J Reprod Med.* 2010;55(7-8):285–295.

45. Herskovits AZ, et al. False-negative urine human chorionic gonadotropin testing in the clinical laboratory. *Lab Med.* 2020;51(1):86–93.

46. Griffey RT, et al. "Hook-like effect" causes false-negative point-of-care urine pregnancy testing in emergency patients. *J Emerg Med.* 2013;44 (1):155–160.

47. Berkowitz RS, Goldstein DP. Current management of gestational trophoblastic diseases. *Gynecol Oncol.* 2009;112(3):654–662.

48. Sebire NJ. The diagnosis of gestational trophoblastic disease in early pregnancy: implications for screening, counseling and management. *Ultrasound Obstet Gynecol.* 2005;25(5):421–424.

49. Benson CB, et al. Sonographic appearance of first trimester complete hydatidiform moles. *Ultrasound Obstet Gynecol.* 2000;16(2):188–191.

50. Fine C, et al. Sonographic diagnosis of partial hydatidiform mole. *Obstet Gynecol.* 1989;73(3 Pt 1):414–418.

51. Savage JL, et al. Sonographic diagnosis of partial versus complete molar pregnancy: a reappraisal. *J Clin Ultrasound.* 2017;45(2):72–78.

52. Zhou Y, et al. Sonographic characteristics of placental site trophoblastic tumor. *Ultrasound Obstet Gynecol.* 2013;41(6):679–684.

53. Okumura M, et al. Sonographic appearance of gestational trophoblastic disease evolving into epithelioid trophoblastic tumor. *Ultrasound Obstet Gynecol.* 2010;36(2):249–251.

54. Parker VL, et al. Computed tomography chest imaging offers no advantage over chest X-ray in the initial assessment of gestational trophoblastic neoplasia. *Br J Cancer.* 2020.

55. Strohl AE, Lurain JR. Postmolar choriocarcinoma: an independent risk factor for chemotherapy resistance in low-risk gestational trophoblastic neoplasia. *Gynecol Oncol.* 2016;141(2):276–280.

56. Braga A, et al. Is chemotherapy always necessary for patients with nonmetastatic gestational trophoblastic neoplasia with histopathological diagnosis of choriocarcinoma? *Gynecol Oncol.* 2018;148(2):239–246.

57. Frijstein MM, et al. Management and prognostic factors of epithelioid trophoblastic tumors: results from the International Society for the Study of Trophoblastic Diseases database. *Gynecol Oncol.* 2019;152(2):361–367.

58. Frijstein MM, et al. The results of treatment with high-dose chemotherapy and peripheral blood stem cell support for gestational trophoblastic neoplasia. *Eur J Cancer.* 2019;109:162–171.

59. Mu X, et al. Comparison of pulsed actinomycin D and 5-day actinomycin D as first-line chemotherapy for low-risk gestational trophoblastic neoplasia. *Int J Gynaecol Obstet.* 2018;143(2):225–231.

60. Petrilli ES, et al. Single-dose actinomycin-D treatment for nonmetastatic gestational trophoblastic disease. A prospective phase II trial of the Gynecologic Oncology Group. *Cancer.* 1987;60(9):2173–2176.

61. Osborne RJ, et al. Phase III trial of weekly methotrexate or pulsed dactinomycin for low-risk gestational trophoblastic neoplasia: a gynecologic oncology group study. *J Clin Oncol.* 2011;29(7):825–831.

62. Schink JC, et al. An international randomized phase III trial of pulse actinomycin-D versus multi-day methotrexate for the treatment of low risk gestational trophoblastic neoplasia; NRG/GOG 275. *Gynecol Oncol.* 2020;158(2):354–360.

63. Lawrie TA, et al. First-line chemotherapy in low-risk gestational trophoblastic neoplasia. *Cochrane Database Syst Rev.* 2016;6, CD007102.

64. Braga A, et al. Comparison of treatment for low-risk GTN with standard 8-day MTX/FA regimen versus modified MTX/FA regimen without chemotherapy on the weekend. *Gynecol Oncol.* 2020;156(3):598–605.

65. Parker VL, et al. Classification systems in gestational trophoblastic neoplasia—sentiment or evidenced based? *Cancer Treat Rev.* 2017;56:47–57.

66. Maesta I, et al. Effectiveness and toxicity of second-line actinomycin D in patients with methotrexate-resistant postmolar low-risk gestational trophoblastic neoplasia. *Gynecol Oncol.* 2020;157(2):372–378.

67. Osborne RJ, et al. Second curettage for low-risk nonmetastatic gestational trophoblastic neoplasia. *Obstet Gynecol.* 2016;128(3):535–542.

68. Sugrue R, et al. Outcomes of minimally invasive versus open abdominal hysterectomy in patients with gestational trophoblastic disease. *Gynecol Oncol.* 2021;160(2):445–449.

69. Clark RM, et al. The evolving role of hysterectomy in gestational trophoblastic neoplasia at the New England Trophoblastic Disease Center. *J Reprod Med.* 2010;55(5-6):194–198.

70. Newlands ES, et al. The management of high-risk gestational trophoblastic tumours (GTT). *Int J Gynaecol Obstet.* 1998;60(Suppl. 1):S65–S70.

71. Jareemit N, et al. EMA vs EMACO in the treatment of gestational trophoblastic neoplasia. *Gynecol Oncol.* 2020;158(1):99–104.

72. Cagayan MS. High-risk metastatic gestational trophoblastic neoplasia. Primary management with EMA-CO (etoposide, methotrexate, actinomycin D, cyclophosphamide and vincristine) chemotherapy. *J Reprod Med.* 2012;57(5-6):231–236.

73. Lurain JR, Singh DK, Schink JC. Primary treatment of metastatic high-risk gestational trophoblastic neoplasia with EMA-CO chemotherapy. *J Reprod Med.* 2006;51(10):767–772.

74. Hartenbach EM, et al. A novel strategy using G-CSF to support EMA/CO for high-risk gestational trophoblastic disease. *Gynecol Oncol.* 1995;56 (1):105–108.

75. Newlands ES, et al. Etoposide and cisplatin/etoposide, methotrexate, and actinomycin D (EMA) chemotherapy for patients with high-risk gestational trophoblastic tumors refractory to EMA/cyclophosphamide and vincristine chemotherapy and patients presenting with metastatic placental site trophoblastic tumors. *J Clin Oncol.* 2000;18(4):854–859.

76. Lurain JR, Schink JC. Importance of salvage therapy in the management of high-risk gestational trophoblastic neoplasia. *J Reprod Med.* 2012;57 (5-6):219–224.

77. Kong Y, et al. Clinical characteristics and prognosis of ultra high-risk gestational trophoblastic neoplasia patients: a retrospective cohort study. *Gynecol Oncol.* 2017;146(1):81–86.

78. Alifrangis C, et al. EMA/CO for high-risk gestational trophoblastic neoplasia: good outcomes with induction low-dose etoposide-cisplatin and genetic analysis. *J Clin Oncol.* 2013;31(2):280–286.

79. Newlands ES, et al. Management of brain metastases in patients with high-risk gestational trophoblastic tumors. *J Reprod Med.* 2002;47(6):465–471.

80. Gadducci A, et al. Placental site trophoblastic tumor and epithelioid trophoblastic tumor: clinical and pathological features, prognostic variables and treatment strategy. *Gynecol Oncol.* 2019;153(3):684–693.

81. Papadopoulos AJ, et al. Twenty-five years' clinical experience with placental site trophoblastic tumors. *J Reprod Med.* 2002;47(6):460–464.

82. Balachandran K, et al. When to stop human chorionic gonadotrophin (hCG) surveillance after treatment with chemotherapy for gestational trophoblastic neoplasia (GTN): a national analysis on over 4,000 patients. *Gynecol Oncol.* 2019;155(1):8–12.

83. Elias KM, Berkowitz RS, Horowitz NS. Continued hCG surveillance following chemotherapy for gestational trophoblastic neoplasia: when is enough enough? *Gynecol Oncol.* 2019;155(1):1–2.

84. Lybol C, et al. Relapse rates after two versus three consolidation courses of methotrexate in the treatment of low-risk gestational trophoblastic neoplasia. *Gynecol Oncol.* 2012;125(3):576–579.

85. Neubauer NL, et al. Fatal gestational trophoblastic neoplasia: an analysis of treatment failures at the Brewer Trophoblastic Disease Center from 1979-2012 compared to 1962-1978. *Gynecol Oncol.* 2015;138(2):339–342.

86. Powles T, et al. A comparison of patients with relapsed and chemo-refractory gestational trophoblastic neoplasia. *Br J Cancer.* 2007;96(5):732–737.

87. Feng F, et al. Prognosis of patients with relapsed and chemoresistant gestational trophoblastic neoplasia transferred to the Peking Union Medical College Hospital. *BJOG.* 2010;117(1):47–52.

88. Kong Y, et al. Management and risk factors of recurrent gestational trophoblastic neoplasia: an update from 2004 to 2017. *Cancer Med.* 2020;9 (7):2590–2599.

89. Alifrangis C, et al. Role of thoracotomy and metastatectomy in gestational trophoblastic neoplasia: a single center experience. *J Reprod Med.* 2012;57 (7-8):350–358.

90. Fleming EL, et al. The changing role of thoracotomy in gestational trophoblastic neoplasia at the New England Trophoblastic Disease Center. *J Reprod Med.* 2008;53(7):493–498.

91. Doll KM, Soper JT. The role of surgery in the management of gestational trophoblastic neoplasia. *Obstet Gynecol Surv.* 2013;68(7):533–542.

92. Wang J, et al. Salvage chemotherapy of relapsed or high-risk gestational trophoblastic neoplasia (GTN) with paclitaxel/cisplatin alternating with paclitaxel/etoposide (TP/TE). *Ann Oncol.* 2008;19(9):1578–1583.

93. Osborne R, et al. Successful salvage of relapsed high-risk gestational trophoblastic neoplasia patients using a novel paclitaxel-containing doublet. *J Reprod Med.* 2004;49(8):655–661.

94. Alazzam M, et al. Chemotherapy for resistant or recurrent gestational trophoblastic neoplasia. *Cochrane Database Syst Rev.* 2016;1, CD008891.

95. Worley Jr MJ, et al. Durable remission for a woman with refractory choriocarcinoma treated with anti-endoglin monoclonal antibody and bevacizumab: a case from the New England Trophoblastic Disease Center, Brigham and Women's Hospital and Dana-Farber Cancer Institute. *Gynecol Oncol.* 2018;148(1):5–11.

96. Bolze PA, et al. PD-L1 expression in premalignant and malignant trophoblasts from gestational trophoblastic diseases is ubiquitous and independent of clinical outcomes. *Int J Gynecol Cancer.* 2017;27(3):554–561.

97. Ghorani E, et al. Pembrolizumab is effective for drug-resistant gestational trophoblastic neoplasia. *Lancet.* 2017;390(10110):2343–2345.

98. Clair KH, Gallegos N, Bristow RE. Successful treatment of metastatic refractory gestational choriocarcinoma with pembrolizumab: a case for immune checkpoint salvage therapy in trophoblastic tumors. *Gynecol Oncol Rep.* 2020;34:100625.

99. Goldfarb JA, et al. A case of multi-agent drug resistant choriocarcinoma treated with Pembrolizumab. *Gynecol Oncol Rep.* 2020;32:100574.

100. Huang M, et al. Complete serologic response to pembrolizumab in a woman with chemoresistant metastatic choriocarcinoma. *J Clin Oncol.* 2017; 35(27):3172–3174.

101. You B, et al. Avelumab in patients with gestational trophoblastic tumors with resistance to single-agent chemotherapy: Cohort A of the TROPHIMMUN Phase II trial. *J Clin Oncol.* 2020;38(27):3129–3137.

102. Lin LH, et al. Multiple pregnancies with complete mole and coexisting normal fetus in North and South America: a retrospective multicenter cohort and literature review. *Gynecol Oncol.* 2017;145(1):88–95.

103. Williams J, et al. Effect of early pregnancy following chemotherapy on disease relapse and fetal outcome in women treated for gestational trophoblastic neoplasia. *J Reprod Med.* 2014;59(5-6):248–254.

104. Garrett AP, et al. Methotrexate infusion and folinic acid as primary therapy for nonmetastatic and low-risk metastatic gestational trophoblastic tumors. 15 years of experience. *J Reprod Med.* 2002;47(5):355–362.

105. Lurain JR, Elfstrand EP. Single-agent methotrexate chemotherapy for the treatment of nonmetastatic gestational trophoblastic tumors. *Am J Obstet Gynecol.* 1995;172(2 Pt 1):574–579.

106. Prouvot C, et al. Efficacy and safety of second-line 5-day dactinomycin in case of methotrexate failure for gestational trophoblastic neoplasia. *Int J Gynecol Cancer.* 2018;28(5):1038–1044.

Index

Note: Page numbers followed by *f* indicate figures and *t* indicate tables.